On loan from   Alastair Weir.

Functional Restoration of Adults and Children with Upper Extremity Amputation

EDITED BY

ROBERT H. MEIER, III, MD
DIANE J. ATKINS, OTR

Demos Medical Publishing, Inc., 386 Park Avenue South, New York, New York 10016

Visit our website at www.demosmedpub.com

Library of Congress Cataloging-in-Publication Data

Functional restoration of adults and children with upper extremity amputation / edited by
  Robert H. Meier, III, Diane J. Atkins.— 1st ed.
      p. ; cm.
  Includes bibliographical references and index.
  ISBN 1-888799-73-0 (hardcover : alk. paper)
    1. Arm—Amputation. 2. Amputees—Rehabilitation. 3. Artificial arms.
    [DNLM: 1. Amputation—rehabilitation. 2. Artificial Limbs. 3.
  Prosthesis Fitting. 4. Treatment Outcome. 5. Upper Extremity—surgery. WE 170
  F979 2004] I. Meier, R. H. (Robert Henry) II. Atkins, D. J. (Diane J.)

  RD557.F865 2004
  617.5′7403—dc22   2004000904

Made in the United States of America

Dedication

I would like to dedicate this book to the many individuals with limb loss whom I have come to know throughout my career. They have truly been my best teachers in so much of what I have learned, now teach, and communicate in writing. These individuals are an inspiration to me. I am grateful for the opportunity to share their knowledge and experience with others.

This dedication would not be complete without acknowledging and thanking my two mentors, Skip Meier, MD and Al Muilenburg, CPO. They were the "seed" that started this learning process for me and have remained an inspiration and the motivation throughout my professional life.

— DJA

This book is dedicated to my wife, Martha and our children, Liesl, Robin, and Christian, who have been marvelously supportive of my chosen career and who have enjoyed having many of my patients become fine family friends. We are immensely grateful for the extraordinary privilege of learning that patients can be wonderful people and not just another clinical case.

— RHM

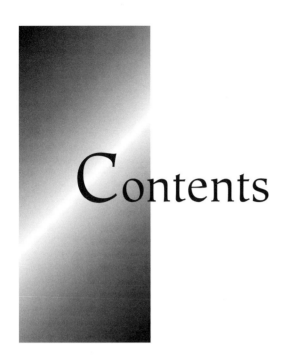

Contents

PROSTHETIC RESTORATION IN ARM AMPUTATION

PEDIATRIC UPPER EXTREMITY AMPUTATION

OUTCOMES IN UPPER EXTREMITY AMPUTATION

HISTORICAL TRENDS AND THE FUTURE

Preface

The incidence of arm amputation is low compared to that of the lower extremity. In addition, the demographics of those who lose an arm are different from those who lose a leg. The arm amputee is usually a young man who sustains a traumatic injury, most often to his right dominant arm. In addition, the functional outcomes without using an arm prosthesis are different from those who lose a leg and do not use a prosthesis. An arm amputee can learn to functional quite well without ever wearing an arm prosthesis. This is not true for the leg amputee who does not use a leg prosthesis.

Because the incidence of arm amputation is low, few health professionals get much experience in providing surgery, therapy, rehabilitation, prosthetic care, or counseling for any significant number of arm amputees. Also, the older literature indicates that not many arm amputees achieve successful function from wearing and using an arm prosthesis.

Because we have had the good fortune to work with a large population of arm amputees and have developed a center that provides comprehensive rehabilitation services, we are editing this new text. We believe that centers of experience and rehabilitation excellence are the most suitable health care settings to provide comprehensive care for arm amputees. This type of center has several attributes. They have a system of service delivery that is specific for persons with arm amputation. In addition, they treat 25 or more arm amputees every year so that the team keeps up their skills for prosthetic fabrication and rehabilitation services. These centers also have systems that provide regular and periodic follow-up for prosthetic maintenance and also measure the outcomes of emotional and physical function, both with and without a prosthesis. These centers are experienced at setting goals with the amputee and in devising comprehensive rehabilitation programs that focus on the needs and desires of the amputee. They are not focused only on making and wearing an arm prosthesis.

A book of this complexity is not brought together without the efforts of many experienced health professionals from many backgrounds and from many parts of the United States. As has been said before, there are few experienced professionals and they are spread out in a few pockets of practice. We wish to thank all of our contributors for their time and effort in helping to produce this new text. It is most generous of them to share their experience and knowledge.

We are also privileged to have worked with a wonderful variety of persons with arm amputation who have taught us so much more than just how to prescribe or make a prosthesis. We have been constantly amazed to witness the human spirit rise above unbelievable types of disability and adversity and to have these disabled persons become newly functioning individuals who resume a productive role in the family, the community, and the workplace. This triumph of the human spirit has been the rule and not the exception.

We have also benefited from being part of a community of rehabilitation professionals dedicated to providing the best possible care for persons with arm amputation. This group of professionals has also shared their years of experience, their knowledge, and their passion for rehabilitation with us. We have learned at the feet of several masters over the lengths of our careers.

Our families have also played a role in our ability to spend time in our professions and to support our efforts in providing the best possible rehabilitation services. They have also learned from our amputee friends and have come to understand our passion for working with this population. They have generously forgiven our lateness in arriving for dinner, the numerous meetings, and the time taken for writing that we might have spent with them instead. We thank them for their understanding and encouragement.

Finally, we wish that this text will fall into the hands of all those who provide services for persons with arm amputation and that it will prove to be most useful.

While we have tried to be comprehensive in the subjects presented, there will always be obvious omissions. We assume responsibility for those gaps in this text. Our goal is to improve the quality of service and to improve the outcomes for those who sustain arm amputation. We hope that you will find useful information in this book for your own education and to enhance the quality of your amputee outcomes. We trust you will find that those amputees with whom you work will contribute to the quality of your life and, through partnership and teamwork, you will contribute to the quality of their future.

Robert H. Meier, III, MD
Thornton, Colorado

Diane J. Atkins, OTR
The Woodlands, Texas

Foreword

Prosthetic devices have been used for countless centuries. From pirates to panhandlers, amputees of yesteryear used crude peg legs and iron hands to replace limbs severed by sword or saw. Fashioned out of forked wood or forged metal, fit was always forsaken for function.

Mankind's profound fascination with the human anatomy in its perfection and endless variation was, arguably, first manifested in the artistic studies of the great masters. Such geniuses as Leonardo da Vinci and Donatello labored to illustrate the flawlessness of the human body, its mobility, its form, and its function. But their mission was only to describe, never to duplicate.

In the spirit of these bygone handicraftsmen and artists, modern-day prosthetists have synthesized their predecessors' discoveries with refined materials, revolutionary componentry, and an element of fashion to create prostheses that perform, provide comfort, and please the eye. Modern technology continues to broaden the range of possibilities for amputees, yet it remains evident that the industrial production of artificial limbs is still influenced by the hand craftsmanship of its origin and its tradition. The industry's aim of a thousand years ago endures— foremost not to rebuild the human part, rather to offer its basic function.

To define prosthetic function for the upper extremity amputee is not to look for exact measurement. It does not allow for calibration. Prosthetic function is neither static nor stationary, but rests on a continuum. Today it presents itself one way, tomorrow another. It is both the journey and the destination. It is attainable, yet it is elusive at the same time. And it is emotional—a source of pain and frustration and still, the rootstock of enjoyment and satisfaction.

Prosthetic function may be best characterized as a product of interdependent relationships, both personal and environmental. Trust and responsibility serve as the foundation for these alliances. Cooperation and sensitivity are the building blocks. The amputee must come to trust that the componentry and materials will meet his or her needs and endeavor to trust in the ability and accountability of the prosthetist to apply that technology. Responsibility, however, is not the burden of the prosthetist alone. Equally important to the quality of the prosthetic product and its fitting is the extent to which the user accepts and controls his or her new limb with its relative diversity of possibilities. This too is a determinant of the reliability of the man–machine connection.

Nonetheless, the prosthetic field, including its allied healthcare team, takes on a formidable task in restoring physical capabilities to the upper extremity amputee. This feat is not accomplished solely by using modern technology. Technology is not always the central issue. Rehabilitation involves a great deal more. It requires an underlying commitment in many essential areas of care: for one, sensitivity to the desires, anxieties, and fears of the individual with amputation. While the prosthetic practitioner has at his or her disposal more technology than ever before, restoring integral function for the amputee involves still more than mechanical application. Interdisciplinary, cooperative efforts in research, development, and treatment between prosthetic practitioners and other constituents of the allied healthcare team is paramount.

To expand on the keystone of relationships, favorable unions between the amputee and medical professionals, therapists, counselors, family members, and peers throughout the "adjustment" time of formal rehabilitation can have tremendous influence on restoration of function, essentially paving the road to greater independence. This rehabilitation process should not only focus on the provision and use of a prosthesis. Issues related to surgical procedures, self-determination, and pain management, for example, are as important to the rehabilitation process as prosthetic preparation, prescription, and training.

When the time arrives for prosthetic restoration for the amputee, it is the co-dependence between practitioner and patient or client that is most incisive in the integration of prosthetic technology into one's personal life and the environment in which they work and play. That environment represents the playing field, where the technology is tested, where the amputee is tried, where that individual wins or loses physically, socially, and psychologically.

As a bilateral, above-elbow amputee for more than 25 years, I have tried and tested a vast array of relationships that define and embody prosthetic function. The physical, social, and psychological playing fields have furnished great rewards. I have experienced tremendous satisfaction in the independence afforded me by my artificial limbs. Conversely, it is now the limits and the susceptibility of the technology that bring about frustration. Moreover, technological relationships involving greater comfort and higher cosmetic fashion have come to supercede former functional concerns and objectives.

The maturation of my responsibility to the practitioner–client relationship now presents new challenges for the prosthetist as I continue to demand more from my prostheses in everyday function and in new recreational and sporting environments. With the achievement of every new functional destination, another unvisited mark is mapped out, as the rehabilitation team and amputee together reach for the desirable end of the continuum of prosthetic function. Despite affinities to fashion, like the pirates of the high seas and the great students of human form before us, function will forswear all else in our ongoing pursuit of life's many delights.

Jeffrey A. Tiessen

Contributors

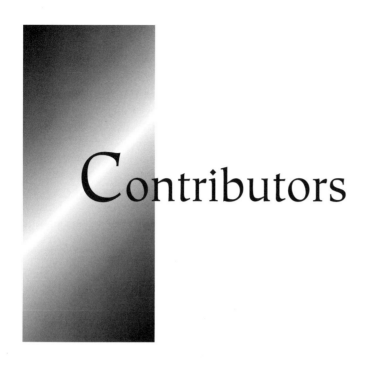

Charlotte B. Alexander, MD
Houston Orthopedic/Sports
    Medicine Associates
Houston, Texas

Randall D. Alley, BSC, CP, FAAOP
Hanger Prosthetics and Orthotics, Inc.
Thousand Oaks, California

Diane J. Atkins, OTR
Clinical Assistant Professor
Department of Physical Medicine
    and Rehabilitation
Baylor College of Medicine
The Woodlands, Texas

James B. Bennett, MD
Chief of Staff
Texas Orthopedic Hospital
Clinical Professor
Department of Orthosurgery
University of Texas-Houston
Clinical Professor
Department of Plastic Surgery
Baylor Medical College
Houston, Texas

William C. Brown, MD
Co-Director, Institute for Limb
    Preservation
Presbyterian/St. Luke's Medical Center
Denver, Colorado

Dudley S. Childress, PhD
Professor
Biomedical Engineering
Northwestern University
Senior Research Scientist
VA Chicago Healthcare System
Chicago, Illinois

Alberto Esquenazi, MD
Chairman and Director
Moss Rehabilitation Center
Philadelphia, Pennsylvania

Annaliese M. Furlong, CP
Owner
Clark and Associates, Prosthetics
    and Orthotics
Marshalltown, Iowa

Elena Grantcharova, MD
Division of Plastic Surgery
University of Texas Medical Center
Houston, Texas

Craig W. Heckathorne, MSc
Research Engineer
Specialist Upper Limb Prostheses
Northwestern University Rehabilitation
    Center
Chicago, Illinois

Mike Hillborn, CP
Owner
Certified Upper Extremity Specialist
Pros-Tech, Inc.
Troy, Michigan

Scott Hompland, DO
Rehabilitation Associates
    of Colorado
Englewood, Colorado

Maurice LeBlanc, MSME, CP
Stanford University
Biomechanical Engineering Division
Stanford, California

James A. Leonard, Jr., MD
Clinical Professor and Department
    Chairman
Department of Physical Medicine
    and Rehabilitation
University of Michigan
Ann Arbor, Michigan

Robert H. Meier, III, MD
Director, Amputee Services
    of America
Manager, the ARMteam
North Valley Outpatient
    Rehabilitation
Thornton, Colorado

John W. Michael, MEd, CPO
President
CPO Services, Inc.
Portage, Indiana

John M. Miguelez, BSc, CP, FAAOP
President and Senior Clinical Director
Advanced Arm Dynamics, Inc.
Rolling Hills Estates, California

Linda Miner, OTR, CHT
Upper Extremity Occupational Therapist
Clinical Specialist
University of Michigan Health System
Department of Physical Medicine
    and Rehabilitation
Ann Arbor, Michigan

Stephen C. Nicolaidis, MD

Mary P. Novotny, RN, MS
Education Consultant and Disability
Advocate
Knoxville, Tennessee

Joanna Grace Patton, OTR/L
Child Amputee Prosthetics Project
Shriners Hospital for Children
Los Angeles, California

Robert Radocy, BS, MS
President/CEO
TRS Inc.
Bouldler, Colorado

Harold H. Sears, PhD
General Manager
Motion Control, Inc.
Salt Lake City, Utah

Yoshio Setoguchi, MD
Medical Director
Child Amputee Prosthetics Project
Shriners Hospital for Children
Los Angeles, California

Saleh M. Shenaq, MD
Professor and Chief
Division of Plastic Surgery
Baylor College of Medicine
Houston, Texas

Joanne Shida-Tokeshi, OTR/L
Child Amputee Prosthetics Project
Shriners Hospital for Children
Los Angeles, California

Gerald Stark, BSME, CP, FAAOP
Director of Education and Technical
    Support
Fillauer Company
Chattanooga, Tennessee

Wendy Stoeker, OTR/L
Salisbury, Maryland

Jack E. Uellendahl, CPO
Hanger Prosthetics and Orthotics Inc.
Phoenix, Arizona

Brent Van Dorsten, PhD
Associate Professor
Department of Rehabilitation
    Medicine
University of Colorado Health Sciences
    Center
Aurora, Colorado

Roger Weed, PhD, CLCP, CRV, CDMS,
CCM, LPC,
    FIALCP, FNRCA
Professor and Coordinator of Graduate
Rehabilitation
    Counseling Training
Georgia State University
Duluth, Georgia

Richard F. ff. Weir, PhD
Research Scientist
VA Chicago Healthcare System
Northwestern University Prosthetics
    Research Laboratory
Chicago, Illinois

Ross M. Wilkins, MD, MS
Medical Director
The Institute for Limb Salvage
Presbyterian/St. Luke's Medical Center
Denver, Colorado

T. Walley Williams, III
Director of Product Development
Liberating Technologies, Inc.
Holliston, Massachusetts

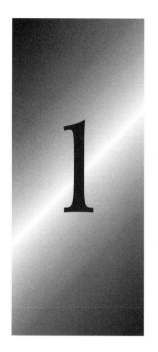

History of Arm Amputation, Prosthetic Restoration, and Arm Amputation Rehabilitation

Robert H. Meier, III, MD

In the United States today, upper extremity amputation is most frequently related to work-related civilian trauma. However, much of the writing on and work with amputation and the restoration of function following limb loss is related to man's inhumanity to man—the progress of war. War has served as the impetus to develop techniques for amputation surgery, prosthetic design improvements, and the development of specialized centers of care and excellence for those who have been victims of war. Amputations of the arm or leg have been recorded over many centuries. Much of the early writing that exists in reference to amputation is related to war injuries sustained by men who were chronicled by now famous authors of those ancient times.

Major General Norman Kirk, Surgeon General of the Army during World War II, provides a broad history of amputation surgery over the centuries in Introductory Survey of the Development of Amputation (1).

Dr. Kirk traces the recorded history of amputation back to Hippocrates, who wrote about amputation in cases of gangrene in the treatise entitled "On Joints," which probably belongs to the latter half of the fifth century, B.C., when Herodotus also was writing. The author recommends amputation of the gangrenous extremity at the joint below "the boundaries of the blackening" as soon as it is "fairly dead and has lost its sensibility."

From Hippocrates through Celsus, amputation seems to be indicated only in gangrene, and only as a last resort. By the time of Archigenes and Heliodorus, under Trajan (c. 100 A.D.), it had become a recognized procedure for ulcers, growths, injuries, and even deformities. Archigenes advises placing a tight circular bandage above the line of severance and cutting down on and tying or sewing the chief blood vessels. If bleeding is nevertheless profuse, he recommends cautery.

Antylus, in the first half of the second century A.D., gives a full and clear description of double ligature to prevent hemorrhage in arteriotomy for aneurysm. Galen, half a century later, adds that the ligatures should be of a material that does not rot too quickly. In view of the frequency with which ligatures are advised in other operations from Celsus onward, it is remarkable that no ancient writer mentions them in connection with amputation.

About the middle of the thirteenth century, a crude anesthetic technique was developed by Hugh of Lucca and adopted by his son and pupil, Theodoric. A sponge was saturated with a soporific solution containing opium and mandrake and dried in the sun. Before the operation, it was soaked in hot water for an hour, then held under the patient's nose. After the operation, the patient was revived by applying a sponge soaked in vinegar.

In 1517, Gersdorff I published *Feldtbuch der Wundt-Artzney,* the first printed book to contain a woodcut illustration of an amputation. He used two circular constricting bands a finger's breadth apart and amputated between them. He prints an elaborate recipe for a styptic to be mixed with egg white and applied to the wound to control the bleeding. If that fails, he suggests that cautery be used.

In the sixteenth century, Ambrose Paré revived several almost forgotten techniques first recorded by Celsus and reintroduced the ligation of vessels in amputation, discounting the use of cautery and burning oil for checking hemorrhage and the treatment of gunshot wounds.

Paré continued to recommend cautery through dead tissue, but not through living tissue because it was too painful and left an eschar. When this eschar sloughed, secondary hemorrhage occurred, the bone was bared, and an incurable ulcer remained.

The reintroduction of the ligature by Paré, and the discovery of the circulation of the blood by Harvey in 1616, led to the invention of Morel's tourniquet in 1674 and Petit's tourniquet in 1718. These means controlled hemorrhage during amputation.

Until the eighteenth century, with the exception of Paré, few physicians gave thought to the condition of the amputation stump for prosthetic appliance. The introduction of anesthesia in 1846–47, and aseptic surgery following the antiseptic period of Lister in 1870, allowed surgeons to take more time to produce a viable amputation stump capable of supporting prosthetics.

With the introduction of sulphuric ether at the Massachusetts General Hospital by Morton and Warren in 1846, a period of rapid progress in general surgery began. Speedy surgery, to lessen the pain, struggles, and distress of the patient, was no longer necessary.

During his early hospital experience (1864–66), Lister had been concerned by his own high mortality in amputations (45% in Syme-level amputations). Unfortunately the antiseptic technique of Lister came too late for the U.S. Civil War and was first used by the military surgeons in the Franco-Prussian War. The closed method of amputation was not a safe procedure until the advent of general asepsis, introduced by Von Bergman (1886–91).

During the Civil War, George Otis, M.D., curator of the Army Medical Museum tallied 253,142 wounded soldiers of whom about 20,559 (8.1%) had significant amputations (2). Of those who sustained gunshot fractures, almost half went on to amputation, and of those, the mortality rate was 35.7%. Chloroform was the anesthetic of choice; infection and suppuration were the rule after operation, and healing was usually by granulation. Hospital gangrene of the stump, a frequent complication, was attributed to overcrowding.

The advent of our understanding of arm amputation and its rehabilitation flows from the high incidence of arm amputation during the Civil War. More amputations in this conflict occurred than in prior wars because of the increased power and accuracy of rifled muskets with a range of 300 to 500 yards. Lead bullets were used; they traveled relatively slowly and, in the process of wounding, flattened out and carried in particles of clothing and skin, with the result that most wounds became infected. The most common major operation of the Civil War was an extremity amputation. The indications for amputation were a badly lacerated extremity or the presence of a compound fracture.

Anesthesia was applied extensively—usually chloroform, which was introduced in 1851. Ether was also used, but more so in the general hospitals because of the hazard of flammability in field usage. Antisepsis and asepsis had not been accepted; Lister's first article on antisepsis was not published until 1867, several years after the war ended. Extremity bleeding was controlled by pressure bandages or silk ligatures.

Samuel Gross (1805–84), a famous Philadelphia surgeon, wrote that the surgeon often is confronted with an incredible dilemma when deciding to salvage an extremity or to amputate it. This decision process today depends on the adequacy of the blood supply, the severity of the trauma, the presence of infection, or the extent or type of tumor. Dr. Gross wrote "while the surgeon endeavors to avoid Scylla, he may not unwittingly run into Charybdis, mutilating a limb that might have been saved, and endangering life by the retention of one that should have been promptly amputated." This dilemma still rings true today, but with newer advances in medicine and surgery, the decision tree has changed and often become much more complex.

In 1949, Dr. Donald Slocum published a comprehensive text, "An Atlas of Amputations," based on experience gained during World War II (3). He indicates that amputation surgery had evolved during the period between the first and second world wars, and that this surgery was "no longer the ghoulish cutting off of a part, but rather it is a phase of reconstruction employing plastic and orthopedic surgery in delicate balance." A chapter on the physical rehabilitation of the upper extremity amputee is included in his work and covers the basic training for activities of daily living and a functional outcomes assessment tool.

Dougherty, in his article on wartime amputations (2), indicates that the improved management of extremity trauma reduced the incidence of amputation from 8.5% at the time of the Civil War to 1 to 2% at the time of the Vietnam War. Similarly, improved treatment of extremity trauma decreased mortality from 35% during the Civil War to 3 to 4% during the Vietnam War. The levels of extremity amputation during the Civil War,

TABLE 1-1
Levels of Amputation

| | CIVIL WAR | WORLD WAR I | WORLD WAR II | | VIETNAM |
			EUROPEAN THEATER	MEDITERRANEAN THEATER	
Shoulder	4.2%	–	–	–	
Above elbow	26.8%	21.8%	13.2%	9.8%	
Elbow	0.9%	1.6%	–	–	13.9%
Below elbow	8.5%	8.4%	11.4%	8.4%	
Wrist	–	1.0%	–	–	
Hip	0.32%	–	–	–	–
Above knee	30.0%	45.1%	27.5%	25.8%	26.6%
Knee	0.94%	3.7%	–	–	–
Below knee	26.8%	12.9%	47.6%	55.9%	47.6%
Ankle	0.78%	5.2%	–	–	–
Multiple	–	–	–	–	16.3%

World War I, World War II, and Vietnam are shown in Table 1-1.

AMPUTATION DEMOGRAPHICS

In a recently published study of extremity amputations in the United States (4), a total of 1,199,111 hospital discharges between 1988 and 1996 was studied for the presence of an amputation ICD-9 code at discharge.

133,235 limb loss–related discharges occurred per year. Amputations secondary to vascular conditions accounted for 82% of limb loss discharges and increased from 38.3 per 100,000 in 1988 to 46.19 per 100,000 persons in 1996 (Table 1-2). Trauma-related amputations, the second most common cause of limb amputation, decreased from 11.37 per 100,000 in 1988 to 5.86 per 100,000 in 1996. Upper limb amputations accounted for the vast majority of the trauma-caused

TABLE 1-2
Adjusted Annual Rates of Limb Loss and Limb Deficiency Per 100,000 US Population: 1988–1996

| CALENDAR YEAR | ETIOLOGY | | | |
	CONGENITAL* N = 9,326 (0.8%)	CANCER N = 10,967 (0.9%)	TRAUMA N = 196,026 (16.4%)	DYSVASCULAR N = 982,792 (82.0%)
1988	24.21	0.62	11.37	38.30
1989	19.44	0.51	11.48	38.22
1990	27.26	0.50	10.85	38.89
1991	26.12	0.58	8.73	38.61
1992	26.55	0.56	8.14	40.19
1993	23.79	0.52	6.90	43.52
1994	30.94	0.39	6.85	45.51
1995	29.08	0.31	6.62	46.42
1996	25.64	0.35	5.86	46.19
Change over study period†	NS	−42.6%**	−50.2%**	26.9%**

* Rates per 100,000 live births.
† Based on linear regression models.
** $P < .01$.
NS = Not statistically significant.
All rates are standardized to the 1988 US population by age, sex, and geographic region.

TABLE 1-3
Number and Adjusted Rates of Newborn Discharges With Congenital Deficiencies by Level

LEVEL	No. (%) 1988–1996	ADJUSTED ANNUAL INCIDENCE PER 100,00 LIVE BIRTHS	
		1988	1996
Upper limb (all)	5,458 (58.5)	14.73	15.74
Transverse	1,398 (15.0)	3.82	3.44
Longitudinal hand	2,532 (27.2)	6.50	7.68
Longitudinal radial	641 (6.9)	2.32	1.81
Longitudinal humeral	104 (1.1)	0.18	0.09
Unspecified	735 (7.9)	1.78	2.71
Lower limb (all)	3,868 (41.5)	9.48	9.90
Transverse	457 (4.9)	0.73	1.01
Longitudinal toe	1,327 (14.2)	3.62	3.47
Longitudinal foot	67 (0.7)	0.25	0.24
Longitudinal fibular	178 (1.9)	0.14	0.44
Longitudinal tibial	158 (1.7)	0.57	0.42
Longitudinal remoral	568 (6.1)	1.32	1.80
Unspecified	1,115 (12.0)	2.84	2.52
All discharges	9,326 (100.0)	24.21	25.64

1996 rates are standardized to the 1988 US population by sex and geographic region. Totals represent all discharges from 1988 to 1996.

amputations (68.6%) during this study period. Limb amputation secondary to malignancy decreased from 0.62 per 100,000 to 0.35 per 100,000 over this same period. Congenital deficiencies remained stable at 25.64 per 100,000 live births in 1996. Of the congenital limb anomalies, upper limb deficiency was the most common and accounted for 58.5% of all newborn limb deficiency discharges (Table 1-3).

According to this study, males were at significantly higher risk for trauma-related amputations than females, with an incidence rate ratio of 4.94. For both males and females, risk of traumatic amputations increased steadily among those ages 85 and older. Blacks, particularly those ages 35 and higher, were generally at a higher risk than non-blacks for trauma-related amputations.

Among non-blacks, the incidence of trauma-caused amputations was essentially constant across age groups at about 7 per 100,000, except for a much lower rate at younger ages and a higher rate among those aged 75 and higher.

Dillingham, et al., also studied the epidemiology of amputation-related to trauma in the state of Maryland during a 15-year period (5). The number and incidence per 100,000 persons for major and minor trauma-related amputations in Maryland from 1979 through 1993 is found in Table 1-4. In this study of trauma-related amputees, the age-specific incidence and the gen-

TABLE 1-4
Number and Incidence Per 100,000 of Major and Minor Trauma-Related Amputations by Amputation Level: Maryland, 1979–1993

AMPUTATION LEVEL	TOTAL NUMBER (PERCENTAGE), 1979–1993	ANNUAL INCIDENCE PER 100,000	
		1979	1993
Major	992 (16.3)	1.88	1.07
Above elbow	95 (1.6)	.10	.04
Below elbow	93 (1.5)	.22	.08
Above knee	267 (4.4)	.31	.30
Below knee	276 (4.5)	.75	.32
Multiple lower extremity	102 (1.7)	.17	.16
Multiple upper extremity	23 (0.4)	.02	.02
Foot	136 (2.2)	.31	.14
Minor	5,077 (83.7)	10.76	4.70
Finger	3,201 (52.7)	7.33	3.19
Hand	696 (11.5)	1.60	0.52
Toe	1,053 (17.4)	1.78	0.91
Multiple	127 (2.1)	.07	.08
Total	6,069 (100.0)	12.65	5.77

TABLE 1-5
Distribution of Major and Minor Trauma-Related Amputee Patients by Age and Gender: Maryland, 1979–1993

AGE GROUP	MAJOR AMPUTATIONS			MINOR AMPUTATIONS			
	MALES	FEMALES	TOTAL (A)	MALES	FEMALES	TOTAL (B)	TOTAL (C)
0–14	43 (6%)	20 (7.4%)	63 (6.4%)	403 (9.3%)	184 (25.2%)	587 (11.6%)	650 (10.7%)
15–24	154 (21.4%)	30 (11.1%)	184 (18.5%)	947 (21.8%)	103 (14.1%)	1,050 (20.7%)	1,234 (20.3%)
25–34	153 (21.2%)	38 (14.0%)	191 (19.3%)	1,002 (23.0%)	122 (16.7%)	1,124 (22.1%)	1,315 (21.7%)
35–44	93 (12.9%)	21 (7.7%)	114 (11.5%)	687 (15.8%)	116 (15.9%)	803 (15.8%)	917 (15.1%)
45–54	83 (11.5%)	21 (7.7%)	104 (10.5%)	567 (13.0%)	82 (11.2%)	649 (12.8%)	753 (12.4%)
55–64	97 (13.5%)	28 (10.3%)	125 (12.6%)	419 (9.6%)	47 (6.4%)	466 (9.2%)	591 (9.7%)
65–74	56 (7.8%)	37 (13.7%)	93 (9.4%)	232 (5.3%)	43 (5.9%)	275 (5.4%)	368 (6.1%)
75+	42 (5.8%)	76 (28.0%)	118 (11.9%)	91 (2.1%)	32 (4.4%)	123 (2.4%)	241 (4.0%)
Total	721 (100%)	271 (100%)	992 (100%)	4,348 (100%)	729 (100%)	5,077 (100%)	6,069 (100%)
% of A or B	72.7%	27.3%	100%	85.6%	14.4%	100%	
% of C	11.9%	4.5%	16.3%	71.6%	12.0%	83.7%	100%

der of major and minor amputations is found in Table 1-5. Males accounted for 72.3% of the major trauma-related amputations, whereas males accounted for 85.6% of minor amputations that were trauma-related.

The leading causes of trauma-related amputations were injuries involving machinery (40.1%), powered tools and appliances (27.8%), firearms (8.5%), and motor vehicle crashes (8%).

The mean length of inpatient hospital stay for an above-elbow amputation was 20 days; 15 days for a below-elbow amputation. It was rare for these patients to be discharged to a rehabilitation facility or other institution.

Many factors may have contributed to the observed decline in the incidence of amputations secondary to trauma. Changes in the aggressiveness of both reconstructive (limb salvage) surgery and the reimplantation of severed digits and extremities may account for part of the decline in amputation rates. The decline may also represent an actual decrease in the incidence of injuries severe enough to result in amputation. Improved occupational safety standards and an increased awareness and enforcement of safety regulations may have led to a decline in injuries resulting in limb amputation. Males dominated among both major and minor traumatic amputee patients for all years of study.

HISTORY OF ARM PROSTHESES

In 61 A.D., Pliny wrote that a Roman general, Marcus Sergius, lost his right hand in the Second Punic War (218–201 B.C.). The general had an iron hand made, which he used to support his shield. Skipping forward to the Middle Ages, in 1509 a classic example of an early artificial hand is a mailed fist that was made for Goetz von Berlichingen (Figure 1-1). This prostheses was equipped with jointed fingers that could passively grip his sword like a vise.

In 1564, Ambrose Paré, the great French military surgeon, published his ten-volume work on surgery. In it, he presented illustrations and descriptions of artificial arms and legs that he claimed could be reproduced by any locksmith of the time. None of these devices had any volitional control and were locked in place passively.

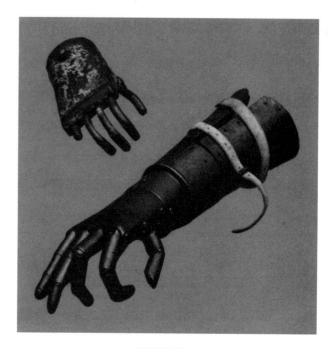

FIGURE 1-1

Medieval arm prosthesis made for Goetz von Berlichingen circa 1509.

In 1818, after the Napoleonic Wars, a Berlin dentist, Peter Baliff appears to have been the first person to introduce the use of the trunk and shoulder girdle muscles as sources of power to flex or extend prosthetic fingers. Baliff reversed the spring action of the Paré and Goetz hands by having the terminal device extend through the action of the sound shoulder. This design was only for a transradial level of amputation.

In 1844, the first transhumeral amputation replacement used Baliff's principle to apply flexion for the elbow joint. This design was from a Dutch sculptor, Van Peeterssen.

In 1860, the Crimean and Italian campaigns of the French Empire left a number of amputees whose needs were provided for by Comte de Beaufort. He provided the amputee control through a shoulder harness. The controlling power started with a strap buttoned into the front button of the trousers, passed through a loop to the opposite axilla, over to the amputated side to a pulley at the elbow, and then to the artificial hand. He also invented a simple hand with a movable thumb and a transhumeral prosthesis in which the elbow was flexed by the pressure of a lever against the side of the chest. He also designed a hand in which the opening and closing of the fingers was effected by repeated pulls on the same cord. A double spring hook was also included for holding objects, similar to that of the well-known split hook.

During World War I, a tremendous loss of manpower arose in all countries because of the large number of casualties. Thus, all countries, by necessity, equipped as many amputees as possible to carry on their accustomed trades by means of mechanical aids. A great effort was made to return amputees to productive work on the farm or in trade occupation. The amputee was given a socket and a universal terminal device that held work tool for his trade; if he did another activity, he needed to change out the terminal device. In Great Britain, a "dummy" hand was also provided in addition to the tool terminal device. In the United States, a split hook was developed that was closed by rubber bands. This terminal device satisfied the American appetite for speed and true universality.

In October, 1917, the Surgeon General of the United States Army issued an invitation to limb makers to meet in Washington, D.C. Following this meeting, the Association of Limb Manufacturers of America was formed, which later became the American Orthopedic Limb Manufacturers Association.

At the conclusion of World War II, a great national need to provide better artificial limbs occured, and in 1945, the National Research Council was established. This later became the Advisory Council on Artificial Limbs, and later the Prosthetic Research Board.

Between 1953 and 1956, courses were presented that focused on the principles and techniques for prescription, fabrication, and training of the upper extremity amputees. These courses were held under the direction of Craig L. Taylor, Ph.D. at UCLA and at New York University under the direction of Sidney Fishman, Ph.D.

In 1958, "A Manual for Occupational Therapists on the Rehabilitation of Upper Extremity Amputees" was written by Thelma Wellerson, an occupational therapist, at the Institute for the Crippled and Disabled in New York City (6). She chronicled a development of prostheses in this manual.

The use of external power was first unveiled by Alderson, with support from the United States government and IBM. He developed the first electrically powered artificial arm about 1949 (7). In 1958, the Russians announced the first myoelectric arm for the below-elbow (transradial) amputee. The Otto Bock company first made versions of the Russian design commercially available for general application.

During the 1980s, electric arm prosthetic components became more universally applicable, and newer electric arm prosthetic developments continue as robotic designs are explored.

HISTORY OF ARM AMPUTATION REHABILITATION

The codification of the practice and history of the physical medicine and rehabilitation specialty, as it was developed in the United States, dates to the founding of the American Academy of Physical Medicine and Rehabilitation in 1938. The founding fathers, Frank Krusen, M.D. and Howard Rusk, M.D., each brought their knowledge and experiences to the developing field. The American Academy of Physical Medicine and Rehabilitation was first known as the Society of Physical Therapy Physicians (8). The American Board of Physical Medicine and Rehabilitation was established in 1947. Following World War I, amputees received therapies in prosthetic use and "centers of excellence" were established for those who had lost arms and legs. However, the codification of an integrated team of health professionals devoted to the comprehensive treatment of the amputee was first established during World War II at specified military hospitals around the United States. Wounded soldiers required physical therapeutic measures for treatment, so military physicians were sent to Rochester, Minnesota for a three-month training program in physical therapy medicine under the direction of Frank Krusen, M.D. Dr. Howard Rusk began his contributions to the field of rehabilitation during World War II, when he came across a large number of inactive wounded soldiers being warehoused following their initial course of acute medical and surgical care. The Rusk approach advocated an interdisciplinary attempt to providing rehabilitative care, and all phases of rehabilitation service were available for servicemen who sustained an amputation. Videotapes of those servicemen being trained and restored to meaningful function show most of the usual vocational and avocational activities that non-amputees perform today.

As schools of Occupational Therapy and Physical Therapy were established, their core curriculum included prosthetic information and the basic skills for prosthetic training.

One of the first texts published to deal with the biomechanics of arm prosthetic use was entitled "Human Limbs and Their Substitutes," by Klopsteg and Wilson in 1954 (9). A most important contribution to the literature of prosthetic fabrication and training was edited by Santschi in 1958 (10). Two texts devoted to the rehabilitation of amputees, with focus on the patient with an arm amputation, were written in the 1970s by Dr. Leonard Bender and Dr. Lawrence Friedmann (11,12). In his introduction, Dr. Friedmann indicates that whereas "treating the patient as a whole has become a platitude, there is no substitute for so doing, if one wishes to provide optimal care rather than partial, fragmented, and inadequate care." He exhorts health professionals "to see the patient from the patient's perspective, and not only from the perspective of our medical specialties."

In 1989, the first extensive text devoted to arm amputation rehabilitation was published (13). In addition, the American Academy of Orthopedic Surgeons has published its *Atlas of Limb Prosthetics* (14), for a number of years. These texts attempt to provide the total approach for prosthetic application and rehabilitation services as practiced in the United States.

CONCLUSION

Although persons have suffered arm amputation for centuries, it is only during the past 500 years that substitutes, no matter how crude, have been fabricated in an attempt to provide a substitute for the amputated part of the arm. Even with the advances made in the electrical control of prosthetic parts, man has not built an excellent substitute for a missing hand, wrist, elbow, or shoulder. We continue to strive for better prosthetic designs, methods of training in their use, and rehabilitation. However, we have made significant strides in decreasing the incidence of arm amputation and improving the reattachment or reconstruction of traumatically damaged hands and arms. Thus, the apparent frequency of arm amputation appears to be decreasing.

*R*eferences

1. Kirk NT. The Development of Amputation, An Introductory Survey. In: Vasconcelos E, *Modern Methods of Amputation*. New York: The Philosophical Library of New York, 1945.
2. Daugherty PJ. Wartime amputations. *Mil Medicine* 158; 1993.
3. Slocum D. An *Atlas of Amputations*. Philadelphia: Mosby, 1949.
4. Dillingham TR, Pezzin LE, MacKenzie EJ. Limb amputation and limb deficiency: epidemiology and recent trends in the United States. *South Med J* 95(8); 2002.
5. Dillingham TR, Pezzin LE, MacKenzie EJ. Incidence, acute care length of stay, and discharge to rehabilitation of traumatic amputee patients: an epidemiologic study. *Arch Phys Med Rehabil* 79, 1998.
6. Wellerson TL. *A Manual for Occupational Therapists on the Rehabilitation of Upper Extremity Amputees*. Dubuque: Kendall/Hunt Publishing Company, 1958.
7. Wilson AB. History of Amputation Surgery and Prosthetics. In: Bowker JH, Michael JW (eds), *Atlas of Limb Prosthetics: Surgical, Prosthetic, and Rehabilitation Principles*. St. Louis: Mosby, 1992.
8. Materson RS. Introduction. In: Grabois M, Garrison SJ, Hart KA, Lehmkuhl LD (eds), *Physical Medicine & Rehabilitation: The Complete Approach*. Malden: Blackwell Science, 2000.
9. Klopsteg PE, Wilson PD. *Human Limbs and Their Substitutes*. New York: McGraw-Hill Book Company, 1954.
10. Santschi WR. *Manual of Upper Extremity Prosthetics*. Los Angeles: UCLA, 1958.
11. Bender LF. *Prostheses and Rehabilitation after Arm Amputation*. Springfield: Charles C Thomas, 1974.
12. Friedmann L. *The Surgical Rehabilitation of the Amputee*. Springfield: Charles C Thomas, 1978.
13. Atkins DJ, Meier RH. *Comprehensive Management of the Upper-Limb Amputee*. New York: Springer-Verlag, 1989.
14. *Atlas of Limb Prosthetics: Surgical, Prosthetic, and Rehabilitation Principles, Second Edition*. Bowker, JH. and Michael, JW (eds). St. Louis: Mosby, 1992.

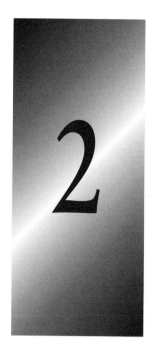

Amputation Levels and Surgical Techniques

James B. Bennett, MD, and Charlotte B. Alexander, MD

Upper-extremity amputation presents a complex loss for the patient. The hand functions in prehensile activities as a sensory organ and as a means of communication. Any loss interferes with the patient's productivity and feeling of completeness, and alters his interactions with his environment.

Amputation surgery encompasses reconstruction for prosthetic fitting and functional use of the extremity. A coordinated team approach includes the patient, surgeon, prosthetist, and rehabilitation specialist. Ideally, the amputation should be approached as a form of reconstructive surgery even in the acute traumatic amputation. An ideal residual limb should be well padded, pain free, functional, and aesthetically acceptable.

Most upper-extremity amputations are secondary to trauma. Initial treatment should consist of preservation of all viable tissues after appropriate debridement of nonviable tissues. Treatment may require more than one surgical procedure, as it is often difficult to assess viability in a severely injured extremity upon initial presentation. Patient needs vary with vocation, avocation, age, and ethnic origin. A working man may prefer an ablative procedure that will allow early functional return to work rather than staged reconstruction requiring multiple surgeries, prolonged rehabilitation, and an uncertain functional result. Single fingertip amputations do not often result in disability unless the hand is used for activities of precision or for keyboard instruments. Among Latin, Asian, and Arabic populations severe social stigma is associated with loss of the hand or of its parts, so that retention of a painful, less functional part may be preferable to amputation for these individuals.

Amputation levels may be predetermined by disease processes such as tumors or infection. Maximum length is preserved, consistent with removing the diseased tissue and prosthetic fit, if desirable. Staged procedures may be indicated to preserve maximum function. In the case of infection or vascular impairment, a guillotine or more limited debridement can be performed at the first surgery. A second look two days later allows the tissues to define themselves. Wound closure can then be planned for maximum function and tissue preservation.

Vascular problems necessitating amputations are less common in the upper extremity when compared with the lower extremity. Irreparable loss of vascular blood supply is an indication for acute amputation. In a patient with peripheral vascular disease, a midforearm amputation may have a higher survival rate than a distal forearm amputation with less perfusion of tissues.

In general, amputation levels are more conservative in the upper extremity than in the lower extremity. In the leg, a below-knee amputation may be a preferred level for prosthetic wear and early return to normal activities. However in the upper extremity, length and function are more critical.

Improved microvascular techniques have allowed for replantations of cleanly severed parts. Where tissues are more traumatized, the limb can be shortened to create clean margins more amenable to primary closure. Elegant delay implantation has been performed in which the amputated part is primarily anastamosed to a distant clean site while the recipient site is being prepared for a final closure. Free flaps have provided an opportunity to preserve length with good quality skin that is often sensate. Muscle can be transferred to improve function. Free bone transfers can facilitate reconstruction of large bone loss areas.

Six components of the amputation stump or residual limb must be addressed: skin, muscle, nerves, vessels, bone, and joints (Figure 2-1).

Skin should be well healed and painless. It should be nonadherent and pliable, but not hypermobile. Soft-tissue padding should be adequate to cover bony prominences but not so bulky or redundant as to impede prosthetic fit. Translation of motion from the residual arm to the prosthetic socket requires fixation of the skin and soft tissues to the underlying bony architecture. Above all it should be sensate. Sensibility makes a partial hand with the ability to pinch superior to any prosthesis. This sensibility can be provided most effectively by similar innervated tissue. Cross-finger flaps, thenar eminence flaps, or split-thickness skin grafts can provide better than 1 cm two-point discrimination, whereas abdominal or distant flaps rarely provide more than protective sensation (1,2). Innervated skin may also be

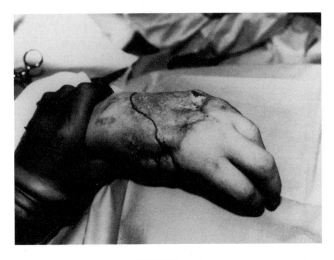

FIGURE 2-1

Crushed, insensitive, nonfunctional hand with poor skin coverage following several reconstructive operations for wrist disarticulation and prosthetic hand unit.

transferred by a free or rotational neurovascular pedicle to key contact areas, such as a partially amputated thumb (1,3). Tissue expansion provides skin that is compatible in color and texture with the surrounding tissue (4).

Muscle provides motor ability, contour, and bulk. Useful motor units require innervation, excursion, and bone or tendinous attachment. Innervation may require appropriate nerve repair. After one year, muscle fibrosis precludes useful recovery of function (5). Excursion must be present for muscle contraction and tendon gliding. Postinjury swelling and edema can create scarring, which limits this excursion. Improper or prolonged immobilization can contribute to contracture. Even nonfunctional muscle can provide coverage for bone, tendon, or nerves, as well as a vascular bed for grafts. Contractile muscle can activate a myoelectric prosthesis.

All cut nerves form neuromas at the proximal stump, which may become painful if they are adherent to skin, contracted in scar tissue, in areas of repetitive trauma, or in close contact with the prosthetic wall. Neuromas can be dealt with in several ways:

- The nerve can be resected or placed proximal to the amputation level in a padded or protected area. Care must be taken not to stretch the nerve unduly in resection, as this can lead to painful neuroma incontinuity formation proximal to the transected nerve.
- The cut nerve can be ligated through a proximal wound, forming a well-protected neuroma.
- Two end nerves can be anastomosed to each other to minimize neuroma formation (1).
- Capping the nerve end with epineural grafts has been shown to be significantly effective in preventing neuroma pain (6).

When possible, vascular supply to remaining tissues should be repaired to preserve maximum tissue coverage and to minimize cold intolerance. Severed major vessels in the stump should be doubly ligated to protect against rebleeding. Tourniquets should be deflated prior to wound closure and meticulous hemostasis obtained. Drains should be used where there is dead space or concern about bleeding and hematoma formation.

If fractures are present, the bone must be stabilized to promote bone healing and to allow early joint motion. Bony prominences should be rounded off and have good soft-tissue padding. Free flaps from a nonsalvageable amputated limb may provide immediate wound coverage and preservation of functional amputation stump lengths (7–9). Spurs may occur at the ends of the bony stump, but these rarely cause problems in

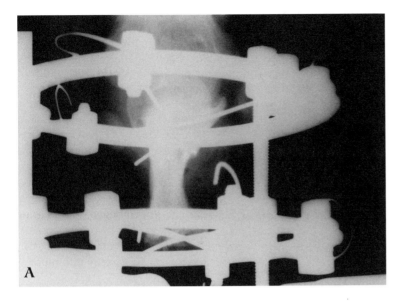

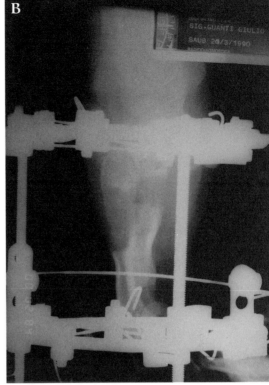

FIGURE 2-2

A. Short below-elbow amputation lengthened by the Ilizarov technique to allow below-elbow prosthetic fit, preoperative cordotomy. B. Ilizarov technique to lengthen the short below-elbow amputation residual limb.

adults with adequate soft-tissue coverage. The cartilage at joint surfaces need not be removed unless there is concern that marginal tissue coverage may lead to a chronic chondritis (8,10).

Joint motion should be preserved and protected. Even short residual bone distal to the joint may be a basis for a reconstructive procedure, such as soft-tissue coverage, bone lengthening, or tendon transfer. The Ilizarov technique has allowed for bone lengthening even through free tissue transfers (11). Retained joint motion can motor a more functional distal prosthesis and provide for a lighter prosthesis (Figures 2-2A and B).

Revision of traumatic amputations because of a painful stump is common. A painful stump may be due to entrapped neuroma, inadequate soft-tissue coverage, bony overgrowth, or a painful scar. Redundant bulky flaps or soft tissue may require thinning or revision. Retained nonfunctional digits may be excised to provide a more functional or cosmetic result in the hand.

The surgical approach to upper-extremity amputation varies somewhat with the amputation levels. Specific amputation techniques are well described in the literature (1,12–15) and will not be repeated in this book. Special concerns referable to each level are mentioned below.

DIGITAL

Digital-tip amputations without exposed bone do equally well with conservative care consisting of dressing changes and healing by secondary intent or operative closure with primary skin or flap coverage. Straight growth of the nail depends on volar support for the nailbed. If this is lost, volar curving of the nail will result.

Amputations more proximally through the nailbed and distal phalanx require soft-tissue coverage of bone. In the thumb, all length should be preserved, even if this requires local or distant flaps (16). Complete loss of the thumb is a 40 to 50% disability of the hand (12,15). In distal amputations in the other digits, shortening of the bone to allow for skin coverage leaves little disability. If the amputation involves the nail matrix, all of this must be excised or horns of nail may appear, which can be painful or disfiguring.

Amputation of the thumb to the midproximal phalanx and the mid-distal phalanx can be treated by a Z-plasty deepening of the web space (5,3,12). In metacarpophalangeal (MP)-level amputations, the thumb can be lengthened by the creation of a skin pocket, Gillies' cocked hat flap, or groin pedicle skin tube into which a bone graft can be inserted (1,3,12).

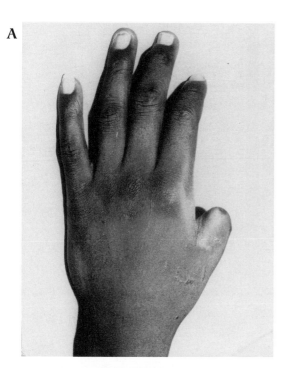

FIGURE 2-3

Metacarpal distraction lengthening of the thumb with a Z-plasty of the thumb index web to improve thumb function after proximal phalanx amputation A. Pre-op, B. Lengthening, C. Z-plasty & STSG.

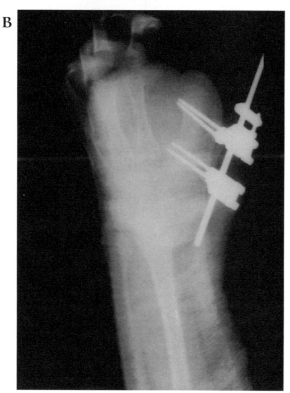

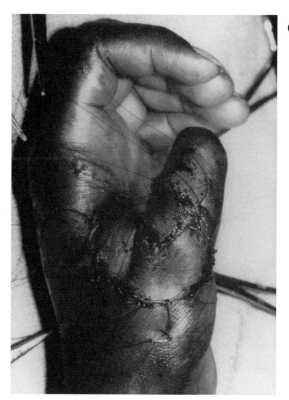

Distraction lengthening of the remaining metacarpal or previous bone graft can be used in a young person with good skin coverage (Figure 2-3A,B,C) (3,7,12). More proximal amputation requires pollicization of an adjacent digit (Figure 2-4A,B) or microvascular toe transfer (Figure 2-5A,B) (1,3,5). Thumb prostheses that provide

a post for the remaining fingers to oppose pinch and grasp are available (Figure 2-6A,B).

In amputations through the distal interphalangeal (DIP) joint of the fingers, the condyles should be contoured for improved cosmesis and function. The tendons should be divided and allowed to retract. Suturing

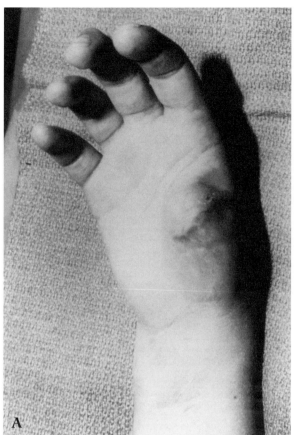

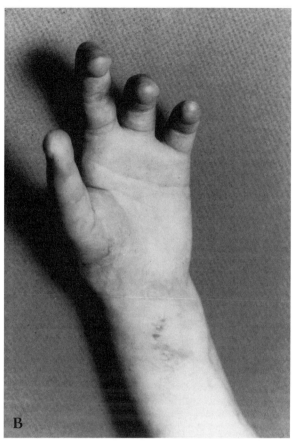

FIGURE 2-4

A. Traumatic amputation of the thumb for reconstructive pollicization of the index finger. B. Postoperative index finger pollicization procedure for thumb reconstruction.

the tendons may lead to tethering of the tendons of the adjacent digits, resulting in limitation of motion (1,10,17,18). Occasionally, division of the profundus tendon creates a "lumbrical plus" deformity, which may be relieved by sectioning the lumbrical tendon (1). The index finger is the prime digit for thumb opposition. However, in amputations proximal to the DIP joint, the thumb readily transfers pinch to the long finger. The residual index finger may impede this motion, and a more cosmetic appearance can be provided with a ray II amputation (10,17). However, the resulting narrowed palm of a ray II amputation leads to a 20% decrease in grip strength (1) and is contraindicated in someone requiring power grip in his vocation. Digital amputations distal to the sublimis insertion allow full proximal interphalangeal (PIP) participation in grip.

In PIP joint amputations, the condyles should also be contoured. Amputations at this level allow 45 degrees of proximal phalangeal flexion to contribute to grip and help maintain objects in the palm (1).

Amputations at the MP level, especially of the central two digits, result in objects dropping through the palm and finger. If the long finger is involved, the long ray may be resected and the index finger transposed. This will lead to a weakness in pinch unless the adductor pollicis is reattached (3). With defects in the ring finger, ray resection and little-finger transposition will narrow the palm (Figure 2.7A–D). Care must be taken to control rotation of the digits, because resection of ray IV increases the normal mobility of ray V (1). Amputation of ray V can be cosmetic and functional, provided the metacarpal base with tendinous attachments is preserved. Reattachment of the hypothenar muscles may create an intrinsic plus deformity of the ring finger and is not necessary. In multiple-digit amputations, special care should be taken to preserve all length and viable tissues. A sensate hand with two-digit pinch will not require a functional prosthesis. Cosmetic prostheses are available for partial finger amputations (Figure 2-8).

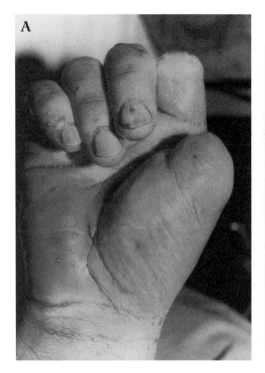

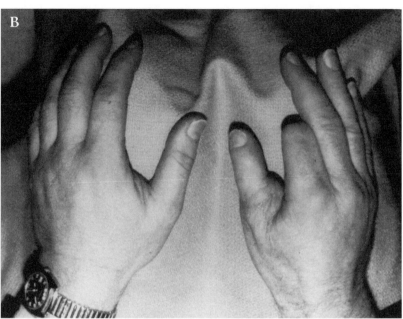

FIGURE 2-5

A. Thumb and index amputations for microsurgical free toe to thumb transfer. B. Postoperative great toe-to-thumb microsurgical free transfer for amputation of thumb in a male patient.

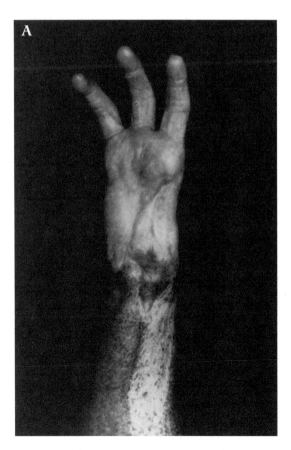

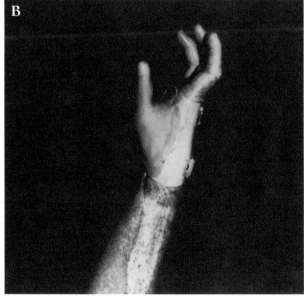

FIGURE 2-6

A. Thumb and index ray resection after burn injury in elderly patient who did not want reconstructive surgery. B. Thumb prosthesis to allow some grip and pinch function to a cosmetic opposition post.

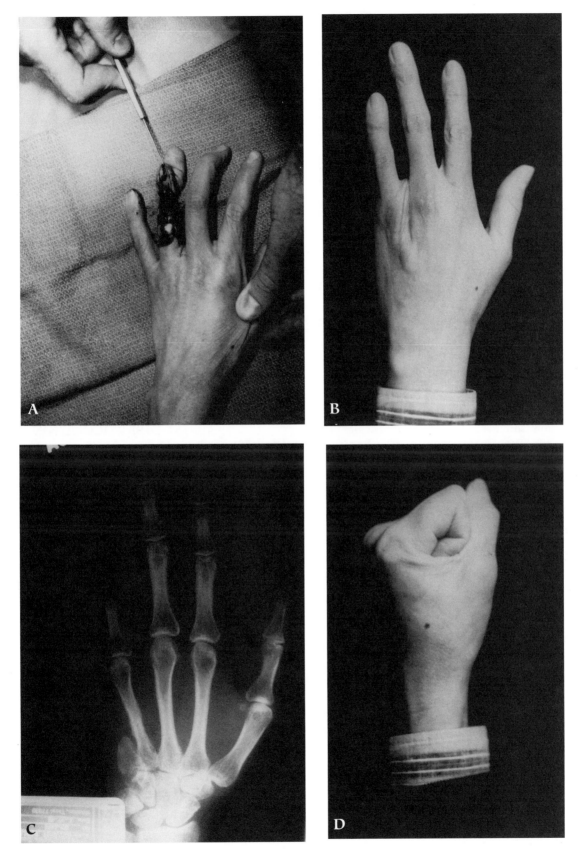

FIGURE 2-7

A. Ring finger avulsion amputation. B. Ringer finger ray amputation with little finger metacarpal shift to close the palm defect. C. X-ray to demonstrate the healed fifth to fourth metacarpal shift to gain length and close the palm defect. D. Full fist closure.

FIGURE 2-8

Prosthetic finger for single digit amputation.

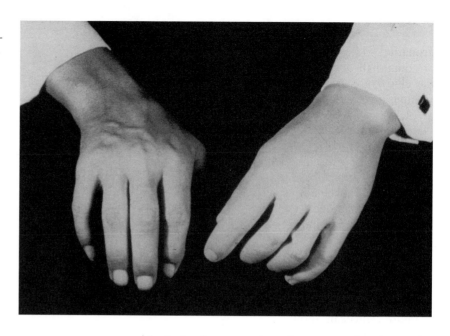

PARTIAL HAND

For multiple digit injuries, the primary goal is to have all viable tissue for reconstruction at a later date. Reconstruction should be planned to provide pinch where possible. Partial phalanges or metacarpals can provide a post for opposition or extension to assist grip. These remnants can often be lengthened or used as bone stock for transfers (19). Even damaged digits with little use in their anatomic position can be moved to provide more function with translocation or microvascular transfer (20).

In a transmetacarpal amputation with the thumb intact, the fifth metacarpal can be phalangized by rotation and separation to provide an opposition post. Fourth metacarpal resection may improve mobility (3,5). With good soft tissue coverage, the ulnar metacarpal can be lengthened acutely by transposition of tissues or by distraction to improve pinch. With accompanying thumb amputation, deepening of the first web space increases mobility and allows for a pincher action (1,3). The efficiency of this can be improved by distraction lengthening of the remaining bone stock. Proximal metacarpal or carpometacarpal amputations do not usually allow for reconstruction of pinch or grasp. More proximal replantation of an amputated finger or toe transfer has been tried in an effort to solve these difficult cases (21,22). A single hook can assist with activities of daily living. A prosthetic paddle or lengthened ulnar pad can provide limited pinch. Even preservation of the radiocarpal joint allows a hook-like action, especially in holding objects against the body. This level of amputation provides poor prosthetic function; better prosthetic function is gained from a wrist disarticulation amputation and

prosthetic hook restoration. A cosmetic hand may be used for social occasions.

WRIST DISARTICULATION

In radiocarpal amputations, flexion and extension are lost but supination and pronation are complete as long as the radioulnar joint and triangular fibrocartilage are preserved (Figure 2-9) (1,14,15). At least 50% of this motion can be transferred to the prosthesis (12,15). The radial and ulnar styloids may be trimmed to facilitate prosthetic fitting. However, this is controversial since not trimming the styloid permits prosthetic self-suspension. The triangular fibrocartilage should be preserved to protect the radioulnar joint. A fish mouth incision with a longer volar flap is used for increased sensitivity and durability of the stump, rather than equal dorsal and volar flaps.

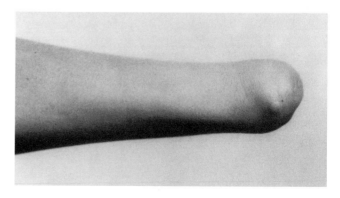

FIGURE 2-9

Wrist disarticulation with preservation of maximum pronation and supination.

BELOW ELBOW

Pronation and supination are lost in amputation of the proximal half of the forearm. Flexion and extension at the elbow are critical, and as little as 1.5 inches of stump is preferable to an amputation through the elbow (1,14,15). With split socket and step-up hinges, the range of motion can be preserved and residual motor function amplified. Functional length can also be increased with a biceps tendon recession, leaving the brachialis and brachioradialis muscles to provide elbow flexion (14,15). The amputation technique is similar to wrist disarticulation, using a fish mouth incision of equal skin flaps fashioned distal to the anticipated final level. These skin edges retract with muscle transsection. The bone edges should be smoothed with a rasp or burr. Fascial closure over the end pads the bone, or residual sublimis muscle can be used to pad the distal stump. Nerves are ligated proximally. A compressive dressing (a figure eight) can allow primary compression distally and diminishes pressure proximally. This provides hemostases, begins stump shaping, and prevents the edema that can be caused by a circumferential dressing. Latissimus dorsi myocutaneous transfer or free tissue transfer should be considered to preserve below-elbow length and coverage, rather than an amputation at a more proximal level for improved prosthetic use with a below-elbow prosthesis. Distraction lengthening has been shown to successfully double residual forearm length, thus facilitating prosthesis fit (23,24).

ELBOW DISARTICULATION

Elbow disarticulations and transcondylar amputations allow the transfer of humeral rotation to the prosthesis.

Anterior exposure allows the identification of brachial artery and veins. Nerves are transsected and allowed to retract proximally. Attachments of flexor to extensor forearm muscle and triceps to anterior musculature can provide good soft-tissue coverage (Figure 2-10A,B). The condyles are not trimmed, because these allow a transfer of rotation to the prosthesis.

ABOVE ELBOW

Above-elbow amputation should preserve all possible length. In more proximal amputations up to the axillary fold, rotation is lost but other shoulder motions are retained. To maintain equal arm length, a 1.5-inch resection of the distal humerus is required to allow space for the elbow turntable mechanism in the prosthesis (14,15). With long above-elbow amputations proximal to the flare, an angulatory osteotomy of the humerus, as described by Marquardt (25), allows humeral rotation to be transferred to the prosthesis. This may be especially helpful in the bilateral amputee (26). Skin flaps of equal size are designed. Anterior and posterior muscle closure will give good bone coverage, although this may be too bulky and require some thinning. Shoulder arthrodesis is recommended if shoulder control is absent but scapular function is intact, as in brachial plexus injury (Figure 2-11).

SHOULDER DISARTICULATION

Amputations proximal to the axillary fold are treated as functional shoulder disarticulations, since abduction and flexion are lost. However, maintenance of any part of the humerus improves the contour of the shoulder

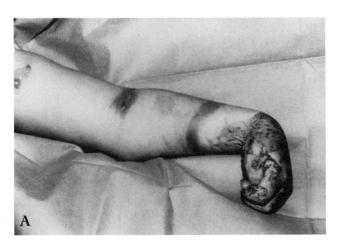
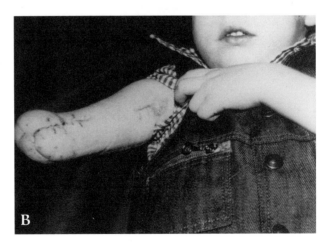

FIGURE 2-10

A. Electrical burn in a child resulting in nonviable hand/forearm to the elbow with burn exit at the axilla. B. Elbow disarticulation in child with an electrical burn.

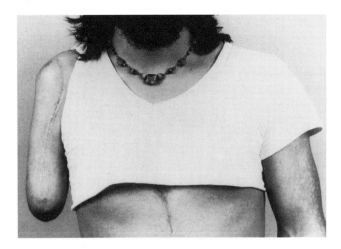

FIGURE 2-11

Above-elbow amputation and shoulder arthrodesis for upper extremity above-elbow prosthetic use.

and provides a better fit for the above-elbow shoulder prosthesis (Figure 2-12). In a shoulder disarticulation, the deltoid is preserved, which maintains some shoulder contour. A latissimus dorsi myocutaneous flap may be utilized to cover skin deficit or open shoulder disarticulation to preserve contour (Figure 2-13A,B).

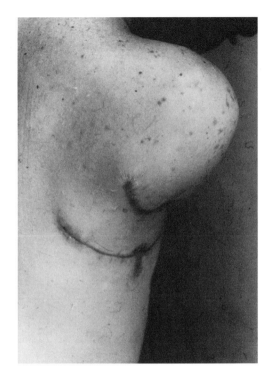

FIGURE 2-12

Proximal humeral amputation with preservation of deltoid muscle and proximal humeral head for shoulder contour.

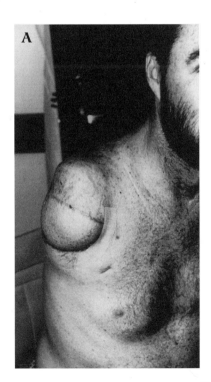
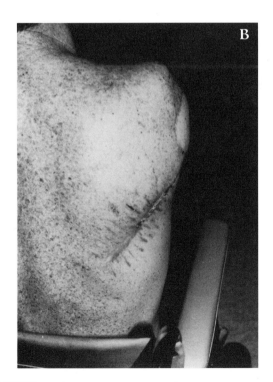

FIGURE 2-13

A. Latissimus dorsi myocutaneous flap following open shoulder disarticulation to provide soft tissue cover and contour to the shoulder. B. Cosmetically acceptable donor site of latissimus dorsi flap.

FOREQUARTER

The forequarter amputation removes the entire shoulder girdle and is usually performed for tumor excision. A posterior approach facilitates the easy isolation of the major neurovascular structures (1,14,15). The interscapulothoracic amputee frequently has a sensitive surgical site that requires fitted padding to allow prosthetic wear. A total volar forearm musculocutaneous free flap harvested from the amputated extremity can facilitate the closure of this large defect (27). In the Tikhor-Linberg procedure, the shoulder girdle is resected while the arm is preserved. The indications are quite limited, especially suited to well-localized tumors of the proximal humerus or scapula. The arm can be suspended from the rib cage or soft-tissue attachments about the hemithorax (1,28).

CHILDREN

Amputations in children follow similar general guidelines, with a few exceptions. Conservation is more important, because the child may develop exceptional use from minimal residual parts. Children's tissues are more forgiving; they heal more reliably and joints tolerate prolonged immobilization. Diaphyseal and metaphyseal amputations in the child are often associated with overgrowth, which may exceed the ability of soft-tissue coverage to compensate, thus producing erosion and possible penetration by the growing bone (29). This oppositional new bone formation is not decreased by epiphysiodesis, which only limits growth at the physis (13,15). Silastic caps and synostosis to adjacent bones have been used with varying success. Transplantation of a metatarsal epiphysis has been successful in animals, but usually this overgrowth requires subsequent revisions until maturity (13,15). For this reason, diaphyseal and metaphyseal amputations should be avoided unless necessary to preserve the proximal joints. As a rule, disarticulations at a more distal level are preferable to metaphyseal or diaphyseal levels, and epiphyseal growth should be preserved.

Congenital amputations may be transverse or longitudinal, and each of these may be partial or complete. Revision amputation is required in 10% of upper extremity congenital amputations, as opposed to 50% of those involving the lower extremity (13). In congenital hands, most of the proximal portions are relatively normal. This is not the case with most other congenital absences, which may involve proximal hypoplasia or dysplasia.

The radial club hand is a radial longitudinal deficiency that varies from thumb hypoplasia to complete absence of the radius and deficiency of the extensor and flexor forearm musculature. The hand may be radially deviated and the thumb and thenar musculature hypoplastic; 50% are bilateral. Treatment is directed at centralization of the hand and reconstruction of the thumb. Prior to correction, elbow and shoulder function must be evaluated, because either elbow flexion or radial deviation of the hand is necessary for hand-to-mouth function. Splinting may help stretch contracted radial structures, but surgical release is usually necessary. Centralization of the carpus on the ulna may then be done. Pollicization of the index finger for thumb reconstruction may be indicated (Figure 2-14). In bilateral involvement, one hand may be placed in slight supination for feeding and the other in slight pronation for perineal care (1). Distraction lengthening of the shortened ulna can enhance the ability to perform activities of daily living, such as reaching the face or perineum, or driving a car (30).

The ulnar club hand presents with ulnar deficiency that can vary from hypoplasia to total absence of the ulna with radiohumeral synostosis. The wrist is usually stable, with ulnar deviation, a bowed radius, and frequently an unstable radiohumeral joint. Stability of the elbow depends on the presence of a proximal ulnar portion, which is common. Treatment consists of the release of hand syndactyly and corrective osteotomy of the humerus. If the proximal radius is unstable, conversion to a one-bone forearm by osteotomy and fusion of the distal radius to the proximal ulna is indicated. If the thumb is syndactylized in the plane of the hand, syndactyly release or rotation osteotomy to allow opposition of the thumb with the remaining digits is indicated (1).

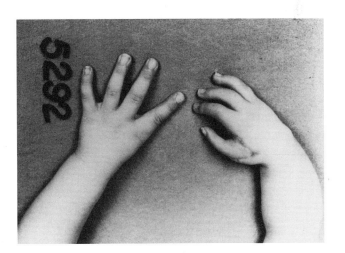

FIGURE 2-14

Radial club hand with pollicization of the index finger. Centalization of the wrist and forearm lengthening may be performed in the unilateral involved child to maximize equal length functional activity.

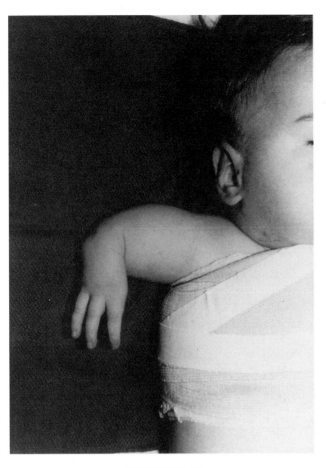

FIGURE 2-15

Phocomelic child with minimally functional digits that will be functional to activate prosthetic switches or myoelectrical sensors in the prosthesis.

The phocomelic patient rarely requires amputation revision. The terminal digits can be used to activate switches or myoelectric sensors in the prosthesis (Figure 2-15) (13–15).

SPECIAL CONSIDERATIONS

Bilateral below-elbow amputations can be reconstructed by means of a Krukenberg procedure, which divides the forearm musculature, allowing the radius to move against a stable ulna to provide pinch. The pronator teres provides the primary closing force, and the biceps or supinator provides the primary opening force. Ideally, the forearm should be 12 to 15 inches long with good soft tissue. Proper planning of skin flaps allows the creation of a sensitive pincher with some degree of stereognosis. This sensation is particularly helpful for the bilateral amputee and indispensable for the bilateral blind amputee. The procedure does not preclude wear-

ing a conventional prosthesis and should be considered a substitute for prosthesis wear, especially in developing countries (31). The major objection is cosmetic (Figure 2-16) (10,17,32).

Many attempts have been made to use residual motor function to power a prosthesis. Historically, the most successful has been the biceps cineplasty, in which a cutaneous tunnel is created through the muscle belly, allowing the insertion of a dowel that can be connected to the opening or closing arm of a distal lever. The movements are natural, and the amputee has the ability to modulate the strength of grasp. Some feedback of object size and position is also possible. The motion provided is weak and the amplitude small. Problems with ulceration can occur with poor flap design, and good hygiene is essential. Cineplasty is contraindicated in children (10,15,17,18).

Currently, electric prosthesis development provides another means of harnessing residual motor function. The prosthesis uses an external source of power triggered by the patient. A bony prominence, such as the acromion or a digit remnant, can activate a switch using a push or pull movement. Myoelectric prostheses can be triggered by muscle contraction. Surface (skin) electrodes record the potential of a muscle contraction as the signal to activate a portion of the prosthesis. The magnitude of the electromyographic (EMG) signal varies with muscle tension and the distance to the electrode. Securing the residual muscle in an amputation stump helps maintain tension as well as provide coverage and preserves the potential for myoelectric use in the future. Any muscle can be used, as long as the electrical potential is great enough and the electrode can be

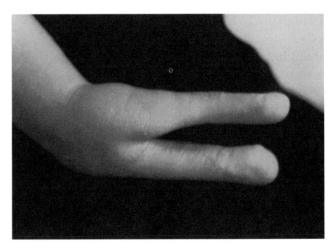

FIGURE 2-16

Krukenberg procedure to create pincher effect in below-elbow amputation patient.

connected to the prosthesis. The muscle should not have other physiologic function, as unwanted movement of the prosthesis will occur. Tenodesis of the transected muscles that cross two joints can remove their participation in adjacent joint motion. An example of this would be division of the biceps origin at the scapula and anchoring to the humerus in an above-elbow amputation. Background noise from other muscles is a problem, so the patient should be trained to do an independent contraction of the trigger muscle or muscle group. Varying the rate and strength of contraction can allow one muscle to initiate more than one function and even motor more than one joint. Work is being done with microcomputers that will allow the programming of EMG activities from multiple muscles in the remaining extremity. Activity associated with common functions will then be projected to the prosthesis. These will also provide for a lighter weight prosthesis with more natural body movements (33–35).

POSTOPERATIVE CARE

The success of an amputation depends, to a large extent, on the postoperative regime. Immediate postsurgical fitting (IPPF) allows the amputee to incorporate his new extremity more rapidly into daily use patterns. A cast or temporary prosthesis can be applied in the operating room. This provides a rigid dressing with uniform contact to help control swelling, encourage tissue healing, and allow early use of the extremity (Figure 2-

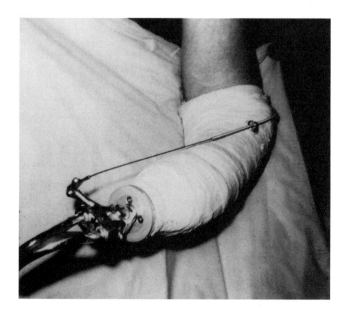

FIGURE 2-17

Immediate fit cast with terminal device applied at the time of the below-elbow amputation.

17). The cast can be revised as swelling decreases. Stump wrapping with elastic compression can be used to mature the stump if soft dressings are used initially. Physical therapy is begun shortly after surgery to preserve motion and gain strength. Early use of the extremity encourages patient acceptance and decreases the risk of developing a chronic pain pattern and a functionless extremity (1,14).

*R*eferences

1. Louis DS. Amputations. In: Green DP (ed), *Operative Hand Surgery*, Vol 1. New York: Churchill Livingstone, 1982, 55–111.
2. Sarrafian SK. Kinesiology and Functional Characteristics of the Upper Limb. In: *American Academy of Orthopedic Surgeons: Atlas of Limb Prosthetics, Surgical and Prosthetic Principles*. St. Louis: Mosby, 1981, 69–258.
3. Porter R. Functional assessment of transplanted skin in volar defects of the digits. *J Bone Joint Surg* 1968; 50A:5:955–963.
4. Wieslander JB. Tissue expansion in functional and aesthetic reconstruction of the trunk and extremities. Case report. *Scand J Plast. Reconstruction Surg Hand Surg* 1991; 25:285–289.
5. Bunnell S, Omer G. Amputation. In: Hunter E et al. (eds), *Rehabilitation of the Hand*. St. Louis: Mosby, 1978, 541–573.
6. Yuksel F et al. Prevention of painful neuromas by epineural ligatures, flaps, and grafts. *Br J Plastic Surg.* 1997; 50:182–185.
7. Chernofsky MA. Upper extremity salvage with free ulnar forearm flap from the amputated part—case report. *J Trauma* 1993; 34:450–452.
8. Foo IT, Malabu CM, Kay SP. Free tissue transfers to the upper limb. *J Hand Surg* 1993; 18:279–284.
9. Hammond DC et al. The free-fillet flap for reconstruction of the upper extremity. *Plast Reconstruction Surg* 1994; 94:507–512.
10. Boyes JH. Amputations. In: *Bunnell's Surgery of the Hand*, 5th ed. Philadelphia: Lippincott, 1970, 566–579.
11. Jupiter JB et al. Limb reconstruction by free tissue transfer combined with the Ilizarov method. *Plast Reconstruction Surg* 1991; 88:943–951.
12. Beasley RW. Amputations and prosthetic considerations. In: *Hand Injuries*. Philadelphia: Saunders, 1981, 344–361.
13. Beasley R. General considerations in managing upper limb amputations. Symposium on management of upper limb amputations. *Orthop Clin North Am* 1981; 12(4):743–842.
14. Tooms R. Amputation surgery in the upper extremity. Symposium on amputation surgery and prosthetics. *Orthop Clin North Am* 1972; 3:2:383–395.
15. Tooms R. The Hand: Amputations. In: Edmonson, Crenshaw (eds), *Campbells Operative Orthopedics*, 6th ed. St. Louis: Mosby, 1980, 231–262.
16. Koshima I et al. Sixty cases of partial or total toe transfer for repair of finger losses. *Plast Reconstruction Surg* 1993; 92:1331–1338.
17. Aitken GT, Pellicore RJ. Introduction to the Child Amputee. In: *American Academy of Orthopedic Surgeons: Atlas of Limb Prosthetics, Surgical and*

Prosthetic Principles. St. Louis: Mosby, 1981, 493–651.

18. Brown PW. Amputations. In: Sandzen S Jr (ed), *The Hand and Wrist.* Baltimore: Williams & Wilkins, 1985, 65–78.

19. Lee JW, Chiu HY, Hsu HY. Distraction lengthening of a replanted digit. *Plast Reconstruction Surg* 1995; 96:1438–1441.

20. Jeng SF, Wei FC. The distally based forearm island flap in hand reconstruction. *Plast Reconstruction Surg* 1998; 102:400–406.

21. Foucher G. The "stub" operation-modification of the Furnas-Vilkke technique in traumatic and congenital carpal hand reconstruction. *Am Acad Med,* Singapore 1995; 24:73–76.

22. Jeng SF, Wei FC, Noordhoff MS. Salvage replantation of two fingers from a nonreplantable midpalm. *Plast Reconstruction Surg* 1993; 91:1147–1150.

23. Kows AK, Seo JS, Pho RW. Combined free flap, Ilizarov lengthening and prosthetic fitting in the reconstruction of a proximal forearm amputation—case report. *Am Acad Med,* Singapore, 1995; 24:135–137.

24. Stricker SJ. Ilizarov lengthening of a posttraumatic below elbow amputation stump—a case report. *Clin Orthop* 1994; 124–127.

25. Marquardt E. The angulation osteotomy of above elbow stumps. *Clin Orthop* 1974; 104:232–238.

26. Milford L. The Hand: Amputations. In: Edmonson, Crenshaw (eds), *Campbells Operative Orthopedics,* 6th ed. St. Louis: Mosby, 1980, 231–262.

27. Cordeiro PG et al. The total volar forearm musculocutaneous free flap for reconstruction of extended forequarter amputation. *Ann Plast Surg* 1998; 40:388–396.

28. Tikhor P. Tumor studies (monograph). Sussia, 1900.

29. O'Neal ML et al. Osseous overgrowth after amputation in adolescents and children. *J Pediatric Orthop* 1996; 16:78–84.

30. Pickford MA, Scheker LR. Distraction lengthening of the ulna in radial club hand using the Ilizarov technique. *J Hand Surg* (Br) 1998; 23:186–191.

31. Visuthikosol V et al. The Kruhenberg procedure in the bilateral amputee after electrical burn. *Am Plastic Surg* 1991; 27:56–60.

32. Krukenberg H. *Ulber die Plastihe Uniwertung von Armamputation Stiempfern.* Stuttgart: Verlag, 1917.

33. Law H. *Advances in External Control of Human Extremities, 1981.* Dubroviuk: Yugoslav Committee for Electronics and Automation, 1981, 549–559.

34. Scott R. Surgical implications of myoelectric control. *Clin Orthop Rel Res* 1968; 61:248–260.

35. Shaperman J. Recent advances in research in prosthetics for children. *Clin Orthop Rel Res* 1980; 148:26–33.

3 Upper Extremity Salvage and Reconstruction for Trauma and Tumors

Ross M. Wilkins, MD, MS, and William C. Brown, MD, MS

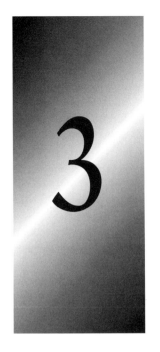

Since recorded history, it is evident that man has been disturbed by the problem of limb loss and its resulting dysfunction. The loss of a limb from either trauma or as a result of a tumorous process can be devastating physically and psychologically. Despite dramatic advances in fabrication and construction, no artificial limb can rival the corresponding natural part, especially in the upper extremity. The possibility of saving diseased limbs or reattaching amputated extremities has fascinated the medical and surgical sciences for centuries.

Legend has it that Saints Cosmos and Damian were brought back from the dead in the Middle Ages to perform surgery on a nobleman of the time who had lost a limb (1). Evidently, these patrons of physicians transplanted the limb of a recently deceased man onto the lower extremity of the nobleman, and with reported success. Similar myths and fables regarding limb preservation and reattachment have arisen from many cultures.

Despite mythology and the best intentions of evolving medical specialties, limb preservation following trauma did not become possible until several surgical innovations came into practice. The first, and probably most important, was Alexis Carrell's tech-

nique of sewing one blood vessel to another and maintaining physiologic flow. Thus it became possible to re-establish circulation to either severely damaged or severed extremities. With the advent of these microsurgical techniques and the further development of sophisticated instruments, such as operating microscopes in the late 1950s and early 1960s, more research was undertaken to employ revascularization techniques in traumatic situations. Following the successful suturing of vessels came the attempt to connect nerve endings to re-establish sensory and motor function to traumatized limbs. As these procedures became more widespread and used on a routine basis, further developments involved the grafting of vessels and nerves. Following the restoration of circulation to limbs that had been without blood supply for long periods, out of necessity came the expertise to combat the metabolic degradation products experienced in these cases. The success rate for extremity replantation and revascularization increased dramatically with the understanding of these traumatic mechanisms. Concomitantly, advances were made in the orthopedic realm regarding the methods of fixation of bony injury and the repair of tendinous and muscular tissues. Once the bony structures are stabilized, full nerve and vessel reconstruction can be obtained and

This chapter is dedicated to Thomas A. Arganese (1947–2000), Co-founder of The Institute for Limb Preservation at Presbyterian/St. Lukes Medical Center, Denver, Colorado.

maintained. With modern-day techniques, it is possible to establish circulation in the majority of cases. Realistically, however, not all these operations are seen as "successful." A number of patients who undergo these extensive, heroic operative attempts still do not regain appropriate use of their extremity and many continue to have problems with chronic pain.

The traditional treatment for malignant tumors of the extremities was immediate amputation. The majority of these patients had malignant mesenchymal tumors or sarcomas and micrometastatic disease at the time of diagnosis. The general approach was to amputate and keep the patient mobile with prosthetic devices, with the expectation that most patients would eventually succumb to their disease. Over the last twenty-five years dramatic improvement has occurred in the treatment of these extremity malignancies, mainly due to advances in chemotherapy regimens, which have dramatically improved the survival of patients with these tumors (2–4). The chance of survival in a patient with an extremity sarcoma 20 years ago was 20% or less. Current survival figures approach 80%, as a result of progressive modern-day treatment. With improved patient survival, attention became focused on preserving limbs rather than performing an automatic amputation. Simple criteria for limb salvage were proposed: 1) the tumor could be surgically removed in its entirety, and 2) the resultant limb with appropriate orthopedic reconstructive procedures could function comparably, or better, when compared to the corresponding amputation. Encouraged by early success, orthopedic oncologists have developed many innovative limb preservation procedures involving prosthetic devices, bone and joint transplantation, and even "growing" prostheses. Currently, approximately 90% of patients with extremity malignancies are candidates for a limb salvage procedure.

The purpose of this chapter is to briefly review and discuss aspects of upper limb preservation in trauma and tumor situations. Although it may be technically possible to "save" an upper limb from amputation, the educational and decision-making process among the medical professionals, the patient, and the patient's family is essential.

UPPER EXTREMITY SALVAGE AND RECONSTRUCTION IN TRAUMA

Extent and Scope of Traumatic Amputations

The first reported arm replantation was done by Malt and McKhann in Boston in 1962 (5). This was followed by a thumb replantation done by Komatsu and Tamai in Japan (6). Since that time, a virtual explosion of interest has occurred in the discipline of microsurgery, with centers of excellence developing worldwide (7). Microsurgery is currently incorporated into training programs, not only in plastic surgery but also in orthopedics, ear-nose-throat surgery, hand surgery, and many other disciplines. The scope of reconstructive surgery for upper extremity limb salvage ranges from replantation of digits distal to the lunula of the nail to entire arm replantations. In orders of magnitude, digital replantation numbers far exceed those of more proximal amputations. The mechanisms of injuries include avulsion and guillotine-type laceration amputations all the way to crush and burn type areas of limb loss. (Limb loss secondary to tumors is covered elsewhere.) Lower extremity limb salvage, including lower extremity replantation, is relatively uncommon given the suboptimal results (with the exception of children).

The criterion for limb salvage depends on a number of factors. As with any trauma, the most important consideration is the entire patient, the mechanism of injury, and associated life threatening problems (8). The first condition that must be satisfied with consideration to any attempt at limb salvage is the advanced trauma life support (ATLS) criteria used in trauma patient resuscitation. Strict adherence to these trauma protocols is critical to the safe conduct of upper extremity limb salvage. Many trauma-scoring systems have been developed to predict which extremities are "worth saving" based on the long-term functional result (9,10). These extremity scoring systems are limited by their significant problems with low sensitivity and low specificity.

In general, the anatomic area or level of injury and the zone of injury (i.e., that area involved directly with the trauma through laceration, crush, avulsion, or burn) significantly impacts the functional result. In general, more proximal amputations and injury tend to be associated with an increased risk of cervical spine injury, thoracic trauma, and significant blood loss plus or minus hemodynamic instability; these require more vigorous resuscitation.

Proximal amputations also tend to involve significant muscle in the amputated part, and problems are compounded by prolonged warm and/or cold ischemia or prolonged de-enervation, which limits the functional results following replantation. In general, replantations across the wrist and digital amputations including the thumb have a more favorable prognosis. The general indications for replantation include replantations of the thumb in any patient who is medically suitable, any amputation in children, and any zone I amputation of the digits other than an isolated border digit (amputations distal to the insertion of the flexor digitorum superficialis [FDS] equals zone I). Multiple digit amputations should always be considered for replantation, as should any amputation proximal to the digits (i.e., hand

and wrist injuries). Contraindications to replantation include severe crush injuries, zone II amputations, amputations distal to the A-1 pulley and proximal to the FDS insertion, any amputation with prolonged warm ischemia, especially with a proximal injury involving a significant amount of muscle tissue in the amputated part, and multiple level amputations such as grain augur injuries. The work status, hand dominance, and motivation of the patient or the patient's guardian must also be considered a significant factor in the decision for replantation. The patient's occupation, level of cognitive functions, and functional expectations are critical in the decision making progress. Patients with multiple system injuries, especially life threatening injuries, or patients incapable of tolerating prolonged operations should not be considered for replantation or limb salvage. Patients with proximal amputations and significant distal crush or tissue destruction and loss may be considered for proximal replantation in an attempt to preserve shoulder or elbow function and allow the better fitting of limb prostheses. Specialized instances include spare part surgery, where a proximal significant tissue destruction allows one to scavenge parts from the distal extremity to preserve length.

The single largest advance relevant to limb salvage has been the understanding of regional blood flow to tissues. The explosion of flap surgery greatly increased the ability to think about limb salvage. This applies not only to the upper extremity but also to the lower extremity. This understanding of blood flow to specific types of tissue whether muscle, skin, bone, or composite tissues involving muscles, bone, and skin has been one of the most critical developments that has allowed aggressive attempts at limb salvage. The ability to place composite tissue segments, including the use of functional muscle transfers, has expanded the horizons of what is possible in limb salvage.

The first clinical free tissue transfer in 1973 (11) for lower extremity salvage, coupled with the advances in surgical instrumentations and microscope optics, has allowed major medical centers to perform replantation. Integral to the ability to offer limb salvage for traumatic amputations has been the development of an emergency medical transport system (EMS) and routine use of the air ambulance for the rapid delivery of these patients to regional centers. There are several requirements for such a system to work.

The development of the replantation team involves a commitment by individuals as well as an institution, and a system must be in place to provide 24-hour, 7-day per week service. In brief, for replantation services to succeed, a significant coordination of efforts by multiple disciplines must occur. Timely patient triage is critical, and this usually occurs in the surrounding hospitals.

The ability to identify life-threatening problems is key to appropriate patient care. The receiving institution must be a level I or level II type facility with a staff of trauma surgeons, full intensive care facilities, and a well-staffed emergency room.

Dedicated operating room personnel who are familiar with the various aspects of the limb salvage and trauma resuscitation are also key before these types of procedures can be performed. Intraoperative staffing includes nursing staff and a microsurgical assistant completely familiar with the operation of the microscopes, fluid warmers, tissue monitoring devices, and the actual conduct of the operation.

Excellent relationships between supporting physicians, intensivists and critical care doctors, infectious disease specialists, hyperbaric medicine physicians, physiatrists, and pain specialists are important not only in the immediate perioperative period, but also to ensure the long term successful outcomes of limb salvage efforts. A psychologist or psychiatrist familiar with dealing with trauma patients is also a beneficial and nearly mandatory member of the limb salvage team.

Nonphysician Members

The importance of a clinical director of the replantation service cannot be overstated. The smooth running of a team that virtually must function at any time of the day or night is critical in the management of patients with complex limb-threatening injuries. The nursing director allows for early decision-making as it concerns the triage of the patient and, in cases of a multiply injured patient, ensures that referral is made to the appropriate physicians.

The multiply injured patient or the patient with the limb-threatening injury quite often is a 20- to 50-year-old male, who may or may not have appropriate insurance coverage. The key work of the social worker in the replantation team is to coordinate available insurance and finances and home and nursing care for the postoperative period. The support of the hospital administrator to the program, as well as strong occupational, hand, and physical therapists is vital to the results of this complex surgery.

Technical Surgical Considerations

As with any trauma-related injury, strict adherence to the ATLS guidelines is vital. Overlooking a critical injury that jeopardizes the patient's life to save a single digit or hand would be absolute folly. The anatomic level of injury and mechanism of injury significantly impact replantation considerations. This, coupled with the general health of the patient and associated diseases, such as arthrosclerosis, coronary artery disease, and peripheral vascular disease, are of prime importance before taking on replantation (12,13).

The anatomic level of injury significantly impacts the outcome of a salvage attempt. More distal injuries—zone I digital amputations, such as those distal to the insertion of the flexor digitorum superficialis with a clean mechanism of amputation such as laceration or guillotine type amputation—are the most favorable (14). Because of the lack of tissues that are susceptible to critical ischemia in these parts, the replantations can be undertaken with delays of up to 36 hours. This must be considered in conjunction with the length of warm and cold ischemia. Minimizing the length of warm ischemia and cooling the part, wrapped in a moistened gauze, by keeping it in a container on ice allows one to proceed in a more leisurely fashion. As the amputation becomes more proximal, the amount of muscle susceptible to ischemia becomes more critical and diminishes the overall result. As one proceeds more proximally up the extremity to distal forearm, elbow, humerus, and shoulder, the long-term results are least optimum. Mitigating factors include the age of the patient, with the results in younger patients being better than older patients. Nerve regeneration in children younger than age 9 is significantly better with respect to sensory and motor recovery than it is in older patients. As mentioned earlier, with more proximal amputations, the preservation of maximum length is important in postoperative prosthesis fitting.

In general, the operative sequence involving the resuscitation of the patient with a full ATLS evaluation and appropriate preoperative work-up, including blood work, electrocardiogram (ECG), and radiology, is important. The amputated part should be carefully assessed to rule out multiple level injury, avulsion, or crush, which may cause the part to be unsuitable for replantation. Quite often with distal amputations, the part is brought to the operating room and prepared while the patient is being stabilized, blood is being prepared, and the appropriate radiological work-up is being performed. This reduces the overall operating time for the patient. The part is cleaned and vital structures are identified. Initial orthopedic stabilization may be accomplished, depending on the part. The patient is then brought to the operating room and the appropriate hemodynamic and physiologic monitoring is accomplished. Gel pads are used liberally on the table to provide pressure dispersal for these relatively lengthy operations. For upper extremity replantation or limb salvage, the use of a tourniquet reduces blood loss. The amputated part has all vital structures (tendons, nerves, artenes, and veins) tagged, and the procedure is commenced.

Aggressive debridement serves to minimize the infectious risk and remove devitalized tissue. The maxim to repair vessels outside the zone of injury holds true and optimizes the results. With avulsion type injuries, such as a roping injury or a ring avulsion injury, the liberal use of vein grafts plus or minus flow-through flaps allows for tissue coverage. The parts are stabilized with orthopedic fixation; tendons are repaired, followed by arterial repairs. This reduces the length of ischemic injury to the part. The veins are then repaired, followed by nerves and loose skin approximation.

During certain replantation efforts, the length of the amputated part must be salvaged to preserve maximum function. The liberal use of acute and subacute free tissue transfers that allow the replacement of composite tissues can be used. Toe-to-hand reconstructions for some losses are typically done in a more delayed fashion once stable wound coverage has been obtained.

Postoperative Care

Hematologic and physiologic monitoring continue during the postoperative period to assess blood supply to the replanted part and the stability of the patient. Depending on the level of complexity of the various teams, postoperative monitoring can be accomplished on a dedicated floor, or if conditions exist that require postoperative anesthesia, ICU monitoring may be instituted. Various flow monitors are utilized as well as clinical assessment for replanted parts.

Laser Doppler temperature, ultrasonic Doppler, and clinical monitoring are vital to the success of replantation.

Postoperative anticoagulation varies depending on physician experience and the extent of injury. Typically, Dextran 40 is utilized to decrease ADP-mediated platelet aggravation and to decrease blood viscosity. Heparin is occasionally utilized. The careful monitoring of hematocrit, electrolytes, and other blood constituents is important to the success of such an undertaking.

Following the early postoperative period, the rehabilitation goals are instituted. Depending on bone fixation, early activity is begun under the direction of a certified hand therapist in order to optimize the outcome. Secondary surgery is often required for capsulotomies and tenolysis. Standard functional protocols are utilized to assess the results of replantation.

Other than failed replantations, long-term complications include those involving rigid internal fixation, aggressive debridement and nerve repair and—in a very few—nonunions and persistent infection.

UPPER EXTREMITY SALVAGE AND RECONSTRUCTION FOR TUMORS

Limb-Threatening Tumors

Three factors must be considered when an extremity tumor appears to put a limb in jeopardy: size, location, and histologic grade. If a tumor is quite small, be it benign or malignant, a local resection can generally be performed without removing major structural or functional components. The goal is to achieve local control and ensure that the tumor will not recur in the limb itself. The tumor and its surrounding tissue, which may be contaminated with micrometastatic disease, must be removed. If the tumor is of small size and doesn't involve the deep major structures, these procedures are usually not difficult, and the patient is left with a limb that functions well. On the other hand, if the patient has a malignant tumor of a large size, or a very aggressive, destructive benign tumor, one must consider both the options of limb preservation and amputation. Multiple factors go into these considerations involving the structures: the extent of tumor invasion; the effectiveness of proposed reconstructive techniques; the patient's age, activity level, and overall prognosis; and family and religious desires and influences.

When considering limb preservation surgery for a patient with a malignancy of the upper extremity, either in bone or soft tissue, the primary concern is the survival of the patient, not the preservation of the limb. If the tumor is not removed in its entirety, it is likely to recur and put the patient's life at risk. A local recurrence decreases the patient's overall prognosis by at least 50%. That is, if a tumor patient has a 70% chance of being cured following resection but has a local recurrence, his chance of disease-free survival is reduced to 35%. Therefore, a critical first step in the decision-making process is the orthopedic oncologist's determination of how extensive the resection will be, or "what has to go."

Once the surgeon has decided how much "has to go," only then can he ponder the need and techniques for reconstruction of the limb. The surgeon should be familiar with all limb preservation techniques so that he can predict the likely functional outcome. At that time he can propose the options with the patient and family and allow them to make an appropriate, educated decision. The decision-making process may be quite difficult due to the varied backgrounds of patients and families, their previous experience with surgery and the medical profession, and often, their preconceptions regarding amputation and surgical reconstruction techniques. It is imperative, however, that time is set aside to educate the patients and families preoperatively so that they may make a cogent decision that they later look back on without regrets.

Biologic and Technical Advances

Three specific advances have made limb preservation for tumors quite feasible. The first advances came in the area of tumor biology. Over the years, following combined specialty center experience, it has become evident which tumors are aggressive, which are less aggressive, and which tumors lend themselves to surgical resection more readily than others. Tumors such as extra-abdominal desmoid tumors routinely underwent radical surgical procedures and even amputation in the past, but are now rarely operated on. Malignant cartilage tumors of bone or chondrosarcomas used to be quite difficult to diagnose, and many patients had amputations or radical surgery for what were probably low-grade or benign lesions. Modern-day techniques and the development of specialty centers for bone sarcomas has greatly improved our understanding of the biology of these processes. Into this realm of tumor biology came improvements in chemotherapy for the treatment of micrometastatic disease in malignant extremity tumors. The prognosis for patients with sarcomas improved dramatically with the advent of postoperative chemotherapy alone, and the current regimen of preoperative and postoperative chemotherapy. Once the diagnosis has been made, many patients undergo an induction course of chemotherapy prior to any definitive surgical procedure (2). This allows immediate attention to possible micrometastatic disease, in addition to allowing an assessment of the resected tumor after it has been exposed to the various chemotherapy drugs. With this "preoperative testing" of chemotherapy drugs, the oncologist then knows if he is giving the appropriate therapy. After the tumor is removed, it is inspected for necrosis. If the majority of the tumor is dead, the implication is that the chemotherapy was effective and the regimen is continued postoperatively. If, however, the majority of the tumor is not necrotic, it is clear that the preoperative chemotherapy was insufficient. The chemotherapy regimen is then altered to another group of drugs. With these improved, aggressive chemotherapy protocols, the overall prognosis and survival for extremity malignancies has improved dramatically.

The last area of advancement to impact upper limb preservation following tumor resection involves the improvement of orthopedic techniques. Before the first half of this century it was not possible to replace the large bony defects created by tumor resections with a material or prosthesis that would be successful. With the advent of new metal alloys, including cobalt-chrome, steel and titanium, and the development of special formulations of polyethylene, artificial bones and joints became possible. In addition, the banking of cadaver bones became more prevalent, and it became possible to

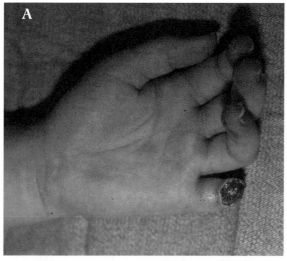

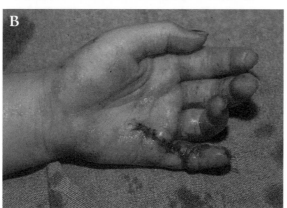

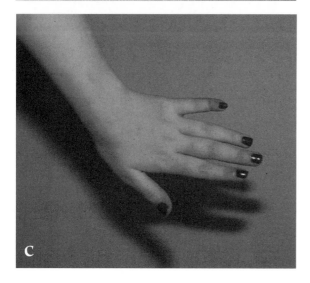

FIGURE 3-1

A. A 16-year-old female with an avulsion amputation of the left small finger secondary to a boat propeller injury. B. Immediate post-replantation. C. Follow-up at 5 months showing normal nail growth and normal appearance of the finger.

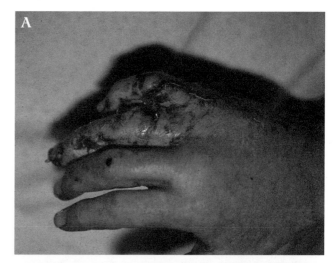

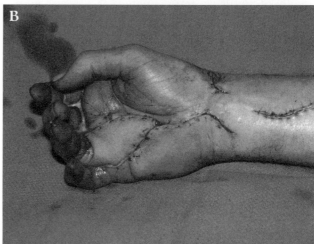

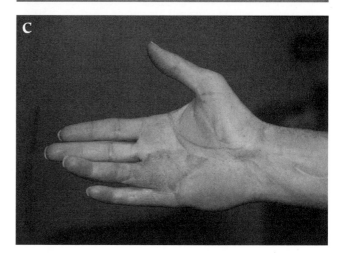

FIGURE 3-2

A. Ring avulsion injury of an oil field worker. B. Extensive palmar and finger devascularization requiring immediate free-tissue transfer with revascularization. C. Long term follow-up showing lateral arm flap, resurfacing of palm, and result at greater than 1 year.

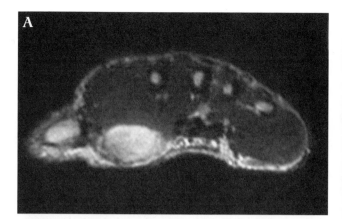

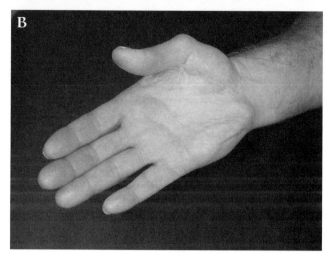

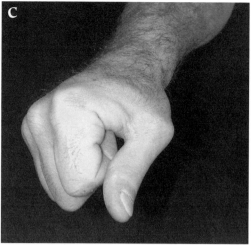

FIGURE 3-3

A. MRI of a 50-year-old male with a large synovial cell sarcoma of his thenar eminence. Rather than amputation, which had been suggested, he underwent a limb preservation procedure. The tumor involved several tendons and the radial artery, which were resected. Tendon transfers were performed and a vein graft was used to reconstruct the artery. B. At one year postoperatively, the patient has an excellent cosmetic appearance and 90% of normal hand function. C. Although there is some decrease in thumb flexion, the patient is able to grasp well and pick up small objects.

literally replace the resected part with a corresponding part from a bone donor. These two techniques, or combinations of these techniques, have been used extensively over the last twenty years and have been quite successful in structurally reconstituting areas where malignant tumors have been removed (15,16). In addition to the orthopedic advances, muscle coverage and skin grafting advances, such as the ability to move bone or muscle to an entirely new site with re-anastomosis of the vessels, has greatly increased our ability to reconstruct skeletal and soft tissue defects involved in these resections. Likewise, nerve and vessel grafts are possible to maintain a viable upper limb when tumor cell contamination of these structures has occurred (Figure 3-3).

One of the greatest challenges facing orthopedic oncologists is the growing child with a malignancy in a long bone, such as the humerus. Most of these patients have undergone amputation, because there were few reconstructive techniques that could reliably maintain length equal to that of the normal contralateral limb through the duration of the child's growth.

The standard methods for limb length equalization can be utilized if the total discrepancy is predicted to be several centimeters. However, many of these children will require between 4 to 10 cm of lengthening, especially if it involves the proximal humerus of a child 7 or 8 years old. Some centers have attempted to equalize length using the Ilizarov technique after completion of chemotherapy. This has met with limited success due to difficulties encountered with infection and contracture in the femur or tibia, and it is a technique rarely employed for the upper extremity. Expandable artificial bones and joints have been used with some success: The prosthesis is implanted at the time of the definitive surgery, and the extremity is usually lengthened acutely by several centimeters. Once the child has had surgery, completed postoperative chemotherapy, and the normal, unaffected humerus resumes active growth, attention is devoted to maintaining equal length by surgically expanding the prosthesis. This may require surgery every 6 months, with the attendant complication risks and reduced function. In recent years, an innovative prosthesis has been developed that can be lengthened without a surgical procedure (Repiphysis, Wright Medical Technology, Arlington TN) (Figure 3-4) (17). Through the application of external forces, either physical or electromagnetic, the prosthesis can be

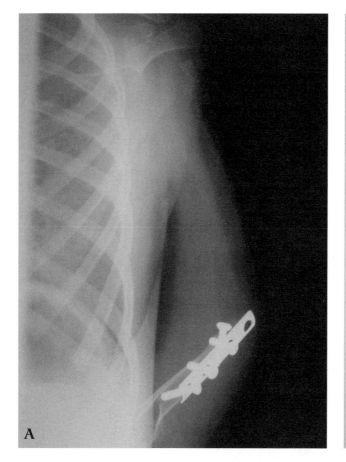

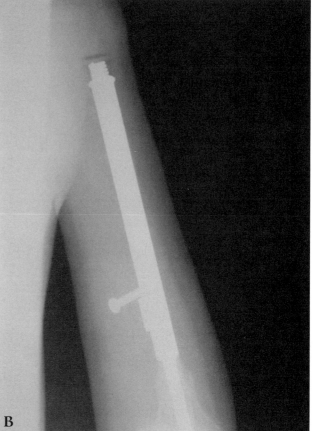

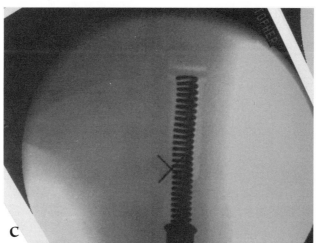

FIGURE 3-4

A. An 8-year-old male with osteosarcoma of his humerus treated at another institution had originally undergone reconstruction with a fibular allograft to save his arm. The graft resorbed, probably due to immunologic factors, leaving him several years later disease free but with a totally flail upper extremity. B. Rather than an amputation, the parents opted for a second limb salvage procedure consisting of reconstruction with the "growing prosthesis." The prosthesis is expanded through application of a controlled magnetic field to the prosthesis. Lengthenings are performed in an outpatient facility without anesthesia, and are measured by the expansion of the spring device (denoted by bracket). A lengthening procedure may be done as often as every month, and maintains equal limb length in a growing child. C. X-ray after four lengthenings. At this point, the patient has gained over 5 cm in length to keep pace with the growth of his contralateral humerus.

lengthened sequentially and major surgery for the patient is avoided. At the present time, this prosthetic technology is undergoing further design refinement and longer follow-up will be needed before it becomes a mainstay in the orthopedic oncologist's armamentarium.

Criteria for Limb Preservation Following Tumor Resection

Faced with a malignant upper extremity tumor, the orthopedic oncologist accumulates all the information necessary to make a reasonable decision regarding the patient's candidacy for limb preservation. Once the diagnosis has been made, staging procedures are performed (18). The purpose for staging is twofold. The first is to discern the local extent of the process; the second is to find out whether there has been distant spread or metastasis. The presence of metastasis is a dire prognostic factor and may influence decisions regarding treatment and surgery. Once staging has been completed, the next step is prognostication. A patient's prognosis is related primarily to the histologic grade or aggressiveness of the tumor. Cancer is generally classified as low-, medium-, or high-grade. Patients with low- to medium-grade cancers have a good prognosis; patients with high-grade sarcoma survive less often. The other important prognosticators are the size and location of the tumor. Tumors that are large and invade multiple local structures have a worse prognosis than those that are either small or superficial. The overall prognosis will also influence decisions made by the medical team and the patient and family.

Once the local and distant extent of the disease is ascertained and the staging performed, the surgical team will be able to predict which structures need to be removed to safely consider limb preservation. In some cases, it is immediately obvious that due to the extent of the tumor, the prognosis, and its aggressiveness, there is no limb sparing option. When the decision has been made as to which structures will be removed, the reconstruction options are reviewed. Should the bony defect be rebuilt with a metal device, a bone transplant, the patient's own bone, or a combination of these materials? Will the patient need vessel or nerve repair or grafting? Will muscle flap coverage be necessary? Can local muscle be used, or will a free muscle transfer need to be performed? After these factors have been considered, the surgical team should then be able to predict with some degree of certainty what functional result can be anticipated. It is only through fairly extensive experience that this preoperative process is completed and an appropriate projection of outcome made. For this reason alone, extremity sarcomas are best treated in specialty centers rather than by a physician who only occasionally encounters these situations.

When these technical considerations have been explored and final decisions regarding the surgical procedure have been made, a frank and open discussion should be held with the patient and family during which the risks and benefits of each procedure are explained, including amputation and prosthetic fitting. It is often extremely helpful to have the patients talk to other patients who have had similar procedures so that they can get a firsthand account of the magnitude of the procedure, recovery time, expected discomfort, and possible complications. It is only then that the patient and family will be truly prepared for the upcoming procedure.

Tumors: A Team Approach

To appropriately diagnose, evaluate, and treat patients with extremity tumors, a multispecialty team is as necessary as it is with replantation patients. The team involves physicians and ancillary health professionals who assist in the educational process. Many of these professionals will be involved in the care of the patient on a routine basis for a period of time. In addition, a tertiary hospital care facility must be available to provide the equipment and personnel necessary to perform these major limb-sparing procedures. Generally, the medical team consists of an orthopedic oncologist, a medical oncologist, a radiologist experienced in bone and soft tissue imaging, a radiation therapist, and a pathologist who has extensive experience in evaluating mesenchymal tissues. In addition to this primary medical team, other members are necessary, including vascular surgeons, hand surgeons, plastic surgeons, and microvascular surgeons, as well as the administrative support necessary for a comprehensive, multispecialty department. Ideally, the mechanism exists whereby all team members meet on a regular basis to discuss the cases and formulate treatment plan protocols and options. A full-time clinical director and a social worker, as well as oncology and orthopedic nurses, are tremendously helpful. A physiatrist who has worked extensively with patients who have undergone limb preservation surgery and amputations is an extremely important member of the team, especially in discussing possible functional outcomes, activity levels, and long-term acceptance of physical dysfunction. A prosthetist or occupational therapist is an essential resource person to discuss prosthetic options preoperatively.

Post-Operative Care and Evaluation

Once the major procedure has been performed, the work has only just begun, not only for the professional team but for the patient and the family. Many postoperative patients continue to undergo chemotherapy, which increases the difficulty of physical rehabilitation. Any strength a patient gains between courses of chemotherapy is quickly lost once subsequent drugs are administered. Patients undergoing chemotherapy become ill, often bedridden and with severe nausea, which can create a frustrating situation for everyone involved. To avoid disappointment and depression in these situations, it may be a good idea to set minimal and more realistic functional goals for the patient. It may require up to two years after surgery for a patient to fully realize his physical capability.

The major complication rate in limb preservation surgery is quite high, approximating 10%. These complications include infection, life-threatening bleeding, nerve damage, healing problems, and recurrent cancer. Any one of these complications could possibly lead to an amputation if uncontrolled. Patients should be prepared for the possibility of these problems before their index procedure. If a complication does occur, the type of treatment depends on many factors. For example, it is a severe problem if a patient develops a surgical complication such as infection or healing problems while they are on postoperative chemotherapy. The prolonged, protracted treatment of these complications delays the administration of the chemotherapy—which is, in fact, what is going to save the patient's life. Therefore, in situations in which the problem cannot be brought under control quickly, an amputation may be necessary. In complications that may occur after a patient is finished with postoperative therapy, such as a delayed infection, prosthetic breakage, or the nonhealing of bone grafts, the treatment can be extensive without jeopardizing the patient's life.

Once a severe complication occurs, it would be expected that future function is at risk. However, in several studies, it has been exhibited that even with multiple surgeries for complications or revisions, patients maintain a high level of activity and function with their extremities despite these problems (15). Psychologically, it can be difficult on patients to anticipate multiple surgical procedures over their lifetime, but most adapt well and continue to function at a high level. The approach should be standardized, comprehensive, and educational, and the patient and family allowed sufficient time to make an informed, educated decision. All options are ideally discussed with the patient: limb preservation, amputation, and even the anticipated results of receiving no treatment. Only under these circumstances is the patient treated appropriately, thus avoiding a "triumph of technique over reason."

Conclusions

In many patients with limbs in jeopardy from cancer or trauma, there is no choice but an amputation procedure.

There have been many dramatic improvements in prosthetic design and use; however, there is no medical replacement for a human hand. The criteria for considering limb preservation in these situations involves the prediction that the limb will function favorably when compared to the corresponding prosthesis. The majority of patients with malignancies of the upper extremity are now candidates for limb preservation due to advances in or knowledge of the disease process, orthopedic reconstructive techniques, and advances in microvascular reconstruction. Because traumatic events may do such substantive damage, in cases of severe trauma, preservation is not a prudent option. As the fields of limb preservation surgery and artificial limb science progress, additional options will be available to patients under these difficult circumstances.

ACKNOWLEDGMENTS

The authors wish to thank Anne Camozzi and Ann Collins for their invaluable assistance in preparing this chapter.

References

1. Kahan BD. Cosmos and Damian in the 20th century? *New Engl J Med* 1981; 305:280–281.
2. Eilber FR, Morton DL, Eckardt J, Grant T, Weisenbuger T. Limb salvage for skeletal and soft tissue sarcomas: Multidisciplinary preoperative therapy. *Cancer* 1984; 53:2579–2584.
3. Marcove RC, Sheth DS, Healey J, Huvos A, Rosen G, Meyers F. Limb-sparing surgery for extremity sarcoma. *Cancer Invest* 1994; 12:497–504.
4. Sim FH, Bowman WE Jr, Wilkins RM, Chao ES. Limb salvage in primary malignant bone tumors. *Orthopedics* 1985; 8:574–581.
5. Malt RA, McKhann CF. The classic replantation of severed arms. *J A M A* 1964; 189:716.
6. Komatsu S, Tamai S. Successful replantation of completely cut-off thumb: case report. *Plast Reconstr Surg* 1968; 42:374–377.
7. Kleinert HE, Jablon M, Tsai TM. An overview of replantation and results of 347 replants and 245 patients. *J Trauma* 19880; 20:390–398.
8. American College of Surgeons Committee on Trauma. *Resources for Optimal Care of the Injured Patient.* Chicago: American College of Surgeons, 1999.
9. Arakaki A, Tsai TM. Thumb replantation: survival factors and re-exploration in 122 cases. *J Hand Surg* 1993; 18B: 152–156.
10. Weiland AJ, Raskin KB. Philosophy of replantation 1976–1990. *Microsurgery* 1990; 11:223–230.
11. Daniel RK, Taylor GJ. Distant transfer of an island flap by microvascular anastomoses: a clinical technique. *Plast Reconstr Surg* 1973; 52:111–117.
12. O'Brien BM. *Microvascular Surgery.* New York: Churchill Livingstone, 1977.
13. O'Brien BM. Replantation surgery. *Clin Plastic Surg* 1974; 1:405–426.

14. Kleinert HE, Juhala CA, Tsai TM, Van Beck A. Digital replantation: selection technique, and results. *Orthop Clin North Am* 1977; 8:309–318.

15. Wilkins RM, Miller CM: Reoperation after limb preservation surgery for sacromas of the knee in children. *Clin Orthop* 2003; 412:153–61.

16. Wilkins RM. Complications of allograft reconstruction for skeletal defects following oncological surgery. In: Simon MA, Springfield D (eds), *Surgery for Bone and Soft-Tissue Tumors.* Philadelphia: Lippincott-Raven, 1997, 487–496.

17. Wilkins RM, Soubeiran A. The Phenix expandable prosthesis: early American experience. *Clin Orthop* 2001; 382:51–58.

18. Wilkins RM, Sim FH. Evaluation of bone and soft tissue tumors. In: D'Ambrosia R (ed), *Musculoskeletal Disorders: Regional Examination and Differential Diagnosis,* 2nd ed. Philadelphia: Lippincott, 1986.

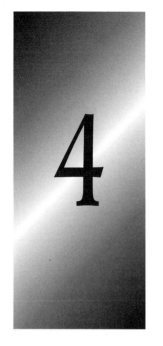

4 Upper Extremity Amputation Revision and Reconstruction

Saleh M. Shenaq, MD, and Elena Grantcharova, MD

pper extremity amputation can result from congenital malformations, traumatic injuries, or malignancies. Hand function is vital in our industrial and highly competitive society. Although recent advances in microsurgery and hand surgery have improved the outcome of the replanted upper extremity, especially in young patients with distal injuries, a number of patients continue to require amputation and subsequent reconstruction and prosthetic fitting (1–4). The development of new sophisticated prostheses (5) has created a need for the advanced surgical reconstruction and salvage of residual limbs (6,7). Higher level amputations result in greater functional loss and, therefore, the preservation of length with new plastic and reconstructive techniques facilitates the rehabilitation process. Reconstruction of the amputated upper extremity, prosthetic fitting, and rehabilitation are major tasks requiring the expertise of a rehabilitation team that includes a reconstructive plastic surgeon, a physical medicine and rehabilitation specialist, a prosthetist, an orthopedic surgeon, a therapist, and a social worker. This chapter provides a review of the current and traditional treatment options available to the plastic surgeon for the reconstruction of the amputated upper extremity so that proper prosthetic fitting can be achieved.

INDICATIONS

The goal of the plastic surgeon in the reconstruction of upper extremity amputations is to create a stump that is well suited for prosthetic fitting while minimizing the number of operations. The characteristics of the ideal stump are excellent skin coverage, minimal scarring, good sensation, and no pain with handling (8). The careful planning of the amputation and reconstruction is necessary for the attainment of a stump that is optimal for prosthetic fitting. A knowledge and understanding of the pressure loading of the prosthesis on the stump (9), familiarity with the different prostheses (2,5,6,10), the needs of the individual patient (11), and the various reconstructive methods available, is crucial. Certain reconstructive pathways narrow future options, and the plastic surgeon has to make a conscious effort not to burn any bridges when deciding on a certain treatment plan (12).

SURGICAL TECHNIQUES

Revision Amputation

Revision amputation is one of the oldest techniques in orthopedics for stump reconstruction, especially when a shortage of soft tissue or stump breakdown and nonhealing occurs (13). This method of reconstruction restores stump contour for prosthetic fitting, but inevitably results in diminished stump length; it should be avoided when revision would involve amputation of a joint or of a functional muscle group. With the recent advances in microvascular techniques, the preservation of length can be achieved with a conservation of parts from the amputated extremity for the coverage and reconstruction of the stump (14,15).

Skin Grafting

Skin grafting is often used for the reconstruction of small or large open superficial wounds with reasonable receptor beds, such as burns and stump breakdown. The technique simply employs the use of split thickness skin grafts harvested from the hips or thighs in the form of sheet or mesh. The advantage of this procedure is that it is simple, fast, and provides primary skin closure (16). However, grafting is plagued by a high rate of skin breakdown with prosthetic use, and it cannot be employed for the coverage of deep wounds with exposed tendons, vessels, nerves, cartilage, or bone. Furthermore, even when skin graft take occurs, a risk of failure exists that results in delayed healing and contractures, with a subsequent inability to wear a prosthesis (13,17). To minimize hypertrophic or keloid scar formation and prevent dessication and ulceration of the skin, grafts should be covered with emollient cream and compressive garments should be worn at all times.

Scar Revision and Local Flap Rotation

Scar revision can be used when ample soft tissue and skin is available. This technique is applied in the presence of painful scars, neuromas, or stump ulceration. Bulky stumps can be treated by the excision of excess skin and soft tissue, and recontouring. Flaps contain several tissue elements and are ideal for the coverage of bony structures, exposed vessels, nerves, bones, and tendons. According to their circulation, flaps can be classified as either random or axial. When designing a flap, the reconstructive surgeon should be well aware of its circulation, so that adequate coverage and healing can be ensured (18).

Fasciocutaneous flaps span the entire length of the brachium and are based on septal and fascial perforators to the skin. These flaps are thin, well vascularized, with a favorable length to width ratio, and permit a single-staged regional tissue coverage.

Unlike fascial flaps, muscle and myocutaneous flaps are bulky and extremely helpful in providing the necessary tissue for the prosthesis. Their excellent blood supply makes them ideal candidates for closing deadspace areas and combating infection.

Local transposition flaps are perfectly suited for resurfacing of the axilla or antecubital defects, areas which are difficult to cover with skin grafts.

Reconstruction Using Pedicled Flaps

Pedicled flaps can be elevated from the groin, thorax, or thoracoepigastrium to cover virtually any defect of the upper extremity (19). The use of pedicled flaps entails at least two surgical procedures for complete reconstruction. The first stage involves raising the flap as a pedicle and bringing the residual limb in close proximity so that the stump can be resurfaced. The upper extremity is immobilized and kept attached to the donor site for approximately 2 to 3 weeks. The pedicle is then divided and the donor site repaired. Examples of pedicle flaps include the chest flap for reconstruction of hand and digital defects, and the groin or inferior epigastric flap for coverage of large defects and exposed vital structures. Another example is the bipedicled groin flap, which is a thin dermal flap raised with bilateral blood supply and used for the resurfacing of digits (20). The major drawback of pedicled flaps is that they require a multistage procedure and prolonged immobilization of the upper extremity, which can lead to stiffness and occasional contractures. In addition, these flaps might require debulking once healed. Since the advent and perfection of microvascular techniques, pedicled flaps have become less desirable.

Reconstruction Using Regional Flaps

The concept of muscle and musculocutaneous flaps as a reconstructive modality was introduced during the early part of the last decade and has gained great importance and utility (21–23). The two most frequently used musculocutaneous flaps for upper extremity reconstruction are the latissimus dorsi and the scapular flap.

The latissimus dorsi myocutaneous flap was proposed by Tansini in 1906 and has a pedicle based on the thoracodorsal artery. With its large tissue volume and excellent vascularity, the latissimus dorsi flap has become the workhorse of the reconstructive surgeon. The flap can be harvested as a myocutaneous or osteomyocutaneous flap and can be rotated from its bed and tunneled subcutaneously to cover defects as far as the elbow and proximal forearm in one surgical setting (Figure 4-1). Functional reconstruction can be attained by preserving the thoracodorsal nerve. If a thin flap is required, the nerve can be divided so that atrophy of the muscle can be achieved.

The scapular flap is the second most commonly used regional flap for upper extremity reconstructions. It was first described by Dos Santos in 1980, and is

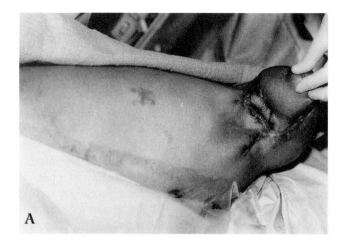

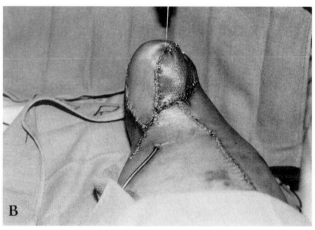

FIGURE 4-1

Latissimus Dorsi Myocutaneous Flap. A. Left above the elbow amputation with chronically open wound. B. Latissimus dorsi myocutaneous flap sutured into place.

based on the circumflex scapular artery. The flap can be harvested as a composite graft in which part of the scapula is also used. This flap has thick skin and no innervation, and it is ideal for medium-sized defects in the forearm and hand.

Free Tissue Transfer

During the last three decades, microvascular free tissue transfers have superceded any other conventional pedicled flap operations. Free flaps are safe, effective, and versatile, with current success rates between 90 and 95%. They have the advantage of a one-stage procedure and a wide selection of donor sites (24,25). In addition, they offer good vascularity and sufficient tissue for coverage, and they allow the limb to be mobilized in the immediate postoperative period. The two major disadvantages of microvascular free tissue transfer are the

need for healthy vessels, which might not be present in the traumatized limb, and the availability of an experienced microvascular surgeon and operating team capable of handling acute vascular thromboses. Absolute indications for microvascular free tissue transfer is trauma in which vital structures such as bone, tendons, nerves, and vessels are exposed (26,27). The free flap is also an ideal candidate for the obliteration of dead space or in the infected patient. The most commonly used free flaps are latissimus dorsi (Figure 4-2), rectus abdominus, gracilis, and scapular flaps. The latissimus dorsi and scapular flaps were previously discussed as pedicled flaps. The scapular flap allows the surgeon to raise a very large flap if both the transverse and the descending branches of the scapular artery are used.

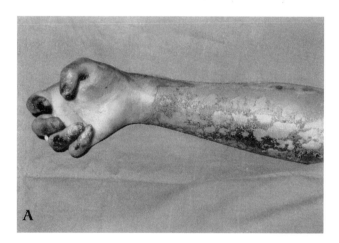

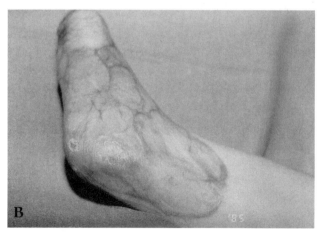

FIGURE 4-2

Free Latissimus Dorsi Flap. A. Fourth degree burns to right upper extremity. B. Following below-elbow amputation and split thickness skin grafting, with evidence of skin ulceration at elbow. C. Resurfacing of grafted skin at right elbow with free latissimus dorsi flap. D. The patient's final result, with adequate use of prosthesis. (*Figure continues*)

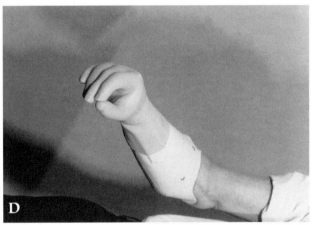

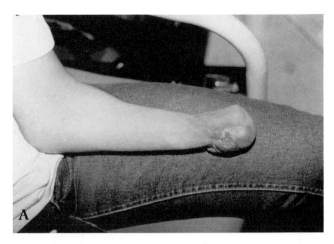

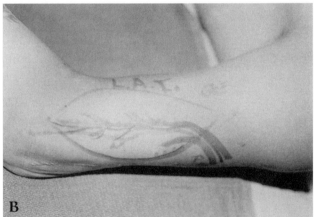

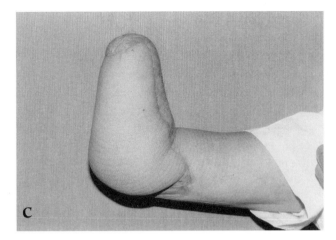

FIGURE 4-2 (continued)

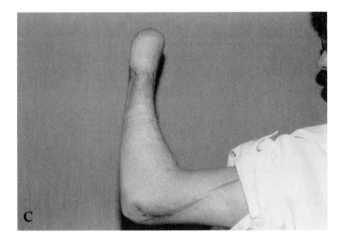

FIGURE 4-3

Lateral Arm Free Flap. A. Patient with ulcerated left wrist stump. B. Design of left lateral arm free flap. (C.) Postoperative result shows stump completely covered with adequate soft tissue.

The rectus abdominis flap is smaller, and its skin paddle is bulkier when compared to the latissimus dorsi. However, its major advantage is the ease of elevation and convenient position; donor morbidity is also significantly small. The gracilis muscle can be used as a free flap based on the medial circumflex femoral artery. This muscle is innnervated by the obturator nerve, and its major advantage is that it can be transferred as a motorized muscle. Furthermore, the donor site morbidity is minimal and the scar is cosmetically very acceptable. Other free flaps that can be used for reconstruction of the upper extremity are the radial, ulnar, and lateral arm fasciocutaneous flaps (Figure 4-3), (28). All can be transferred as sensate flaps, and the donor site morbidity is very similar to local pedicle flaps.

Vascularized Bone Grafts

A new advance in microvascular techniques is the ability to transfer autogenous composite tissue, such as vascularized bone grafts (29,30). The first vascularized bone graft performed was a free fibula used by Taylor for the reconstruction of long bone defects. Its long straight and corticle structure and low donor site morbidity make the fibula the first choice for long bone reconstruction. It can be transferred as composite graft including skin, bone, muscle, and innervation. Other vascularized bone grafts include ileum, scapula, rib, radius, and femur (31). Toe transfer has also been used extensively for hand reconstruction. Vascularized bone grafts are indicated in the reconstruction of large soft tissue defects of the upper extremity caused either by severe trauma or tumor resections. They are ideal for intractable nonunions, pseudoarthroses, and osteonecrosis. Vascularized bone grafts are very effective because they do not require prolonged immobilization, maintain their characteristics, heal from both ends, and increase in structural strength with time. After the fibula, the rib and iliac crest are the most commonly used vascularized bone grafts. Unlike the fibula, these grafts are curved and their principal advantage is the ability to transfer adjacent skin, muscle, and nerves.

Tissue Expansion in the Upper Extremities

Skin expansion as a reconstructive surgical technique was first introduced by Radovan in 1976. Since then it has been hailed as one of the most significant advances in reconstructive surgery, along with musculocutaneous flaps and microsurgical free tissue transfer (32). Its main use in the reconstruction of amputated extremities has been for skin resurfacing of the stump. The method entails the insertion of a tissue expander under the skin in proximity to the deficient area. The skin is then expanded by serial injections of saline into the reservoir over a period of 2 to 3 months. At that point, the tissue expander is removed and the skin used to resurface the stump (Figure 4-4), (33). The disadvantage of this technique is that it requires several surgical procedures, although it is useful when there are no other alternatives. New advances in tissue expansion include expansion in the hand and fingers, arterial and peripheral nerve elongation, intraoperative sustained limited expansion, and osteodistraction (34).

Other Reconstructive Methods

Several other methods for increasing the functional capabilities of the stump have been described, such as kinematic operations (14,35), neurosensory free flaps (36,37), and functioning free-muscle transplantation (38). Although the author had no personal experience with such techniques, familiarity with these procedures, and with their advantages and disadvantages in comparison with other techniques already described, is encouraged.

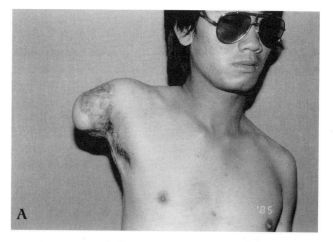

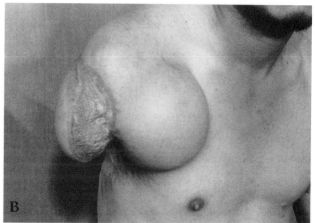

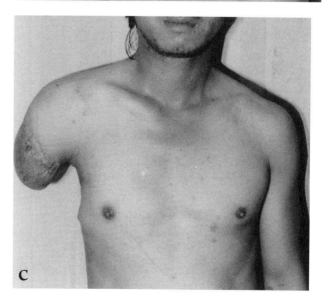

FIGURE 4-4

Tissue Expansion. A. Patient with right above-elbow amputation, with ulcerated skin-grafted stump, unable to wear prosthesis. B. Tissue expander placed in adjacent area. C. Following expansion of normal skin and coverage of stump. D. The patient with adequate use of prosthesis. *(Figure continues)*

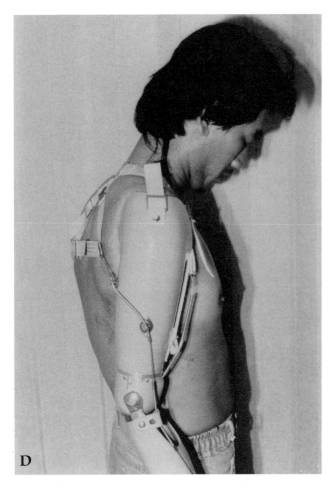

FIGURE 4-4 (continued)

CONCLUSIONS

The development of new functional prosthetic devices has been paralleled by an explosion in microvascular techniques and has made the resurfacing and prosthetic fitting of the upper extremity stump a viable option for most patients. To gain a satisfactory function in the amputated upper extremity, the combined efforts of a rehabilitation team led by a reconstructive plastic surgeon is needed. Familiarity with the variety of reconstructive options presented in this chapter will provide the plastic surgeon with flexibility when dealing with complex upper extremity injuries. It will also enable the plastic surgeon to choose the most suitable option for coverage in accordance with the individual patient's requirements, medical status, and the injury itself so that a well functioning and aesthetically pleasing result can be achieved.

References

1. Graham B, et al. Major replantation versus revision amputation and prosthetic fitting in the upper extremity. *J Hand Surg* 1998; 23A: 783.

2. Beasley RW, de Bese GM. Upper limb amputations and prostheses. *Orthop Clin North Am* 1986; 17:395.

3. Ober JK. Upper limb prosthetics for high level arm amputation. *Prosthet Orthot Int* 1982; 6:17.

4. Steinbach TV. Upper limb amputation. *Prog Surg* 1978; 16:224.

5. Lamb DW. State of the art in upper-limb prosthetics. *J Hand Ther* 1993; 13:1.

6. Pinzur MS et al. Functional outcome following upper limb amputation and prosthetic limb fitting. *J Hand Surg* 1994; 19A: 836.

7. Hierner R, Berger A, Brenner F. Considerations on the management of subtotal and total macro-amputation of the upper extremity. *Unfallchirurg* 1998; 101:184.

8. Louis DS, Hunter LY, Keating TM. Painful neuromas in long below-elbow amputees. *Arch Surg* 1980; 115.

9. Sanders JE. Interface mechanics in external prosthetics: review of interface stress measurement techniques. *Med Biol Eng Comp* 1995; 33:509.

10. Leow ME et al. Aesthetic life-like finger and hand prostheses: presciption and factors influencing choices. *Ann Acad Med Singapore* 1997; 26:834.

11. Krebs DE, Edelstein JE, Thornby MA. Prosthetic management of children with limb deficiencies. *Phys Ther* 1991; 71:920.

12. Barwick WJ, Riefkohl R, Georgiade G. Skin coverage in occupational injuries. *Hand Clin* 1986; 2:533.

13. Kerstein MD. Management of amputation-stump breakdown. *Am Surg* 1975; 41:581.

14. Anderl H, Hussl H, Papp CH, et al. Actuelle rekonstruktive verfahren zur defektdeckung an den extremitaten. *Der Cirurg* 1982; 53:235.

15. Weinberg MJ, Al-Qattan MM, Mahoney J. "Spare part" forearm free flaps harvested from the amputated limb for coverage of amputation stumps. *J Hand Surg* 1997; 22B: 615.

16. Ablove RH, Howell RM. The physiology and technique of skin grafting. *Hand Clin* 1997; 13:163.

17. Levy SW. Amputees: skin problems and prostheses. *Cutis* 1995; 55:297.

18. Birbeck DP, Moy OJ. Anatomy of upper extremity skin flaps. *Hand Clin* 1997; 13:175.

19. Ikuta Y, Kimori K. Flap reconstruction in the upper limb. *Ann Acad Med Singapore* 1995; 24:124S.

20. Mih AD. Pedicle flaps for coverage of the wrist and hand. *Hand Clin* 1997; 13:217.

21. Russell RC, Zamboni WA. Coverage of the elbow and forearm. *Orthop Clin North Am* 1993; 24:425.

22. Vasconez HC, Oishi S. Soft-tissue coverage of the shoulder and brachium. *Orthop Clin North Am* 1993; 24:435.

23. Sherman R. Soft-tissue coverage of the elbow. *Hand Clin* 1997; 13:291.

24. Shenaq SM, Krouskop T, Stal S, Spira M. Salvage of amputation stumps by secondary reconstruction utilizing microsurgical free-tissue transfer. *Plast Reconstr Surg* 1987; 79:861.

25. Kay S, Coady M. The role of microsurgery and free-tissue transfer in the reconstruction of pediatric upper extremity. *Ann Acd Med Singapore* 1995; 24:113.

26. Katsaros J. Indications for free soft-tissue transfer to the upper limb and the role of alternative procedures. *Hand Clin* 1992; 8:479.

27. Lutz BS, Klauke T, Dietrich FE. Late results after microvascular reconstruction of severe crush and avulsion

injuries of the upper extremity. *J Reconstr Microsurg* 1997; 13:423.

28. Brown DM, Upton J, Khoury RK. Free flap coverage of the hand. *Clin Plast Surg* 1997; 24:57.

29. Gerwin M, Weiland AJ. Vascularized bone grafts to the upper extremity. *Hand Clin* 1992; 8:509.

30. Yajima H et al. Vascularized bone grafts to the upper extremities. *Plast Reconstr Surg* 1998; 101:727.

31. Wood ML. Composite free flaps to the hand. *Hand Clin* 1997; 13:231.

32. Radovan C. Adjacent flap development using expandable silastic implants. Annual Meeting. American Society of Plastic and Reconstructive Surgeons. Boston. September 30, 1976.

33. Radovan C. Development of adjacent flaps using a temporary expander. *ASPRS Plast Surg Forum* 1979; 2:62.

34. Meland NB, Smith AA, Johnson CH. Tissue expansion in the upper extremities. *Hand Clin* 1997; 13:303.

35. Filatov VI, Voinova LE. Reconstructive surgery in the preprosthetic period. *Acta Chir Plast* 1982; 3:140.

36. Halbert CF, Wei FC. Neurosensory free flaps: digits and hand. *Hand Clin* 1997; 13:251.

37. Brunelli GA, Brunelli F, Brunelli GR. Microsurgical reconstruction of sensory skin. *Ann Acad Med Singapore* 1995; 24:108.

38. Chuang DC. Functioning free-muscle transpalntation for the upper extremity. *Hand Clin* 1997; 13:279.

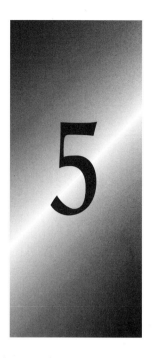

Surgical Options for Brachial Plexus Injury

James B. Bennett, MD, and Stephen C. Nicolaidis, MD

Trauma to the brachial plexus is a devastating injury to the individual. It renders the involved upper extremity partially or totally functionless and with impaired sensation. The recovery period may range from several months to several years, during which time the patient must learn to adapt and function with a disabled upper extremity. Additionally, one must tolerate a significant amount of pain associated with the plexus disruption or the phenomenon of rein- nervation of the damaged plexus. Recovery is unpredictable, and the surgical approach to the brachial plexus injury has ranged historically from "do nothing, wait and see," to a more aggressive approach involving accurate assessment of the degree of injury and early surgical intervention in selected cases (1–3). The surgical approach encompasses reconstruction of major vessel disruption, nerves of the brachial plexus, reconstructive orthopedic procedures that include bony and musculotendinous procedures, and, in some cases, ablative amputation surgery and prosthetic fitting (3). The management of severe pain requires various modalities: psychological with support therapy; pharmacologic through various medications; electrical through nerve stimulation; and, at times, surgical through sympathectomy, dorsal column stimulation, thalamotomy, cordotomy, and rhizotomy (4–6).

Brachial plexus injuries may involve closed traction or stretch injuries; open direct lacerations with life-threatening vascular compromise; or a combination of explosion and contusion injury as is seen in gunshot wounds. Accurate initial assessment of the injury and subsequent follow-up with reproducible documentation are required to determine the level of lesions, the degree of injury, and the potential for recovery. Initial evaluation will outline the mechanism of the injury and whether the injury involves associated fractures, head injury, or cervical spine or cord injury. The patient's profession and his dominant extremity are important in the evaluation and rehabilitation process.

A thorough knowledge of brachial plexus anatomy and its variations is required to assess these injuries (Figure 5-1).

OBSTETRIC BRACHIAL PLEXUS PALSY

Although obstetric brachial plexus palsy (OBPP) is not the focus of this chapter, a brief description is given. The incidence of OBPP in the U.S. ranges from 0.038 to 0.26% of full term births (7,8). The etiology involves fetal malposition, cephalopelvic disproportion, and the use of forceps at delivery. Seventy-three percent of OBPP cases involve a pure upper plexus injury to C5 and C6, also known as Erb's palsy, presenting with

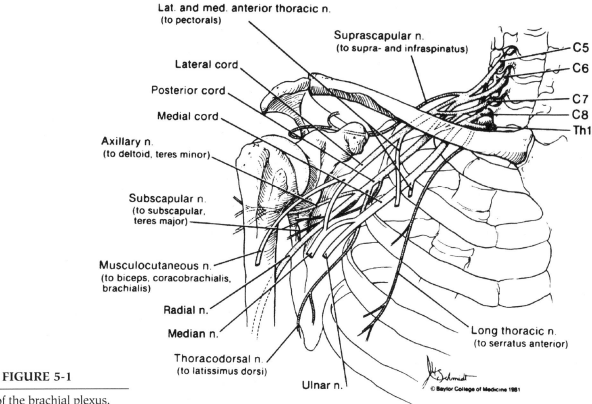

FIGURE 5-1

Anatomy of the brachial plexus.

shoulder and elbow dysfunction. Total plexus injury occurs in 20% of OBPP cases and presents with a flail arm. The least common presentation involves paralysis of the hand with function at the shoulder and elbow, secondary to a pure lower plexus injury to C8 and T1, also known as Klumpke's palsy.

Infants are initially treated with physical therapy. Reevaluation is performed at 3, 6, and 9 months of age, by which times significant improvement is expected. Failing this, *primary brachial plexus exploration* with microsurgical reconstruction of the plexus must be considered (Figure 5-2). Beyond 12 to 18 months of age, microsurgical reconstruction becomes less of an option because of the prolonged denervation period that will take place. Consideration must then be given to contracture releases and tendon transfers (Figure 5-3).

PHYSICAL EXAMINATION

The physical examination must include a complete neurologic evaluation for sensation, active and passive motion of all joints, and manual muscle testing with strength grading. These must be recorded in a reproducible fashion so that each subsequent examination may be compared with the initial and previous examinations. Only through such comparison can a determination of prognosis and recovery be ascertained. Pertinent clinical

signs are important to determine the level of the lesions and to differentiate a nerve root avulsion (a preganglionic lesion with a poor prognosis for recovery or reconstruction) from a postganglionic lesion that has the potential for recovery or surgical intervention and reconstruction.

Loss of the posterior cervical muscles, rhomboids, and serratus anterior, or an elevated hemidiaphragm suggest a nerve root avulsion of the upper trunk in the C5–6 distribution and a poor prognosis. Evidence of a Horner's syndrome indicates a lower root lesion of the C8–T1 distribution and a nerve root avulsion. The absence of a Tinel's sign in the face of a brachial plexus injury suggests nerve root avulsion, and the presence of "long tract signs" suggests that a significant spinal cord injury has occurred and the possibility of nerve root avulsion exists (9).

In the severe brachial plexus injury a common finding is one of a mixed preganglionic and postganglionic distribution. Clinical findings can be somewhat altered in those cases that have a prefixed plexus in which C4 contributing the upper portion of the plexus, or in those cases that have a postfixed plexus pattern in which T2 contributes to the lower portion of the plexus.

Peripheral circulation must be documented as well as the presence of bruits or palpable pulsation in the plexus region, which may suggest disruption or false aneurysm from a major vascular injury.

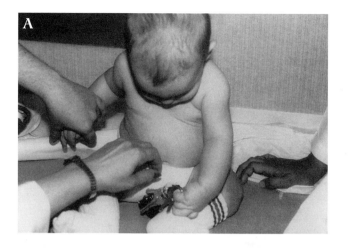

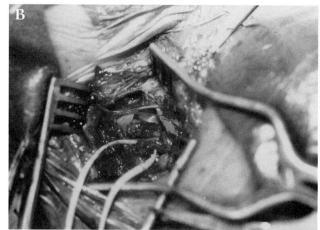

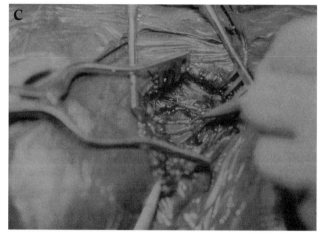

FIGURE 5-2

A. Obstetrical brachial plexus palsy, clinical. B. Intra-operative lesion of the plexus palsy. C. Intraoperative reconstruction of the plexus with nerve grafts.

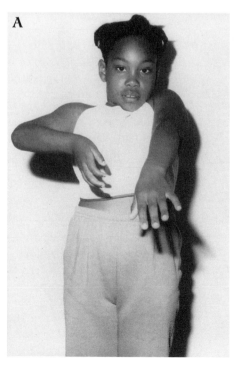

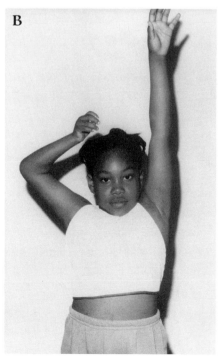

FIGURE 5-3

A. Latissimus dorsi transfer to provide shoulder elevation and external rotation preoperatively. B. Postoperative shoulder elevation and external rotation.

INVESTIGATIONS

Initial evaluation should also include plain radiographs of the head, cervical spine, ipsilateral shoulder girdle, and any other region of the extremity that is suspicious for either fracture or dislocation. Cervical spine injury must be documented and treated appropriately. Fractures of the transverse processes of the cervical spine carry a poor prognosis, suggesting nerve root avulsion secondary to the significant force necessary to produce such a fracture.

INITIAL MANAGEMENT

After stabilization of the patient and initial documentation, the closed brachial plexus injury is supported in a sling and wrist support for comfort and evaluated at approximately 4-week intervals. The open injury, whether it is a laceration or an avulsion, must be addressed immediately using bony stabilization; vascular reconstruction; and primary nerve identification and repair, or tagging of the disrupted nerve fibers for secondary repair. In those cases that have an acute transection of the brachial plexus, primary repair of the transected plexus is recommended. This is a time-consuming, exacting technique and generally requires the vascular reconstruction to be completed prior to the plexus reconstruction. If accurate plexus repair cannot be performed, then the plexus is tagged by suture to prevent retraction and to maintain some orderly arrangement of the plexus fibers. This allows secondary

neurorrhaphy or grafting procedures after approximately 2 to 4 weeks, at which time the wound and the vascular reconstruction are healed. Proximal nerve injury level is also differentiated by this time to allow accurate neuroma resection to viable proximal nerve fascicles.

FURTHER INVESTIGATIONS

A cervical myelogram is performed at approximately 1 month if no improvement of the closed brachial plexus traction injury has occurred. Myelogram is generally not performed initially because of the possibility of producing arachnoiditis and the difficulty in interpretation due to bleeding, blood clot formation, and tearing of the nerve root sleeves (all of which produce a false study). At one month, however, a myelogram may demonstrate the presence of traumatic pseudomeningoceles in areas of nerve root avulsion (Figure 5-4) (10). It must be noted that false-positives and false-negatives exist in the interpretation of the myelogram; however, two or more meningoceles suggest multiple nerve root avulsions, a poor prognosis and, in some institutions, a contraindication to brachial plexus exploration. Myelography can be combined with a computed axial tomography (CAT) scan to improve diagnostic accuracy (11). An increasing number of articles have described the use of magnetic resonance imaging (MRI) to diagnose nerve root avulsions (2,12,13).

Electromyography and nerve conduction velocity studies are performed at approximately 3 to 4 weeks,

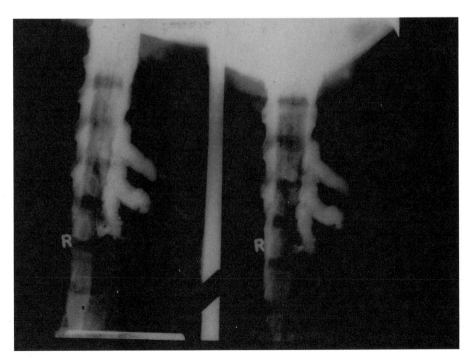

FIGURE 5-4

Cervical myelogram showing pseudomeningoceles or nerve root avulsion.

when denervation potentials have been established. The sensory nerve action potential will be normal in a preganglionic lesion since the sensory arch of axon and cell body is maintained. Similarly, posterior cervical muscle denervation by electromyography (EMG) is suggestive of a preganglionic lesion. Such a lesion carries a poor prognosis for recovery. As regeneration occurs in incomplete lesions, serial EMGs should demonstrate decreasing denervation potentials and the appearance of reinnervation potentials that predate clinical muscle activity.

The axon reflex test or histamine test may be used to differentiate preganglionic and postganglionic lesions. A triple response consisting of an area of vasodilatation, wheel formation, and flair will be demonstrated in the preganglionic lesions in which the sensory fibers are intact.

In the postganglionic lesions, the patient will demonstrate only vasodilatation and wheel formation, but no flair will occur.

DEFINITIVE MANAGEMENT

Timing

The potential for regeneration and recovery should be determined between 3 and 6 months postinjury. In the face of recovery, based on clinical and electrodiagnostic testing, the patient is treated conservatively, using the modalities of physical medicine, joint mobilization, and orthopedic support.

If no recovery can be detected by 3 months, or if recovery has plateaued before 6 months, surgical intervention should be considered. If surgical reconstruction of the brachial plexus is delayed past 6 months, the prognosis of maximum recovery is reduced. Delays past 1 year offer little motor return and only partial sensory recovery. Nerve root avulsion, despite reconstruction, carries the poorest prognosis, followed by supraclavicular lesions. After reconstruction of the plexus, the best prognosis for recovery is offered by infraclavicular lesions that have begun to differentiate into the individual peripheral nerves.

Microsurgical Reconstruction of the Brachial Plexus Injury

Brachial plexus exploration and reconstruction is a time-consuming procedure, which may take 8 to 12 hours in the performance of the operation. Reconstruction may involve neurolysis, primary or secondary neurorrhaphy, nerve grafting, and nerve transfers with or without nerve grafts (Figure 5-5). Any or all of these procedures may be required in reconstruction of the plexus. Motor components of the cervical plexus, spinal

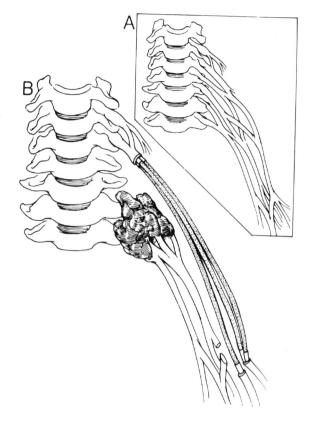

FIGURE 5-5

Neurotization at C5 with cable grafts to suprascapular and musculocutaneous nerves.

accessory nerve, and intercostal nerves may also be utilized for complete reconstruction. Intraoperative nerve action potential evaluation of neuroma incontinuity is performed to determine whether simple neurolysis is indicated or section of the neuroma and cable grafting is required (14,15). Sensory-evoked potential response helps to determine intraforaminal or intraspinal nerve root avulsion from the spinal cord.

Priority for upper-extremity functional recovery consists of reconstruction of elbow flexion, wrist stabilization, and finger flexion and extension. Shoulder arthrodesis will satisfactorily stabilize an unstable shoulder (Figure 5-6). The recovery of intrinsic hand function has not been demonstrated in adults after lower root brachial plexus reconstruction.

Neurolysis

Neurolysis of the intact plexus from external scar or bony compression offers the best prognosis. Decompression of a thoracic outlet or callus about a clavicular fracture is indicated in incidences of external compression of the plexus.

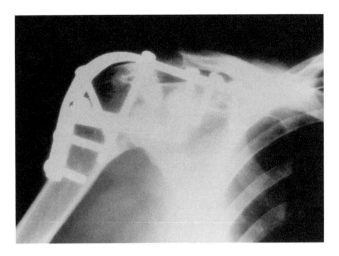

FIGURE 5-6

Shoulder arthrodesis using compression plate fixation to alleviate the need for shoulder spica cast immobilization.

Neurorrhaphy

For purposes of discussion, we will define *primary neurorrhaphy* as direct nerve repair performed at the time of injury, and *secondary neurorrhaphy* as direct repair in a delayed fashion. Primary and secondary neurorrhaphy provide predictable and measurable motor and sensory return, except for C8–T1 repair on adults. Regeneration at that level has not been reported for adults but seems worthwhile in children who have improved regeneration potential.

Nerve Grafting

Nerve grafting is indicated when direct repair is not possible, because of either a large gap between nerve ends or nerve root avulsion. We do not yet have the medical knowledge to reconstruct an avulsed nerve root. For example, an OBPP patient might be found to have C5 avulsion and C6 rupture (disruption distal to the nerve root) at the time of exploration. In this case, a reasonable approach would involve auricular nerve grafting from C6 proximally to both C5 and C6 distally. Nerve-grafting procedures restore muscle function and sensation to a lesser degree than neurorrhaphy, and have a more guarded prognosis (Figure 5-7) (11). Donor sites for nerve grafts in adults include sural, medial cutaneous, medial antebrachial cutaneous, and sensory branches of the cervical plexus. The ulnar nerve may be used as a donor in complete C8–T1 root avulsion

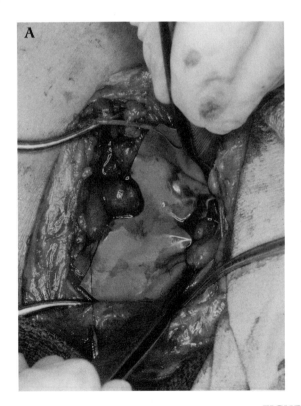
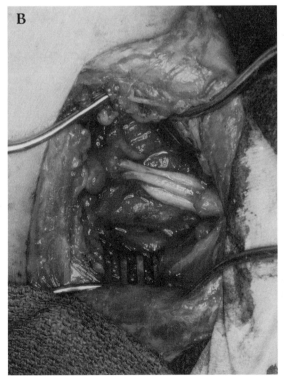

FIGURE 5-7

A. Ressected C5 and C6 postganglionic plexus neuromas for cable graft reconstruction. B. Multiple nerve cable grafts of C5–6 postganglionic plexus rupture injury.

lesions, as ulnar nerve recovery with these injuries in adult patients has not been documented.

Nerve Transfers

As the number of avulsed nerve roots increases, nerve grafting to the remaining nonavulsed nerve roots becomes less of an option. In this case, components of the cervical plexus or the spinal accessory nerve can be transfered into the distal nerve ends (corresponding to the avulsed nerve roots) (16). Intercostal nerves utilizing three intercostal nerves may be grafted into the musculocutaneous nerve for elbow flexion (17). These two techniques may be utilized in the total root avulsion of the C5, 6, 7 group to allow elbow flexion and components of finger flexion and extension activities.

Neural deficits in postganglionic plexus disruption are bridged by several nerve cable grafts to establish the continuity of the plexus. More recent articles have described the transfer of part of the ulnar nerve, or transfer of the medial pectoral nerves, to the musculocutaneous nerve in an attempt to restore elbow flexion as early as possible (18–20). For complete avulsion of the brachial plexus, transfer of the contralateral C7 nerve root via nerve grafts provides a greater number of axons to the denervated region (21,22).

Rehabilitation

Following plexus reconstruction, the patient's repair is protected for approximately 1 month. Subsequent physi-cal medicine modalities, mobilization of joints, and orthotic devices are again used to preserve position and function until the results of the reconstruction can be assessed. Regeneration following microsurgical recon-struction of the brachial plexus may require 1 to 2 years before maximum function is achieved. In addition to the results of the reconstructive procedures, the patient's pain pattern may be significantly altered to a much more toler-able level following the resection of neuromas, release of scar tissue, and reconstruction of the brachial plexus (18).

Electrical Stimulation

Denervated muscles in a brachial plexus injury will undergo progressive atrophy and fibrosis until reinner-vation takes place. If the denervation period is pro-longed, the muscles may never regain adequate function. Therefore, preservation of denervated muscle groups using electrical stimulation appears desirable. However, transcutaneous muscle stimulation is inade-quate, and it is impractical to maintain the daily level required to be of significant benefit.

The preservation of denervated muscle using an implantable electrode stimulator has recently been described. The implantable pulse generator (IPG) is the size of a pacemaker device and connects to two stimula-tor leads that are placed in the denervated muscle. The IPG fires for 1.5 seconds every 25.5 seconds, 24 hours a day, and can be programmed externally. Clinical results have been encouraging; however, the system awaits FDA approval (Figure 5-8) (23–25).

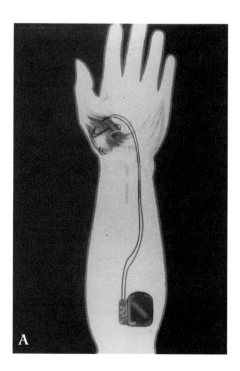 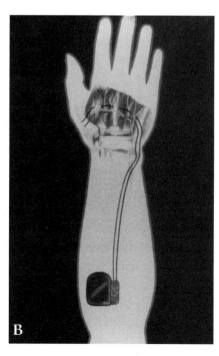

FIGURE 5-8

A. Implantable electrode stimulator for muscle stimulation with nerve regeneration occurs in intrinsic muscles of the hand–thenar muscles. B. Ulnar innervated intrinsic muscles with electrode stimulator.

Transcutaneous nerve stimulation may be of use in reducing the pain of nerve regeneration during this period. The mobilization of all joints and strengthening as muscle units recover are required for ultimate maximum return.

Orthopedic Reconstruction for Brachial Plexus Injury

Orthopedic reconstructive procedures are used following plexus reconstruction or in selected cases in which isolated nerve avulsion injuries are not reconstructed.

Shoulder

The trapezius muscle can be transfered to the proximal humerus to improve shoulder abduction (26). The L'Episcopo procedure (in which the insertions of the latissimus dorsi and teres major are transposed posterolaterally) enhances active lateral rotation and is particularly useful in OBPP (1,27–29).

Shoulder arthrodesis and derotational osteotomy of the humerus are indicated for total loss of shoulder control without scapular motors and when transfers are not possible. These are acceptable procedures to position the shoulder and arm while allowing increasing strength patterns of the muscles that must motor the elbow and the fingers. Absence or significant weakness of scapular motor strength is a contraindication to the shoulder arthrodesis.

Elbow

Major tendon transfers to the elbow for flexion or extension are likewise utilized during the recovery phase. Transfer of the pectoralis major, as described by Clark (in which a portion of the pectoralis is used) (30), or Schottstaedt (in which the entire pectoralis muscle is used on its neurovascular bundle) (31) (Figure 5-9A,B) has been particularly useful. Similar transfers of the latissimus dorsi may be utilized to restore elbow flexion or extension (32). In the individual with strong forearm and hand musculature, transfer of the forearm flexor mass, as described by Steindler (33) may produce adequate elbow flexion pattern. Triceps transfer to biceps tendon is an excellent transfer to regain elbow flexion; however, the resulting loss of elbow extension is undesirable in the paraplegic patient, for example, who depends on such function (34) for transfer and crutch walking.

Wrist and Hand

Once the shoulder is stabilized and the elbow allows position with active flexion and gravity extension, hand

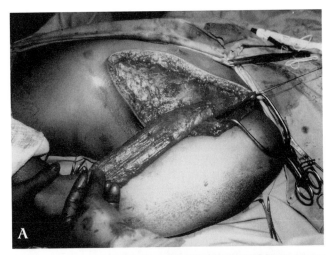

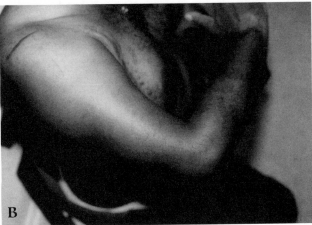

FIGURE 5-9

A. Pectoralis major flexorplasty to restore elbow flexion. B. Clinical elbow flexion postoperative flexorplasty.

reconstruction may be considered. Reconstruction of a usable hand may utilize various forms of tendon transfers, tenodeses, or arthrodeses. Specific techniques are well described in the literature and will not be discussed, but the surgeon must use muscles of good grade and strength (4/5) before any tendon transfers can be successful. If the muscles present are felt to be inadequate motors, consideration can be given to the use of free muscle transfers to deliver stronger motors. Doi has described a double free-muscle transfer technique to restore prehension in patients following complete avulsion of the brachial plexus (35).

Wrist arthrodesis is indicated when two tendons of adequate power are not available for wrist flexion and extension, or preservation of wrist motion will make it impossible to adequately reconstruct a functional hand. Tenodesis and arthrodesis are not indicated if there is no potential for utilization of the hand or if its insensitivity allows repeated injury, fractures, lacerations, or infection. With complete avulsion of the brachial plexus, intrinsic hand function is unlikely to return despite neural reconstructive procedures (36).

Sensibility

Sensibility is, of course, required on the prehensile surface of the hand; therefore, its restoration is particularly important in median and ulnar nerve injuries. Surgical options include nerve grafts, with or without a vascular supply; digital nerve translocation, for example, of ring finger ulnar proper digital to thumb ulnar proper digital nerve for isolated median nerve injury; and neurovascular cutaneous island flaps, for example, from dorsum to palm (36).

Amputation

If the hand is insensitive and has no potential for recovery, the patient with elbow function may elect below-elbow amputation and prosthetic fit as a form of reconstruction that will allow two-handed function (Figures 5-10 and 5-11). Such patients will almost always obtain adequate elbow flexion. Likewise, the rare patient with irreparable total brachial plexus root avulsion injury and a flail arm may elect above-elbow amputation (37). Shoulder arthrodesis (Figure 5-12) is

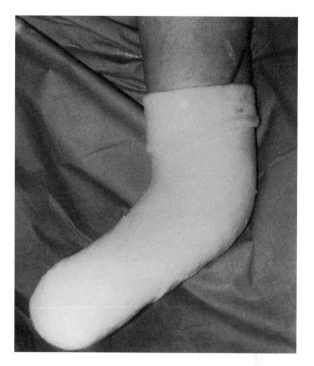

FIGURE 5-11

Immediate fit rigid cast dressing in below-elbow amputation for terminal device application.

indicated for improved prosthesis control if some scapular control is present. Amputation at the wrist is only indicated in the patient with an insensate hand with recurrent ulcers or infections.

Psychological support as well as medical management, physical and rehabilitation therapy, and orthopedic and prosthetic options must be available to the patient to ensure maximum functional recovery (38,39).

Pain Management

To date, the greatest problem confronting the brachial plexus injured patient, in addition to a flail, anesthetic limb, is the management of pain. This must be approached in an orderly fashion utilizing a multidiscipline professional approach to the maximum benefit of the patient. Medication and electrical stimulation are used in the management of pain. In cases of severe pain, neurosurgical intervention must be considered, although the prognosis is guarded and ultimate results often are poor. Cordotomy, rhizotomy, sympathectomy, dorsal column stimulation, and other forms of neurosurgical intervention have been used (6). Coagulation of the dorsal root entry zone (DREZ) is perhaps one of the most efficient techniques (40,41).

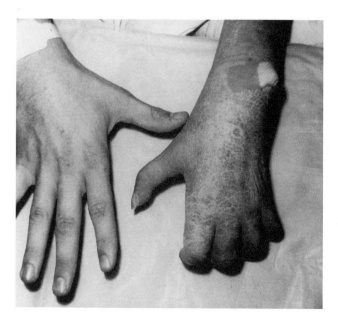

FIGURE 5-10

Insensitive rigid claw hand deformity in C7-8–T1. Nerve root avulsion injury with elbow flexion for below-elbow amputation.

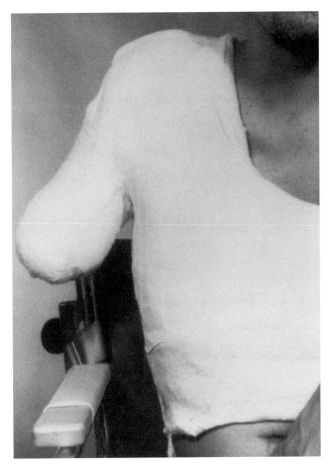

FIGURE 5-12

Total C5–T1 nerve root avulsion of the brachial plexus treated with above-elbow amputation and shoulder arthrodesis.

CONCLUSIONS

With the advent of microsurgical procedures and a better understanding of the microneural anatomy of the brachial plexus, reconstruction of brachial plexus injuries is possible. This approach can produce a functioning extremity as well as decrease the pain associated with this injury. In cases of complete plexus disruption, if elbow control is gained, the nonfunctional hand may be amputated at a below-elbow level and undergo useful prosthetic fit. It is our opinion that this gives more useful function to the patient than either a flail, anesthetic limb or an above-elbow amputation in which the patient has little to limited use of a conventional above-elbow prosthesis. Hand and upper extremity transplantation have been performed with limited success. Current multicenter evaluation of these results and recommendation for future investigation surgery are ongoing. These procedures are not addressed in this chapter (42,43).

References

1. L'Episcopo JB. Restoration of muscle balance in the treatment of obstetrical paralysis. *NY State J M* 1939; 357–363.
2. Muth CP, Biemelt F, Kamenz M. Significance of MRI diagnosis for imaging traumatically induced cervical root avulsions. *Rontgenpraxis* 1996; 49 (11): 283–285.
3. Yeoman P, Seddon H. Brachial plexus injury: treatment of the flail arm. *J Bone Joint Surg* [Br] 1961; 43B(3):493–500.
4. Stanwood J, Kraft G. Diagnosis and management of brachial plexus injuries. *Arch Phys Med Rehabil* 1971; 52:52–61.
5. Wynn Parry CB. The management of traction lesions of the brachial plexus and peripheral nerve injuries of the upper extremity: A study in teamwork. *Injury* 1980; 11(4):265–285.
6. Zorub D, Nashold B, Copok W. Avulsion of the brachial plexus: a review with implication on the therapy of intractable pain. *Surg Neurol* 1974; 2:347–353.
7. Laurent JP, Lee R, Shenaq S, Park JT, Solis IS, Kowalik L. Neurosurgical correction of upper brachial plexus birth injuries. *J Neurosurgery* 1993; 79:197–203.
8. Sjoberg I, Erichs K, Bjerre I. Cause and effect of obstetric (neonatal) brachial plexus palsy. *Acta Paediatr Scand* 1988; 77:357–364.
9. Rorabeck CH, Harris W. Factors affecting the prognosis of brachial plexus injury. *J Bone Joint Surg* (Br) 1981; 63B (3):404–407.
10. Murphey F, Hartung W, Kirklin JW. Myelographic demonstrations of avulsion injury of the brachial plexus. *An J Roentgen* 1947; 58:102–105.
11. Roger B, Travers V, Laval-Jeantet M. Imaging of posttraumatic brachial plexus injury. *Clin Orthop* 1988; 237:57–61.
12. Ochi M, Ikuta Y, Watanabe M, Kimori K, Itoh K. The diagnostic value of MRI in traumatic brachial plexus injury. *J Hand Surg* (Br) 1994; 19(1):55–59.
13. Uetani M, Hayashi K, Hashimi R, Nakahara N, Aso N, Ito N. Traction injuries of the brachial plexus: signal intensity changes of the posterior cervical paraspinal muscles on MRI. *J Comput Assist Tomogr* 1997; 21(5):790–795.
14. Kline DG. Physiologic and clinical factors contributing to the timing of nerve repair. *Clin Neurosurg* 1977; 24:425.
15. Kline DG. Timing for exploration of nerve lesions and evaluation of neuroma incontinuity. *Clin Orthop Rel Res* 1982; 163:42–49.
16. Brunelli G. Neurotization of avulsed roots of the brachial plexus by means of the anterior nerves of the cervical plexus. *Int J Microsurg* 1980; 2(1):55–58.
17. Suzuki N, Yamaji K, Tajima A, et al. Brachial plexus injuries. Experience with intercostal nerve grafting and root avulsions. *Nagoya Med J* 1972; 18(2):91–103.
18. Brandt KE, Mackinnon SE. A technique for maximizing biceps recovery in brachial plexus reconstruction. *J Hand Surg* 1993; 18A:726–733.
19. Leechavengvongs S, Witoonchart K, Uerpairojkit C, Thuvasethakul P, Ketmalasiri W. Nerve transfer to biceps muscle using a part of the ulnar nerve in brachial plexus injury (upper arm type). *J Hand Surg* 1998; 23A:711–716.
20. Oberlin C, Beal D, Leechavengvongs S, Salon A, Dauge MC, Sarcy JJ. Nerve transfer to biceps muscle using a part

of ulnar nerve for C5-C6 avulsion of the brachial Plexus. *J Hand Surg* 1994; 19A:232–237.

21. Gu YD, Chen DS, Zhang GM, Cheng XM, Xu JG, Zhang LY, Cai PQ, Chen L. Long-term functional results of contralateral C7 transfer. *J Reconstr Microsurg* 1998; 14:57–59.

22. Gu YD, Zhang DS, Chen JG, Yan JG, Cheng XM, Chen L. Seventh cervical nerve root transfer from the contralateral healthy side for treatment of brachial plexus root avulsion. *J Hand Surg* (Br) 1992; 17B; 518–521.

23. Nicolaidis SC, Williams HB. Preservation of denervated muscle following nerve injury using an implantable electrode stimulator. *Plast Reconstr Surg* (submitted 1999).

24. Williams HB. The value of continuous electrical muscle stimulation using a completely implantable system in the preservation of muscle function following motor nerve injury and repair. *J Microsurg* 1996; 17:589–596.

25. Williams HB. A clinical pilot study to assess the functional return following continuous muscle stimulation after nerve injury and repair in the upper extremity using a completely implantable electrical system. *J Microsurg* 1996; 17:597–605.

26. Aziz W. Singer RM, Wolff TW. Transfer of the trapezius for flail shoulder after brachial plexus injury. *JBJS* 1990; 72B:701–704.

27. Hoffer MM, Phipps GJ. Closed reduction and tendon transfer for treatment of dislocation of the glenohumeral joint secondary to brachial plexus birth Palsy. *JBJS* 1998; 80A:997–1001.

28. L'Episcopo JB. Tendon transplantation in obstetrical paralysis. *Am J Surg* 1934; 25:122–125.

29. Terzis JK, Shiamishis G. Outcome of scapula stabilization in obstetrical brachial plexus palsy. Presented at American Association for Hand Surgery Meeting, January 1999.

30. Clark JMP. Reconstruction of biceps brachii by pectoral muscle transplantation. *Br J Surg* 1946; 34:180.

31. Schottstaedt ER, Larsen LJ, Bost FG. Complete muscle transposition. *JBJS* 1955; 37A:897.

32. Leffert RD. *Brachial Plexus Injuries*. New York: Churchill Livingstone, 1985.

33. Steindler A. *Orthopedic Operations*. Springfield: Charles C. Thomas, 1940, 129.

34. Hoang Ph, Mills C, Burke FD. Triceps to biceps transfer for extablished brachial plexus palsy. *J Bone Joint Surg* (Br) 1989; 71B:268–271.

35. Doi K. New reconstructive procedure for brachial plexus injury. *Clin Plast Surg* 1997; 24(1):75–85.

36. Omer GE. Reconstruction of the forearm and hand after peripheral nerve injury. In: Omer, Spinner, Van Beek (eds), *Peripheral Nerve Problems*. 1998, 675–705.

37. Wright TW, Hagen AD, Wood MB. Prosthetic usage in major upper extremity amputations. *J Hand Surg* 1995; 20(4):619–622.

38. Perry J, Shu J, Barber L, et al. Orthosis in patients with brachial plexus injuries. *Arch Phys Med Rehabil* 1974; 55:134–137.

39. Wynn Parry CB. Rehabilitation of patients following tractions lesions of the brachial plexus. *Clin Plast Surg* 1984; 11(1):173–179.

40. Carvalho GA, Nikkhah G, Sammi M. Pain management after post-traumatic brachial plexus lesion. *Orthopade* 1997; 26:621–625.

41. Emery E, Blondet E, Mertens P, Sindou M. Microsurgical drezotomy for pain due in brachial plexus avulsion. *Stereotact Funct Neurosurg* 1997; 68:155–160.

42. Breidenbach WC, Tobin GR, Gorantla VS, Gonzalez RN, Granger DK. A position statement in support of hand transplantation. *J Hand Surg* 2002; 27:771.

43. Owen F, Dubernard JM, et al. First Modern Hand Transplant Performed in France. News release. September 23, 1998.

6

Rehabilitation Planning for the Upper Extremity Amputee

Robert H. Meier, III, MD, and Alberto Esquenazi, MD

The person with an amputation is likely to receive the most relevant and cost-effective array of rehabilitation services if a specific rehabilitation plan is developed that has time-stated and objectively measurable goals. This plan is best undertaken using a team approach and with a thorough evaluation and understanding of the amputee's needs and desires. A useful framework has been developed that divides the stages of amputee rehabilitation into nine phases (Figure 6-1). Although these phases are rather artificial and may overlap at times, the framework does provide useful goals and treatment focuses for each relevant phase of amputee rehabilitation.

NINE PHASES OF AMPUTEE REHABILITATION

Because of the obvious disability of amputation, a team approach is essential to the restoration of full function and emotional well-being for the person with an amputation. Amputee rehabilitation should include more than an amputating surgeon and a prosthetist. In developing a plan for rehabilitation with the person with an arm amputation, it is helpful to divide the entire program into phases based on the time sequencing before and following an amputation. A schema that is useful for setting appropriate goals provides for nine distinct phases (Table 6-1) (1):

1. Preoperative
2. Amputation with surgical reconstruction
3. Acute postoperative
4. Preprosthetic
5. Prosthetic prescription and fabrication
6. Prosthetic training
7. Community reintegration
8. Vocational rehabilitation
9. Functional follow-up.

This schema assists in organizing the rehabilitation team and treatment planning. This format can be utilized in almost any team and rehabilitation setting and modified to develop team efficiency and comprehensive amputee rehabilitation. Using these phases also assists in developing the types of outcome measures that the team wishes to use to assess the benefits of their system of amputee rehabilitation and when each component of that system should be administered.

Preoperative Phase

The preoperative phase is an appropriate time to discuss phantom limb sensation, phantom pain, and residual limb pain with the patient. The staging of the rehabilita-

- Preoperative
- Amputation Surgery
- Acute Postsurgical
- Preprosthetic
- Prosthetic Prescription and Fabrication
- Prosthetic Training
- Community Integration
- Vocational/Avocational
- Follow-up

FIGURE 6-1

Nine phases of amputee rehabilitation.

tion plan, the potential for prosthetic use, and the approximate timetable for the rehabilitation program should be presented. A discussion of the emotional adaptive process is also helpful during the preoperative phase. During this phase, the focus should be placed on maintaining the scapulothoracic and glenohumeral motion and, if remaining, elbow flexion and forearm pronation and supination. In addition, this is an excellent time to work on changing hand dominance, if necessary and also

to teach one-handed activities. This is an excellent time to introduce the use of a rocker knife, a button hook, and other one-handed adaptive equipment.

Amputation with Surgical Reconstruction

It cannot be stated strongly enough that the careful reconstruction of the amputated limb at the time of surgery is the *sine qua non* for optimal functional outcomes. Those techniques that seem to determine successful prosthetic fit and comfort are related to:

- Identification of a level of tissue viability that will heal primarily
- Formation of a cylindrical residual limb
- Myoplastic closure for prevention of undesirable movement of the residual limb soft tissues over the bone
- Beveling of the ends of the residual bones
- Control of postoperative edema with immediate postoperative rigid dressings
- Burying the ends of major peripheral nerves. This is the ideal time to begin to discuss what outcomes, both emotional and functional, are possible for the amputee. This is also the best time for the professional team members to decide which outcomes are most likely to be achievable for the individual amputee.

TABLE 6-1
Phases of Amputee Rehabilitation

PHASE	HALLMARKS
1. Preoperative	Assessment of body condition, patient education; discussion of surgical level, postoperative prosthetic plans
2. Amputation with surgical reconstruction	Length, myoplastic closure, soft tissue coverage, nerve handling, rigid dressing
3. Acute postoperative	Wound healing, pain control, proximal body motion, emotional support
4. Preprosthetic	Shaping and shrinking of amputation stump, improvement of muscle strength, restoration of patient as locus of control
5. Prosthetic prescription and fabrication	Team consensus on prosthetic prescription, experienced limb prosthetic fabrication
6. Prosthetic training	Increased wearing of prosthesis and mobility skills
7. Community reintegration	Resumption of roles in family and community activities; regaining of emotional equilibrium and healthy coping strategies; pursuit of recreational activities
8. Vocational rehabilitation	Assessment and planning of vocational activities for future; possible need for further education, training, or job modification
9. Functional follow-up	Lifelong prosthetic, functional, medical, and emotional support; regular assessment of functional level and prosthetic problem solving

Acute Postoperative Phase

At the conclusion of the amputation, the residual trans-radial or lower level limb stump is best placed in an immediate postoperative rigid dressing to diminish postoperative edema, enhance wound healing, and decrease pain. Various postoperative rigid dressing protocols have been proposed and are part of a comprehensive coordinated amputee management system (2). If a soft dressing is applied at the conclusion of the surgery, no attempt should be made to use elastic compression to shrink the stump until the wound shows evidence of primary wound healing (at least 3 weeks on average). Edema control can be initiated immediately if there is no evidence of vascular compromise.

After skin sutures or staples have been removed (usually between days 14 to 21), a more aggressive program of residual limb shaping and shrinking can begin. Suture removal marks the beginning of the preprosthetic phase if the patient has the potential for using a prosthesis. The important components of rehabilitation during this phase consist of controlling pain; promoting wound healing; and increasing upper limb, trunk, and remaining limb muscle strength. During this acute postoperative time, the rehabilitation emphasis should be placed on the remaining body segments that will substitute for the part that has been amputated. These activities enhance mobility before use of a prosthesis is desirable or practical. This is an ideal time for the patient to adjust to the new appearance of the body and to learn functional skills without using a prosthesis.

Preprosthetic Phase

Once the wound has developed adequate tensile strength, the stump must undergo a process of shaping and shrinking. A rigid dressing or Unna boot dressing changed weekly, compression with a shrinker garment, or elastic rolled bandages can be utilized (3). If elastic rolled bandages are used, they must be applied in a figure-eight fashion. The elastic bandages are anchored by incorporating the next proximal joint, and bandages should be rewrapped every 4 hours, or more frequently if the dressing becomes loose. When these elastic bandages are removed, they should not remain off for more than 15 minutes so that extracellular fluid does not reaccumulate. Usually, 2 weeks of shaping and shrinking should produce enough residual limb shrinkage and shaping to permit creation of a cast for the initial prosthetic socket.

During this phase, increasing the strength of the residual and opposite limb muscles is of paramount importance. These remaining muscles must compensate for those lost in the amputation. In addition, trunk and upper limb strengthening is essential during this phase. This is also a time to improve cardiovascular fitness and endurance with the use of aerobic training, unless this is medically contraindicated.

Psychosocial issues are of great importance during the preprosthetic period. All rehabilitation team members play important roles in the patient's psychosocial adaptation to limb loss. A psychologist or social worker experienced in the process of adaptation to limb loss and change in body image is essential for optimal rehabilitation. Often these aspects of rehabilitation—and not simply the provision of the prosthesis—are the basis of a successful outcome. Psychological counseling enhances the coping mechanisms of the amputee in adapting to altered body image and function, with or without a prosthesis. Those team members responsible for psychosocial issues should interact with the amputee throughout all phases of the rehabilitation program. This phase of rehabilitation is concluded when the patient is ready for prosthetic fabrication.

Prosthetic Fabrication

The prosthetic fabrication phase should be brief, beginning with the decision regarding whether the amputee is to be fitted with a prosthesis. Whenever possible, component options should be tried before the final prosthetic prescription is developed. This flexibility requires a willing prosthetist and third-party payer. Third-party sponsorship for the prosthesis should be obtained as quickly as possible. Experienced prosthetists should be able to fabricate any type of arm prosthesis within 2 weeks of casting of the prosthesis, once financial responsibility for prosthetic payment has been approved.

It is important to discuss the length of time that it takes to fabricate the prosthesis. In addition, it is essential to educate the amputee regarding the steps in fabrication and the approximate number of visits that will likely be required to the prosthetist's laboratory before the prosthesis is ready to wear and prosthetic training can begin.

Prosthetic Training

The prosthetic training phase begins with the delivery of the prosthesis from the prosthetic laboratory and ideally begins within 4 to 12 weeks of the amputation surgery. This phase ideally should not be delayed more than 6 months. Literature available indicates that an increased rate of acceptance of the prosthesis occurs when fitting takes place before the end of this time frame. Training should occur under the guidance of an experienced physician, therapist, and prosthetist, all of whom understand the biomechanics and principles of prosthetic use and are available for frequent evaluations. Short periods of wearing the prosthesis and instruction in donning and doffing should be the initial focus. Exploring the use of the prosthesis for activities of daily living (ADLs) driving, recreation, and vocational needs should also be part of this phase.

An assessment should be made of the amputee's perception of the prosthesis, its meaning to the quality of life, the effort needed to use it, and how closely it simulates the lost arm. Often the artificial limb does not meet the fantasized expectations of the amputee in regard to what a prosthesis should look like, what function it provides, and how it feels to be seen with it compared to the arm before the amputation.

This training phase is completed when the amputee achieves full use of the prosthesis. To assess the patient acceptance of his prosthesis, a proficient team experienced in amputee rehabilitation and knowledgeable about prosthetic function is required. An assessment of the outcomes, both functional and emotional, at the completion of this phase of rehabilitation should be accomplished.

Community Reintegration

Re-entering society with an altered body image and a change in functional ability is often an emotionally stressful time for an amputee. Identifying a meaningful support structure in the community is one of the most important roles of the rehabilitation team. The individual's function in society, although changed, should be made as meaningful and satisfying as possible. This integrative model really draws on all persons and resources in the community: spouse, family, merchants, employer, clergy, social workers, health professionals, municipal government, and the federal government, working in concert to assist in restoring the individual to his rightful place in society. Whenever possible, previous community supports must be enlisted. This phase of rehabilitation will influence the amputee for the remainder of his life.

Vocational Rehabilitation

A careful discussion of vocational plans should occur. Knowledgeable vocational services should be provided for the arm amputee who has questions about his future vocational options. In such cases, an understanding of the amputee's maximal prosthetic functional skills should help in proper vocational rehabilitation planning. For most arm amputees, this phase is an essential part of the entire rehabilitation process.

In most cases, the arm amputee should be able to return to some type of one-handed work within several weeks of the arm amputation. It is anticipated that, with good primary wound healing and prompt prosthetic fitting and training, a unilateral arm amputee should be back at work within 10 to 16 weeks of the amputation, with or without use of a prosthesis.

Follow-Up

Careful patient follow-up remains the single most important phase of amputee rehabilitation following completion of the initial phases of rehabilitation. During this lifelong phase, attention to functional outcome, with or without a prosthesis, follows the quality of life achieved by the amputee. Emphasis should not be placed on the prosthesis but instead on the ultimate functional capability achieved by the amputee. The emotional well-being, and the patient's role in the family and community are continually assessed and enhanced whenever possible by the rehabilitation team. Follow-up visits to the physiatrist should be frequent enough to maintain a sense of continuity of care. Any prosthetic fitting problem should receive prompt attention, and any decrease in the level of function should be investigated for its cause. Often, correcting the problem requires more than just a visit to the prosthetist, and the problem should be discussed with the rehabilitation team. Only with a comprehensive array of amputation rehabilitation services can the wide variety of amputee issues be dealt with thoroughly and in a coordinated fashion. This highly structured system provides health care to the amputee in the least frustrating and most cost-effective manner. Such a system results in the best functional outcome and quality of life following an amputation

PYRAMID SCHEMA OF AMPUTEE EVALUATION AND CARE PLANNING

The pyramid schema bases the rehabilitation program on the initial history and physical examination (Figure 6-2). Such a system is thus based on the needs and desires of the amputee. It then progresses through the established details of the preamputation lifestyle and interests. These patient history details are outlined in Chapter 10 regarding the patient evaluation. Comorbid factors also contribute to the complexity of rehabilitation issues that confront the amputee and the rehabilitation team. These factors must be carefully assessed, and the team must decide how they will be approached therapeutically. In addition, a decision should be made whether the comorbid factors are likely to influence prosthetic use and functional outcome.

The pyramid points upward to the assessment of the other, so-called, "normal" remaining extremities. This system of care focuses on the remaining extremities, since they will always be more functional than the

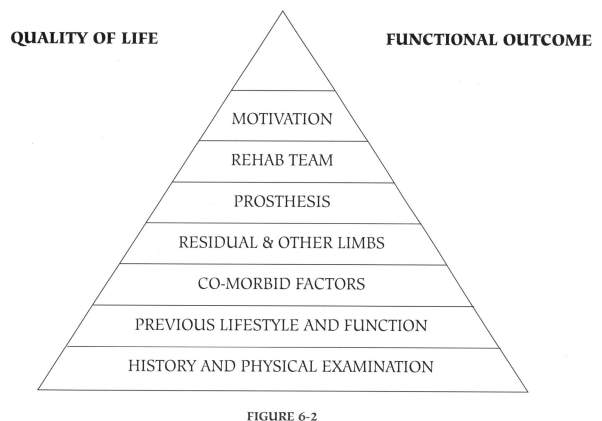

QUALITY OF LIFE **FUNCTIONAL OUTCOME**

MOTIVATION

REHAB TEAM

PROSTHESIS

RESIDUAL & OTHER LIMBS

CO-MORBID FACTORS

PREVIOUS LIFESTYLE AND FUNCTION

HISTORY AND PHYSICAL EXAMINATION

FIGURE 6-2

Pyramid Schema.

amputated extremity. The team will make a decision regarding whether a prosthesis should be fitted, when it should be fitted, and which components will achieve the desired function and cosmesis. Also, a decision should be made on the essential members of the team needed for this individual patient. Not all rehabilitation disciplines are necessary for every arm amputee, and individualizing the make-up of the team for each patient should help to realize a cost-effective system of care.

Amputee motivation is an important component of this pyramidal algorithm. If the amputee's needs and interests have been the focus of the plan, then chances are excellent that they will succeed. However, if the amputee has not had a thorough education about prostheses and prosthetic realities, there may be conflicts that arise between the amputee and the team. Disappointment may also arise during the early prosthetic fitting and training phases, because no prosthesis is a good cosmetic or functional substitute for the arm that has been lost. If conflict arises, or the amputee shows negative emotional changes or drops out of the treatment program, it is likely that disillusionment with the prosthetic result will occur. This type of conflict or disappointment does not necessarily reflect a lack of patient

motivation, thus it is essential that the team assess the situation with the patient and call him back in for an open discussion of his impression of what is happening to him. This provides an opportunity to provide further education, change the focus of the rehabilitation program, modify the prosthesis, or consider further emotional support or counseling. It is never enough to just blame the amputee's motivation as the cause of the treatment plan breaking down. When a conflict arises, this is an appropriate time to assess whether the patient truly feels empowered to resume the locus of control in his life.

Using the pyramid model should also assist the amputee achieve the best possible quality of life and functional outcomes. If there is a problem with achieving the desired quality of life or prosthetic function, the team can trace back down the pyramid to see where the system has not functioned in the best interests of the patient.

SYSTEMS OF AMPUTEE REHABILITATION

Any system of rehabilitation developed for working with an amputee must be based on two essential tenets.

The first is a definition of rehabilitation for the amputee program. The second is a system of amputee education that covers a wide variety of issues. Education provides a means to empower the person with the amputation. *Rehabilitation,* in our discussion, means independence for the amputee from systems of health care. Certainly, following the healing of an amputation, the person is not ill because of the amputation. Therefore, other than scheduled follow-ups with a physician and therapist and periodic visits for prosthetic maintenance, the amputee is free of a health care system.

However, for the person to function as well as possible in an able-bodied society, the amputee must be educated about his prosthesis, its maintenance, the potential problems of prosthetic use, the expected level of function, emotional well being, his return to work options, and the benefit of periodic follow-up.

A standardized educational program for all amputees is a means of empowerment so that the amputee can make the best possible decisions for his life and future needs (4,5). The educational program should be developed by a core team of rehabilitation professionals with a clear understanding of which team member has responsibility for the specific components of the educational program. These educational programs can be more difficult to coordinate in the outpatient setting, and the fragmentation of outpatient service provision makes the delivery of coordinated patient education more important. Much of the essential education of an amputee can be developed as an education manual and reviewed with the patient once he has read the material.

The care team should be designed to meet the individual needs of the amputee. The team may include only some of the team members (i.e., amputee, physician, prosthetist, and therapist), or all team members may be included in the rehabilitation process. Obviously, if significant emotional issues are involved, a psychologist can be utilized, and if there are questions regarding future vocational options, a vocational rehabilitation professional should be included. If surgical revision is contemplated, the appropriate surgeon will join the team also. Regular outpatient team conferencing should occur if three or more professional disciplines are actively participating in the implementation of the treatment plan.

TEAM CONCEPTS

Perhaps of all types of limb amputation, the arm amputee is least likely to work with an integrated system of rehabilitation that includes a traditional multidisciplinary team. Most frequently, the arm amputee interacts with a surgeon and a prosthetist, but seldom interacts with the larger group of rehabilitation team professionals. This lack of coordinated service provision may account for the reported low use rates and acceptance of upper extremity prostheses (about 50%).

In centers that deal with a large number of arm amputees each year, the preference continues to be a core multidisciplinary treatment team approach that includes a surgeon, a physiatrist, a rehabilitation nurse, a prosthetist, a psychologist, an occupational therapist, and a physical therapist. Some centers also include a recreational therapist, a case manager, and a vocational rehabilitation counselor. Most upper extremity amputee services are delivered on an outpatient basis unless other comorbid factors require an inpatient stay, such as bilateral arm loss, triple or quadruple amputations, or significant medical comorbidities.

Even when the rehabilitation program is provided on an outpatient basis, it is preferable to hold regular team conferences that include the amputee. These conferences, held with the amputee and family members, assist in measuring the treatment plan goals and also allow participants to modify the treatment plan as it progresses. This team meeting process provides the opportunity for team members to know what each member has implemented in the complicated process of amputation rehabilitation. These meetings also help to identify patient issues that may have been missed, and provides the opportunity to clarify issues between team members and the amputee, in particular. This is an excellent opportunity to incorporate a case manager, if one is assigned, into the treatment plan and its implementation. This type of meeting provides an opportunity to work through any points of disagreement or lack of clarity in the treatment plan.

ECONOMIC ISSUES

In today's health care environment, cost containment is a major focus. In rehabilitative care, the concept of teamwork has been fragmented because of this emphasis on cost. This seems to be especially true as we move from the days of inpatient rehabilitation stays and treatment to predominantly outpatient models. We have not transposed our excellent systems of inpatient comprehensive service and team cohesion to the outpatient mode. Most rehabilitation patients, and amputees in particular, find themselves lost in a maze of services, going from one professional office to the next, with little coordination of communication or recommendation among professionals. In addition, more therapy services are provided in the home, where little attention is paid to the professional skills offered by the in-home therapist. In addition, no direct supervision of the home health provider is undertaken by the prescribing physician.

CONCLUSIONS

For many reasons, it is essential for the arm amputee to receive his treatment in a center that has experience with arm amputation rehabilitation. Arm amputee rehabilitation is more than a visit to the amputating surgeon and the prosthetist and the delivery of a prosthesis.

Using a carefully chosen team of arm amputee rehabilitation professionals is most likely to ensure the appropriate functional outcomes in the shortest time following the amputation. Because so few new arm amputees occur in the United States each year, the disabling process of losing an arm and restoring function with a prosthesis is one that is best treated in a "center of excellence," where many arm amputees receive rehabilitation services through an experienced specialized treatment team.

References

1. Esquenazi A, Meier RH. Rehabilitation in limb deficiency. 4. Limb amputation. *Arch Phys Med Rehabil* 1996: 77:S 18–28.
2. Malone, JM, Childers SJ, Underwood, J et al. Immediate postsurgical management of upper extremity amputation. Conventional, electric and myoelectric prosthesis. *Orthot Prosthet* 1981: 35:1.
3. Meier RH. Upper limb prosthetics. In: Pemier C (ed), *Surgery of the Hand and Upper Extremity.* New York: McGraw-Hill, 1996. 2453–2468.
4. Meier RH. The physiatrist's role in patient empowerment. Proceedings of the 8th World Congress of the International Rehabilitation Medicine Association. Monduzzi Editore, 1997, 21–24.
5. Purtilo R, Meier RH. Regulatory constraints and patient empowerment. *Am J Phys Med Rehabil* 1993: (72) 327–330.

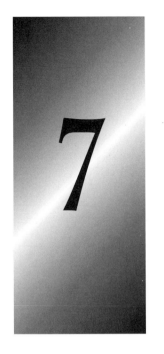

Self-Determination of the Person with an Upper Extremity Amputation

Mary P. Novotny, RN, MS

The concept of self-determination encompasses the right of an individual to make decisions without external constraints and the freedom to select from several options. The process of decision-making or selecting implies the existence of information and active participation in a judgment; this chapter addresses the self-determination movement and its related legislation, the literature and associated research, case histories, and professional guidelines.

Historically, consumer decisions in matters regarding limb loss were unheard of. Patients had little or no choice in health care issues or treatment, technology was extremely limited, and professionals were perceived as "experts." Today, individuals can exhibit self-determination in the manner in which they become informed about options, seek alternatives to traditional models, and advocate for involvement in care. Essentially, self-determination involves an individual confronting the crisis and actively participating in decision-making issues. Factors inherent in this process may be the individual's perception of himself as capable, access to information, knowledge of resources, an awareness of individual rights and responsibilities to aid in decision-making, a willingness to become a self-advocate, and a willingness to collaborate in goal setting and accept responsibility for outcomes.

In conjunction with the consumerist movement, self-determination has been gaining momentum in the United States over the past several decades. The Patient Self Determination Act (PSDA) of 1990, which went into effect December 1991, was federally legislated to empower the public with the right to make end of life decisions. This law applies to all health care facilities receiving any federal reimbursement for services, including hospitals, nursing homes, home health agencies and clinics (1). The PSDA requires institutions to establish mechanisms for the dissemination of information about advance directives and patient rights and to designate persons responsible for discussing these directives with patients and document the information in the patient record.

In 1995, the Americans with Disabilities Act (ADA) was passed by Congress. This broad legislation encompassed extensive regulations prohibiting discrimination against persons with a disability and enhancing access to public buildings, transportation systems, educational institutions, and agencies receiving federal funds.

Although patient's rights bills and accessibility guides are posted everywhere, evidence of national acceptance by providers to fully implement the intent of patient advocacy legislation is questionable (2). Several important issues affecting compliance include adequate funding to comply with laws and shifting paradigms from a medical model to a consumer model. The traditional medical model involves a superior (medical personnel) and an inferior (the consumer). The superior takes charge of the inferior and provides the care that the superior believes is needed. In the consumer model, health care professionals work under a contractual relationship in which the patient has autonomy, empowerment, and cooperative responsibility. This promotes reciprocal responsibility, with an onus on consumers to seek information, engage in extensive self-determination, and use available resources.

A further development in the patient advocacy movement is the establishment of new foundations, publications, and electronic bulletins to highlight progress and to provide a forum for networking. The self-determination movement has several goals:

- to empower people with physical differences to have more control over the goods and services provided;
- to build upon partnerships between patient consumers, families, service providers, advocates, and state and local governments;
- to lower the cost of current services; and
- to assist people and families who are awaiting services.

The self-determination movement was founded on four American principles: the freedom to exercise the same rights as all other citizens; the authority to control whatever sums of money are needed or designated for one's own support; access to the support and resources of organizations determined necessary by persons with disabilities and their allies; and the responsibility to carefully allocate public dollars for appropriate health-care needs (3).

RELATED LITERATURE AND STUDIES

Many theories exist about self-determination, motivation, and empowerment, including a vast array of books on the topic. Although volumes have been written about ways to achieve self-actualization, optimize performance, and become your own self-advocate, limited data supports most of this literature. Hence, it is a complex challenge to predict who will develop greatness or a precise formula for self-determination. To address this challenge and to establish professional guidelines, the author has identified several theories and case studies that have a relationship to self-determination, including the holistic model, adaptation theory, and body image theory. Hopefully, the concepts included support a rehabilitative model that can foster

independence and promote self-determination in persons experiencing limb loss.

Holistic Models

Whereas traditional Western thinking divides man into separate, essentially noninteracting domains of soma (body) and psyche (mind), newer theorists emphasize the mind–body connection in balancing physical and psychological factors.

Holism focuses on the whole person, with attention to the physical, psychologic, and social needs of each individual. The physical domain includes health and wellness, level of functioning, skill mastery, physical ability, and medical condition. The psychologic domain encompasses body image, self-esteem, emotional well-being, attitudes, and beliefs. The social domain includes family relationships, significant others, vocation, peer support, and available resources (including finances, community agencies, services, and technology). Taken together, the three domains comprise what some refer to as the "bio-psycho-social" aspects of man, which must be addressed in order to treat the whole person—a concept that has been described in medical, psychology, and nursing literature as well as other disciplines (4,5).

In 1977, Dr. Kenneth Pelletier wrote a book that brought together information about the mind–body connection. In *Mind as Healer, Mind as Slayer,* he presented a wide range of compelling evidence that the mind indeed was a major participant in illness and contributing factor in health as well (6). Later, Norman Cousins' book, *Anatomy of an Illness as Perceived by the Patient,* detailed his successful effort to overcome a degenerative collagen disease using, among other things, large doses of self prescribed laughter therapy (7). This shift demonstrates a progression away from traditional medical models, which focused mainly on the illness or presenting problem, to a more holistic patient-oriented focus considering the mind and body as parts of the process.

Adaptation Theory

In *Future Shock,* Toffler postulated that adaptation to change is based on the individual's need to develop and later discard a series of different core selves. Each crisis or change provides one with the opportunity to define the concept of self, learn new behaviors, and master new tasks (8). Evolving for decades as a prevailing perspective, this theory presents life as a balancing act of adaptation for survival amid the absolute certainty of change.

A correlate to this idea in nursing literature is Roy's Adaptation Theory, which views man as a bio-psycho-social being in constant interaction with an ever-changing environment. Depending on the situation, man adapts to changes in the environment within four basic modes, according to his physiologic needs, self-concept, role functions, and system of interdependence. Individuals have the capability to demonstrate an adaptive positive response to new situations when circumstances are within the realm of their personal "zone of experience." Maladaptive or negative responses generally occur when the situation is outside an individual's scope of highly individualized experience. Positive adaptation occurs when the individual can develop and integrate useful strategies for coping using effective behaviors (5).

Body Image Theory

Another theory closely linked to self-determination is the concept of body image, defined by Schilder as "that picture or scheme of our own body which we form in our minds as a tridimensional entity, having interpersonal, environmental, and temporal factors." He describes the development of body image as a continuous active process, constantly affected by physical, psychological, and social factors including:

- sensory experiences that begin in infancy and occur through multiple objective and subjective perceptions;
- internal psychological factors that arise from personal emotional experiences;
- social factors and feedback received via interactions with significant others, coupled with one's own interpretation of these interactions; and
- attitudes toward one's body from past experiences, perceptions, comparisons, and identifications with others.

Emphasizing the dynamics of body image development, Schilder notes that we constantly construct, dissolve, and reconstruct our body image and the body images of others. He contends that body image incorporates or spreads itself into space. Given the dynamic capacity to adapt to changes such as prosthetic devices, individuals are capable of integrating alterations over time. Thus, a firm object, rigid in its connection with the body, such as a prosthesis, cane, or crutch can be incorporated into one's body image (9).

Relative to body image, positive adaptation occurs when individuals incorporate physical changes into all aspects of life, achieve control and autonomy, set realistic goals, and generally improve the situation at hand.

Maladaptation is manifested when an individual continues to cling to a previous image or displays denial or a distorted self-concept. These individuals are often incapable of integrating changes and fail to adapt following an amputation or other significant change.

Additional threats to the body image occur throughout the lifespan because of continual changes, growth, and development. These threats include the physical and metabolic alterations associative with puberty, pregnancy, menopause, and aging. Less predictable external threats to body image occur when surgery is required, medical problems develop, or trauma is experienced. Based on this information, we can predict that an individual's response to limb loss depends on a myriad of factors including:

- individual meaning of amputation;
- developmental stage of amputee;
- cultural, ethnic, and spiritual orientation;
- communication style, ability to grieve, life experience, and coping style;
- availability and response of support system;
- presence or absence of concurrent medical problems and additional stressors;
- timely access to information and resources; and
- availability of competent, caring, health care team members.

PERSPECTIVES ON SELF-DETERMINATION

It can be gleaned from various theoretical frameworks and current literature that a number of factors play a significant role in the amputee's ability to participate in decision-making plans following limb loss. Because each person is complex, so too are the factors to be considered in any attempt at successful rehabilitation.

These factors include the amputee's ability to communicate feelings and successfully reformulate alterations in body image, the ability to identify supportive role models, access to experienced rehabilitation professionals who initiate early intervention, the ability to gain knowledge about options and resources for enhancing skill mastery, and the willingness to adapt positively to changes incurred by limb loss.

In each situation, the health care team must maintain a consumer-centered holistic focus that considers previous experiences, values family dynamics, self image, and adaptive resources. Rehabilitative efforts to replace a limb driven by professionals rather than the amputee are often doomed to failure.

"A man convinced against his will, is of the same opinion still."

Unknown

Early Intervention

There is no doubt that rehabilitation should be undertaken during the acute phase of loss and follow up should be immediate and comprehensive (10). Literature suggests that whether an individual receives rehabilitative services early is the most critical determinant of his ability to return to work. Many studies stress that effective rehabilitation should be initiated early, to decrease or eliminate the problems of immobility, long-term inactivity, and depression. Additional evidence supports the idea that early response to disability may include a period of heightened anxiety as the individual responds to new stressors.

In *The Sky is the Limit,* Wayne Dyer discusses five stages encompassing inertia, striving, coping, mastery, and finally self actualization. Using the health–illness continuum, he demonstrates how individuals move from maladaptive behavior or erratic fluctuations of mental illness through normalcy and finally achieve "no-limits" living or above-average self-actualization (11).

Studies also demonstrate that the prognosis for people experiencing a short acute stage of stress is more optimistic than for those who experience stress over longer periods. For this reason, it is very important to initiate early intervention, which facilitates positive responses, brings immediate success, diminishes depression, and sustains self-determination (12,13). This can be done by initiating early training and assessment for skills and vocational interests, and beginning a program of physical training, sports, or exercise. These activities have been associated with higher self-esteem and decreased levels of depression as well as a reduction in stress across all ages and both genders (14,15).

Meaningful Activities

Most literature reinforces the fact that fulfillment and a positive sense of identity come from awareness that one is becoming everything within one's capacity. Self-determination is a way of moving toward the realization of one's full potential. Viktor E. Frankl noted in *Man's Search for Meaning,* that to be truly happy, man needs a clear sense of direction. Worthy goals and ideas are based on the fact that one of man's deepest subconscious drives is to find meaning in life (16).

Numerous studies have emphasized that early return to work can have a positive effect on rehabilitation due to a variety of factors. Work can function as a source of identity, self-esteem, standing, or respect in the community. It can provide social support, companionship, and role fulfillment in the family. Essentially, work can provide structure, meaning, and purpose for life and enhance psychological well-being (17).

Additionally, early return to work helps people focus on adaptive activities thereby de-emphasizing the secondary gains of disability, which lower motivation and encourage the individual to settle into disability as a way of life (18).

Social Support System

The effect of families and significant others as they impact on the new amputee is also remarkable. One study showed a significant correlation between the social discomfort of amputees and depression (19). With young amputees, it is vitally important to focus efforts not only on the child, but also on the family. In almost every situation, the parent of a child with a limb deficiency feels a tremendous amount of guilt. All too frequently, attempting to recreate the dream of the perfect child has led to enforcing the constant use of prosthetics for their sometimes-unwilling children. Others spend huge amounts of time and resources to find a perfect technological solution, only to feel additional frustration as the child reaches adolescence and rejects the mechanical devices. Clearly, family history and environment directly impacts the child's response to stress and has been shown to correlate with anxiety, lowered self esteem, and depression in juveniles and adolescents (20).

Families can enhance or inhibit communication as well as in impede or facilitate adaptation to crises. A family can either promote social support or enhance isolation, thus serving in either a protective or problematic function. McCubbin and his colleagues indicated ten resiliency factors that enhanced recovery in the family setting including family hardiness, truthfulness, flexibility, problem solving, communication, the equality of spouses, spirituality, togetherness, social support, and over-all health (21). As evidenced here, promoting inclusion rather that exclusion of significant others is a real key to teamwork in rehabilitation of amputees.

Adaptive Options

As many possible outcomes for adaptation are possible as there are people with limb differences. Although one cannot always predict who will succeed and who will fail, a few predominant patterns arise, dependent on amputee needs, desires, and resources. Many arm amputees learn alternative approaches to performing the activities of daily living through therapy, ingenuity, and assistive devices, thereby adapting well to a satisfying life. Some ignore the absent limb and function single handedly. In these cases, the impairment created by the missing limb is coupled with a positive adaptive response and does not equal a disability.

Others seek the "perfect prosthetic replacement" for their missing limb, often a challenging search for both the patient and professionals due to the impossibility of replicating the complex functions of the hand with an aesthetically acceptable device. Still another group of amputees perceive themselves as truly "handicapped." They choose neither alternative resources nor available technology. Their impairment, coupled with a maladaptive response pattern of reliance on others and failure to reconstruct a new self image with appropriate goals and opportunities for full participation in life, creates a permanent physically and emotionally disabling condition that equates to a failure for the rehabilitation system.

In any situation, attention to the cosmetic desire of the consumer, as well as to functional needs, is a primary consideration. As with all developmental changes taking place in an individual's self-image, the need for a specific technology, training, prosthetic device, or components evolve with the individual's lifestyle. An important concept to understand is that a prosthesis is much like a tool or makeup kit. It can be used to enhance not only function, but also acceptance of one's self image, which is subject to change in a variety of situations. Conversely, a large number of upper limb amputees achieve very functional, satisfactory lifestyles aided only by ingenuity and minor environmental modifications, thus testifying to the fact that consumers are our greatest teachers.

EXAMPLES OF SELF-DETERMINATION

The use of examples often vividly demonstrates a concept. The following are highlights of several exemplary individuals who this author believes demonstrated unusual self-determination in their quest to adapt to upper extremity limb loss. Through studying their self-determination, we may derive some truths to apply to our efforts.

Success is almost always preceded by multiple attempts to find the right solution.
                                        Vince Lombardi

An accident that caused Bob Radocy to lose part of his left arm in 1971 initiated a series of events that demonstrate how the power of self-determination in one individual led to the revolution of an industry. Incorporating his desire for function and participation in sports and recreation with an interest in engineering motivated him to develop an entire line of new terminal devices. In addition, his success expanded the expectations about the functional abilities of upper extremity amputees everywhere.

Once Bob's initial depression after losing his arm turned to determination, he began to focus on how he could overcome the impairment and accomplish all the activities he had performed before his accident. Initially he was comforted by a surgeon who told him "Don't worry about that, they've got everything you need." After being fitted with a standard split hook, Bob soon realized that he was more disabled by technology than by his missing hand. Unable to function at his normal work and everyday activities (not to mention the wide variety of sports and recreation interests that he liked), Bob realized that the first prosthetic device he had not only didn't match his life style, it didn't even match his naturally sun-tanned skin tone. With tremendous optimism and great expectations for his new prosthesis, Bob acknowledged later that the surgeon's attempts to reassure him delayed him at least 5 years before he could finally focus realistically on designing an adequate prosthesis to meet his needs.

Bob's self-determination was assisted by his engineering knowledge, experience as a recreational therapist, and his desire for a device that would be more than a passive partner to his healthy right hand, allowing him to participate in a variety of sports and other favorite activities. As an environmental field engineer he wanted to actively use his arm muscles to be able to grip ladders and other items without fear of falling. He also wanted a tool with an opposing thumb.

Using information gained from his studies of biology, engineering, and drafting, Bob combined his ideas into a rough sketch of the kind of prosthesis he hoped would enable him to resume his normal activities. His goal was a device that would allow wearers an opportunity to compete and participate in sports without worrying about injury to self or others. In his final year as a graduate student, his idea materialized into a terminal device with a three-point grip utilizing a metallic imitation thumb, index, and middle fingers. The grip allowed him to hold small things like safety pins, as well as larger items like a hammer or a board. Mechanically, it operated like the brake on a bicycle; the harder he pulled on the harness the greater the closing force.

Because similar designs had failed in the past, many professionals were not excited about Bob's first ideas. In retrospect, he believed that an industry-wide bias existed against voluntary closing devices because of these failures. They were not widely prescribed or disseminated, and most patients were not appropriately instructed in how to use them.

Slow response to the ideas he presented did not lessen Bob's determination. He continued using his knowledge gained as an amputee to work on his concept. Bob's original idea was to use the device personally. He had not planned to begin producing prosthetic devices. It was only after 3 years of utilizing his first GRIP that he realized he really had discovered something that could be generally applicable for other amputees. Finally, in 1979, Bob forged a partnership with a former professor, creating his own company, known as Therapeutic Recreation Systems (TRS).

Since Bob's design of the original GRIP, his determination to improve function has evolved into a wide variety of terminal devices for upper extremity amputees. First were the Super Sports, anatomically proportioned with a cupped hand and constructed of an unbreakable flexible polymer material to act as a shock absorber. Super Sports are intended to enable the active participation of upper extremity amputees in a wide variety of recreational and athletic activities where player contact and collision could occur including basketball, soccer, football, volleyball, skating, jogging, aerobics, dance, and martial arts.

Later, ADEPT prehensors emerged as a series of child-sized voluntary closing (VC) devices that provide a strong prosthetic grip. ADEPTs allowed young amputees to be more competitive and active participants in activities such as swinging, jogging, bicycle riding, climbing, baseball, and dressing. Today, TRS produces a variety of terminal devices that afford the upper extremity amputee a wide variety of options for increasing participation, including a golf grip, a high-fly fielder, a freestyle swimming device, an AMP-u-POD for photography, bicycle brake levers, skiing devices, a hockey adaptor, and even the Hustler TD for playing pool and billiards. Each of these tools can maximize an amputee's function in adaptation to limb loss (22).

Bob Radocy's self-determination also proved to be an exemplary model for other amputees. As a businessman, salesman, and advocate for consumers, he travels around the country marketing his devices and speaking to other amputees. Bob's goals have as much to do with education as sales. He perceives amputees as customers and urges them to shop around for the best designs, prices, and quality care from physicians and prosthetists. Bob recognizes that assertive, well-educated amputees are placing an increased demand on professionals for improved prosthetic designs, a trend that he believes will continue (23).

Bob's informative style of teaching makes him an effective peer counselor who can actively demonstrate not only the importance of self-advocacy but also positive adaptation after losing an arm. He stresses the importance of maintaining physical condition as well as the collaboration required with professionals to supplement good prosthetic usage. In numerous presentations and articles, he emphasizes the need for a team effort between patients, therapists, physicians, and other rehabilitation professionals as a prerequisite for amputee success in sports and recreation. With appropriate technology, a proper design and comfortable socket, and appropriate suspension, components, exercise, and conditioning, Bob believes amputees can excel in most sports without injury to themselves or others (24).

Clearly, Bob's determination to succeed at his quest for a better replacement for his hand revolutionized not just prosthetic design but, more important, the philosophy and ideology about function and quality of life for upper extremity amputees everywhere.

If a man advances confidently in the direction of his dreams and endeavors to live the life he has imagined, he will meet with success unexpected in common hours.

Henry David Thoreau

In remarkably different circumstances, the story of Harold Wilke, born in 1914 of German immigrant parents in a farm home nestled in the hills near Washington, Missouri, is a miraculous story of self-determination. The success of his life, despite the complete absence of both arms, documents the value of supportive family, deeply ingrained core values, faith, and a persistent zeal to accomplish his goals.

In his book, *Using Everything You've Got*, Harold unashamedly describes himself as a missionary for independence and a perpetual seeker of how old materials and patterns can be used in new ways. His premise in writing a book was not to produce a how-to guide but to share ideas on utilizing resources. Harold tells readers to "think new" and "to try over and over again." At a time when no role models were available, Harold was forced to learn independence one step at a time.

> I was two or three years old, sitting on the bedroom floor of our home, having an extraordinarily difficult time getting a shirt over my head and around my shoulders. I grunt against sweat, while my mother just stood there and watched. Her arms must have remained riveted to her side even though every instinct in her wants to reach out and do it for me. Finally, a neighbor friend turned to her in exasperation said, "Ida why don't you help that child?" My mother responded through gritted teeth, "I am helping him!"
>
> Her pain in withholding help was actually a granting of help, an assurance that even though the pain and sweat level was high in the short run, it would be reduced to the long run ... expressing for me most graphically her own feeling that I must learn by myself. She helped me by not helping me (25).

As each opportunity presented itself in everyday living Harold, guided by his parents, was forced to confront the challenges of having no hands. Persistence paid off as he tried a variety of ideas to encorporate independence in dressing and other activities of daily living. When he needed increased functionality for foot use because freedom of his toes was essential, he began using Japanese tabi socks, with a separated toe. Harold also adapted loafer-style shoes for daily wear so that he can easily slip in and out of them to use his feet.

His ideas for travel include such things as placing his tickets and correct change in a pocket nearby so that he does not have difficulty in retrieving a wallet with his feet while standing in line at a bus or subway stop. Carrying wood to the fireplace, Harold is aided by a "log carrier," which is a piece of canvas with handles at each end. He inserts a wooden hook up into the handles and secures it to a 5-foot long strap on his shoulder.

Although handling children could pose difficulties for any parent, Harold handled it with little difficulty by placing his children on a blanket grasped between his chin and shoulder, which he pulled from room to room. In hindsight he confessed, if this had been a regular activity, he would have developed a roller cart or table with casters and high sides for added efficiency and safety (26).

Harold's adaptive activities go far beyond daily work to sports and hobbies. He describes his full participation in swimming, moderate mountain climbing, croquet, photography, and shooting. For those who are wondering, he accomplished this with the gun butt against his shoulder in a regular position, right foot soundly on the ground, while his left foot holds and balances the rifle using his second toe as a trigger finger.

Perhaps one of the most pivotal lessons of self-determination learned from Harold Wilke is that opportunities and decisions to adapt positively or negatively occur repeatedly throughout our lives. He sees *cope* as a four-letter word along with, love, pray, work, and play. Each are tools to use in the face of disability, problems, anxiety, or other trouble, to find strength deep inside and develop new ways of fulfilling tasks when old ways have been closed.

In one of his writings, Harold Wilke eloquently contrasts Shakespeare's King Richard III and his own life. Drawing parallels between two individuals with physical differences, he clearly demonstrates the role of faith and religion in his perspective on life.

The opening words of Shakespeare's Tragedy of King Richard III, "Now is the winter of our discontent..." are followed by Richard's self introduction "I, that am rudely stamped ... deformed, unfinished, sent before my time, into this breathing world, scarce half made up, and so lamely and unfashionable that dogs bark at me as I halt by them." His statement of being emphasizes his birth deformity, not that he was born a Duke of Gloucester, a brother to the King. Rather related to being "cheated of feature" unable even "to court in amorous looking glass" or "struck before an ambling wanton nymph." Later his negative response to being, "I am determined to prove villain," does indeed become reality.

In contrast to Richard III, Harold (perhaps even more "unfinished" since he had no hands at all) believed he was much more fortunate. As a faithful Christian, he saw himself a child of God, even without the royal trappings of dukedom and palace. He perceived his parents were king and queen of their home, which was his palace. He had no need to rail against fate and defy others more pleasing than himself because he did not feel cheated! Wilkes's central core of faith and spiritual home made him feel accepted, beloved, and deeply wanted regardless of any physical differences (27).

You have to act to actualize.

Guy Falkes

Another remarkable case of a guitar teacher who returned to his original career after the subtotal and total finger amputation of his left hand emphasizes that the motivation a person brings with him to rehabilitation can also be a key deciding factor in overall outcome. With consistent exercise on his instrument, he used his partial hand for gripping chords, thus compensating for the loss of his digits. He even won a lawsuit against his employer, who claimed the teacher lacked the ability to continue playing classical guitar. This success clearly demonstrates the joint responsibility and tremendous potential of both the amputee and rehabilitation team in determining goals as well as collaborating on a program to achieve them (28).

IMPLICATIONS FOR PROFESSIONAL PRACTICE

Recognize Keys to Success

As rehabilitation professionals, it is important to identify the key factors that affect outcomes and to create environments that promote meaningful, quality lives, facilitate self-determination, and encourage the freedom to take an active role in decision making for the individual with an amputation. If years of experience have taught us anything about upper extremity limb loss, it is that a hand is a complex appendage, carrying great emotional value and providing complex functions that are difficult to replicate.

Body image theory demonstrates that we are not merely replacing an appendage. We are rebuilding a life. Reconstructing that life and new self-image cannot be accomplished in a clinical laboratory without design input from the main character. Any artificial replacement for a hand will be accepted only if it meets the amputee's personal criteria for comfort, cosmesis, and function in everyday life. Facilitating the acceptance of the limb difference and an involvement in the decision making process is a task requiring a thorough knowledge of the patient's levels of coping, his psychosocial perspectives, and his life goals.

Goal setting must be consistent with the patient's ability to cope with and adapt to new situations. Communication, self-determination, and empowerment cannot be forced. If deficiencies or maladaptive behaviors are evident, focus on the patient's priorities and seek his counsel in setting reasonable goals.

To optimize opportunities for success, professionals must assess and communicate information on an individual's physiology and function, psychological issues, and self-image as well as technical requirements to address all needs for care, education, and support. These are key to amputee adaptation, self-determination, and a successful outcome following the loss of an upper extremity. Without the coordination of these issues, even the best systems can fall short, as evidenced by the following case history.

If you think you can't, you are correct.

Anonymous

This case involves a 46-year-old father of three teenagers who underwent a forequarter amputation to remove a malignancy. He was blue-collar worker with a family from a middle-class black neighborhood. Six weeks postoperatively, he appeared for outpatient follow up in a serious state of depression and anger. Expressing complete disgust with his altered self-image, he stated that no one had prepared him for this high-level amputation. He was disturbed that he couldn't even get a shirt to hang properly. He felt his wife should not bother talking to "half a man" and thought his children had no respect for him because he wasn't able to maintain his provider and father role. While no objective evidence existed that his family was unwilling to be supportive, he had apparently alienated himself from them in anticipation of their rejection. The lack of a complete preoperative team conference, including both the patient and his family, left a serious gap in understanding, knowledge, and acceptance of the amputation. It also led to a void in anticipatory planning postoperatively.

Lacking peer support, he had no knowledge of prosthetic options, or that a temporary device could have been made available for cosmetic purposes prior to his hospital discharge. Justifiably, he felt isolated, angry, and confused. Surgery may have eradicated his malignancy, but his perception of the quality of his existence diminished any desire to continue living.

The clinic team assessed the problems as a combination of inadequate communication and information sharing between professionals, patient, and family; loss of self-esteem; lack of pre- and postoperative care coordination; and a failure to use resources, particularly peer support. Although surgery was successful, the absence of preoperative preparation, peer support, and an assessment of psychosocial needs delayed this patient's overall rehabilitation. Had he not vented his feelings loudly, the team may have never been aware of his severe depression and maladaptive response (29).

This situation emphasizes the need to assess the amputee information base, support system, and resources to adapt to the loss. Lacking experience or information about amputation and rehabilitation, the new amputee faces a tremendous challenge and may be overwhelmed when confronted with decisions. Lacking education, peer support, and a knowledge of the resources or available options, the development of adaptive behavior, self-determination, and realistic goal setting is unlikely to occur.

Practice Holistic Consumer-Oriented Teamwork

Professionals who embrace a holistic, patient-centered approach generally complement each other's abilities to achieve desired outcomes for their patients through:

- Enhancement of physical functioning and the promotion of wellness, mastery, and coping mechanisms
- Acknowledgment of the mind–body connection, particularly the development of adaptive responses
- Facilitation of social networks through peer referral, utilization of community resources, educational programs, and family involvement

In some cases, ancillary skills can also be developed to assist in adaptation if these aren't already present. These include relaxation techniques, new physical abilities, and improved communication skills. Additionally, some individuals' recovery may be complicated by significant premorbid psychologic and emotional problems that may require counseling or skills training before real progress can be made with rehabilitation (30).

Divided into achievable tasks, these are not impossible challenges if one considers the great opportunity for success. The economic value of teamwork and a holistic consumer-centered approach—versus the loss of time, money, and resources to move an individual through rehabilitation training and prosthetic fitting, only to have the device discarded on a shelf or in a closet—is unquestionable. By addressing the entire spectrum of amputee needs as a team, professionals have a much greater chance to facilitate positive adaptation, maximize function, and promote self-determination, which results in improved outcomes for all involved.

Enhance Support Systems and Resources

Providing a role model who has made a successful adjustment to limb loss is one of the most essential ingredients to facilitating self-determination. Well-adjusted peers can assist the new amputee in seeking information, identifying what is a normal response to limb loss, decreasing feelings of isolation, facilitating adaptation, and learning appropriate assertive and self-advocacy skills.

A corollary to this is promoting the active involvement of family and significant others throughout each phase of rehabilitation. Families are the primary point of reference in adapting to life experiences. It is essential to assess the family's abilities to increase motivation, enhance communication, and support independence and self-determination. Without these abilities, family members can become protective and overly helpful, thus promoting disability rather than encouraging the independence of the amputee.

If family or significant others are unavailable or unwilling to become involved, locate a surrogate support system. Volunteers and community agencies are rich resources dedicated to working with rehabilitation patients. They are natural bridges back to mainstream activities, effective complements to the efforts of professionals, and economical resources for patients and families.

Set Timely Achievable Goals

One of the greatest obstacles in rehabilitation is overcoming inertia and avoiding unnecessary delays in treatment. The longer an individual remains immobile, the greater the effort required to regain movement, energy, and motivation. Taking advantage of the initial reactions to stress and momentary disequilibrium, which occurs within the first several weeks after injury, can focus the amputee on change and learning new activities, and retraining skills. Assess the amputee's level of ability, and what she values and hopes to achieve. Maximize every opportunity for participation, always keeping the patient at the center of the team.

Identify goals that have meaning and are achievable within a reasonable time to increase success and promote positive adaptation. Be flexible regarding plans and options as situations change, remaining open to new learning situations from experienced teachers—particularly other amputees. Goals are integral to increase skill mastery, build confidence, and enhance self-determination. Finally, maintain a positive attitude regarding the possibilities, rather than the parameters, of what you as a professional anticipate can or cannot be done. Too often, lowered expectations lead to minimal achievement. Meeting challenges is inherent in self-determination and paramount to success.

Maintain Team Communication and Follow-up

As evidenced by the case described earlier, persistence in overcoming adversity through joint problem solving with the patient and family is a primary role of the health care professional. We cannot rehabilitate any amputee in isolation or by focusing only on the missing extremity. Psychologic issues require communication, affirmation, and the dissolution of previous self-image in order to adapt to change and identify new goals. Ignorance and preconceived ideas generally require information sharing.

Achieving an acceptable functional level for the new amputee demands a combination of medical input, prosthetic expertise, and follow-up training. Acknowledging prior experiences and expectations can help the patient move on to acquire needed skills and utilize available resources.

The ability to demonstrate self-determination may vary from time to time. Optimistic professionals can provide invaluable assistance in facilitating positive moves toward an amputee's optimal rehabilitation when they work together. Sustaining this quality requires ongoing reinforcement by peers, family members, and society.

CONCLUSIONS

Self-determination is a complex experience, affected by a unique set of forces acting on an individual at a given time to respond to a change or crisis. Confronted with profound challenges, survival necessitates a response, which can be adaptive or maladaptive. Where we stand in life can indicate how, or if, we mobilize these forces and subsequently, what the outcome will be.

Adaptive response to a crisis, loss, or change allows one to see beyond crisis and assimilate it into the big picture of life experience. Whether we rail against difficulties, anxiety, pain, and loss or not implies a decision. Immobility, denial, and flight are also decisions that generally delay or preclude a positive outcome. Inherent in self-determination is a willingness to face a crisis and take responsibility for directing our future outcomes. Individuals can choose to seek alternatives; withhold response; or become submissive, assertive, attacking, understanding, or accepting, or a combination of these.

In every situation, health care providers have a responsibility to be knowledgeable about the forces affecting an individual at any given time and to proactively cooperate in facilitating the amputee's involvement in developing and achieving goals that have meaning. Self-determination is fueled by challenge, fostered by supportive, significant others, or extinguished by provincial paradigms of professional control. Successful outcomes are truly a team endeavor.

ADDITIONAL RESOURCES

The Center for Patient Advocacy
1350 Beverly Road # 108
McLean VA 22102
(800) 846-7444
www:patientadvocacy.org
National Program Office on Self Determination
Self Determination Bulletin
npnd@cs.net (University of New Hampshire)
www.self-determination.org,
National Limb Loss Information Center
900 East Hill Avenue Suite 285
Knoxville TN 37915
(888) AMP-KNOW
www:amputee-coalition.org

References

1. Federal Patient Self Determination Act (PSDA) of 1991.
2. Crego PJ. When, how and why of advance directives: tools for the cardiovascular nurse. *Prog Cardiovasc Nurs* Summer 1999; 14:3 92–96.
3. Self Determination Foundation. We hear the words, but what does it mean? *Self-Determination Bull* 1999; 1: July.
4. Romano MD. Psychosocial diagnoses and social work services. In: Kottke FJ, Lehman JF (eds), *Krusen's Handbook of Physical Medicine and Rehabilitation Second Edition.* Philadelphia: WB Saunders, 1990.
5. Roy C. *Introduction to Nursing: An Adaptation Model.* Englewood Cliffs, New Jersey: Prentice-Hall, 1976.
6. Pellitier K. *Mind as Healer, Mind as Slayer.* New York: Delta/Lawrence, 1977.
7. Cousins N. *Anatomy of an Illness as Perceived by the Patient.* New York: Norton, 1979.
8. Toffler A. *Future Shock.* New York: Bantam, 1970.
9. Schilder P. *The Image in Appearance of the Human Body.* New York: International University Press, 1950.
10. Smith D. Implementing disability management: a review of basic concepts and essential components. *Employee Assistance Quarterly* 1997; 12:4, 37–50.
11. Dyer W. *The Sky is the Limit.* New York: Simon & Schuster, 1981.
12. Boschen KA. Early intervention and vocational rehabilitation. *Rehabilitation Counseling Bulletin* 1989; 32:255–265.
13. Young MA. Crisis intervention in the aftermath of disaster. In: Roberts AR (ed), *Contemporary Perspectives on Crises Intervention and Prevention.* Englewood Cliffs, New Jersey: Prentice-Hall, 1991, 83–103.
14. International Society of Sport Psychology. Physical activity and psychological benefits: a position statement from the International Society of Sport Psychology. *J Applied Sport Psychology* 1992; 4:1, 94–98.
15. McAuley E. Physical activity and psychosocial outcomes. In: Bouchard C, Shepard RJ, Stephens T (eds), *Physical Activity Fitness and Health: International Proceedings and Concensus Statement.* Champaign Ill.: Human Kinetics Publishers, 1994, 551–568.
16. Frankl VE. *Man's Search for Meaning.* Beacon Press, 1988.
17. Quick JC, Murphy AR, Hurrell JJ, Orman D. The value of work, the risk of distress, and the power of prevention. In: JC Quick et al, *Stress and Being Well at Work.* Washington D.C.: American Psychological Association 1992, 3–13.
18. Boschen KA. Early intervention and vocational rehabilitation. *Rehabilitation Counseling Bulletin* 1989; 32:255–265.
19. Varni JW, Rubenfeld LA, Talbot D, Setogucci Y. Stress, social support and depressive symptomatology in children with congenital/acquired limb deficiencies. *J Pediatric Psychology* 1989; 14:4, 515–530.
20. Rybarzek BD et al. Social discomfort and depression in a sampling of adults with leg amputations. *Arch Physical Med Rehabil* Dec 1992: 73:12, 1169–1173.
21. McCubbin HI, McCubbin MA, Thompson AI, Han SY, Allen CT. Families under stress: what makes them resilient? *J Family Consumer Sciences* Fall 1997; 2(11).
22. Therapeutic Recreation Systems (TRS) product information.
23. Swartz M. *Esquire Register* 1984, 94–97.
24. Radocy B. Upper extremity prosthetics: considerations and designs for sports and recreation. *Clin Prosthetics Orthotics* 1989; 2:3, 131–153.
25. Wilke HE. *Reflections on Managing Disability.* Harold H. Wilke, 1984.
26. Wilke HE. *Using Everything You've Got.* Harold H. Wilke 1977, 1984; reprinted Amputee Coalition of America, 1998.
27. Wilke HE. *The Healing Congregation Newsletter,* used with permission of author.
28. Neuber M, Joist A, Probst A. Klinik und Poliklinik fur Unfall und Handchirurgie, Westfalischen Wilhelms-Universitat Munster. *Chirurg* 1998 May; 69:5, 581–584.
29. Novotny MP. Psychosocial issues affecting rehabilitation. *Phys Med Rehabilitation Clin N Am* May 1991 2:2, 373–393.

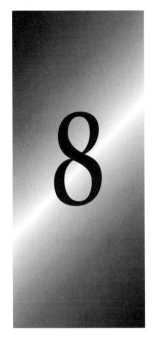

Integrating Psychological and Medical Care: Practice Recommendations for Amputation

Brent Van Dorsten, PhD

Traumatic physical injury and chronic illness have long been anecdotally recognized as precipitants of inevitable degeneration in emotional functioning. However, until recently, little empirical attention has been devoted to clarifying the emotional consequences of traumatic physical injury. In fact, less than 20 years ago, Kleiber et al. (1) reported the astonishing finding that a literature review of nearly 100,000 "trauma" references produced only two that specifically addressed the psychosocial sequelae associated with the events. Over the past decade, published articles have identified various emotional features that may complicate recovery from motor-vehicle accident injuries (2–5), burns (6), myocardial infarction (7,8), and traumatic hand injuries (9,10). Several authors have examined the specific emotional challenges following medical trauma and limb loss (11–13). Multidisciplinary care systems have accentuated the need to recognize amputation as both a significant physical and emotional event, and some have recommended the provision of psychological services beyond the acute postsurgical period (14,15). This chapter recognizes the advances in medical treatment over the past two decades that have decreased mortality and increased the number of individuals who survive limb loss to confront changes in physical appearance, lifestyle activities, life goals, and self-esteem. Unfortunately, few innovations have been developed to guide the psychosocial management of the person with limb loss. Shalev, Shreiber, and Galai (16) suggest that whereas medical approaches to traumatic injury have evolved into a pseudostandardized format, psychosocial interventions have lagged in the clear identification of treatment goals and standardized management approaches. A comprehensive review of the current literature failed to identify specific published recommendations regarding the integration of psychological and medical evaluation and treatment efforts for those who have lost limbs. Further, no treatment pathways have been published to specify a format for the provision of psychosocial services following traumatic physical injury or the loss of a limb. This chapter offers guideline recommendations for comprehensive psychosocial management for people with amputation. While necessarily limited in scope, these recommendations will address the unique interplay of emotional and medical factors encountered during multidisciplinary rehabilitative management for those with limb loss.

As contrasted with congenital limb deficiency, traumatic loss of limb and surgical amputation are considered "acquired amputation." Although a minority of upper extremity amputations are attributable to tumor or disease complication, accidents constitute the predominate etiologic factor (17). Healthy, young adult males sustain the greatest number of upper extremity amputations, typically related either to work injuries or motor vehicle events (18). Consequently, the following guidelines address both the medical sequelae of the injury and the heterogeneity of emotional responses following a traumatic medical injury. Clinical experience with traumatic limb loss formulates the basis of the following recommendations. However, these strategies may be readily adapted for use with other traumatically injured patient populations. Since few randomized clinical studies have been completed with limb loss populations, many of the following recommendations have been adapted from research conducted with comparable patient populations and await the scrutiny of further study on their direct applicability with amputation.

PSYCHOSOCIAL EVALUATION AND TREATMENT GOALS

The goals for psychologic evaluation and treatment are necessarily consonant with those developed by other members of the rehabilitation team; these include the stabilization of acute emotional symptoms and enlisting patient and family participation with treatment efforts. Psychosocial goals should include specific evaluation, treatment, and relapse prevention components, and must be developed via collaboration with the patient, family members, health care providers, and community resources throughout the rehabilitative process.

Psychologic assessment goals following limb loss include the identification of acute emotional responses to maintain the patient's active participation with the necessary acute medical treatments. This is not to imply that all potential emotional obstacles will be present in the immediate post-injury interval, but to emphasize the importance of thoroughly assessing the patient and family's initial response to limb loss. This initial evaluation data provides a post-injury baseline measure of functioning and allows for the implementation of emotional "triage" strategies. A thorough initial evaluation allows the rehabilitation team to identify and minimize the impact of emotional issues on acute medical care and to promote initial reintegration of family, recreational, or avocational interests. Other evaluation goals include clarifying the patient's past emotional history, pre-morbid coping repertoire, personal strengths and characteristics, initial misconceptions regarding his condition, and incidences of previous trauma.

Given the heterogeneity of emotional responses to trauma and limb loss, psychologic treatment goals may be multiple and include the development of adaptive cognitive and behavioral coping strategies, behavioral pain management, emotional exploration, structuring of consistent patient participation with medication and therapy efforts, managing acute changes in sleep or appetite, managing lethargy or apathy, instructing relaxation strategies to manage aversive physiologic sensations, and facilitating effective communication with treating professionals and social supports. Treatment efforts should naturally include family members and other available care providers to address their emotional issues throughout the recovery process.

Finally, relapse prevention goals should encapsulate rehearsing problem solving strategies to manage long-term emotional vacillations, and identifying and preparing for "high-risk" situations that might reasonably precipitate emotional degeneration. Training in appropriate assertiveness skills should allow the patient to effectively enlist assistance when needed.

COMMON EMOTIONAL CONCERNS FOLLOWING LIMB LOSS

A variety of emotional issues associated with limb loss are identified in the medical and psychologic literature. Most anecdotal writings propose severe emotional compromise and limited long-term adjustment as either modal or "expected" following amputation. In fact, although some may struggle indefinitely in their attempts to adapt to the challenges of limb loss, most individuals make timely psychologic adjustments and resume at least a modified level of premorbid functioning. Although an exhaustive review of potential emotional challenges is well beyond the scope of this chapter, brief discussion of some common concerns is warranted.

Phantom and Residual Limb Pain

Pain is an obvious frequent experience following traumatic physical injury and poses a considerable threat to long-term emotional functioning, independent of other factors associated with recovery. The substantial chronic pain literature suggests a variety of emotional struggles associated with intractable pain. In the case of amputation, the presence of residual limb or phantom pain may provide a constant stimulus for the intrusive recall of events associated with loss of one's limb. Given a historical psychiatric implication associated with the experience of phantom pain, previously published prevalence estimates are highly variable, ranging from 5 to 85% of cases (19–21). Historically, patients have been understandably reluctant to acknowledge phantom pain or sensation, and without specific training, have been unsophisticated in differentiating phantom pain, phantom sensation, and residual limb pain. Previous studies have failed to support the hypothesis of phantom pain as purely a psychologic event, rather implicating psychophysiologic mechanisms in the production of these symptoms (22). Consistent with the existing pain literature, it is accepted that phantom pain sensations may be adversely affected by any of a variety of cognitive and behavioral stimuli (21). However, treating providers should avoid conceptualizing persistent phantom pain complaints as being solely psychologic in nature. Previous authors (23,24) have reported the incidence of acute postoperative phantom pain to be over 70%, with only a minimal 5% decrease observed at 6 months. Jensen et al. (23) reported phantom sensation in nearly 85% of cases in the acute postsurgical phase, with an *increase* to over 90% 6 months after amputation. In one study, the acute incidence of phantom pain in upper extremity amputation was found to be over 80%, compared with a 54% incidence in lower extremity amputation cases (25). Several recent reports suggest little to no impact of phantom pain on prosthetic use (17,26–28). However, aside from prosthetic use, chronic phantom limb pain has been shown to pose a significant obstacle to the recovery of premorbid vocational and avocational activities. For example, Sherman and Arena (29) reported that patients with phantom pain frequently acknowledged pain-related limitations in their ability to work and participate in social activities, sleep difficulties, and problems in completing activities of daily living.

Residual limb discomfort, or "stump pain" as it is unfortunately known, poses a particular concern given the potential interference with preprosthetic exercise and graded prosthesis use—threatening delays in the acquisition of rehabilitation goals. Jensen, Kregs, Neilsen, and Rasmussen (30) report that 22% of 58 amputees experienced marked residual limb pain at 6 months post amputation, with a decrease to approximately 10% at 2 years. In contrast, in a valuable recent study, Kooijman et al. (17) conducted a thorough assessment of 99 people with upper extremity amputation an average of 19 years post limb loss. Fifty-one percent of those surveyed indicated experiencing daily phantom pain, with a 76% prevalence of phantom sensation, and 49% prevalence of residual limb pain. This study suggested that nearly all phantom pain sufferers (36 of 37) also reported experiencing phantom sensation (i.e., cold, "electrical" sensations, and "movement" of the phantom limb). Further, the relative risk of having phantom pain was twice as high in those with residual limb pain as compared to those without. Residual limb pain must be closely assessed and managed via medication, injection, or surgical revision if necessary to allow the individual to comfortably resume progress towards prosthesis mastery.

The necessity for adequate pain management is apparent in all stages of limb loss rehabilitation, including presurgery, if possible. It has been proposed that the risk for phantom pain is greater in cases where severe presurgical pain is present (31). However, available data suggests that this relationship may only hold true for the immediate postoperative period and does not support presurgical pain as predictive of long-lasting phantom pain (30,32). Following a review of multiple pain management strategies, Katz (33) concluded that epidural anesthesia started before, and continuing during and after the amputation, may offer the best buffer against the development of phantom pain. Accordingly, successful acute postsurgical pain management might diminish the likelihood of chronic pain for patients with limb loss (20). Although it is often proposed that phantom pain will gradually diminish over time, available empirical data fail to support this contention (17,28,34). In a review of nearly 70 phantom pain treatments, few were found to be even modestly successful for a minimal number of phantom pain sufferers (35,36). Opioid management of phantom limb pain has shown to be quite controversial regarding demonstrated efficacy. A number of authors have reported medication efficacy in approximately 50% of patients without a clear consensus as to the most desirable agents for specific subgroups of patients (37–40). More recently, Huse, Larbig, Flor, and Birbaumer (41) reported a "clinically relevant" response (i.e., more than 50% pain reduction) in five of twelve patients with phantom limb pain taking oral retarding morphine sulfate. Unfortunately, this study also suggests that 50% of the participants received less than a 25% reduction in pain using this same medication. Consequently, considerably more work appears indicated to clarify the efficacy of opioid agents in the battle against phantom limb pain. In the Kooijman study (17), 64% of the participants reported suffering from daily pain "moderately" to "very much," yet less than 5% were receiving any treatment for discomfort. The authors hypothesize that the absence of active pain treatment was likely attributable to the apathetic belief of both patients and physicians that medical treatment is inherently ineffective for phantom pain. Considering the apparently limited medical arsenal available to effectively control phantom pain, all efforts should be expended in the preoperative and immediate postoperative environments to reduce the likelihood of phantom pain development.

Depression

As is evidenced by a massive existing literature, depression has long been identified as a significant barrier to recovery from illness or injury. Underdiagnosis, or delay in diagnosis and treatment of neurovegetative symptoms (e.g., sleep, appetite, and lethargy), frequently occurs, given the similarity to the behavioral sequelae of pain and exertional fatigue. Despite the considerable depression literature involving other medical populations, comparatively little attention has been directed to the standardized assessment of depression following amputation. Available data suggests that people with amputation experience considerable levels of depression, with published estimates ranging from 21 to 35% (42–46). In other patient populations, elevated levels of depression have been associated with impaired rehabilitation and social adjustment (47), increased medical utilization (48), and relapse (49). Following limb loss, an ongoing evaluation of the impact of financial, parental, marital, sexual, vocational, and personal issues on depression and suicidal ideation status must occur. Threats to personal integrity and efficiency, including the loss of functional independence, altered life goals, and loss of the spontaneous ability to perform activities are all significant factors encountered by this patient population. Serial, multimodal efforts at depression detection should be incorporated into standard protocol when working with a traumatically injured population. Certainly, some initial depressive response is common and not considered pathologic in the acute stages of recovery. These acute episodes are typically alleviated with education, support, and actively involving the patient in a comprehensive rehabilitative goal setting. A restoration of the locus of control and enhancement of body function—with or without prosthetic restoration—is usually effective in reducing initial depressive symptoms. If depressive features become sufficiently pervasive to interfere with treatment participation, rehabilitation efforts may necessarily need to be pared until intensive intervention allows the patient to resume active participation.

Anxiety

According to Grunert and colleagues (9), generalized anxiety may be present in as many as 50% of traumatic hand/arm injury cases in the acute phase following surgery. Anxiety is considered a reasonable response for any individual facing the most unique challenge of their life, and which for most there is ultimately no preparatory event. Anxiety is commonly reported by amputation patients in response to fears of uncontrolled disease progression, potential revision surgeries, prosthesis failure, or anticipated severe pain. Further, a variety of interpersonal anxieties may exist related to uncertainty of one's personal ability to cope with the multitude of challenges thrust forth after amputation, or to anticipating family embarrassment at one's altered body appearance. Learning the phases and goals of the rehabilitation process may actually delay progress unless these issues are thoroughly reviewed by treating professionals with

clarification of each party's responsibilities, reasonable timeframes, and specific outcome measures. Previous literature suggests that anxious health care patients are commonly unable to retain up to half of the information presented at routine physician visits (50). Consequently, all treatment providers must be vigilant of the potential significant interference of anxiety and pain with learning novel information in an amputation circumstance. Repetition and review of both verbal and written information is likely necessary for complete learning.

Finally, feelings of vulnerability and fear of reinjury are commonly verbalized by patients following amputation. This fear of injury involves perceived threat of reinjury to their body, fear of injury to their unaffected limb, or injury to spouses or family members whom they feel either responsible for or dependent upon. Each of these concerns is reasonable considering the reality of one's decreased ability to provide resistance to falls or other physical challenges, sudden dependence upon one's unaffected limb for virtually all fine-motor activities, and heavy reliance upon spouse or family to provide needed care to them or dependent children. Graded participation with daily rehabilitation and the acquisition of new skills to address these areas is necessary to minimize concerns.

Posttraumatic Stress Disorder

Over the past decade, the rapidly expanding trauma literature reflects the considerable professional attention devoted to the evaluation of traumatic stress symptoms in victims of violence, rape, and natural disaster. Considerably less investigation exists addressing the presence of posttraumatic stress disorder (PTSD) symptoms in people experiencing aversive medical events. The specific prevalence of PTSD in medical patients is unknown, with only preliminary reports existing for the presence in a variety of conditions (51). For example, isolated reports exist regarding PTSD symptoms associated with Guillan-Barre syndrome (52), obstetric and gynecologic conditions (53), myocardial infarction (7), burn injuries (6,54), and cerebral vascular accident (55). A comprehensive review of the literature investigating PTSD and amputation revealed only two citations, with one describing the vicarious development of posttraumatic stress symptoms in the mother of a child who sustained a bilateral upper extremity amputation due to burns from high voltage electrical shock (56). Grunert and colleagues (9) reported the acute prevalence of flashbacks and event-specific nightmares in a traumatic hand injury population to be 81% and 70%, respectively. Interestingly, while the percentage of nightmares decreased to about 10% at 18-month follow-up, flashbacks remained a troubling concern for nearly 40% of this population. Most would agree that the circumstances surrounding traumatic limb loss are quite sufficient to promote high levels of trauma-related stress, and unpublished data on traumatic amputation patients from our clinic suggests diagnostic rates of posttraumatic stress as high as 30 to 35%. The characteristic phobic avoidance of trauma-related stimuli can pose a substantial challenge to rehabilitative progress following limb loss. Many features of the rehabilitation environment may either directly or symbolically represent aspects of the traumatic injury event to patients. Avoidance of physical conditioning equipment (e.g., weight machines, treadmills, certain diagnostic machines) may occur in individuals who sustained their injuries on machines with similar hydraulic press or belt- or wheel-drive components. Further, treatments that call for restriction of movement or being confined to an aparatus (e.g., traction, certain weight machines) are frequent sources of acute anxiety for patients. In severe cases, even the prosthesis itself has served as a stimulus for severe anxiety in patients who are actively avoiding even symbolic reminders of their injury event. As it is virtually impossible to premeditate the complete range of potential anxiety-producing stimuli one might encounter in postinjury rehabilitation, each member of the treatment team should be sensitized to the possibility of iatrogenic medical retraumatization, and asked to remain vigilant of symptoms of progressive emotional compromise or treatment avoidance.

Considering the potentially chronic, degenerative nature of undiagnosed or untreated posttraumatic stress disorder, and the sincere threat this condition might pose to timely treatment improvements, the ongoing evaluation of PTSD symptoms is highly advised. Patients and families should be educated regarding symptoms and treatments and encouraged to remain vigilant of anxiety symptoms. To use a medical analogy, if patients were determined to be at heightened risk for a medical condition (e.g., stroke) that would threaten treatment outcome after amputation, a protocol would obviously be established to serially assess for this condition. As it would be prudent to develop a proactive management strategy in this hypothetical circumstance, it is equally prudent to develop proactive strategies to detect and minimize PTSD symptoms at any point in the rehabilitative process.

Of probable interest to those without extensive knowledge of the PTSD literature is the phenomenon of delayed symptom onset. Several event-specific factors have been implicated as either preventing or delaying the onset of posttraumatic stress symptoms, including loss of consciousness or impaired arousal levels secondary to alcohol or drug intoxication at the time of injury. Although no literature exists to verify this contention in traumatic amputation, the premise is consistent with both our clinical experience and reports of lack of traumatic stress development for motor vehicle accident patients who either lost consciousness or were amnesic for the event (57). Certainly it seems reasonable that some vulnerable patients may not demonstrate stress symptoms until they encounter the specific environment in which their injury occurred (e.g., their work site of injury). Although these cases may be considered delayed onset, behavioral theory suggests that certain symptoms or behaviors might be situation-specific, and not observed in environments that bear little resemblance to that in which the injury occurred. Symptoms that develop at the time of return to work are often severe enough to prohibit reintegration efforts without targeted treatment. The few published papers encouraging the preparation of patients for return to work in the original environment as a component of their recovery have offered promising results.

Grunert and associates (58) reported successful work reintegration training for 90% of a patient population who developed PTSD after traumatic hand injury. This cognitive-behavioral exposure program, designed to reintroduce the individual to the work environment in which he was traumatically injured, also demonstrated gradual decrease of injury-related flashbacks over the first 6 months after reintegration. Unfortunately, no reliable methods exist for assessing the vulnerability of patients to develop delayed onset PTSD. Similar efforts to determine predictors in Vietnam veterans yielded disappointing results. Watson et al. (59) were unable to identify differences in acute versus delayed onset PTSD in combat veterans by evaluating psychosocial stress history, personality factors, or "repression" scale scores. Their results also failed to support the contention that the delayed onset of symptoms were attributable to the magnitude of the trauma event or the severity of existing symptoms. Even had this investigation identified promising results, the generalizability of much of the PTSD literature to amputation populations is suspect. Bernstein (60) failed to identify unique characteristics in those trauma patients who necessitated longer-term treatment (i.e., over 12 months) from those demonstrating successful resolution with 3 months of therapy. Perhaps the strongest rationale in support of serial evaluation of posttraumatic stress symptoms is the apparent decline in treatment efficacy associated with delayed detection and treatment. For example, Bernstein reported dropout rates exceeded 80% for those entering treatment after 40 weeks.

Body Image

The majority of theoretical discussion and empirical study regarding body image exists in the eating disorder literature, with little consensus regarding the applicability of these models to the altered body appearance and self-image experienced following limb loss. As long as 50 years ago, authors emphasized the importance of body image to the long-term emotional adjustment of people with amputation, and they have anecdotally suggested that people with limb loss need develop three subjective, interchangeable body image constructs. Barker, Wright, and Gonick (61) recommended the development of three body images including the preinjury body image, postamputation image of body with missing limb, and postamputation image of body with prosthesis in place. Clinical experience suggests that it is common for limb loss patients to glamorize their premorbid body image, and this tendency might pose a considerable obstacle in their accepting a revised image. Although no data supports the assertion for three body images, it is conceivable that the development of comfortable body images with and without prostheses would assist the individual's transition with intimacy issues, personal acceptance and self-care, or projecting a more positive public image. This flexible body image development might actually contribute to healthier adjustment for patients conceptualizing prosthesis use as a means of "hiding" disfigurement from the public.

Body image has been minimally studied in amputation, and most published material is entirely anecdotal. No data exists to clarify whether body image challenges might be greater for persons without a limb for congenital reasons, due to a traumatic accident, or due to dysvascular disease. In an investigation of the relationship between body image and psychosocial adaptation, Rybarczk et al. (44) found ratings of body image to be a significant predictor of depression and reduced quality of life in 112 persons following lower extremity amputation. Further, perceptions of social stigma (i.e., that others held negative attitudes about them related to their amputation) were found to be an independent predictor of level of depression. Rybarczyk and associates (43) earlier reported that individuals with limb loss who acknowledged discomfort related to social interactions in which their amputation or prosthesis were mentioned, were also at greater risk for depression. In this study, social discomfort (i.e., perceived appearance) was a significant independent predictor of depression in amputees without regard for age, sex, social support, time since amputation, reason for amputation, or perceived health recovery. Grunert et al. (9) identified similar concerns in 173 people who underwent upper extremity crush injury, amputation, or replantation surgeries. Serial evaluation measures taken from baseline to 18 months postinjury revealed significant aesthetic concerns endorsed by this patient group. Specifically, 51% of patients acknowledged difficulty with personal acceptance of the physical appearance of their injured limbs acutely post injury, with 14% maintaining concern at 18 months. Of these same patients, 62% endorsed baseline concerns regarding their perceptions of social acceptance (i.e., their perception of the acceptance of the appearance of their affected limb by others), with 32% maintaining this concern at 18-month follow-up. This data well exemplifies the potential body image threat to social adjustment.

Given the nomenclature of amputation medicine, it seems most unlikely that efforts to "normalize" or desensitize concerns with altered physical appearance might actually begin during the acute medical care and prosthetic fitting phases. Poorly derived terms such as "stump" for residual limb, or "hook" to describe a terminal prosthetic device, are commonly used in the early rehabilitation stages—precisely the time when the individual is making difficult efforts to minimize the shock of their physical alteration and to glean hope for a sense of normality and recovery. The use of these terms quite likely serves only to hypersensitize patients to the salience of the change in their physical being.

PROPOSED PSYCHOLOGIC EVALUATION AND TREATMENT INTERVALS

The following psychosocial assessment and treatment intervals are offered with regard to the relative time periods in which amputation patients might reasonably encounter specific medical and rehabilitative milestones and their associated emotional and adaptational challenges. The procedure of outlining this discussion in intervals is clearly *not* intended to imply a linear relationship between time since injury and emotional adjustment. To the contrary, empirical research has not supported the "common sense" assumption that passage of time promotes emotional healing. Rather, despite the apparent popularity of stage theories of adjustment, several authors (47,62,63) have emphasized the lack of a clear relationship between time since injury and emotional adjustment. Prolonged emotional assessment is strongly indicated, given that only a portion of amputation patients might be acutely symptomatic. This proposition obviates the provision of both long-term medical and psychologic treatment resources for patients following limb loss. It matters little when one might consider it appropriate for a person with amputation to begin "getting on with life." Treatment providers can only attempt to create an atmosphere that promotes the graded exploration of emotional issues and encourages incremental adjustment to changes.

It is not the opinion of this chapter that individuals with amputation follow any standard course of emotional adjustment or that they must reliably progress through any identifiable coping stages to successfully recover. Emotional adjustment must be conceptualized as a product of a complex interaction of premorbid personality, life experiences, postsurgical health complications, available social and community resources, and the acquisition of amputation-specific coping skills. Meier (64) proposed nine rehabilitative phases following amputation, with associated hallmark features for each phase. These nine phases comprehensively address the medical and functional management of patients with amputation, and psychosocial concerns are anticipated in each phase. Because a comprehensive understanding of the postsurgical rehabilitation process is highly desirable for psychosocial providers working in amputation, the phases proposed by Meier appear in Table 8-1.

A framework for psychologic assessment and intervention for patients with limb loss follows, and those psychosocial factors of utmost importance are discussed. This schema provides ready delineation of the emotional and behavioral factors that parallel the rehabilitation milestones proposed by Meier. For the sake of convenience, the psychosocial framework is divided into three intervals: survival, recovery, and reintegration. In addition to assessing for prominent psychosocial challenges in each interval, recommendations for the frequency of contact, and those family and community issues that correspond to each interval, are included. Current rehabilitation medicine textbooks suggest that, in specific cases, patient assessments should be extended from days to weeks postinjury. Due to the high variability in emotional expression following amputation, and the prolonged rehabilitative nature of the injury, this proposed framework recommends making psychologic providers standard long-term collaborators with the rehabilitation team, with at least episodic ongoing patient contacts. These serial evaluations are recommended even for those patients who do not demonstrate acute emotional symptoms. A comparison of the proposed psychosocial framework using the medical rehabilitation phases is provided in Table 8-2.

Survival Interval

Patient and Family Issues

The survival interval includes presurgical psychosocial contacts (when possible), immediate postsurgery hospital contacts, and outpatient visits during the first 6 to 8 weeks after hospital discharge. This interval derives its name from the near complete focus by patients and families on mortality and survival, and the priority of intensive medical management at this time. Any intensive efforts to facilitate psychologic adjustment or acceptance are relegated to secondary priority during the presurgical or immediate postsurgical period. Nonetheless, rehabilitation psychology consults should be initiated at the earliest patient contacts. A critical care pathway for amputation patients developed by our hospital staff recommends psychology consultation preoperatively whenever possible, and immediately post surgery (i.e., post-op day one) in all other cases (65). The benefit of presurgical patient preparation for a vari-

TABLE 8-1 *Phases of Amputee Rehabilitation*	
PHASE	**HALLMARKS**
1. Preoperative	Assessment of body condition, patient education, surgical level discussion, postoperative prosthetic plans
2. Amputation surgery, reconstruction	Length, myoplastic closure, soft tissue coverage, nerve handling, rigid dressing
3. Acute postsurgical	Wound healing, pain control, proximal body motion, emotional support
4. Preprosthetic	Shaping, shrinking, increase muscle strength, restore patient locus of control
5. Prosthetic prescription and fabrication	Team consensus on prosthetic prescription
6. Prosthetic training	Increase in prosthetic wearing and functional utilization
7. Community integration	Resumption of roles in family and community activities Emotional equilibrium and healthy coping strategies Recretional activities
8. Vocational rehabilitation	Assessment and planning of vocational activities for future. May require further education, training, or job modification.
9. Follow-up	Life-long prosthetic, functional, medical assessment, and emotional support

TABLE 8-2

Van Dorsten's Proposed Psychosocial Intervals with Associated Rehabilitation Phases, Prominent Psychosocial Objectives, and Recommended Frequency of Psychosocial Contact

PSYCHOSOCIAL INTERVAL	REHABILITATION PHASE	PSYCHOSOCIAL OBJECTIVES	FREQUENCY OF CONTACT

Survival	Preoperative
	Amputation Surgery And
	  Reconstruction
	Acute Postsurgical
	Preprosthetic
		Crisis Intervention
		Support and Information
		Family/Spouse Assessment
		Self-Management Strategies
		Cognitive Distraction
		Peer Visits
		Initial Home Re-integration
			Patient:
			  In-Hospital: Daily
			  Outpatient: 1–2 × week
			Family:
			  2–4 × month

Recovery	Prosthetic Prescription And
	  Fabrication
	Prosthetic Training
	Community Reintegration
		Psychometric Testing
		Autonomic Assessment
		Emotional Management
		Self-Stigma/Expectations
		Relaxation Training
		Family Role Re-integration
		Social Re-integration
		Adherence Monitoring
		Peer Support Group
			Patient: 1 × week; then fade
			  to 1 × month or as
			  needed by interval end.
			  May require bouts of
			  intensive sessions to
			  address acute symptoms
			Family: 1–2 × month; Fade
			  to as needed over
			  interval

Re-Integration	Vocational Rehabilitation
	Follow-up
		Emotional Management
		Work Re-integration
		Independent Driving
		Insurance Case Closure
		Intimacy/Sexuality Issues
		Fear of Re-injury
		Peer Support Group
		Relapse Prevention Training
			Patient: As needed; may
			  need short-term intensive
			  sessions for acute issues
			Family: As needed

ety of general medical conditions has been demonstrated and can form a solid therapeutic foundation for future work (66–68). Specific to amputation, Frierson and Lippman (69) demonstrated a reduction in hospital stay associated with psychiatric consultation in 86 subjects with limb loss. Results showed that 14 subjects who received preamputation counseling averaged 2.5 fewer hospital days, and 45 subjects receiving postamputation consultation averaged 1.5 fewer days.

The primary emphasis of inhospital psychosocial contacts should be providing information, stabilizing acute emotional responses, providing support, and training cognitive distraction however possible. While clearly accepting the benefits of early assessment and treatment, an overly aggressive approach with acute psychologic efforts aimed at any sort of "acceptance" or "resolution" is not recommended. Attempts to begin actively processing one's loss or initiating a psychosocial agenda to "work through" issues is not recommended at this time. Experience has taught us patience, because the patient and family's primary focus at this time is on survival, not contemplation of long-term life changes. Our informal surveys of people with amputation have offered interesting insights concerning the most helpful services or comments they received in the acute injury phase. Simple statements of reassurance that patients are in good care, realistic statements regarding prognosis for long-term independent functioning, and assurances that a skilled treatment team will be available to them throughout their recovery are the most frequently identified pieces of comforting information offered at this time. In short, psychosocial providers are encouraged to provide accurate information and supportive therapy. Providers must take care to avoid overwhelming the patient with in-depth discussions of grief and loss, since their cognitive resources need largely be devoted at this acute point to intensive medical care. Brief, frequent visits conducted in conjunction with the medical staff to provide information as to the acute medical treatment process and strategies patients can use to maintain composure are helpful. In-hospital contacts also offer the opportunity to desensitize the patient and family to the presence of the medical and psychologic treatment team, specify the role of psychologic providers on the team, and to enlist family members as active observers for evidence of cognitive or emotional deviation from normal.

Acute medical attention and the hospital environment provide a milieu that supports or even promotes emotional constriction and avoidance of consideration of the impact of limb loss on one's life. Several features of the hospital environment provide distraction from self-assessment, including pain medication or patient-controlled anesthesia (PCA), medical triage care and revision surgeries, and daily physical and occupational therapist contacts for passive ranging and wound care. Around-the-clock nursing contact and an initial hyper-response from friends and family to the injury leave the patient with little time alone to contemplate. As length of hospital stay is commonly less than 1 week post injury, it is typical that the individual with limb loss has not begun taking an "internal inventory" of their circumstance until some time after hospital discharge.

Although seemingly obvious, treatment staff should avoid "interpreting" the patient's affect or behavior as deviating from premorbid functioning until family can provide detailed information regarding the individual's typical characteristics. Providers also need to resist the temptation to begin developing prognostic impressions of recovery potential based upon anecdotal factors with little empirical support. For example, there is scant support that any of the following factors have been associated with poor emotional adjustment after limb loss: age or developmental stage at time of amputation, passage of time since amputation, cause of amputation, level of amputation, or initial physical impairment (43–46,70,71). Conversely, the presence of significant phantom pain has been implicated as a threat to recovery and again emphasizes the need for aggressive acute pain management efforts (72,73).

Many rehabilitation services recommend peer visits—often at the patient's request—either presurgically or immediately postsurgically. Peer visitors are typically well received by patients, and the importance of peer similarity has been previously reported (74,75). Nosek and colleagues (76) reported that people with mobility impairments rated counselors with like disabilities as more credible than able-bodies counselors, and disabled peers without professional academic training as substantially more credible on specific topics (e.g., requesting personal assistance). Of course, amputation peers should not be requested to provide professional advice, and need to be prepared for these visits to provide support, validation, and personal impressions of their course of recovery. Families should be encouraged to attend peer visits and to ask questions and partake in the discussion as well.

Adaptation to amputation and the lifestyle challenges imposed by limb loss often occurs at differing rates for family members, spouses, or significant others than for the patient himself. Family anxieties often produce a desire to accelerate the recovery process so as to limit their contemplation of the severity of injury or the very real brush with mortality their loved one may have encountered. To find positive outlets for this anxiety, family members can be recruited along with the patient in providing information about the premorbid characteristics of the patient and family, verbalizing fears or concerns about recovery, and providing comfort or wound care assistance. Patients and family should be familiarized with digital readings or sounds produced by monitors or other devices attached to the patient (e.g., PCA beeps, pulse oxygen monitors) whenever possible to avoid undue anxiety. Regular contacts with primary family members should be conducted in-hospital to evaluate their current and historical emotional status, unrealistic fears, challenges they anticipate in the early stages of home reintegration, and to obtain information on the family's pre-morbid emotional and coping characteristics.

Proposed Frequency of Contact

The frequency of contact necessary to manage different amputation issues throughout each psychosocial interval is highly variable and depends on a host of extenuating factors, including the patient and family's premorbid emotional and coping characteristics, previous trauma exposure, availability of quality social supports, history of substance misuse, postsurgical medical complications, pain intensity, and the need for additional invasive procedures. In this survival interval, brief daily in-hospital visits should allow providers to effectively meet the postsurgical psychosocial goals for initial assessment and emotional stabilization. A timely follow-up appointment is strongly indicated within the first 3 days postdischarge to reconfirm the presence of a coordinated care plan from inpatient to outpatient. As the outpatient environment provides a more standardized opportunity for comprehensive psychologic assessment, one to two weekly visits in the first month postdischarge are suggested. Once patients demonstrate a suitable transition to the home environment, weekly to twice per month visits may be sufficient.

Family contact should be maintained on a weekly to twice per month basis in this acute interval to allow psychosocial providers to provide support and discuss family impressions of the patient's initial adjustment. A host of new concerns may confront the patient and family in the early stages of returning home, including need for additional equipment or reinstruction in wound care, uncontrolled pain, medication side effects, or insurance coverage issues. Those persons sustaining traumatic limb loss should be closely assessed at this time for evidence of anxiety or depression, nightmare activity, sleep disruption, or excessive medication use. Multiple calls and cards from concerned friends and extended family can be prioritized as time allows. All of these items require time and energy from patients and families who are likely fatigued from the anxiety of the injury and hospital regimen.

Recovery Interval

Patient and Family Issues

The recovery interval encompasses outpatient psychosocial care from several weeks to approximately 9 months postdischarge. The primary emphasis of medical rehabilitation in this interval is designing and training prosthesis use. Consequently, it is inevitable that in this interval, psychosocial providers will confront any discrepancy between the reality of prosthetic limitation and the potentially grandiose expectation patients might have held for prosthesis function. Although it is standard protocol for health care providers to offer reasonable caveats regarding prosthesis limitations, it is also common for patients to make "self-promises" of full functional recovery with prostheses as a means of self-soothing. The greater the discrepancy between these private promises and the ultimate reality, the greater the emotional challenge likely to be encountered.

Appreciating their potential threat to treatment outcome, depression, anxiety, anger, self-acceptance, social reintegration, pain management, and consistent compliance with treatment recommendations are all psychosocial priorities throughout this recovery interval. Any number of pitfalls may be encountered in even a relatively uncomplicated course of prosthetic preparation, purchase, fitting, and training. For example, an amputation patient may at any time encounter difficulties with performing preprosthesis strengthening or stretching exercises, pain, or skin problems associated with initial prosthesis fitting or the initial wear schedule. If these setbacks are avoided, patients then face potential prosthesis revision or failure, with training necessarily halted until repairs can be ordered and completed. Next, the challenge of mastering bodily movements to efficiently operate the prosthesis may take considerable time, and when patients and therapists have successfully navigated the rehabilitation course to this point, insurance challenges regarding the purchase of desired componentry may be confronted. Depending

on the patient's urgency for prosthesis mastery as a means of symbolically conquering the emotional and physical "dragon" of amputation, wide swings in emotional stability or marked emotional compromise may occur. Episodically, patients may become apathetic and be less devoted to their recommended therapies. All resources need be expended to ensure active, consistent participation with ongoing therapies throughout the prolonged rehabilitation course.

Williamson and Schulz (77) reported that a perceived level of activity restriction following amputation was found to be a significant predictor of depression. These authors suggested that the loss of certain activities related to self-worth (e.g., self-care, employment, social interaction), was associated with increased depression. The degree of deviation from premorbid personal interests, family roles, or recreational hobbies threatens successful adjustment after amputation. Consequently, serial assessment of emotional flexibility, and the development of an active, distractive coping repertoire are the primary psychosocial targets of this recovery interval.

It is recommended that psychometric testing of emotional functioning, pain, and coping style be conducted at 6 to 8 weeks postinjury to establish a posthospital, yet relatively acute baseline measure of functioning. The postinjury timeframe is recommended for testing, because the family will most likely have begun to re-establish preinjury lifestyle patterns including a return to work for the spouse, back to school for children, transition of frequency of medical care contacts to an outpatient schedule, and titration of medication doses. This gradual return to normal for the family provides the person with limb loss increasing independent time to contemplate the loss of their limb and the potential resultant impact on their life. As the acute distractions diminish, this is often the first time that the person with limb loss has begun to contemplate their future, and their future "normalcy" after amputation. Psychometric testing should be delayed to this logical period to capture some measure of response to these deliberations, rather than being conducted at an earlier point before this introspection might naturally begin.

Although rarely a standard evaluation component of comprehensive rehabilitation programs, the tendency of people with disabilities to pejoratively self-label or stigmatize should be assessed (44,62). It is generally accepted that our society may hold certain prejudicial biases against those with physical disabilities, and therefore it seems quite conceivable that the person with amputation himself may have possessed premorbid misconceptions about others with physical impairment. Van Dorsten (62) recommended direct exploration of a patient's personal history of experience with amputation (e.g., friends, family, acquaintances), and premorbid perceptions of others with disability, since these preconceptions likely provide the foundation for their expectations for recovery. Distorted preamputation beliefs may negatively frame the individual's expectations as to how others might perceive them and interfere with social reintegration efforts. As no standardized means of assessing these preinjury disability biases are known, clinical interviews must be tailored to address this specific topic.

Psychophysiologic assessment can be conducted to assess muscle tension that produces pain or to assess symptoms of autonomic arousal associated with any traumatic etiology producing loss of limb. Biofeedback-assisted relaxation training is a common treatment for pain, insomnia, and anxiety issues. Also, the diagnosis of PTSD is strengthened with the verification of hyperphysiologic arousal to stimuli associated with one's injury. Available research suggests that the presence of PTSD symptoms at 3 months is prognostic of poor adjustment at 1 year (78). As previously discussed, anxiety symptoms may not be acutely apparent and may develop weeks to months postinjury. Rocca, Spence, and Muster (79) reported that whereas only 7% of 31 burn patients studied met the diagnostic criteria for PTSD at hospital discharge, 22% met the criteria at 4-month follow-up. Psychosocial providers working with individuals with traumatic amputation hold an inherent responsibility to be familiar with PTSD and the treatment options for this condition. Given the imposition of physical injuries and the threat of emotional compromise, it is often difficult for patients to tolerate exposure treatment attempts early in this interval. Decisions to engage in either implosion or in-vivo exposure regimens should be conducted on a case-by-case basis, and carefully take into account the patient's emotional resources and threat of exacerbation of depression, suicidal ideation, or pain concerns. If a patient is deemed a tenuous candidate for exposure therapies at a particular time, psychosocial providers may develop an initial hierarchy of anxiety-producing features of the accident, and reconsider this treatment when the patient has suitable resources to tolerate more intensive treatment. Certainly training the individual to use multiple types of relaxation strategies to promote enhanced self-management can be completed early on.

As has been noted, psychosocial providers must facilitate a graded exploration of lifestyle changes secondary to limb loss. Patients should be encouraged to identify those areas of their life that might be least affected after limb loss. Identifying and emphasizing areas in which limb loss may have minimal impact (e.g., certain life goals, work experience, recreational interests, specific parenting duties) can help to maintain perspective that several areas of one's life remain as before. We find the common starting point for reintegration is within the family, and it is encouraged that the patient assumes whatever previous family roles possible (i.e., that are not limited by physical injury) at the earliest possible time. Often patients are able to resume most roles as parent, sibling, and spouse in the first months after injury, and thus build confidence for initial efforts at community reintegration.

Just as peer visitors may be a valuable resource in the acute phase of recovery, ongoing support from peer groups is highly recommended as an adjunct to individual and family therapy throughout the recovery interval. Amputation support groups can offer unique benefits, including education about a variety of community resources for those with amputation, emotional support and validation of concerns, skilled problem-solving insights from others who have faced similar challenges, and targeted resources for bibliotherapy. Winchell (13) has written a valuable amputation patient resource regarding adjustment to traumatic limb loss. This author's first-hand experience with traumatic amputation addresses the common thoughts, feelings, and coping challenges unique to this population. Family and spouse participation in support group activities is again encouraged. Spouse attendance can promote family cohesiveness by demonstrating support for the patient and emphasizing the impact of this injury on the entire family group. On "group nights," support groups specifically for spouses and families may meet concurrently to provide opportunities for family members to address the specific challenges they encounter in their interactions with their injured loved one. The formulation of these family-only groups is often requested by individuals with limb loss in recognition of the impact their injury has on their family. As a caveat, support group meetings can easily become "gripe sessions" without adequate direction. Peer support groups should initially be facilitated by a person experienced in leading groups, and who has had extensive rehabilitation experience with amputation. Once the group members become cohesive and skilled in the group process, it is encouraged that they then assume responsibility for the group's activities and invite speakers or consultants that meet their needs. Successful support groups typically share the common features of being peer- or patient-directed toward the identification of items of mutual educational interest, and public and government resources, and being devoted to problem-solving the specific challenges the group members encounter. Experienced group members serve as both mastery and coping models of rehabilitative success for others who might be at different phases of recovery.

Frequency of Contact

On a continuum from the survival interval, weekly to twice per month visits may be utilized in the early portion of this interval for completing assessments and initiating targeted interventions. Once patients demonstrate emotional stabilization and the acquisition of lifestyle management skills, psychosocial treatments can reasonably be pared to one meeting per 2 to 3 months, or even "as needed" by the end of this interval. Again, the estimated frequency of contacts remains highly dependent upon resumption of premorbid activities and responsibilities, capacity for self-observation, knowledge of emotional risk factors, and willingness to engage available services for assistance if needed. Some patients experience few struggles after the acute period and will not require consistent contact by the end of this interval. Others may demonstrate limited adjustment over time, and require frequent, intense psychosocial intervention contacts throughout this interval. Family contact should be maintained on a one to two times per month basis at the outset of this interval to facilitate reintegration into the home, premorbid family roles, and to keep them abreast of rehabilitative challenges being faced by the patient. Decreasing family visits to as-needed is appropriate thereafter.

Reintegration Interval

Patient and Family Issues

The reintegration interval encompasses psychosocial contacts provided after approximately 9 months postinjury. The essence of the reintegration interval is complete modified independence by the patient to resume driving, employment, family roles and responsibilities, and recreational activities and hobbies. If physical or emotional issues prohibit resumption of certain premorbid vocational or avocational interests, the development of new activities to meet financial and self-esteem purposes should be eagerly pursued. A return to work after traumatic injury may involve vocational rehabilitation services to facilitate return to a modified work position with one's previous employer, or re-education for a job change either with the previous or new employer. Driving evaluations can be completed at this time to verify the safe, independent operation of a car, and to ascertain mastery of driving with modifications to the automobile as one's injury may require.

Psychosocial providers must remain vigilant for any delayed-onset emotional challenges, since many may be environment-specific and present only at this time of site reintegration. Desensitization to a specific work environment may be necessary, and this has been shown to be successful in facilitating a return to employment (58). Anger issues may be more prominent in the reintegration interval than previous. During this interval, patients are completing rehabilitative care and will undergo evaluation to determine maximum medical improvement (MMI), permanent impairment ratings (IR), and case closure (i.e., if injury occurred at work or in a motor vehicle and produced any sort of litigation). Injured patients often express anger and resentment with insufficient insurance settlements or the lack of progress with litigation regarding damages and compensation. A patient's active involvement in litigation matters can produce increased anxiety and anger, with the constant recall of their loss and life change. Fortunately, Grunert et al. (80) suggested minimal effect of litigation on psychologic symptoms or PTSD if limb injury patients were provided early psychologic intervention. As previously discussed, patients may continue to experience considerable concerns regarding self-acceptance of their altered body, and face negative social encounters during initial efforts at public reintegration. Consequently, long-term efforts to assess the ramification of body image issues must continue during this important interval. By 1 year, most patients will have experienced adequate emotional adjustment to allow for at least modified resumption of their premorbid lifestyle. Others, however, may have made little emotional progress, and continue with postinjury lifestyles that are markedly deviant from those to which they were accustomed. These cases are not to be considered "psychosocial failures." They are simply harrowing reminders of the significance of individual differences, and many may require at least episodic long-term contact for emotional "maintenance" if successful recovery is not achieved. During the reintegration interval, amputation patients are expected to make an important transition by replacing rehabilitation team contacts for support and "security" with their own personal, social, and community supports. For many, this transition may have occurred long ago, but for others, the "finality" of MMI and the paring of medical contacts to a maintenance schedule is an emotional event. The determination of MMI does not imply that patients will need no future medical care, because it is accepted that these patients will need episodic medical and prosthetic adjustment for a potentially infinite future. The more difficult distinction involves the determination of the vague concept of "maximum psychologic improvement." Although accepted that long-term intensive psychologic intervention is not necessary in most amputation cases, it remains wise to similarly consider the reasonable need for many to have infrequent long-term "maintenance" psychosocial visits to maintain independent functioning. It should be emphasized to patients that while the rehabilitation team is an available resource for extenuating circumstances, the hallmark of successful recovery is general independence from the treatment team.

Although the majority of family reintegration challenges have been encountered by this point, several important potential issues remain in the reintegration interval. Families frequently express fears of reinjury as the patient becomes increasingly independent using adaptive modifications. Concerns may be expressed for both the patient's safety and future family functioning should reinjury occur. These concerns must be anticipated and efficiently addressed, because they may pose a considerable threat to reintegration efforts. Also at this time, marital affection, intimacy, and sexuality issues should be discussed. These issues are usually assigned secondary importance in the survival and recovery phases, and may be somewhat uncomfortable for partners to discuss. However, care providers need to initiate conversations regarding the patient's and spouse's acceptance of altered physical appearance so as to determine obstacles to maintaining physical attraction and resuming premorbid sexual practices. Sexual desire and performance may naturally be altered following such a significant injury as loss of limb, and further affected by a variety of modifiable factors including medication side effects or pain issues. Physical appearance perceptions or aesthetic concerns are not corrected with medical treatment and merit specific therapy sessions devoted to desensitizing a couple's reluctance to discuss and overcome such private issues.

Continued support group interaction is encouraged so long as the person and family feel they are deriving benefit from participation. Patients must be reminded that by this time, they have valuable experience to share with others newly injured, and that they now serve as the same models for recovery that they previously observed in their initial group interactions. Well-designed groups are empowering and invaluable for their abilities to promote organizational patient advocacy and community resource identification. Interestingly, several of our clinic's patients have retrained after sustaining their traumatic injuries to become experienced physical therapists and prosthetists to share their unique knowledge with others.

Frequency of Contact

Although infrequent long-term medical and prosthetic reevaluations are expected, contact with psychosocial providers should gradually be transferred to personal and community resources unless extenuating circumstances or instances of emotional degeneration occur. Meetings from twice per year to simply as needed may be sufficient for those demonstrating adequate independent functioning. The person with limb loss should now utilize the psychosocial provider as a community resource having expertise in their specific health and emotional issue. Only those with extenuating circumstances (e.g., major emotional issues, chronic PTSD) might be expected to need more intensive care at this time. However, as these troubled cases occur, the desire to "wean" patients from the rehabilitation team should not allow them to be relegated to community mental health or private practitioners without amputation experience. This relationship is considered unlikely to resolve amputation issues or foster recovery. It simply must be accepted that some individuals, for any of a variety of reasons, demonstrate limited recovery and necessitate long-term specialized psychosocial maintenance care.

CONCLUSIONS

The recommendations proposed throughout this chapter are not made without conscious appreciation for cost containment and parsimonious resource utilization. Some parties might in fact question the utility of such a standard approach to psychosocial care following traumatic physical injury. They might assume a "why plant the seed…" or "We will deal with these issues if they arise…" posture from which to assess the impact of emotional features on recovery. This raises perhaps the most difficult-to-demonstrate benefit of psychologic intervention—indirect cost savings. As per the comprehensive review by Friedman and associates (81), published data exists to demonstrate cost savings associated with the provision of psychologic services. Patients with psychologic conditions have demonstrated an increased utilization of the medical care system. For example, Kroenke et al. (82) reported a strong correlation between the number of physical complaints reported by general medicine patients and the prevalence of diagnostic mood disorders. Further, Shalev, Bleich, and Ursano (83) reported that veterans with PTSD had a significantly greater number of physical complaints than non-PTSD patients; however, they did not differ in the number of actual physical findings upon physical examination or laboratory test findings. Given the threat of emotional compromise after amputation, it seems unwise to limit psychologic care as part of a multidisciplinary treatment approach in hopes of saving dollars. As early emotional symptoms are addressed and minimized, the probability of a patient necessitating long-term chronic psychosocial contact is reduced.

Finally, in many amputation treatment programs, the term "rehabilitation" is synonymous with "prosthetic and orthotic fitting." Amputation treatment may be myopically focused on the prosthesis and what function it might restore for the patient. In these programs, little attention may be devoted to the losses the person has experienced. In the proposed treatment schema, the person with limb loss, and his unique response to the alterations in his body, is the focus of the therapeutic program. A loss of limb attacks the very concept of wholeness and often promotes emotional distancing of one's self from a prosthesis. Individuals will often distantly refer to a prosthesis as *"the* arm," and not *"my* arm." Mental health professionals are fully aware that no emotional prosthesis is available to patients as they struggle with the emotional conceptualization and functional limits of prostheses. Prostheses do not replace a lost limb, but are in fact only an adaptive attachment that may improve functional independence by increasing the pace and range of specific activities at specific times. Many amputees elect not to use prostheses after failing to adjust to the physical sensation with use, or to the inherent meaning they attach to wearing a "false limb." In modern multidisciplinary programs, prosthesis use should not constitute the *sine qua non* of rehabilitation success. It is the acceptance of new self, and the recovery of premorbid personality, activities, and interests, which constitute the true measure of rehabilitation success.

References

1. Brom D, Kleiber RJ, Hoffman MC. Victims of traffic accidents: incidence and prevention of post-traumatic stress disorder. *J Clin Psych* 1993; 49:131–140.

2. Blanchard EB, Hickling EJ. *After the Crash: Assessment and Treatment of Motor Vehicle Accident Survivors.* Washington D.C.: American Psychological Association, 1997.

3. Blanchard EB, Hickling EJ, Taylor AE, Loos WR. Psychological morbidity associated with motor vehicle accidents. *Behav Res Ther* 1994; 32: 3:283–290.

4. Blanchard EB, Hickling, EJ, Taylor AE, Loos WR. Psychiatric morbidity associated with motor vehicle accidents. *J Nerv Ment Dis* 1995; 183: 8:495–504.

5. Green MM, McFarlane AC, Hunter CE, Griggs WM. Undiagnosed post-traumatic stress disorder following motor vehicle accidents. *Med J Austr* 1993; 159: 8:529–534.

6. Baur KM, Hardy PE, Van Dorsten B. Post-traumatic stress in burn populations: a critical review. *J Burn Care Rehab* 1998; 19: 3:230–240.

7. Kutz I, Garb R, David D. Post-traumatic stress disorder following myocardial infarction. *Gen Hosp Psych* 1988; 10:169–176.

8. van Driel RC, Op den Velde W. Myocardial infarction and post-traumatic stress disorder. *J Traum Str* 1995; 8:151–159.

9. Grunert BK, Divine CA, Matloub HS, Sanger JR, Yousif NJ, Anderson RC, Roell SM. Psychological adjustment following work-related hand injury: 18-month follow-up. *Ann Plas Surg* 1992; 29: 6:537–542.

10. Johnson RK. Psychologic assessment of patients with industrial hand injuries. *Hand Clin* 1993; 2:221–229.

11. Dise-Lewis JE. Psychological adaptation to limb loss. In: Atkins DJ, Meier RH (eds), *Comprehensive Management of the Upper Limb Amputee.* New York: Springer-Verlag, 1989.

12. Gerhards F, Floren I, Knapp T. The impact of medical, reeducational and psychological variables on rehabilitation outcome in amputees. *Int J Rehab Res* 1984; 7: 3:283–292.

13. Winchell E. *Coping with Limb Loss: A Practical Guide to Living with Amputation for You and Your Family.* Garden City Park, N.Y.: Avery Publishing Group, 1995.

14. Whatley-Brown, LK: Traumatic amputation: mechanisms of injury, treatment, and rehabilitation. *AAOHN J* 1990; 38:483–486.

15. Bradway JK, Malone JM, Racy J, Leal JM, Poole J. Psychological adaptation to amputation: an overview. *Orth Prosth* 1984; 38: 3:46–50.

16. Shalev AY, Shreiber S, Galai R. Early psychological responses to traumatic injury. *J Traum Str* 1993; 6: 4:441–450.

17. Kooijman CM, Dijkstra PU, Geertzen JHB, Elzinga A, van der Schans CP. Phantom pain and phantom sensations in upper limb amputees: an epidemiological study. *Pain* 2000; 87:33–41.

18. Kay HW, Newman JD. Relative incidence of new amputations: statistical comparison of 6,000 new amputees. *Orthot Prosthet* 1975; 29: 2:3–16.

19. Ehde DM, Czerniecki JM, Smith DG, Campbell KM, Edwards WT, Jensen MP, Robinson LR. Chronic phantom sensations, phantom pain, residual limb pain, and other regional pain after lower limb amputation. *Arch Phys Med Rehab* 2000; 81:1039–1044.

20. Davis RW. Phantom sensation, phantom pain, and stump pain. *Arch Phys Med Rehab* 1993; 74:79–91.

21. Jensen MP, Ehde DM, Hoffman AJ, Patterson DR, Czerniecki JM, Robinson LR. Cognitions, coping, and social environment predict adjustment to phantom limb pain, *Pain* 2002; 95:133–142.

22. Sherman RA, Arena JG, Sherman CJ. The mastery of phantom pain: growing evidence for psychophysiological mechanisms. *Biof S Reg* 1989; 14:267–280.

23. Jensen TS, Krebs B, Nielsen J, Rasmussen P. Phantom limb, phantom pain, and stump pain in amputees during the first 6 months following limb amputation. *Pain* 1983; 17:243–256.

24. Carlen PL, Wall PD, Nadvorna H, Steinbach T. Phantom limbs and related phenomena in recent traumatic amputations. *Neuro* 1978; 28:211–217.

25. Shukla GD, Sahu SC, Tripathi RP, Gupta DK. Phantom limb: a phenomenological study. *Brit J Psych* 1982; 141:54–58.

26. Geraghty TJ, Jones LE. Painful neuromata following upper limb amputation. *Prosthet Orthot Int* 1996; 20:176–181.

27. Jones LE, Davidson JH. The long-term outcome of upper limb amputees treated at a rehabilitation centre in Sydney, Australia. *Dis Rehab* 1995; 17:437–442.

28. Wartan SW, Hamann W, Wedley JR, McColl I. Phantom pain and sensation among British veteran amputees. *Brit J Anaes* 1997; 78:652–659.

29. Sherman RA, Arena JC. Phantom limb pain: mechanisms, incidence, and treatment. *Crit Rev Phys Rehab Med* 1992; 4:1–26.

30. Jensen TS, Krebs B, Nielsen J, Rasmussen P. Immediate and long-term phantom pain in amputees: Incidence,

clinical characteristics and relationship to pre-amputation limb pain. *Pain* 1985; 21:267–278.

31. Katz J, Melzack R. Pain "memories" in phantom limbs: review and clinical observations. *Pain* 1990; 43:319–336.

32. Nikolajsen L. Ilkjaer S, Kroner K, Christensen JH, Jensen TS. The influence of preamputation pain on postamputation stump and phantom pain. *Pain* 1997; 72:393–405.

33. Katz J. Prevention of phantom limb pain by regional anaesthesia. *Lancet* 1997; 349:519–520.

34. Flor H, Elbert T, Knecht S, Wienbruch C, Pantev C, Birbaumer N, Larbig W, Taub E. Phantom limb pain as a perceptual correlate of cortical reorganization following arm amputation. *Nature* 1995; 375:482–484.

35. Sherman RA, Sherman CJ. A comparison of phantom sensations among amputees whose amputations were of civilian and military origins. *Pain* 1985; 21:91–97.

36. Sherman RA, Sherman CJ, Gall NG. A survey of current phantom limb pain treatment in the United States. *Pain* 1980; 8:85–99.

37. Krames ES, Lanning RM: Intrathecal infusional analgesia for nonmalignant pain: analgesic efficacy of intrathecal opioid with or without bupivicaine. *J Pain Symp Man* 1993; 8:539–548.

38. Portenoy RK, Foley KM, Inturrisi CE. The nature of opioid responsiveness and its implications for neuropathic pain: new hypotheses derived from studies of opioid infusions. *Pain* 1990; 43:273–286.

39. Urban BJ, France RD, Steinberger EK, Scott DL, Maltbie AA. Long-term use of narcotic/antidepressant medication in the management of phantom limb pain. *Pain* 1986; 34:191–196.

40. Zeng M, Strumpf M, Tryba M. Long-term oral opioid therapy in patients with chronic nonmalignant pain. *J Pain Symp Man* 1992; 7, 69–77.

41. Huse E, Larbig W, Flor H, Birbaumer N. The effects of opioids on phantom limb pain and cortical reorganization. *Pain* 2001; 90:47–55.

42. Kashani JH, Frank RG, Kashani SR, Wonderlich SA, Reid J. Depression among amputees. *J Clin Psych* 1983; 44:256–258.

43. Rybarczyk BD, Nyenhuis DL, Nicholas JJ, Schulz R, Alioto RJ, Blair C. Social discomfort and depression in a sample of adults with leg amputations. *Arch Phys Med Rehab* 1992; 73:1169–1173.

44. Rybarczyk BD, Nyenhuis DL, Nicholas JJ, Cash S, Kaiser J. Body image, perceived social stigma, and the prediction of psychosocial adjustment to leg amputation. *Rehab Psych* 1995; 40:95–110.

45. Rybarczyk BD, Nicholas JJ, Nyenhuis DL. Coping with leg amputation: integrating research and clinical practice. *Rehab Psych* 1997; 42: 3:243–256.

46. Williamson GM, Schulz R, Bridges MS, Behan AM. Social and psychological factors in adjustment to limb amputation. *J Soc Beh Pers* 1994; 9:249–268.

47. Frank RG, Elliott T, Corcoran J, Wonderlich S. Depression following spinal cord injury: is it necessary? *Clin Psych Rev* 1987; 7:611–630.

48. Forrest AJ, Wolkind SN. Masked depression in men with low back pain. *Rheum Rehab* 1974; 13:148–153.

49. Kerns RD, Haythornthwaite JA. Depression among chronic pain patients: cognitive-behavioral analysis and effect on rehabilitation outcome. *J Cons Clin Psych* 1988; 56:870–876.

50. Belar CD, Deardorff WW. *Clinical Health Psychology in Medical Settings: A Practitioner's Guidebook.* Washington D.C.: American Psychological Association, 1995.

51. Shalev AY, Schreiber S, Galai, R, Melmed RN. Post-traumatic stress disorder following medical events. *Brit J Clin Psych* 1993; 32:247–253.

52. Chemtob CM, Herriott MG. Post-traumatic stress disorder as a sequela of Guillan-Barre syndrome. *J Traum Str* 1994; 7: 4:705–711.

53. Menage J. Post-traumatic stress disorder in women who have undergone obstetric and gynaecological procedures: a consecutive series of 30 cases of PTSD. *J Rep Inf Psych* 1993; 11: 4:221–228.

54. Silva JA, Leong GB, Ferrarri MM. Posttraumatic stress disorder in burn patients. *South Med J* 1991; 84:531.

55. Cassiday KL, Lyons JA. Recall of traumatic memories following cerebral vascular accident. *J Traum Str* 1992; 5: 4:627–631.

56. White S. Hidden posttraumatic stress disorder in the mother of a boy with traumatic amputation. *J Ped Psych* 1991; 16: 1:103–115.

57. Mayou R, Bryant B, Duthie R. Psychiatric consequences of road traffic accidents. *Brit Med J* 1993; 307: 6905:647–651.

58. Grunert BK, Divine CA, Smith CJ, Matloub HS, Sanger JR, Yousif NJ. Graded work exposure to promote work return after severe hand trauma: a replicated study. *Ann Plas Surg* 1992; 29:532–536.

59. Watson CG, Kucala T, Manifold V, Vasser P, Juba M. Differences between posttraumatic stress disorder patients with delayed and undelayed onsets. *J Nerv Ment Dis* 1988; 176: 8:568–572.

60. Bernstein, A. Treatment length in post-traumatic stress disorder. *Psychosom* 1986; 27: 9:632–637.

61. Kohl SJ: Psychosocial stressors in coping with disability. In: Krieger DW (ed), *Rehabilitation Psychology: A Comprehensive Textbook.* Rockville. M.D.: Aspen Systems Corporation, 1984.

62. Van Dorsten B. Amputation. In: Radnitz CL (ed), *Cognitive-Behavioral Therapy for Persons with Disabilities.* Northvale, N.J.: Jason Aronson Inc. 2000.

63. Wortman, C, Silver R. The myths of coping with loss. *J Cons Clin Psych* 1989; 57:349–357.

64. Meier RH III. Upper limb amputee rehabilitation. *Arch Phys Med Rehab: State of the Art Rev* 1994, 8: 1:165–185.

65. Esquenazi A, Meier RH. Limb amputation. *Arch Phys Med Rehab* 1996; 77:S18–S28.

66. Deardorff WW, Reeves JL. *Preparing for Surgery: A Mind-Body Approach to Enhance Healing and Recovery.* Oakland, Cal.: New Harbinger Publications, 1997.

67. Devine EC. Effects of psychoeducation care for adult surgical patients: a meta-analysis of 191 studies. *Pat Educ Coun* 1992; 19:129–142.

68. Johnston M, Vogele C. Benefits of psychological preparation for surgery: a meta-analysis. *Ann Behav Med* 1993; 15:245–256.

69. Frierson RL, Lippman SB. Psychiatric consultation for acute amputees. *Psychosom* 1987; 28: 4:83–189.

70. Bieliauskas LA, Glantz RH. Depression type in Parkinson's disease. *J Clin Exp Neuro* 1989; 11:597–604.

71. Frank RG, Kashani JH, Kashani SR, Wonderlich SA, Umlauf RL, Ashkanazi GS. Psychological response to amputation as a function of age and time since amputation. *Brit J Psych* 1984; 144:493–497.

72. Katz J. Psychophysiological contributions to phantom limb. *Can J Psych* 1992; 37:282–298.

73. Pell JP, Donnan PT, Fowkes FG, Ruckley CV. Quality of life following lower limb amputation for peripheral arterial disease. *Euro J Vasc Surg* 1993; 7:448–451.

74. Atkinson DR, Maruama M, Matsui S. Effects of counselor race and counseling approach on Asian Americans' perceptions of counselor credibility and utility. *J Couns Psych* 1982; 25:76–83.

75. Porche LM, Banikiotes PG. Racial and attitudinal factors affecting the perceptions of counselors by black adolescents. *J Couns Psych* 1982; 29:169–174.

76. Nosek MA, Fuhrer MJ, Hughes SO. Perceived counselor credibility by persons with physical disability: influence of counselor disability status, professional status, and the counseling content. *Rehab Psych* 1991; 36:153–161.

77. Williamson GM, Schulz R. Activity restriction mediates the association between pain and depressed affect: a study of younger and older adult cancer patients. *Psych Aging* 1994; 10:369–378.

78. Meichenbaum D. *A Clinical Handbook/Practical Therapist Manual for Assessing and Treating Adults with Post-Traumatic Stress Disorder (PTSD)*. Waterloo, Ontario, Canada: Institute Press, 1994.

79. Rocca RP, Spence RJ, Munster AM. Posttraumatic adaptation and distress among adult burn survivors. *Amer J Psych* 1992; 149:1234.

80. Grunert BK, Matloub HS, Sanger JR, Yousif NJ, Hetterman S. Effects of litigation on maintenance of psychological symptoms after severe hand injury. *J Hand Surg* 1991; 16A:1031–1034.

81. Friedman R, Sobel D, Myers P, Caudill M, Benson H. Behavioral medicine, clinical health psychology, and cost offset. *Health Psych* 1995; 14:509–518.

82. Kroenke K, Spitzer RL, Williams JB, Linzer M, Hahn SR, deGruy FV, Brody D. Physical symptoms in primary care: predictors of psychiatric disorders and functional impairment. *Arch Fam Med* 1994; 3: 9:774–779.

83. Shalev AY, Bleich A, Ursano RJ. Posttraumatic stress disorder: somatic comorbidity and effort tolerance. *Psychosom* 1990; 31: 2:197–203.

9 Pain Management for Upper Extremity Amputation

Scott Hompland, DO

This chapter is an attempt to provide the reader with the currently available information regarding the history, pathogenesis, and management of post amputation pain syndromes (PAPS). The exact pathogenesis of this process is incompletely understood, although the current theories will be discussed. The research in the field of PAPS is quite vast, but unfortunately double-blind, placebo-controlled clinical trials are rare. Numerous treatments have been attempted over the years (Table 9-1); however, most of these treatments are empiric rather than supported by research data. PAPS is a general term and includes residual limb pain (RLP) and phantom limb pain (PLP). The studies reviewed in the preparation of this chapter seldom discriminate between upper and lower extremity amputation treatments; consequently, the information is a collection of available data regarding amputation regardless of location. In addition, the lack of specificity of the entity being treated made it difficult to evaluate the studies. Treatments were frequently applied to PAPS rather than to residual limb or phantom pain specifically. Phantom pain has been described for nearly all body parts including limbs, which are the most common and are the focus of this chapter. Phantom pain has been reported in the eye (1), tongue (2), teeth (3), breast (4–8), uterus (9), and penis (10). Phantom limb sensa-

tions are extremely common and must be differentiated from residual limb pain and phantom limb pain when making the diagnosis; phantom sensation is not the focus of this chapter. Phantom limb sensation seldom causes significant disability unless the sensation is that of severe contortion of the phantom limb.

HISTORIC PERSPECTIVE

The earliest notations concerning phantom pain date back to a French military surgeon, Ambroise Paré (1510–1590) (11). Paré noted, "following the loss of a limb, the victim may continue to be conscious of the lost part with the same or ever greater clarity than the real one." Descartes made mention of a girl whose arm had been amputated at the elbow and complained about pain in the phantom fingers (12). Charles Bell (1774–1842) who also made mention of phantom limbs in his monograph entitled *The Nervous System of the Human Body* in 1830 (13,14). Gueniot (1861) was the first to formally give systematic detailed description of phantom sensations (15). Silar Weir Mitchell (1829–1914) is given credit for the development of several terms including "ghost limb," "sensory ghost," and "phantom limb," which is still used today (16). The first published account of phantom sensation was in the short story, "The Tale of George Dedlow," which appeared in *The Atlantic*

Monthly Magazine. This story was written about a soldier who loses his arm during the Civil War and later awakens in the hospital where his legs have also been amputated and stated, "I was suddenly aware of a sharp cramp in my left leg. I tried to get at it with my single arm, but, finding myself too weak, hailed an attendant. Just rub my left calf … if you please." "Calf? … you ain't got none, pardner. It's took off." Historians believe Mitchell was using this story to test the acceptance of his colleagues to the concept of pain in an absent limb. "Nearly every man who loses a limb carries about with him a constant or inconstant phantom of the missing member, a sensory ghost of that much of himself, and sometimes a most inconvenient presence, faintly left at times, but ready to be called up to his perception by a blow, a touch, or a change of the wind (17)."

DEFINITIONS

Residual Limb Pain

Residual limb pain (RLP) is a chronic pain syndrome localized to the residual limb after surgical or traumatic amputation. Jensen followed 58 amputees for 2 years and found 57% complained of residual limb pain 8 days after the amputation; 22% complained of RLP 6 months after surgery; and 10% complained of RLP after 2 years (18). Sunderland (19), Carlen (20), and Abramson (21) claim the incidence of residual limb pain is between 10 and 25%.

Phantom Sensation

Phantom sensations are sensory perceptions thought to occur in virtually all patients with amputations (22–28). Wilkins studied phantom sensation in 25 children and found the most common sensations perceived are tingling (60%), numbness (52%), tickling (32%), itching (40%), and "feels as if asleep" (40%) (29). Telescoping (movement of the distal phantom limb into the residual limb) and formication (the feeling of ants walking on the skin) of the limb is more pronounced at the distal aspect of the extremity. This phenomenon is thought to fade during the first year but may last indefinitely or may reoccur. Common triggers of phantom sensation include residual limb stimulation; not wearing a prosthesis; feeling happy, cheerful, or frightened; loud noises; or regional anesthesia (30). Phantom sensation is more likely to occur in the dominant extremity than the nondominant, perhaps due to more intricate neural interconnections (31).

Phantom Pain

Phantom pain is chronic pain syndrome that is perceived in the amputated or absent part of the body. This type of pain may be mild to severe in intensity, and may completely disrupt the function and quality of an individuals' life. The incidence of phantom pain is reported between 0 to 100%, based on the description of the pain experienced (32–36). Individuals with amputations may have single pain syndromes, or they may manifest a mixed type of PAPS including combinations of residual limb, phantom sensation, and phantom pain. A clear diagnosis is crucial, because the treatment paradigm is different for these specific types of pains.

PATHOPHYSIOLOGY: RESIDUAL LIMB PAIN

Residual limb pain occurs in all individuals having had an amputation, secondary to the stimulation of the peripheral nociceptors and their respective A-delta and C-fiber sensory fibers. Fortunately, this pain usually resolves over a 4- to 6-week period, although it occasionally it becomes long lasting and unrelenting. The primary cause of RLP is an ill-fitting prosthesis (37). Others causes include residual limb ischemia, inflammation, infection, bone spurs, neuromata, deafferentation, sympathogenic pain, referred pain, and scarring (38,39). Meticulous physical examination of the residual limb is necessary in an effort to diagnose the etiology or combination of contributing factors. Diagnostic testing may become necessary in the search for the proper diagnosis. Angiography is useful when looking for vascular abnormalities. Roentgenograms, bone scans, and magnetic resonance imaging (MRI) may be helpful if considering infections, bone spurs, or other bony abnormalities. Autonomic nervous system testing is useful to determine the degree of abnormal sympathetic nervous function. The symptoms of residual limb pain can be varied in terms of its frequency, intensity, character, location, radiation, and exacerbating factors. Clinicians must pay close attention to the descriptions of the quality of the pain used during the pain interview. These descriptions of the characteristics of the pain may be helpful in determining the etiology and treatment options. Common descriptors such as shocking, shooting, lancinating, and burning are common for patients with neuropathic pain. Cramping and spasms are common in patients with muscular contractions and can be paroxysmal or constant, creating the pains through a mechanical stimulation. Sympathogenic pain is usually described as a burning, hypersensitivity of the skin, and these descriptors are frequently accompanied by vasomotor and sudomotor changes. Referred pain is usually associated with changes secondary to abnormal gait patterns although this pain can be referred from a herniated disc, facet, sacroiliac joint, or a myofacial pain generator (40–42).

Treatment Considerations

Russell and Spalding report that one of the earliest therapies used for the treatment of postamputation pain was striking the offending residual limb with a wooden mallet several times each day (43). They report that short-term results were good; unfortunately, less than half of their patients had long-term relief. A meticulous physical examination accompanied with diagnostic testing is necessary to diagnose the cause of the residual limb pain, although occasionally the etiology cannot be determined. Residual limb pain should be evaluated by the prosthetist for signs and symptoms of a poor fitting prosthesis, and the prosthesis should be revised accordingly. The treatment of infections, bone spurs, skin ulceration, and ischemia will require appropriate medical and surgical therapies not commonly employed for phantom pain management. The sympathetic nervous system may be involved in creating a complex regional pain syndrome. Possible treatments include physical therapy, medication, peripheral nerve or spinal cord stimulation, sympathetic blockade or, in rare cases, sympathectomy. Neuromata of the residual limb are frequently blamed for the ongoing pain: "I have elsewhere said that many residual limbs are extremely sensitive, and this is especially true of the arm. In these cases it will almost always be found, upon careful examination, that certain nerves are enlarged, hardened, and tender. I have relieved a number of such cases by cold, repeated leeching, and by general irritation of the surface of the residual limb (44)." Neuromas are treated in the most conservative method possible; treatment options include mechanical padding, membrane-stabilizing medications, cryotherapy, neurolytic treatments, and surgery as a last resort. White recommends that the following procedures *not* be performed: repeated resection of neuroma, higher level amputation for pain, periarterial sympathectomies, dorsal rhizotomy, and intrathecal alcohol (45–47). Davis felt that injecting the neuroma with phenol under computed tomography (CT) guidance resulted in the most satisfying long-term results (48). White considered as possibly helpful cordotomy, single resection of a neuromata, and, occasionally, sympathectomy following a positive response to appropriate diagnostic injections (49–51). It must be remembered that surgical resection of a nerve will always result in further neuroma formation. Neuromata cannot be prevented; the new neuroma, which forms as a result of surgical management, may cause more pain than the original presurgical neuroma pain.

Medical Management

Medications may be the mainstay for treatment of residual limb pain not due to an ill-fitting prosthesis. The treatments used should be rational and directed toward the possible mechanism for the pain, based on the symptoms experienced. Unfortunately, few controlled clinical trials have linked treatments to specific symptoms and their subsequent outcomes. Medication trials should be utilized in a controlled sequential fashion in an effort to provide rational reproducible outcomes and to prevent drug interactions and excessive side effects. Pharmacologic therapies found to be effective include non-narcotic analgesics, muscle relaxants, antidepressants, anticonvulsants, local anesthetics, hormonal therapies, vasodilators, beta-blockers, NMDA receptor antagonists, and opioids. The details of these treatments are discussed later in the section under phantom pain medical management.

Physical Therapy

The literature is scarce regarding the outcome of residual limb pain when physical therapy is utilized. It is, however, without significant risk. Modalities such as heat, cold, ultrasound, transcutaneous nerve stimulation (TENS), massage, manipulation, and desensitization have been utilized with some reports of efficacy (52–54). Berger and Lundeberg believe that vibration is an effective treatment for residual limb and phantom pain (55,56).

Alternative Therapies

Alternative therapies such as acupuncture, magnets, nutritional supplements and vitamins, and "natural remedies" continue to be used although no clinical trials demonstrate their efficacy.

Summary of Treatment for Residual Limb Pain

Residual limb pain is common and appears to be a completely different diagnosis than phantom limb pain, although they can occur in concert and one may affect the other. The etiology of residual limb pain can more easily be explained anatomically and may therefore be more amendable to standard treatments such as prosthesis modifications, surgical revisions, and improved gait mechanics. Unfortunately, RLP caused by neuropathic etiologies continues to be a diagnostic and treatment challenge.

PATHOPHYSIOLOGY OF PHANTOM PAIN

The proposed theories of causation for pain can be divided into either peripheral- or central-based mechanisms.

Peripheral Theory

The theory of the peripheral nerve and its generation of phantom pain is based on the belief that a decrease in afferent input to the spinal cord can lead to a decrease in descending inhibitory influences from the central nervous system (CNS) (57,58). These decreasing descending inhibitory influences can result in the generation of phantom sensation and probably pain as well. The application of a local anesthetic block to a wide area of the body, and the subsequent development of the sensation of a phantom, best demonstrate this phenomenon (59,60). When a tourniquet is inflated on the limb, the A-delta afferent nerves are blocked, but not the smaller unmyelinated C-fibers (61). In this situation, using an incomplete anesthetic block will not produce phantom sensation. Thus, one would believe that the maintenance of afferent nerve impulses are important in the prevention of phantom sensation and possibly phantom pain as well.

Amputation is a result of a surgical intervention or a traumatic experience. As a consequence, anatomic and physiologic changes occur in the tissue nociceptors, residual nerve tissue, and the CNS. In the periphery, a nerve injury may stimulate the peripheral nociceptors and result in peripheral receptor sensitization. Once sensitization of these polymodal receptors in the damaged tissues occurs, the receptor threshold decreases. Therefore, less than the normal chemical or mechanical stimulation is required to cause excitation of the receptor, leading to depolarization of the nerve tissue and subsequent conductance to the spinal cord. This sensitization phenomena may contribute to the development of the allodynic (pain induced by a normally nonpainful stimulus) and hyperalgesic (enhanced sensation of pain from a normally painful stimulus) characteristics in patients with PAPS.

Transection of a peripheral nerve results in an immediate explosive discharge of afferent impulses into the spinal cord and can be blocked by prior application of local anesthetic. Soon after transection, the early injury discharges decrease and the nerve becomes silent. Interestingly, transection of the nerve results in a much more violent barrage than does a crush injury (62). Shortly after the injury, the cell body receives a message from the point of injury that causes the synthesis of substances in the cell body to change. This alteration in the chemical composition of the cell body then alters the axonal transport of substances to the terminal afferent, resulting in sprouting. Following this initial excitation phase, the nerve becomes silent until sprouting occurs within the first 24 hours. Sprouting (up to 50 sprouts per axon) is the act of attempting peripheral nerve regeneration. Sprouts will grow in a random and chaotic fashion in an effort to re-establish a connection with the distal, injured component. In the case of amputation, in which there is no distal component, sprouts will invade the connective tissue, blood vessels, or may grow back into the proximal central residual nerve. This creates an alteration in the normal blood–nerve barrier (similar to the blood–brain barrier) that exists around normal healthy nerves. The cut terminal end (even if ligated) can be exposed to chemical influences such as epinephrine, norepinephrine, and acetylcholine elaborated from the sympathetic or motor nerve terminals. The impulses generated by the sympathetic or motor efferents to the distal terminal can chemically stimulate the distal injured sensory afferent nerve. This interaction between efferent nerves and sensory afferent nerves may be perceived as pain. This cross talk between the efferent and afferent terminal ends is referred to as *ephaptic stimulation*. Peripheral nerve sprouts can become permanently established, may spontaneously degenerate. The sprouts that do not degenerate or re-establish connection consolidate and become a stable neuroma, which allows for the potential generation of abnormal discharges into the CNS. Cajal demonstrated that nerves, which are partially transected and immediately resutured, contain a large number of sprouts that will progress to form a partial neuroma around an intact nerve (63).

Microneurographic studies performed by Nystrom and Hagbarth identified spontaneous activity in the axons of transected nerves (64). Neuromas have three functional options: 1) they can be silent and create no pain, 2) they generate abnormal nerve impulses that may be perceived as pain, or 3) they can be susceptible to the influences of cross talk. This proposal is more likely to explain residual limb pain and may be a contributor to phantom pain. Peripheral nerve resections proximal to the area of injury, such as dorsal ganglionectomies or dorsal root resections, do not relieve the phantom pain. Anesthetic blockade of the peripheral nerve or the spinal cord has on occasion initiated or magnified the phantom pain problem (65–68).

A series of changes occur centrally following peripheral nerve injury including:

- A decrease in fluoride-resistant acid phosphatase in lamina I and II (69);
- a decrease in the substance P concentrations in the afferent nerve fibers (70);
- anatomic changes in the substantia gelatinosa and dorsal horn (71); and
- sympathetic invasion of the dorsal root ganglion (72,73). These anatomic changes result in an alteration in the receptive fields of the injured and noninjured nerves in the proximity of injury. Dorsal

column nuclei adopt a new receptive field once they lose their original receptive field (74). These changes have also been observed to occur in the spinal cord, thalmus, and cortex. The changes in the CNS and periphery following nerve injury are referred to as *plastic* changes. (Plasticity refers to an ability to change from one form to another.) No method is known to reverse these changes once they have occurred.

PERIPHERAL THEORY PHYSIOLOGICAL CONSIDERATIONS

Biochemically, afferent nerve transmission occurs from the periphery to the CNS primarily by the fast-conducting myelinated A-delta fibers and the slower unmyelinated C-fibers. When these fibers are stimulated, or damaged, they release neurotransmitters, which are chemicals that stimulate or modulate nerve conduction. The neurotransmitters are divided into two families, the excitatory amino acids (EAA) and the neurokinins (75–79). The EAA of concern are L-aspartate, L-glutamate, and L-homocysteate, all of which are released in response to stimulation by the A-delta fibers. The neurokinins are polypeptides like substance P, neurokinin A, neurokinin B, and are released by the stimulation of the C-fibers. The other important non-neurokinin neuropeptide released by the C-fiber is calcitonin gene related peptide (CGRP). The release of these chemicals results in complex interactions with their respective CNS receptors. The primary glutamate receptor in the CNS is the N-methyl-D-aspartate (NMDA) receptor, of which there are several subtypes (80–82). It is theorized that stimulation of this receptor results in the clinical manifestations of allodynia, hyperalgesia, expansion of receptive fields, and opioid tolerance. Agents that block this receptor subtype may then cause a decrease in allodynia (pain with nonpainful stimuli), hyperalgesia (excessive pain to painful stimuli), phantom pain, and the spread of pain (increased receptive fields) in diseases such as complex regional pain syndrome. For an excellent review of the CNS cascade, please refer to Devor (83) or Blumenkop (84).

In summary, this massive alteration in normal physiology can result in the creation of spontaneous pain generators in the periphery, spinal cord, and brain without having ongoing peripheral nerve stimulation. The exact biochemistry of phantom pain specifically has yet to be completely elucidated; however, the above discussion most likely plays a large role in the generation of phantom pain. Therefore, the goal should be to prevent these changes by aggressive medical and surgical treatments rather than attempt to correct the neural plasticity once it has occurred.

The Central Theory of Phantom Pain

In 1978 Loeser and Melzack described the development of a phantom body in paraplegics with complete spinal cord transection and proposed a central pain generating mechanism (85). In 1989 Melzack concluded, "you don't need a body to feel a body" and that "the brain itself can generate every quality of experience which is normally triggered by sensory input (86)." At least two competing central theories exist: one consists of the body engram (87,88); the other of the concept of dynamic reverberation (89). An *engram* is defined as a pattern of nervous activity established in the performing a skilled act. Wall, in the 1980s, began exploring the possibility that the adult brain was capable of physiologic and functional changes (90). Prior to that time, it was assumed that once connections were made in early life (an engram) they could never be changed, thus very little functional restoration was possible after an injury to the CNS. Researchers diverge at this level into essentially two theoretic camps: those who believe that the CNS maintains an "active body-neuromatrix" or "neurosignature" (91), and those who subscribe to the idea that reorganization of receptive fields occur and this "reorganization" contributes to phantom sensation and pain (92).

Recently, it has become evident that the CNS is capable of an incredible amount of functional change following an injury to a peripheral nerve (93). Kaas demonstrated that after amputation or peripheral nerve denervation in adult mammals, the brain could undergo massive reorganization of the somatosensory cortex (94). Pons et al. discovered that 12 years after deafferentation of one limb in an adult primate, the cortical area of the brain corresponding to the limb was responsive to stimulation of the lower face (95). This data has now been confirmed and reproduced in human beings after amputation (96,97). After peripheral nerve transection the receptive fields (those areas of the CNS corresponding to a specific sensory location) of large areas in the dorsal columns, thalamus, and cortex begin receiving input from surrounding intact tissue. Interestingly, this is demonstrated by stimulating tissue far away from the amputation site and having the patient perceive stimulation of the phantom limb. This is termed *remodeling*. Remodeling can be demonstrated both clinically—for example, by stroking the ipsilateral face and having the sensation referred to the amputated limb (98)—or with the use of neuromagnetic imaging techniques (99). Somatotropic reorganization (remapping) in the human is thought to take considerable time, although the same changes in animal models seems to occur in weeks (100,101). This may suggest that these connections were present prior to the injury and were simply dormant, or that more rapid plastic changes occur in an effort to "fill in the gaps" of the receptive fields left by parts of the CNS not experiencing afferent input. The above theory then suggests that phantom pain and sensation is maintained by other tissues in the body somatotropically filling in for the lost part as a form of normal compensation in the CNS. It appears that the CNS is attempting to keep all areas active and functioning, if not through their original location then through another possibly shared area. Canavero suggests a second central theory: He proposes the presence of a localized corticothalamic reverberatory loop in the brain that may serve to maintain central and phantom pain (102). It has been reported in the literature that some cases of phantom pain disappears after brain lesions (103). These brain lesions typically involve the thalamus or corticothalamocortical fibers contralaterally to the phantom pain. It is postulated that lesions of the corona radiata, deep to the frontoparietal sensorimotor strip, or electroconvulsive therapy may block or cancel the reverberations in both central and phantom pain syndromes.

In summary, the pathogenesis of phantom pain still eludes us. Neither the central nor the peripheral theories alone account for all the physiologic and anatomic changes. More research clearly needs to be completed if we are to clearly understand and prevent the occurrences of these pain syndromes.

Treatments of Phantom Pain

Well-controlled clinical trials regarding the treatments of phantom pain are rare and complicated by our lack of understanding regarding the etiology of phantom pain. Sherman provides us with an extensive review of possible treatment strategies; unfortunately most are prone to failure (104). Sherman suggests that if medications are to be considered, they need to be matched to the appropriate pain descriptor. For example, cold sensation is treated with vasodilating agents; cramping sensations are treated with agents to relieve muscle spasms, and the like. Clinicians must use rational judgment when pursuing a treatment algorithm and use the most conservative methods available before progressing to potentially harmful, more aggressive interventional management. Extensive research is now being directed toward the prevention of PAPS, because PAPS is frequently refractory to treatment modalities once established.

Neurostimulation Therapy

Mitchell was the first to use electricity in the treatment of phantom pain and referred to this as *faradism*. Unfortunately, this technique frequently resulted in the re-emergence of the phantom pain rather than an improvement

(105). Shealy reported that use of transcutaneous electrical nerve stimulation (TENS) was effective in reducing the incidence of phantom pain after 4 months, but not after more than 1 year (106). Finsen et al. reported that when TENS had been applied, the results were short lived at best; no long-term improvements could be found (107,108). Klinger and Kepplinger reported that in 25 patients who were treated with a variety of devices and stimulation patterns, no differences in effectiveness were observed (109). Katz reported the use of contralateral TENS application in an effort to facilitate inhibitory control and decrease or eliminate pain when ipsilateral application exaggerates the pain (110).

Peripheral nerve stimulation or the application of the stimulating electrode directly to the nerve has been utilized in the treatment of various pain syndromes. The basis for this type of treatment may involve an alteration in neurotransmitters or possibly neuromodulation of inhibitory fibers, either peripherally or centrally (111,112). Recanzone et al. observed that ulnar nerve stimulation increased the receptive field size in the primary somatosensory cortex in cats contralateral to the side of stimulation. The widespread analgesic response was reversed by administration of naloxone (113). Campbell implanted peripheral nerve stimulators in thirty-three patients; seventeen patients were treatment failures, eight patients had excellent results, and seven had intermediate results (114). The most dramatic success occurred in patients with peripheral nerve trauma. Picaza implanted twenty-three patients and followed them for 6 to 20 months. Twenty patients estimated their relief between 50 and 100%, with reduced drug intake and improved social performance (115). A potential problem with this technique may be the inadvertent stimulation of motor as well as sensory axons when applied to a mixed nerve for analgesic purposes [personal communication with J.Law M.D (116).]

Spinal cord stimulation is a technique in which electrodes are implanted in the epidural region of the spinal canal either surgically or percutaneously. Krainick and Thoden reported good initial results (26 to 100% pain relief), which unfortunately decreased from 52% in two years to 39% at 5-year follow-up (117). Kumar et al. implanted two PLP patients; neither patient obtained relief of pain (118). Hunt et al. reported excellent relief in one of five PLP patients, with a follow-up of 3 years (119). These investigators reported good results related to the relief of burning and sharp pain in the residual limb and phantom, but severe episodic throbbing pains were not suppressed.

Deep brain stimulation has been reported by Mundinger to result in an 86% improvement in 30 patients afflicted with PLP (120). The procedure requires that the stimulation be applied to the thalamus, periventricular gray matter, and/or internal capsule. The results of using brain stimulation combined with transcutaneous stimulation resulted in a 93% success rate in 14 patients treated (121). Neurosurgeons believe the results are better when single stimulation is applied to the thalamic structures rather than to the periaqueductal gray areas. For a more complete review of the proposed mechanism of brain stimulation, refer to Bonica (122). In summary, neurostimulation is most effective when combined with pharmacologic or other techniques to control both baseline pain and severe episodic pain. Although the available studies are few, the result is frequently good short-term relief. Unfortunately, long-term improvement is less encouraging.

Surgery Considerations

The utilization of surgical interventions in the treatment of phantom pain has been tried for over a century, but the results are dismal for long-term success (123). White and Sweet described at least eleven possible surgical options for the treatment of phantom pain (124). These surgical treatments can be divided into those directed either at the peripheral nervous system (PNS) or the CNS. Cerebral vascular accidents have in some cases resulted in a loss or a decrease in the phantom sensations; for this reason it was thought perhaps destruction of a part of the brain could improve PAPS. Unfortunately, prefrontal lobotomy, anterior cingulate lesions, parietal lobotomy, ablation of the post central gyrus, thalamic surgery, cervical tractotomy, rhizotomy, midbrain lesions, and anterolateral chordotomy have all been attempted with variable degrees of success; they are seldom used today (125).

Nashold developed a new approach for the treatment of pain utilizing radiofrequency thermocontrolled coagulation of the spinal substantia gelatinosa, referred to as dorsal root entry zone (DREZ) surgery (126). The rational for this approach is that the integration of multiple sensory input in this area can produce abnormal neuronal discharges and can be perceived as pain when sent to higher levels. Nashlod and Ostadahl used DREZ surgery in 21 patients with phantom limb pain associated with brachial plexus avulsions and claimed good relief in 67% (127). Saris et al. used DREZ in 22 patients with amputation for more conventional reasons (cancer, trauma, and vascular insufficiency). The results in these patients was not as satisfying, with only 33% obtaining alleviation of their pain after 6 months to 4 years of follow-up. The subjects in this group then underwent a more "refined" technique and received good results in 60% of cases (128). The most common complications of DREZ were cerebrospinal fluid leak, persistent postoperative weakness or numbness, or sphincter dysfunction.

In summary, DREZ surgery has been helpful in a number of cases of phantom pain; it is more therapeutic in the treatment of brachial plexus avulsion and cannot be accepted as the universal cure of phantom pain. Surgery techniques for residual limb pain have been used since the time of Mitchell, but, for the most part, are not useful for the treatment of phantom pain (129). Resection of a single painful neuroma or revision of the bone has been useful when symptoms are due to mechanical pressure and confirmed by diagnostic injections. The subsequent nerve resection will result in the formation of new neuromata that may be better, worse, or the same as the existing condition. Therefore, repeated neuroma resections are discouraged since they are not likely to be beneficial long term for residual limb or phantom pain.

Injection Therapy

Injections have long been utilized in the treatment of residual limb and phantom pain; the benefits are short term and more diagnostic than therapeutic. The injection is usually made with a combination of local anesthetic and steroid and may decrease the inflammation around the irritable focus of a neuroma that has taken on a pacemaker-like function. Potentially helpful injections include bone injections, peripheral nerve blocks, spinal injections, trigger points, sympathetic nerve blocks, neurolytic, motor point blocks, and (possibly) botulism toxin injections. Sporadic reports exist of injections being helpful; however, the benefits are generally transient at best unless a clear diagnosis of sympathetic dystrophy or myofacial pain can be determined. Continuous peripheral nerve infusion therapy, or utilizing a catheter to deliver local anesthetic to eliminate preoperative, intraoperative, and postoperative pain, has been considered helpful in an effort to prevent phantom pain. This concept is discussed later under preventive techniques. Gross injected mepivacaine into the hyperalgesic regions of the contralateral limb of four patients with phantom and residual limb pain. All patients reported good relief in 6-month to 2-year-follow-ups; one patient had a return of pain 3 years after initial injection (130). Davis reports good results in reducing residual limb pain by injecting phenol into the neuroma with CT guidance (131). The use of regional anesthesia after phantom pain has once been established is adequate for the transient anesthetic effect, but it may increase or have no effect on the overall phantom pain experience.

Medication

The use of medications in the treatment of phantom pain has been extensive. No single drug regime or combination therapy has been found to universally cure or palliate this syndrome (132). A review of the various treatments and potential future medication management is presented. No drug dosages will be suggested since the patient's age and general medical condition governs the dosages, frequency, and method of dose escalation.

Nonsteroidal Anti-Inflammatory Drugs (NSAIDs)

NSAIDs are used in the treatment of virtually all pain syndromes. The pharmacology is primarily through the prevention of prostaglandin formation by inhibition of cyclooxygenase II (133). Prostaglandins have the ability to stimulate inflammation in the tissues and increase pain. Wartan et al. found NSAIDs to be helpful especially when combined with TENS in controlling phantom pain (134). Vasko suggests that prostaglandins have a direct effect at the level of the spinal cord to enhance nociception primarily through substance P release (135). This substance P release was abolished by intrathecal ketorolac, probably through the inhibition of prostaglandin production. NSAIDs may have both a peripheral and central action and can be analgesic when administered in the spinal fluid (136). Unfortunately, no NSAID is approved for intrathecal use.

Antidepressants

Tricyclic antidepressants (TCAs) have been used extensively over the years for the treatment of depression as well as for chronic pain (137,138). These medicines seem to work best in the treatment of neuropathic pain states because of their ability to alter the relative state of the neurotransmitter around nerve tissue by inhibiting the membrane pump mechanism responsible for the uptake of norepinephrine and serotonin (139). Serotonin is thought to modulate the descending inhibitory influences to the dorsal horn and suppress pain transmission. The most studied TCA type drug is amitriptyline, but others in this class may be better choices because of a decreased side effect profile. These include nortriptyline, desipramine, or imipramine. The adverse reactions of most concern are anticholinergic, cardiovascular, and neurologic. The side effects of TCA medication can limit their usefulness as the primary agent; they may, however, be used as adjuvant medications in smaller and better-tolerated doses. It is also thought that amitriptyline is an NMDA receptor antagonist drug in vitro and may inhibit the NMDA receptor activation–induced neuroplasticity associated with nerve injuries. Recently, it is thought that use of amitriptyline intraspinally may be more effective for pain relief, but more studies need to be performed (140).

Selective serotonin reuptake inhibitors (SSRIs) are effective for the treatment of depression and are relatively devoid of cardiac toxicity and anticholinergic and antihistaminic effects. SSRIs are less effective in the treatment of pain syndromes than TCAs but can be used to treat the common ancillary comorbidities associated with PAPS. In controlled studies, paroxetine has been shown to provide analgesia in patients with painful neuropathy (141). In one case report, fluoxetine was used to cure a 71-year-old man with a 5-year history of phantom limb pain manifested as severe itching, stabbing cramps, and "hit by lightening sensation" (142).

Anticonvulsants Medications

Anticonvulsants, as a class of drug, have been used extensively in the treatment of phantom and other neuropathic pain states with variable results. The most commonly used anticonvulsant is carbamazepine (143), although phenytoin, valproic acid, and clonazepam have also been tried with varying results (144–146). The mechanism of carbamazepine, phenytoin, and valproic acid appears to be through slowing the rate of recovery of voltage-activated sodium channels, which prolongs depolarization of the neural tissue (147). A proposed mechanism of clonazepam is through its ability to mimic the effects of glycine, which is thought to result in an inhibition of CNS neurotransmitters (148).

Gabapentin is a newer antiseizure medication that acts by an unknown mechanism (possibly via calcium channel modulation) to release gamma amino butyric acid (GABA) CNS. It is being used extensively in the treatment of pain disorders (149).

Topiramate, lamotrigine, zonisamide, tigabine, and felbamate are all new anticonvulsants and are being tried for the treatment of various neuropathic pain disorders; as of this writing, no clinical trials for PAPS are available at this time. The sole use of these medications or combinations do not generally abolish the postamputation pain, but they are useful as adjuvant agents.

Antihypertensive Therapy

Propranolol is a beta receptor-blocker that decreases the effects of circulating catecholamines and is thought to increase serotonin levels in ways similar to benzodiazepines and TCAs (150). Medications in this class may be helpful as adjuvants in the treatment of pain syndromes that have an increased sympathetic tone or signs of vasoconstriction and cold extremities (151–154).

Clonidine hydrochloride stimulates the alpha-2 adrenoreceptor in the brain stem and results in a decrease in sympathetic outflow from the CNS, then a decrease in peripheral vascular resistance and improved blood flow (155,156). Clonidine has been helpful in various pain syndromes, especially in those conditions with high sympathetic tone (157). Clonidine preparations are available for oral, transdermal, and intraspinal use. When instilled into the spinal canal along with diamorphine and bupivacaine, clonidine was found helpful in the prevention of PLP (158,159).

HORMONAL THERAPY

Calcitonin is a polypeptide hormone secreted by the parafollicular cells of the thyroid gland and involved in the regulation of calcium and phosphate metabolism. Calcitonin has been reported of benefit in some patients with phantom pain (160). The mechanism of calcitonin in the treatment of pain problems is still not clear. Mertz first recognized the analgesic qualities of salmon calcitonin in humans in 1986 (161). Calcitonin has been shown to elevate the levels of B-endorphins in humans. However, it is thought to act independently from the normal endogenous opioid system (162). Animal studies suggest that the analgesic effect are independent of the opiate receptors (163,164). Clementi and Candeletti hypothesize that the effects are mediated through central serotoninergic pathways (165–167). Therefore, calcitonin may act by way of the serotoninergic mechanism to increase descending inhibitory influences and suppress phantom pain. Jaeger, in a double-blind study, concludes that I.V. infusion of salmon calcitonin resulted in the significant relief and prevention of PLP after amputation if administered early (168). Fiddler reports the abrupt elimination of spinal anesthesia–induced PLP with the infusion of I.V. calcitonin (169). Intrathecal or epidural calcitonin does produce analgesia, but unfortunately tolerance did occur and safety is a concern (170–173). Calcitonin is not approved for the treatment of PLP by the FDA and may be associated with side effects such as nausea, vomiting, allergic reaction, and hypocalcemia.

In summary, calcitonin has been administered via numerous routes with various successes. However, the most effective dose and route is still unknown.

SUBSTANCE P MEDICATION

Capsaicin, a substance P depletion agent, has demonstrated efficacy for PAPS when applied to the skin of the residual limb (174–176). Capsaicin is thought to trigger membrane depolarization by opening ion channels permeable to sodium and calcium. Application is usually accompanied with an initial intense burning sensation followed by nociceptor desensitization and subsequent analgesia. Application to the skin must be continued indefinitely to maintain the beneficial effects. Successes with this treatment are usually limited, due to lack of patient compliance to the recommended treatment regime. Sporadic reports suggest the application of very high potency capsaicin to patients with the assistance of regional anesthesia (177). Theoretically, this depletes the greatest amount of substance P with the least amount of pain. Substance P will accumulate after emergence from anesthesia if less potent doses are not continued to maintain the depleted state. The optimal concentration and time of application for this treatment needs further study.

ANTI-ARRHYTHYMIC MEDICATION

Mexiletine, like lidocaine, is a class IB antiarrhythmic with sodium channel-blocking capabilities. It is normally prescribed for the treatment of cardiac ectopy (178). Blockade of the fast sodium channels results in a decrease in the activation potential and an increase in the refractory period of neurons (179). Amputation patients are known to develop hyperirritable foci in the wide dynamic range neurons of the dorsal horn and thalamus. These are called "bursting cells" (180–185). This ongoing nociceptive activity of the wide dynamic range neurons can become self-sustaining and is directed centrally via the lateral spinal thalamic track (186). Mexiletine could block the sodium channels of the damaged neurons in the dorsal horn and thalamus after amputation and modulate the ongoing neuronal activity. Davis reports excellent results in eighteen of thirty-one patients with PLP; eleven of the other patients responded favorably to a combination of mexiletine and clonidine; two patients had no response (187). Mexiletine is contraindicated in patients with second- and third-degree heart block and is associated with reversible gastrointestinal symptoms that may prevent adequate dosing (188).

MUSCLE RELAXANT MEDICATIONS

Baclofen is a centrally acting agent reported to result in pain relief because of its similarity to GABA. The primary indications for baclofen are for the treatment of spastic disorders found in spinal cord injuries, multiple sclerosis, or amyotrophic lateral sclerosis. Baclofen has been reported beneficial in patients suffering from trigeminal neuralgia (189). Iacono et al. found baclofen helpful when combined with propranolol and phenytoin in two patients with autonomous shoulder movement and phantom pain (190). Spasms are common in the residual limbs of amputees, and thus baclofen may reduce this type of pain.

Tizanidine hydrochloride (Zanaflex®) is a recently released centrally acting alpha 2 adrenergic agonist that theoretically decreases spasticity by increasing the presynaptic inhibition of motor neurons (191). The effect of these actions is thought to decrease facilitation of spinal motor neurons. The primary indication of tizanidine is for the acute and intermittent management of increased muscle tone or muscle spasms. Muscle spasms or cramping is a common feature of individuals suffering from both phantom and residual limb pains. A recent Russian review suggested that tizanidine was helpful especially when administered as an adjuvant medication with beta-blockers and a TCA (192,193).

ANTIPSYCHOTICS MEDICATION

Neuroleptic agents such as phenothiazines and butyrophenones are primarily used in the treatment of psychoses but can also alter central interpretation of pain. Logan reports a dramatic improvement using chlorpromazine in a patient with 30 years of persistent PLP (194). The outcome reports produced by these agents, including the benzamides, suggest 40 to 100% improvement, although no time frame was available (195–197). Neuroleptic agents are seldom used in the treatment of PAPS because of the side effects of tardive dyskinesia, sedation, or impaired mental functioning. The newer medications such as olanzapine and risperidone may hold promise due to reduced side effects; clinical trials will need to be performed.

NMDA RECEPTOR ANTAGONIST

Ketamine is classified as an arylcycloalkyamine and is related to the street drug phencyclidine (PCP). The primary use of ketamine in the last 30 years has been as a dissociative anesthetic. Ketamine activates the limbic system and depresses the cerebral cortex, producing profound analgesia and amnesia. Ketamine has gained popularity because of its antagonist effect on the NMDA receptor. Hyperactivity of the NMDA receptor for glutamate has been theorized to be involved in the maintenance of neuropathic pain and PAPS. This hyperactivity is believed to be an adaptive response of the spinal cord and perhaps brain to peripheral nerve injury. Ketamine is used as a noncompetitive antagonist of the NMDA receptor to prevent or decrease those CNS plastic changes that occur with some nerve injuries (198). Nikolajsen treated eleven patients with well-established PAPS with intravenous ketamine; all patients responded with a decrease in pain rating (199). Stannard successfully treated three cases of PLP with intravenous ketamine; all required ongoing infusions to maintain the improved state, and had complications (200). Ketamine is poorly absorbed orally and hence is given in very large oral doses, or compounded for transcutaneous, parenteral, or intraspinal administration. The NMDA receptor area is a very active field of research at this time not only because of the CNS implications, but also because of the relationship of this receptor to the development of opioid tolerance.

Amantadine (Symmetrel®) is an antiviral agent that inhibits the replication of Influenza A virus. Interestingly,

it also acts as an NMDA receptor antagonist and has been reported to be effective in the treatment of neuropathic pain (201). Eisenberg describes three patients who reported complete relief of chronic neuropathic pain after intravenous administration of amantadine, presumably due to termination of the CNS wind-up phenomena (202). No clinical trials were found regarding the use of amantadine in the treatment of PAPS, specifically, although it is probably worth trying.

Dextromethorphan (DM) is the D-isomer of levorphanol (levo-dromoran); unlike the L-isomer there is no analgesic and minimal addictive effects, and the effects are not mediated through the opioid receptors system (203,204). Dextromethorphan is primarily regarded as an antitussive, but recently DM and its demethylated derivative, dextrorphan, have been studied for their neuroprotective and antiepileptic properties (205). The theoretical advantage of dextromethorphan is in regard to the noncompetitive blockade of the NMDA receptor the potential benefits of reduced wind-up and CNS plasticity, and in the prevention of opioid tolerance (206).

Dextromethorphan is undergoing clinical trials in the treatment of neuropathic pain disorders of diabetic neuropathy and postherpetic neuralgia (207,208). The dosages required to affect the NMDA receptor and outcomes are yet to be determined. Dextromethorphan at this time is either being purchased over the counter, or it is compounded and used as an adjuvant medication to opioid treatments. The optimum ratio of dextromethorphan to opioid is yet to be determined in an effort to decrease opioid tolerance. No clinical trials regarding the use of dextromethorphan in the treatment of PAPS were found, although a new fixed combination of morphine and dextromethorphan is being studied for all opioid-responsive pain syndromes.

OPIOID MEDICATION

Opioid medications have long been used in the treatment of virtually all pain syndromes. The classic belief is that opioids are very effective in the treatment of somatic but not neuropathic pains (209), and that opioids should be reserved for short-term use only because of the potential for addiction. These beliefs are gradually fading as more recent studies suggest that the incidence of addiction with the long term use of opioids ranges from 5 to 20% (210–212). Urban safely and successfully managed five consecutive patients with intractable phantom pain using a combination of narcotic and antidepressants with no signs of addiction (213). Opioids will result in physical dependency; when stopped abruptly or when an antagonist is administered, patients will experience physical withdrawal symptoms. However, addiction is a psychiatric diagnosis and is associated with the use of chemicals despite harm and accompanied by other drug seeking behaviors. Addiction is seldom seen in pain patients taking stable doses of opioid analgesics under close monitoring. Obviously, the pain being treated must be opioid responsive, and the World Health Organization (WHO) Guidelines should be followed, using an analgesic ladder and incorporating the use of adjuvant medications (214).

Medical societies across the country are developing opioid treatment guidelines that, when followed, should allow the treating physician the option to use opioids in a responsible manner without the interference of regulatory agencies. Opioids can be useful for the treatment of PAPS, especially when utilized with other adjuvant medication; the primary risks are sedation, constipation, nausea, and possible addiction. It is known that individuals with previous histories of substance abuse or bipolar disorder stand a much greater risk of developing addiction problems (215). The management of these individuals can be very taxing and should be directed to a specialized pain clinic. In my opinion, if opioid medications are to be utilized, the patient should be carefully monitored and should clearly demonstrate improved function as a result of these medications. Monitoring may require frequent visits, with careful documentation of pain levels, side-effects, functional change, utilization of emergency rooms, random urine testing, and a well designed treatment plan.

Informed consent and a contract should be utilized explaining the risks, benefits, and pros and cons of pain treatment using opioids. This contract should lay out treatment guidelines and contingencies for uncontrolled pain. Continuous release medications are preferred for chronic daily therapy in an effort to keep constant pain under control; rescue medications can be added if necessary between long-acting doses. Opioids can be prescribed as needed with short-acting medications if the pain is episodic and of short duration. Methadone is the opioid of choice if tolerated in my opinion because it is inexpensive, has an analgesic duration of 6 to 8 hours, has an onset rapid enough to act as a rescue medication, and possesses NMDA receptor antagonist properties.

Methadone comes as a racemic mixture with the L-isomer acting as the analgesic and the D-isomer acting as the opioid inactive form; both isomers exhibit low affinities to the NMDA receptor (216). Caution regarding the use of methadone for analgesia is necessary, and the clinician must become familiar with the idiosyncrasies of the drug. Although the analgesic effect of methadone usually last 6 to 8 hours, it can be used as a long-acting medication and as a rescue medication. Methadone can accumulate as the dosing regime continues resulting in catastrophic overdose effects if one is not totally familiar with the specific half-life of the drug. If methadone is chosen as the analgesic of choice, increase the dose slowly to allow for the accumulation effect.

Use caution when converting from other opioids to methadone because of the differences in absorption, half life, and possible change in opioid tolerance.

Theoretically, an opioid with an NMDA receptor antagonist may act to partially inhibit the development of opioid tolerance and perhaps block the CNS plasticity changes that may contribute to PAPS (217–219). The unique characteristics of methadone may make it the opioid of choice for neuropathic pain of all types if the side effects are tolerable. Trials of other opioids are reasonable if pain is severe, and long-acting morphine, oxycodone, hydromorphone, or fentanyl should be used when necessary because patients differ in their response to analgesic therapy (220).

The advent of epidural and subarachnoid infusion devices has rapidly advanced the treatment of acute and chronic pain and lessened systemic side effects. Numerous medications are now delivered by this method, including baclofen, clonidine, opioids, local anesthetics, and buprenorphine (221), and infusion devices may become the method of choice in the future.

BENZODIAZEPINES

Benzodiazepines (e.g., diazepam, lorazepam, alprazolam) are mentioned only to condemn their routine use in the treatment of pain syndromes. Patients using these medications generally do poorly and frequently develop depressive symptoms and cognitive impairment (222). Benzodiazepines used concomitantly with opioids may result in a progression of tolerance that makes higher doses necessary for adequate analgesia (223)

MISCELLANEOUS MEDICATION

Sporadic case reports arise in the literature regarding the use of lysergic acid diethyl amide (LSD) (224–226) and the oral form of tetrahydro-cannbinol (THC), marketed as marinol (227), although no clinical trials are available. Zeltser believes that the enantiomeric form of THC, which is not psychotropic, has NMDA receptor antagonist properties and has potential to reduce pain (228).

Psychological Aspects and Interventions

Sherman surveyed 2,700 amputees and reported that these individuals were fearful to confide in their physicians about their phantom pain (229). Patients fear being labeled as crazy and creating conflict with their physician. Kolb and Riddoch view phantom pain as due in part to emotional problems such as fear, fatigue, insomnia, grief, and stress (230,231). Melzack reported that amputees have no more tendencies toward neurosis than the normal population (232). Shukla reported that only 1% of the amputee study group was categorized as psychotic (233). When amputees from surgical and rehabilitation hospitals are evaluated, 20 to 60% are diagnosed as clinically depressed or psychosomatic in nature (234,235). Sherman concludes "that there is no convincing evidence that major personality disorders are important in the etiology of phantom pain nor that they are more prevalent among those amputees reporting phantom pain than among those not reporting it (236)."

Post traumatic stress disorder (PTSD) is periodic or continuous rumination regarding a traumatic event. PTSD is common in PAPS patients and can be a source of tremendous anxiety and fear. It should be treated aggressively by psychiatrists and psychologists familiar with the syndrome. Should depression, anxiety, or psychosis be diagnosed, it should be treated as if it occurred in an individual in the general population. Depression, anxiety, or psychosis may be an exacerbating factor of the pain but is not the etiology. Education, reassurance, and patient empowerment are the most useful tools when utilized prior to an amputation to ameliorate the constellation of symptoms surrounding the loss of a limb.

Sleep Disorder Therapy

Sleep disturbances are universal in the chronic pain population. An individual's ability to cope with the daily rigors of a chronic pain syndrome requires adequate hours and quality of sleep. Therefore, a necessary first step in the treatment process of any pain syndrome mandates providing the medication and sleep instruction/hygiene to minimize insomnia.

Biofeedback

Biofeedback is a training program designed to develop the individual's ability to control muscle tone and the autonomic (involuntary) and somatic nervous system. Electromyographic studies suggest that major muscles of the residual limbs may reveal increased tone and exacerbate the symptoms of phantom pain (237,238). Sherman has demonstrated that the burning sensation frequently felt in the residual limb is related to a decrease in blood flow (239). Biofeedback can be an effective treatment in the management of phantom limb pain, especially when temperature and muscle tension monitors are used. This type of treatment has been utilized successfully when the character of the pain is described as burning or cramping, which may indicate evidence of vasospasm or abnormal muscle tension as a contributing factor (240).

Relaxation Training and Hypnosis

Sherman reports that twelve of fourteen patients derived benefit from relaxation and imagery training, which has been utilized in the treatment of many forms of chronic pain (241). This technique may be especially helpful if evidence exists of high stress or an anxiety disorder. Hypnosis has been reported helpful in receptive individuals who can practice the technique themselves (242).

Acupuncture and Magnetic Therapy

Acupuncture treatments have been utilized in an attempt to control both phantom pain and residual limb pain. Unfortunately, no well-controlled studies are available (243,244). Chong-Cheng found that acupuncture not only failed to relieve phantom pain but actually exacerbated it; he recommended acupuncture be used as a research tool only (245). Further investigation is necessary. Freed (246) presented a review of acupuncture for the treatment of phantom pain and related the effectiveness to the resulting body "stillness." The stillness was thought to be related to alpha rhythm prominence on EEG, deep general relaxation, an increased pain threshold, and total body involvement. When acupuncture is utilized, the improvement is short term only. Clearly this technique requires a more critical evaluation.

Tovsa treated ten patients with phantom leg pain using the application of magnets to the skin of the thorax and the ipsilateral cranial ends of the Yin meridians, which originate in the leg. Eight of the patients obtained some relief; two patients were nonresponders in the 1-day to 26-month follow-up (247).

Visualization

Ramachandran has studied the effects of visual input on phantom sensations using a device referred to as a "virtual reality box" to visually reconstruct the phantom limb to study sensory effects. A mirror is placed beside the intact limb, thus creating a mirror image that looks like the phantom limb. In six patients in whom the normal hand was moved, the eye saw the phantom limb move; these sensations were felt in the phantom hand. In five patients with painful clenching sensation in the phantom hand, the mirror was utilized to project opening the hand; this relieved the sensation in four of the patients. In three patients, touching the normal hand evoked exact localized touch sensation in the phantom hand (248). In summary, a great amount of interaction exists between the visual system and proprioception; this technique may be helpful to alter sensations of the phantom limb in a contorted and painful position.

PHANTOM PAIN IN CHILDREN

Diverse literature documents the incidence of phantom pain in children. Historically it was believed that children with amputations or congenital limb deficiencies did not experience phantom pain or sensations. This now has come into dispute, and it is now recognized that children with congenitally absent limbs can have the experience of phantom sensation, although not vivid or precise in its quality (249,250). Krane and Heller found the prevalence on phantom pain in pediatric amputees to be 92%, although no age parameters were listed (251). Simmel gathered information regarding the occurrence of phantom limb pain in pediatric amputees (252). She found that phantom pain is rare in children before the age of 4. In children 8 years of age or older, the frequency of PAPS is equal to that of the adult population. Smith et al. believes that biomedical risk factors, such as cancer or chemotherapy, predispose children to phantom pain (253). The above information, although interesting, is not precise; it does, however, seem to show a correlation between the incidence of phantom pain and age. The development of kinaesthetic and deep pressure sensitivity prior to the amputation is felt to be the governing factor regarding the incidence of PAPS (254), thus it is reasonable to utilize all modalities to prevent and treat PAPS in children as one would in an adult.

PHANTOM PAIN IN REPLANTATION

It is thought that PAPS is caused by an elaborate response involving the peripheral nerve, spinal cord, and brain secondary to deafferentation of a body part. Replantation is the reattachment of a body part through the use of microsurgical techniques. Transplantation, also referred to as *cross transfer,* involves surgery to attach the undamaged part of an irreparably damaged limb to the undamaged limb with irreparably injured part. The procedure involves connecting the blood vessels, nerves, muscles, soft tissues, and then stabilizing the bony structures. Price evaluated three patients in an effort to determine the incidence of a phantom response: one patient with reattachment and two with the cross transfer of a hand. The replant patient was injured in a motorcycle accident and had his right arm disarticulated; soon after the accident the arm was replanted. Initially this patient did not recognize the arm had been amputated but shortly after replantation he began feeling various phantom sensations including formication (the sensation of ants crawling on the skin), itching, and occasional shocking in various parts of the arm. He could not localize them precisely. Eight weeks post replantation this patient had eight nerves transplanted from his leg to his arm; the feelings of formication, itching, and shocking continued, and, in addition, the arm began sweating. This replant patient has never regained complete muscular control of the limb; he continues to dream about missing a leg but has never dreamed about his arm.

The first transplant patient was crossing a railroad yard when his foot got caught in the rails. The train ran over both arms damaging and disarticulating the left arm but leaving the left hand undamaged. The right hand was crushed and severed from the right arm which was left intact. The undamaged left hand was transplanted on to the right wrist residual limb. Shortly after surgery, the patient began feeling a severe burning in his left shoulder and a sensation of his left arm lying beside his body.

With concentration, he feels he can move his phantom left arm, and there has been no shrinking or telescoping of this phantom. The patient states that all sensation felt in the right arm he also feels in the left phantom. He began moving the fingers of his cross-transferred hand at 8 months post-transfer and has developed sensation in the palmer aspect but not the dorsum.

The next case, involving a naturally left-hand dominant patient, reports getting his arms caught in a grinding machine with the result that his left arm was severed above the elbow and the middle three fingers of his right hand were amputated. Initially, the left arm was reattached and the right hand was debrided. Post-surgical vascular problems developed in the left arm, which could not be repaired. An above elbow amputation was performed. It was determined that the existing right hand was not functional, so the left hand and forearm were cross transferred to the right side, which had recently been amputated at the same level. Some time later this patient developed phantom sensation without pain and felt he could move the phantom fingers of the left hand. He never developed any phantom sensation in the right hand (255). Shukla hypothesized that the phantom limb sensation or pain may be more common when amputation occurs to the patient's dominant limb (256). As newer surgical techniques allow for the attachment or tranplantion of essentially any lost structure with substitutes, the future will provide us with critical information regarding PNS and CNS adaptation techniques.

PAPS PREVENTION

The adaptive responses of the peripheral nerve, spinal cord, and the brain to either a decrease in input (deafferentation) or an increase in input (spontaneous repetitive firing of neuromata) are truly remarkable. We are only beginning to understand these anatomic and physiologic responses; as our understanding progresses, we will be better able to direct our surgical and medical treatment at the specific etiology or process. An exhaustive review to the literature fails to uncover a fail safe technique to treat phantom pain once established. Sherman reviewed fifty techniques and concluded that none of the treatments (described earlier) were universally helpful: Some may even exacerbate the condition (257). The perfect technique would reverse the normal adaptive responses and then provide the CNS with input similar to that of the nonamputee state.

Clinicians are now looking at prevention as the best method of phantom pain control, rather than the treatment of the adaptive response. However, these suggestions are not fail-safe. Multiple surgical techniques have been tried in an effort to provide minimal trauma to the nerve: Surgeons avoid abnormal positioning of the sectioned nerve ends, burying the sectioned nerve in muscle, and applying a rigid dressing immediately after amputation. All these techniques seem logical, although no published studies show significantly improved results on long term follow-up.

Bach et al. performed lumbar epidural anesthesia prior to amputation on eleven of twenty-five elderly patients and found after 1 year that three of the controls had developed phantom pain, whereas none of the pre-blocked patients developed PLP (258). Fisher studied eleven patients scheduled to have an above- or below-knee amputation. These patients had an epidural catheter placed along the nerve sheath intraoperatively and were infused with postoperative bupivacaine for 72 hours. Nine of these patients had no phantom pain at 1-year follow-up (259). Malawer et al. evaluated continuous postoperative regional analgesia in twenty-three patients; twelve were amputees and none developed phantom pain. However, no duration of follow-up was given (260). Ovechkin et al. studied 152 patients and concluded that preventive analgesia reduced the incidence of phantom pain syndrome after amputation in patients with preamputation pain from 63.3% to 25.1% (261).

The premise of these treatments involves the concept that phantom pain is of central origin and is actually a memory of the pain prior to amputation. Regional anesthesia temporily blocks the sensory bombardment of surgery or trauma to the CNS, but it does not last indefinitely. The anesthetic agent will ultimately be discontinued, and it is hoped that because the sensory bombardment is lessened, it will ultimately have a less unsettling effect on the CNS. The type of conduction anesthesia is probably of little consequence, as long as the sensory input is decreased for a period of time. The time for optimal sensory blockade is not known, although 3 days seems to be used by convention, per-

haps in an effort to reduce the incidence of infection from an indwelling catheter in a surgical site. Regional anesthesia does little to alter the healing process or neuroma formation; consequently neuromata irritability may still activate CNS plastic changes.

Nikolajsen determined that preamputation pain significantly increased the incidence of residual limb and phantom pain at 1 week and 3 months (262). Nikolajsen et al. later determined that perioperative epidural blockade started approximately 18 hours before amputation and continued into the postoperative period does not prevent phantom or residual limb pain (263). The conclusions regarding the use of preemptive analgesia in the prevention of PAPS are still unclear. However, it seems prudent to use the above techniques when reasonably possible (264).

General anesthesia does not block the sensory input to the CNS, but rather affects the brain in still unknown ways. No studies are available regarding the use of general anesthesia as either reducing or promoting the incidence or severity of PAPS.

Numerous surgical techniques for managing nerve transection have been tried in an effort to prevent phantom pain. The most appealing technique is to provide local anesthesia to the nerve prior to transection. The perineurium is incised longitudinally, the axons are then cut back transversely, and the perineurium is then closed in a pouchlike fashion around the axons in an effort to control neuromata formation. The nerve stump is then placed in muscle for soft tissue protection; as yet no data supports this technique as superior to others.

PHANTOM PAIN ALGORITHM

The principle of pain management stresses the utilization of the least invasive first (those techniques with the fewest potential risks) and advance to the more invasive techniques as treatments fail to provide adequate management of the pain problem (See Figures 9-1 and 9-2). Medication management principles require medications to be started low and slow, titrated to effect, or reduced or discontinued if ineffective or accompanied by intolerable side effects.

A balanced analgesia, in which a combination of treatments is provided in smaller doses, can frequently result in improved relief with fewer side-effects than would a high doses of any single agent. The combinations may include such options as medications, psychiatric and psychologic interventions, injections, and surgery.

In the process of writing this chapter it became clear that no treatment is universally effective for every patient. The converse also was true; all treatments mentioned seemed to work for a limited number of patients. The majority of amputees with pain have a

Residual Limb Pain Algorithm

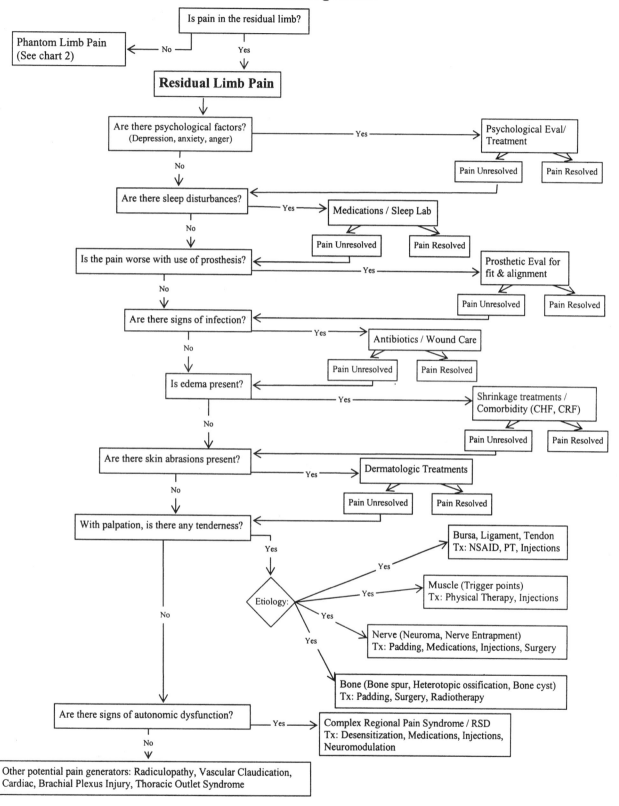

FIGURE 9-1

Residual Limb Pain Algorithm.

Phantom Limb Pain Algorithm

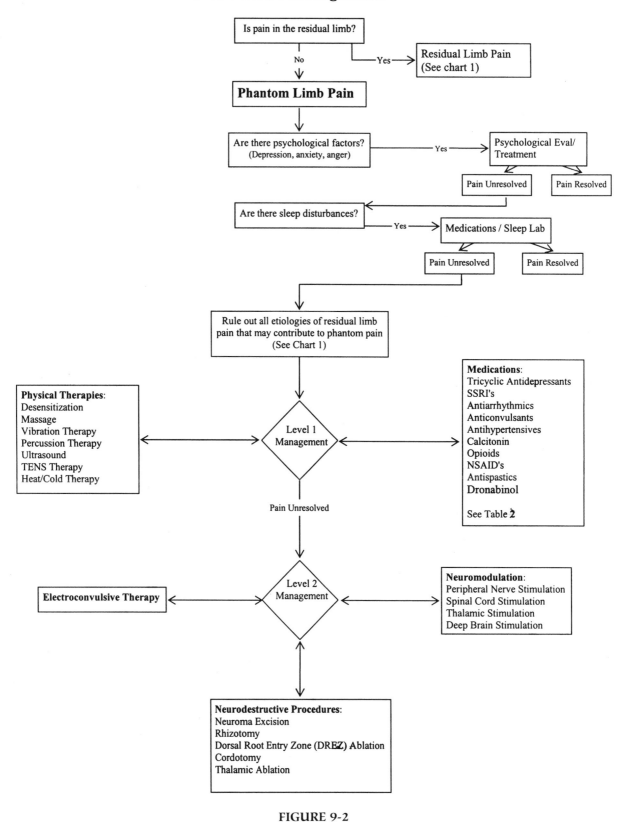

FIGURE 9-2

Phantom Limb Pain Algorithm.

combination of residual limb and phantom limb pain that can vary dramatically between the two forms throughout a lifetime. The proposed algorithms can be utilized at any point where treatment has previously failed and should be used in consideration with the individual patient's comorbid medical condition. The doses and costs of each treatment were intentionally not mentioned. The clinician should use the standards of medical care in dose adjustments, with consideration of cost whenever possible.

CONCLUSIONS

The pathophysiology of PAPS remains a mystery; theories about its origin encompass both the CNS and PNS and their adaptations to amputation. The treatment of PAPS vary depending on the consultant's specialty. Historically, no surgical technique, therapy, medicine, or alternative treatment universally results in amelioration of all symptoms. The treatment paradigm should begin with the simplest treatments first and advance toward the more complicated and risk-prone procedures only after failure of an adequate response.

The same common sense approach applies to the use of medication, with the safety and side-effect profile being a priority—the dosage of medication is advanced until therapeutic benefit is obtained or side effects develop. In the event of an adequate response with excessive side effects, the next most appropriate medication can be chosen for trial, or the dose of medication being used can be reduced and used as an adjuvant treatment. The choice of medication is based on the intensity of the pain, precise symptoms experienced, and the associated factors (such as depression) involved in each case. Frequent follow-up visits and the use of a pain and side-effect diary can be helpful when initially evaluating the dose and response to a given treatment.

In most cases, combinations of treatments will be necessary to control multifactorial pain complaints and maintain optimal function. In summary, PAPS, once established, usually is not curable. The symptoms are frequently manageable with diligent and conscientious use of education, self-empowerment, and the treatment paradigm.

R*eferences*

1. Mitchell SW. *Injuries of Nerves and their Consequences.* Philadelphia: J.B. Lippincott, 1872.
2. Hanowell ST, Kennedy SF. Phantom tongue pain and causalgia: Case presentation and treatment. *Anest Analg* 1979;5:436–438.
3. Reisner H. *Phantom and Stump Pain.* Phantom tooth. New York: Springer-Vergag, 1981;81–83.
4. Ackerly W, Lhamon W, and Fitts WT. Phantom breast. *J Nerv Ment Dis* 1955;121:177.
5. Bressler B, Cohen SI, Magnussen F. Bilateral breast phantom and breast phantom pain. *J Nerv Ment Dis* 1955;122:315.
6. Simmel ML. A study of phantoms after amputation of the breast. *Neuropsychologia* 1966;4:331.
7. Jarvis JH. Post-mastectomy breast phantoms. *J Nerv Ment Dis* 1967;144:266.
8. Weinstein S, Vetter RJ, Sersen EA. Phantoms following breast amputation. *Neuropsychologia* 1970;8:185.
9. Dorpat TL. Phantom sensations of internal organs. *Compr Psychiatry* 1971;1:27–35.
10. Heusner AP. Phantom genitalia. *Trans Am Neurol Assoc* 1950;75:128–131.
11. Keynes G (ed.). *The Apologie and Treatise of Ambroise Paré.* Chicago: University of Chicago Press, 1952.
12. Reise W. In Poynter. F.N.L. *The History and Philosophy of Knowledge of the Brain and Its Function:* An Anglo-American Symposium. Blackwell: Oxford, 1957;115.
13. Furukawa T. Charles Bell's description of phantom phenomenon in 1830. *Neurology* 1990;40:1830.
14. Bell C. The nervous system of the human body embracing the papers delivered to the Royal Society on the subject of nerves. London, Longman, 1830.
15. Gueniot. De l'Homme-et-des Animaux (Phantom experience following amputation in childhood). *J Physiol* 1861;4:416.
16. *See reference 1.*
17. *See reference 1.*
18. Jensen TS, Drebs B, Nielsen J, et al. Immediate and long-term phantom pain in amputees: incidence, clinical characteristics and relationship to pre-amputation limb pain. *Pain* 1985;21:267–78.
19. Sunderland S. *Nerves and Nerve Injuries.* 2nd edition, Edinburgh: Livingstone, 1978.
20. Carlen PL, Wall PD, Nadvorna H, Steinbach T. Phantom limbs and related phenomena in recent traumatic amputations. *Neurology* 1978;28:211.
21. Abramson AS, Feibel A. The phantom phenomenon: its use and disuse. *Bull N Y Acad Med* 1981;57:99.
22. Sherman RA, and Sherman CJ. A comparison of phantom sensations among amputees whose amputations were of civilian and military origins. *Pain* 1985;21:91.
23. Cronholm B. Phantom limbs in amputees: study of changes in integration of centripetal impulses with special reference to referred sensations. *Acta Psychiatr Neurol Scand* (Suppl.) 1951;72:1.
24. Solonen KA. The phantom phenomenon in amputated Finnish war veterans. *Acta Orthop Scand* (Suppl.) 1962;54:7.
25. Livingston KE. *Pain Mechanisms.* Springfield, IL: Charles C Thomas, 1976;150–168.
26. *See reference 1.*
27. Sunderland S. *Nerves and Nerve Injuries.* 2nd edition. Edinburgh: Livingstone, 1978.
28. Abramson AS, Feibel A. The phantom phenomenon: Its use and disuse. *Bull N Y Acad Med* 1981;57:99.
29. Wilkins KL, McGrath PJ, Finley GA, Katz J. Phantom limb sensations and phantom limb pain in children and adolescent amputees. *Pain* 1998;78:7–12.
30. Sherman RA, Sherman CJ. A comparison of phantom sensations among amputees whose amputations were of civilian and military origins. *Pain* 1985;21:91.
31. Livingston KE. The phantom limb syndrome. A discussion of the role of major peripheral neuromas. *J Neurosurg* 1945;2:251.

32. Shukla G, Saitu SC, Gurta DK. A psychiatric study of amputees. *Br J Psychiatry* 1982;141:50–53.

33. Pitres A. Etude sur les sensations illusiores des amputes. *Ann Med Psychol (Paris)* 1897;5:1.

34. *See reference 30.*

35. Cronholm B. Phantom limbs in amputees: Study of changes in integration of centripetal impulses with special reference to referred sensations. *Acta Psychiatr Neurol Scand* (Suppl.) 1951;72:1.

36. Solonen KA. The phantom phenomenon in amputated Finnish war veterans. *Acta Orthop Scand* (Suppl.) 1962;54:7.

37. Haber WB. Observations on phantom-limb phenomenon. *Arch Neurol Psychiatr* 1956;75:624.

38. Golbranson FL, Wirta RW, Kuncir EJ, et al. Volume changes occurring in post-operative below knee residual limbs. *J Rehabil Res Dev* 1988;25:11–18.

39. Sunderland S. *Nerves and Nerve Injuries.* 2nd edition. Edinburgh: Livingstone, 1978.

40. Canty TJ, Bleck EE. Amputation stump pain, U.S. Armed Forces Med J 1958;9:635.

41. Katz J, Melzack R. Referred sensation in chronic pain patients, *Pain* 1987;28:51–59.

42. Lipton DE, Nagendran T. A rare case of stump pain-herniated lumbar disc: a case report. *Ala Med* 1989;58:39–40.

43. Russell WR, Spaulding JMK. Treatment of painful amputations stumps. *Br Med J* 1950;2:68–73.

44. Mitchell SW. *Injuries of Nerves and their Consequences.* Philadelphia: J.B. Lippincott, 1872.

45. White JC. Pain after amputation and its treatments. *JAMA* 1944;124:1030.

46. Battista AF. *Advances in Pain Research and Theory.* Pain of peripheral nerve origin: fasicle ligation for the prevention of painful neuroma. New York: Raven Press, 1979;3:167–172.

47. Samii M. *Phantom and Stump Pain.* Centrocentral anastomosis of peripheral nerves: A neurosurgical treatment of amputation neuroma. New York: Springer-Verlag, 1981;123–125.

48. Davis RW. Phantom sensation, phantom pain, and stump pain. *Arch Phys Med Rehabil* 1993;74:79–91.

49. White JC. Pain after amputation and its treatments. *JAMA* 1944;124:1030.

50. *See reference 46.*

51. Samii M. *Phantom and Stump Pain.* Centrocentral anastomosis of peripheral nerves: a neurosurgical treatment of amputation neuroma. New York: Springer-Verlag, 1981;123–125.

52. Gillis L. The management of the painful amputation stump and new theory for the phantom phenomena. *Br J Surg* 1964;51:87.

53. Anderson M. Four cases of phantom limb treated with ultrasound. *Phys Therp Rev* 1958;38:419–20.

54. Finsen V, Persen L, Lvlien M, et al. Transcutaneous electrical stimulation after major amputation. *J Bone Joint Surg [Br]* 1988;70:109–112.

55. Berger SM. Conservative management of phantom-limb and amputation-stump pain. *Ann R Coll Surg Engl* 1980;62:102.

56. Lundeberg T. Relief of pain from a phantom limb by peripheral stimulation. *J Neurol* 1985;232:79.

57. Noordenbos W. (ed.). *Pain.* Amsterdam: Elsevier, 1959.

58. Hodge CJ, Apkarian AV, Owen MP, et al. Changes in the effects of the stimulation of the locus coeruleus in the nucleus raphe magnus following dorsal rhizotomy. *Brain Res* 1983;288:325–329.

59. Simmel ML. The reality of phantom sensation. *Soc Res* 1962;29:337–356.

60. Melzack R, Bromage PR. Experimental phantoms limbs. *Exp Neurol* 1973;39:261–269.

61. Wall PD. *Phantom and Stump Pain.* On the origin of pain associated with amputation. Berlin: Springer-Verlag, 1981:2–14.

62. Wall PD. *Phantom and Stump Pain.* On the origin of pain associated with amputation. Berlin: Springer-Verlag, 1981:2–14.

63. Cajal SR. *Degeneration and regeneration in the nervous system.* New York: Hafner, 1959.

64. Nystrom B, Hagbarth KE. Microelectrode recordings from transected nerves in amputees with phantom limb pain. *Neurosci Lett* 1981;27:211.

65. DeJong RH, Cullen SC. Theoretical aspects of pain: Bizarre pain phenomena during low spinal anesthesia. *Anesthesiology* 1963;24:628.

66. Prevoznik SJ, Eckenhoff JE. Phantom sensations during spinal anesthesia. *Anesthesiology* 1964;25:767.

67. Melzack R, Bromage PR. Experimental phantom limbs. *Exp Neurol* 1973;39:261.

68. Mackenzie N. Phantom limb pain during spinal anaesthesia. *Anesthesia* 1983;38:886.

69. Devor M, Claman D. Mapping and plasticity of the acid phosphatase afferents in rat dorsal horn. *Brain Res* 1980;190:17–28.

70. Barbut D, Polak JM, Wall PD. Substance P in spinal cord dorsal horn decreases following peripheral nerve injury. *Brain Res* 1981 Feb 2;205(2):289–98.

71. Csillik B, Knyihar E. Degenerative atrophy and regeneration proliferation in the rat spinal cord. *Z Mikros Anat Forsch* 1975;89:1099–1103.

72. Kim HJ, Na HS, Nam HJ, Park KA, Hong SK, Kang BS. Sprouting of sympathetic nerve fibers into the dorsal root ganglion following peripheral nerve injury depends on injury site. *Neurosci Lett* 1996 Jul 19;212(3):191–194.

73. Janig W, Levine JD, Michaelis M. Interactions of sympathetic and primary afferents neurons following nerve injury and tissue trauma. *Prog Brain Res* 1996;113:161–184.

74. Dostrovsky JO, Millar J, Wall PD. The immediate shift of afferent drive of the dorsal column nucleus cells following deafferentation: A comparison of acute and chronic deafferentation in gracile nucleus and spinal cord. *Exp Nerurol* 1976;52:480–495.

75. Aanonsen LM, Lei S, Wilcox GL. Excitatory amino acid receptors and nociceptive neuro-transmission in rat spinal cord. *Pain* 1990;41:309–321.

76. Pernow B. Substance P. *Pharmacol. Rev* 1984;35:85–141.

77. Schneider SP, Perl ER. Selective excitation of neurons in the mammalian spinal dorsal horn. *J Neurosci* 1988;8:2062–2073.

78. Mayer ML, Westbroook GL. The physiology of excitatory amino acids in the vertebrate central nervous system. *Prog Neurobiol* 1987;28:197–276.

79. King AE, Thompson SWN, Urban L, et al. An intracellular analysis of amino acid induced excitation of deep dorsal horn neurons in the rat spinal cord slice. *Neurosci Lett* 1988;89:286–292.

80. Dubner R. *Neuronal plasticity and pain following peripheral tissue inflammation or nerve injury.* In: Bond M.R., Charlton, J.E., Woolf, C.J., eds. Proceedings of the 5th World Congress on Pain. Amsterdam: Elsevier BV, 1991:263–276.

81. Jeftinija S. Excitatory transmission in the dorsal horn is in part mediated through APV sensitive NMDA receptors. *Neurosci Lett* 1989;96:191–6.

82. Woolf CJ, Fitzgerald M. The properties of neurons recorded in the superficial dorsal horn in rat spinal cord. *J Comp Neurol* 1983;221:313–28.

83. Devor M. *Textbook of Pain.* Pathophysiology of damaged peripheral nerves. 2nd ed, New York: Churchill Livingstone, 1989:63–81.

84. Blumenkopf B. *The General Aspects of Neuropharmacology of Dorsal Horn Function.* Deafferentation pain syndromes: pathophysiology and treatments. New York: Raven Press, Ltd, 1991.

85. Melzack R, Loeser JD. Phantom body pain in paraplegics: evidence for a central "pattern generating mechanism" for pain. *Pain* 1978;4:195–210.

86. Melzack R. Phantom limbs, the self and the brain. (The D.O. Hebb memorial lecture.) *Canad Psychol* 1989;30:1–14.

87. Frederiks JA. Occurrence and nature of phantom limb phenomenon following amputation of body parts and following lesions of the central and peripheral nervous system. *Psychiatr Neurol Neurochir* 1963;66:73–79.

88. Jensen TS, Rasmussen P. *Textbook of Pain* Phantom pain and related phenomena after amputation. 2nd edition, New York: Churchill Livingstone, 1989:508–521.

89. Canavero S. Dynamic reverberation. A unified mechanism for central and phantom pain. *Med Hypotheses* 1994 Mar;42(3):203–207.

90. Wall PD. *Phantom and Stump Pain.* On the origin of pain associated with amputation. Berlin: Springer-Verlag, 1968.

91. Melzack R. The John Bonica distinguished lectures. *The gate control theory 25 years later: New perspectives on phantom limb pain.* In: Bond, M.R., Charlton, J.E., Woolf, C.J., eds. Proceedings of the 6th World Congress on Pain. Amsterdam: Elsevier BV, 1991:9–21.

92. Flor H, Elbert T, Knecht S, Wienbruch S, Pantev C, Birbaumer N, Larbig W, Taub E. Phantom-limb pain as a perceptual correlate of cortical reorganization following arm amputation. *Nature* 1995 Jun 8;375(6531):482–484.

93. Merzenich MM, Jenkins WM. Reorganization of cortical representations of the hand following alterations of skin inputs induced by nerve injury, skin island transfer, and experience. *J Hand Ther* 1993 April–June;89–104.

94. Kaas JH. Plasticity of sensory and motor maps in adult mammals. *Annu Rev Neurosci* 1991;14:137–67.

95. Pons TP, Garraghty PE, Ommaya AK, Kaas JH, Taub E, Mishkin M. Massive cortical reorganization after sensory deafferentation in adults macaques. *Science* 252:1857–1860.

96. Doetsch GS. Progressive changes in cutaneous trigger zones for sensation referred to a phantom hand: a case report and review with implications for cortical reorganization. *Somatosensory and Motor Research* 1997;14(1):6–16.

97. Ramachandran VS. Behavioral and magnet encephalographic correlates of plasticity in the adult human brain. *Proc Natl Acad Sci USA* 1993;90:10413–10420.

98. Ramachndran VS, Stewart M, Rogers-Ramachandran D.C. Percentual correlates of massive cortical reorganization. *Neuroreport* 1992 Jul;3(7):583–586.

99. Flor H, Elbert T, Knecht S, Wienbruch S, Pantev C, Birbaumer N, Larbig W, Taub E. Phantom-limb pain as a perceptual correlate of cortical reorganization following arm amputation. *Nature* 1995 Jun 8;375(6531):482–484.

100. Merzenich MM, Kaas JH, Wall JT, Nelson RJ, Sur M, Felleman D. Topographic reorganization of somatosensory cortical areas 3b and 1 in adult monkeys following restricted deafferentation. *Neurosci* 1983 Jan;8(1) 33–35.

101. Jenkins WM, Merzenich MM, Recanzone G. (1990) *Neuropsychologia* 1991;28:573–584.

102. Canavero S. Dynamic reverberation. A unified mechanism for central and phantom pain. *Medical Hypotheses* 1994;42:203–207.

103. Yarnitsky D, Barron SA, Bentl E. Disappearance of phantom pain after focal brain infarction. *Pain* 1988;32:285–287.

104. Sherman RA. Phantom limb pain mechanism based management. In: *Clin Podiatr Med Surg* 1994;11(1):85–106.

105. Mitchell SW. *Injuries of Nerves and their Consequences.* Philadelphia: J.B. Lippincott, 1872.

106. Shealy CN. Transcutaneous electrical stimulation for control of pain. *Clin Neurosurg* 1974;21:269–277.

107. Finsen V, Persen L, Lulien M, et al. Transcutaneous electrical stimulation after major amputation. *J Bone Joint Surg [Br]* 1988;70:109–112.

108. Sherman RA. Published treatments of phantom limb pain. *Am J Phys Med* 1980;59:232.

109. Klingler D, Kepplinger B. *Phantom and Stump Pain.* Transcutaneous electrical nerve stimulation (TNS) in the treatment of chronic pain after peripheral nerve lesions. New York: Springer-Verlag, 1981;103–106.

110. Katz J, France S, Melzack R. An association between phantom limb sensation and stump skin conductance during transcutaneous electrical nerve stimulation. *Pain* 1989:36:367–377.

111. Miles J, Lipton S. Phantom limb pain treated by electrical stimulation. *Pain* 1978;5:373.

112. Men SD, Matsui Y. Peripheral nerve stimulation increases serotonin and dopamine metabolites in rat spinal cord. *Brain Research Bulletin* 1994;33(6):625–632.

113. Recanzone GH, Allard TT, Jenkins WM, Merzenich MM. Receptive-field changes induced by peripheral nerve stimulation on SI of adult cats. *J Neurophysiol* 1990 May;63(5):1213–1225.

114. Campbell JN, Long DM. Peripheral nerve stimulation in the treatment of intractable pain. *J Neurosurg* 1976 Dec;45(6):692–699.

115. Picaza JA, Cannon BW, Hunter SE, Boyd AS, Guma J, Maurer D. Pain suppression by peripheral nerve stimulation. Part II. Observations with implanted devices. *Surg Neurol* 1975 Jul;4(1): 115–126.

116. Law JD, Swett J, Kirsch WM. Retrospective analysis of 22 patients with chronic pain treated by peripheral nerve stimulation. *J Neurosurg* 1980 Apr;52(40);482–485.

117. Krainick JU, Thoden U. *Phantom and Stump Pain.* Spinal cord stimulation in post amputation pain. New York: Springer-Verlag, 1981;63–166.

118. Kumar K, Nath R. Treatment of chronic pain by epidural cord stimulation: A 10-year experience. *J Neurosurg* 1991;75:402–407.

119. Hunt WE, Goodman JH. Dorsal column stimulation for phantom limb pain. *J Neurosurg* 1975;43:250–251.

120. Mundinger F, Salamao J. Deep brain stimulation in mesencephalic lemniscus medialis for chronic pain. *Acta Neurochir* Suppl (Wien) 1980;30:245.

121. Mundinger F, Neumuller H. *Phantom and Stump Pain.* Programmed transcutaneous (TNS) and central (DBS) stimulation for control of phantom pain and causalgia: a new method for treatment. New York: Springer, 1981;164–178.

122. Bonica, JJ. *The Management of Pain.* Philadelphia: Lea & Febinger. 1990:1106.

123. Sherman RA. Published treatments of phantom limb pain. *Am J Phys Med* 1980;59:232.

124. White JC, Sweet WH. *Pain and the Neurosurgeon.* A forty-year experience. Springfield: Thomas. 1969:50–86.

125. Sherman RA. Published treatments of phantom limb pain. *Am J Phys Med* 1980;59:232.

126. Nashold BS, Jr., Ostdahl RH. Dorsal root entry zone lesions for pain relief. *J Neurosurg* 1979;51:59–69.

127. *See* reference 126.

128. Saris SC, Lacono RP, Nashold BS. Dorsal root entry zone lesions for post amputation pain. *J Neurosurg* 1985;62:72–76.

129. Sherman RA. Published treatments of phantom limb pain. *Am J Phys Med* 1980;59:232.

130. Gross D. Contralateral local anesthesia in the treatment of phantom limb and stump pain. *Pain* 1982;13:313–320.

131. Davis RW. Phantom sensation, phantom pain and stump pain. *Arch Phys Med Rehabil* 1993;74:79–91.

132. *See* reference 129.

133. Dahl JB, Kellet H. Nonsteroidal anti-inflammatory drugs: rationale for use in severe post-operative pain. *Br J Anesth* 1991;66:703–12.

134. Wartan SW, Hamann W, Wedley JR, McColl I. Phantom pain and sensation among British veteran amputees. *Br J Anaesth* 1997 June;78(6): 652–9.

135. Vasko MR. Prostaglandin-induced neuropeptide release from spinal cord. *Progress in Brain Research* 1995;104:367–80.

136. Malmberg AB, Yakash TL. Pharmacology of spinal action of ketorolac, morphine, ST-91, U50488 H and L-PIA on the formalin test and an isobolographic analysis of the NSAID interaction. *Anesthesiology* 1993 Aug;79(2): 27–81.

137. Spiegel K, Calb R, Pasternak GW. Analgesic activity of tricyclic antidepressants. *Ann Neurol* 1983;13:4b 2–5.

138. Rogers AG. Use of amitriptyline (Elavil) for phantom limb pain in younger children. *J Pain Symptom Manage* 1989;3:96.

139. Douglas WW. *The Pharmacological Basis of Therapeutics.* Histamine and 5-hydroxytryptamine (serotonin) and their antagonist. 7th edition. New York: MacMillan, 1985;605–638.

140. Eisenach JC, Gebhart GF. Intrathecal amitriptyline acts as an N-methyl-D-asparate receptor antagonist in the presence of inflammatory hyperalgesia in rats. *Anesthesia* 1995 Nov;83(5): 1046–54.

141. Sindrup SH, Gram LF, Brosen K, et al. The selective serotonin reuptake inhibitor paroxetine is effective in the treatment of diabetic neuropathy symptoms. *Pain* 1990:42:135–144.

142. Power-Smith P, Turkington D. Fluoxetine in phantom limb pain. *Br J Psychiatry* 1993;163:105–106.

143. Patterson JF. Carbamazepine in the treatment of phantom limb pain. *South Med J* 1988;81:199–2.

144. Elliott F, Little A, Milbrandt W. Carbamazepine for phantom limb phenomena. *N Engl J Med* 1976;295:687.

145. Swerdlow M. Anticonvulsant drugs and chronic pain. *Clin Neuropharmacol* 1984;7:51–82.

146. Swerdlow M, Cundhill JG. Anticonvulsant drugs used in the treatment of lancinating pain: A comparison. *Anesthesia* 1981;36:1129–1132.

147. Woodbury DM, Fingle E. *The Pharmacological Basis of Therapeutics.* Drugs effective in the therapy of the epilepsies. 5th edition, New York: Macmillan, 1975:201–226.

148. Woodbury DM. Fingle E. *The Pharmacological Basis of Therapeutics.* Drugs effective in the therapy of the epilepsies. 5th edition, New York: Macmillan, 1975:201–226.

149. McNamara JO. *The Pharmacological Basis Therapeutics.* Drugs effective in the therapy of the eplepsies. 9th edition, New York: Mcgraw-Hill, 1996;480–481.

150. Nickerson M, Collier B. *The Pharmacological Basis of Therapeutics* 5th edition, New York: MacMillan, 1975;547–552.

151. Ahmad S. Phantom limb pain and propranolol. *Br Med J* 1975;4:96.

152. Ollie VA. Beta-adrenergic blockade and the phantom limb. *Ann Intern Med* 1970;73:1044–5.

153. Marsland AR, Weekes JWN, Atkinson RL, Leong MG. Phantom limb pain: A case for beta-blockers? *Pain* 1982;12:295.

154. Scadding JW, Wall PD, Wynn-Parry CB, Brooks DM. Clinical trials of propranolol in posttraumatic neuralgia. *Pain* 1982;14:283.

155. Hoffhian BB, Lefkowitz RJ. Alpha adrenergic receptor subtypes. *N Engl J Med* 1980;302:1390–1396.

156. Hoffman BB, Lefkowitz RJ, Taylor P. *The Pharmacological Basis of Therapeutics.* Neurotransmission: The autonomic and somatic motor nervous systems. 9th edition, New York: McGraw Hill, 1996;133.

157. Goldstein J. Clonidine as an analgesic, *Bio Psych* 1983;18:1339–1340.

158. Jahangiri M, Jayatunga AP, Bradley JW, Dark CH. Prevention of phantom pain after major lower limb amputation by epidural infusion of diamorphine, clonidine, and bupivacaine. *Ann R Coll Surg Engl* 1994 Sept;76(5):324–6.

159. Miles J. Prevention of phantom pain after major lower limb amputation by epidural infusion of diamorphine, clonidine, bupivacaine, (Let) *Ann R Coll Surg Engl* 1994 Sep:76(5):324–6.

160. Jaeger H, Maier C. Calcitonin in phantom limb pain: a double blind study. *Pain* 1992, June;48(l):21–7.

161. Mertz DP. Neue therapeutische Versuche gegen Phantom-schmerzen. *Dtsch Arzteblat* 1986;83:348–354.

162. Braga PC. Calcitonin and its antinociceptive activity: animal and human investigations 1975–92. *Agents Actions* 1994;41:121–31.

163. Braga PC, Ferri S, Santagostine A, Olgiati VR, Pecile A. Lack of opiate receptor involvement in centrally

induced calcitonin analgesia. *Life Sci* 1978;22:971–978.

164. Yamamoto M, Kumagai F, Tachikawa S, Maeno H. Lack of effect of levallorphan on analgesia induced by intraventricular application of porcine calcitonin in mice. *Eur J Pharmacol* 1979;55:211–213.

165. Clementi G, Prato A, Conforto G, Scapagnini U. Role of serotonin in the analgesic activity of calcitonin. *Eur J Pharmacol* 1984;98:449–451.

166. Clementi G, Amico-Roxas M, Rapisarda E, Caruso A, Prato A, Trobadore S, Priolo G, Scapagnini U. The analgesic activity of calcitonin and central serotonergic system. *Eur J Pharmacol* 1985;108:71–75.

167. Candeletti S, Romualdi P, Spadaro C, Spampinato S, Ferri S. Studies on the antinociceptive effect of intrathecal salmon calcitonin. *Peptides* 1985;6:273–276.

168. Jaeger H, Maier C. Calcitonin in phantom limb pain: a double blind study. *Pain* 1992, Jn;48(1):21–7.

169. Fiddler DS, Hindman BJ. Intravenous calcitonin alleviated spinal anesthesia induced phantom limb pain. *Anesthesiology* 1991;74:187–189.

170. Chrubasik J, Falke KF, Zindler M, Volk B, Blond S, Meynadier J. Is calcitonin an analgesic agent? *Pain* 1986;27:273–276.

171. Shaw HL. Subarachnoid administration of calcitonin: a warning (letter). *Lancet* 1982;2:390.

172. Eisenach JC. Demonstrating safety of subarachnoid calcitonin: Patients or animals? (letter). *Anesth Analg* 1981;67:298.

173. Candeletti S, Ferri S. Clinical use of subarachnoid neuropeptides: An experimeetal contribution (letter). *Anesth Analg* 1989;69:41b.

174. Rayner HC, Atkins RC, Westerman RA. Relief of local stump pain by capsaicin cream. *Lancet* 1989;251:1276–7.

175. Weintraub M, Golik A, Rubio A. Capsaicin for treatment of post traumatic amputation stump pain. *Lancet* 336:1003–1004.

176. Cannon ST, Wu Y. Topical capsaicin as an adjuvant analgesic for the treatment of traumatic amputee neurogenic residual limb pain. *Arch Phys Med Rehabil* 1998 May;79(5):591–593.

177. Robbins WR, Staats PS, Levine J, Fields HL, Alien RW, Campbell JN, Pappagallo M. Treatment of intractable pain with topical large dose capsaicin: preliminary report. *Anesth Analg* 1998 Mar;86(3):579–83.

178. Snyder DW. Class Ib antiarrhythmic drugs: tocanide, mexilitine and moricizine. *Journal of the St. Louis Medical Society* 1989;141(5):21–25.

179. Costard-Jackle A, Franz MR. Frequency-dependent antiarrhythmic drug effects on post repolarization refactoriness and ventricular conduction time in canine ventricular myocardium in vivo. *J Pharmacol Exp Ther* 1989;251(1):39–46.

180. Dubner R. *Neuronal plasticity and pain following peripheral tissue inflammation or nerve injury.* In: Bond M.R., Charlton, J.E., Woolf, C.J., eds. Proceedings of the Fifth World Congress on Pain. Amsterdam: Elsevier BV, 1991:263–76.

181. Albe-Fessard D, Lombard M.C. *Advances in Pain Research and Therapy.* Use of an animal model to evaluate the origin of and protection against deafferentation pain. New York: Raven Press, 1983;5:691–700.

182. Lombard MC, Nashold BS. Jr., Albe-Fessard D. Deafferentation hypersensitivity in the rat after dorsal rhizotomy; a possible animal model of chronic pain. *Pain* 1979;6:163–174.

183. Davar G, Maciewicz RJ. Deafferentation pain syndromes. *Neurol Clin* 1989;7:289–304.

184. Pagni CA. *The Textbook of Pain.* Central pain due to spinal cord and brainstem damage. New York: Churchill-Livingstone, 1989;634–655.

185. Tasker RR, Dostrovsky JO. *The Textbook of Pain.* The Deafferentation and central pain. New York: Churchill-Livingstone; 1989;634–655.

186. Craig AD. *Pain in Central Nervous System Disease:* The Central Pain Syndromes. Supraspinal pathways and mechanisms relevant to central pain. New York: Raven Press, 1991;157–170.

187. Davis RW. Successful treatment for phantom pain. *Orthopedics* 1993 Jun;16(6): 691–5.

188. Roden DM. *The Pharmacological Basis of Therapeutics.* Antiarrhythmic Drugs. 9th edition, New York: McGraw-Hill, 1996;857.

189. Portenoy, RD, Kanner RM. Nonopioid and adjuvant analgesics. *Pain Management: Theory and Practice, Contemporary Neurology Series.* Philadelphia: FA Davis, 1996;219–247.

190. Iacono RP, Linford J, Sandy K. Pain management after lower extremity amputation. *Neurosurg* 1987;20:496–500.

191. Wagstaff AJ, Bryson HM. Tizanidine, A review of its pharmacology, clinical efficacy and tolerability in the management of spasticity associated with cerebral and spinal disorders. *Drugs* 1997 Mar;53(3):435–452.

192. Vorobeichik IaM, Kukushkin ML, Reshetniak VK, Ovechkin AM, Gnezdilov AV. Treatment of phantom pain syndrome with tizanidine/Lechenie fantomno-bolevogo sindroma tizanidinom. *Zhurnal Nevropatologii I Psikhiatrii Imeni S-S-Korsakova* 1997;97(3):36–39.

193. Kukushkin ML, Ivanova AF, Ovechkin AM, Gnezdilov AV, Reshetniak VK. Differential combined drug therapy of phantom pain syndrome after amputation. *Anesteziologiia I Reanimatologiia* 1996 Jul-Aug;(4): 39–42.

194. Logan T. Persistent phantom limb pain: dramatic response to chlorpromazine. *South M J* 1983;76:1585.

195. Sherman RA. Published treatments of phantom limb pain. *Am J Phys Med Rehabil* 1980;59:232.

196. Benezet P, Cochet C. Tiapride et douleur chez l'amputé. *Sem Hop Paris* 1982:58:2203–2205.

197. Sherman RA, Sherman CJ, Gall NG. A survey of current phantom pain treatment in the United States. *Pain* 1980:8:85–89.

198. Fallen MT, Welsh J. The role of ketamine in pain control. *Europ J Palliative Care* 1996;3(4):43–146.

199. Nikolajsen L, Hansen CL, Nielsen J, Keller J, Nielsen LA, Jensen T. The effect of ketamine on phantom pain: a central neuropathic disorder maintained by peripheral input. *Pain* 1996:67:69–77.

200. Stannard CF, Porter GE. Ketamine hydrochloride in the treatment of phantom limb pain. *Pain* 1993;54:227–230.

201. Pud D, Eisenberg E, Spitzer A, Adlor R, Fried G, Yarnitsky D. The NMDA receptor amantadine reduces surgical neuropathic pain in cancer patients: a double blind randomized placebo controlled trial. *Pain* 1998 Apr;75(2–3):49–54.

202. Eisenberg E, Pud D. Can patients with chronic neuropathic pain be cured by acute administration of the

NMDA receptor antagonist amantadine? *Pain* 1998 Feb;74(2–3):337–339.

203. Tal M, Bennett GJ. Neuropathic pain sensations are differentially sensitive to dextrorphan. *Neuroreport* 1994 Jul 21;5(12): 1438–1440.

204. Tal M, Bennet GJ. Dextrophan relieves neuropathic heat-evoked hyperalgesia in the rat. *Neurosci Lett* 1993 Mar 5;151(1): 107–110.

205. Trube G, Netzer R. Dextromethorphan: cellular effects reducing neuronal hyperactivity. *Epilepsia* 1994:35 Suppl 5:S62–67.

206. Elliott K, Hyansky A, Inturrisi C. Dextromethorphan attenuates and reverses analgesic tolerance to morphine. *Pain* 1994;59:361–368.

207. Nelson KA, Park MM, Robinovitz E, Tsigo C, Max MB. High dose oral dextromethorphan versus placebo in painful diabetic neuropathy and post herpetic neuralgia. *Neurology* 1997 May;48(5) 212–218.

208. Klepstaad P, Borchgrevink PC. Four years treatment with ketamine and trial of dextromethorphan in a patient with severe post-herpetic neuralgia. *Acta Anesthesiol Scand* 1997 Mar;41(3): 422–6.

209. France RD, Urban BJ, Keefe FJ. Long term use of narcotic analgesics in chronic pain. *Sci Med* 1984;19:1379–1382.

210. Houde RW. *Advances in Neurology*. The use and misuse of narcotics in the treatment of chronic pain. New York: Raven Press, 1974;4:527–536.

211. Jaffe JH. *The Pharmacological Basis of Therapeutics.* Drug addiction and drag abuse. New York: McMillian, 1974;538–584.

212. Chabal C, Erjavec MK, Jacobson L, Mariano A, Chaney E. Prescription opiate abuse in chronic pain patients: clinical criteria, incidence and predictors. *Clin J Pain* 1997;13:150–155.

213. Urban BJ, France RD, Steinberger EK, Scott DL, Maltbie AA. Long term use of narcotic/antidepressant medication in the management of phantom limb pain. *Pain* 1986;24:191–196.

214. Jacox A, Carr DB, Payne R, et al. *Management of Cancer Pain. Clinical practice guidelines* No. 9. AHCPR Publication NO. 94-0592. Rockville, MD. Agency for Health Care Policy and Research, U.S. Department of Health and Human Services, Public Health Service, March 1994.

215. Dunbar SA, Katz NP. Chronic opioid therapy for nonmalignant pain in patients with a history of substance abuse: report of 20 cases. *J Pain and Sympt Manage* 1996 Mar;11(3): 163–171.

216. Gorman AL, Elliot KJ, Inturrisi CE. The D and L isomers of methadone bind to the non-competitive site on the N-methyl-D-aspartate (NMDA) receptor in rat forebrain and spinal cord. *Neurosci Lett* 1997 Feb 14;223(1): 5–8.

217. Dickenson AH. NMDA receptor antagonist: interactions with opioids. *Acta Anaesthesiol Scand* 1997 Jan;41(1p+2): 112–5.

218. Herman BH, Vocci F, Bridge P. The effects of NMDA receptor antagonists and nitric oxide synthase inhibitors on opioid tolerance and withdraw. Medication development issues for opiate addiction. *Neuropsychopharmacology* 1995 Dec;13(4): 269–293.

219. Elliott K, Kest B, Man A, Koa B. Inturrisi CE. N-methyl-D-aspartate (NMDA) receptors, mu and kappa opioid tolerance and perspectives on new analgesic drug development. *Neuropsychopharmacology* 1995 Dec;13(4): 347–356.

220. Miaskowski C, Levine J. Does opioid analgesia show gender preference for females? *Pain Forum Spring* 1999;8(1):34–45.

221. Omote K, Ohmori H, Kawamata M, Matsumoto M, Namiki A. Intrathecal buprenorphine in the treatment of phantom limb pain. *Anesth Analg* 1995 May;80(5): 1030–1032.

222. Max MB, Schafer SC, Culmame M, et al. Amitriptyline, but not lorazepam relieves post herpetic neuralgia. *Neurology* 1988;38:1427–1452.

223. Gear RW, Miaskowski C, Heller PH, et al. Benzodiazepine mediated antagonism of opioid analgesia. *Pain* 1997;71:25–29.

224. Sherman RA. Stump and phantom limb pain, Pain mechanisms and syndromes. *Neurol Clin* 1989 May;7:2.

225. Fanciullacci M, et al. Brief report: phantom limb pain: sub-hallucinogenic treatment with lysergic acid diethylamide (LSD-25). *Headache* 1977 Jul;17(3): 118–119.

226. Kuromaru S, et al. The effect of LSD on phantom limb pain phenomenon. *J Lancet* 1967 Jan;87(1): 22–27.

227. Grinspoon L, Bakalar J. *Marihuana, the Forbidden Medicine,* Yale University Press New Haven and London, revised and expanded edition; 1997;200–202.

228. Zeltser R, Seltzer Z, Eisen A, Feigenbaum JJ, Mechoulam R. Suppression of neuropathic pain behavior in rats by a non-psychotropic synthetic cannabinoid with NMDA receptor blocking properties. *Pain* 1991 Oct;47(1): 95–103.

229. Sherman R, Sherman C, Parker L. Chronic phantom and stump pain among American veterans: results of a survey. *Pain* 1984;18:83–95.

230. Kolb L. Psychiatric aspects of treatment of painful phantom limb. *M Rec Anal* 1952;46:370–374.

231. Riddoch G. Phantom limbs and body shape. *Brain* 1941;64:197–222.

232. Melzack R. Phantom limb pain: implications for treatment of pathologic pain. *Anesthesia* 1971;35:409–419.

233. Shukla G, Sahu S, Tripathi R, Gupta D. A psychiatric study of amputees. *Brit J Psychiatry* 1982;141:50–53.

234. Kashani J, Frank R, Kashani S, Wonderlich S. Reid, J. Depression among amputees. *J Clin Psychiatry* 1983;44:256–258.

235. Randall G, Ewalt J, Blair H. Psychiatric reaction to amputation. *JAMA* 1945;128:645.

236. Sherman RA, Sherman SJ, Bruno GM. Psychological factors influencing chronic phantom limb pain: an analysis of the literature. *Pain* 1987;28:285–295.

237. Sherman RA, Griffin C, Evans C. Temporal relationships between changes in phantom limb pain intensity and changes in surface electromyogram of the residual limb. *Int J Psychophysiol* 1992 Jul;13(1):71–77.

238. Sherman R, Sherman C. Physiological parameter that change when pain changes: approaches to unraveling the "cause or reaction" Quandary. *Bulletin of the American Pain Society* 1991;1(4): 11–15.

239. Sherman R, Bruno G. Concurrent variation of burning phantom limb and stump pain with near surface blood flow in the stump. *Orthopedics* 1987;10:1395–1402.

240. Sherman RA, Gall N, Gormly J. Treatment of phantom limb pain with muscular relaxation training to disrupt the pain-anxiety-tension cycle. *Pain* 1979;6:47.

241. *See* reference 240.

242. Sherman RA, Sherman CJ, Gall NG. A survey of current phantom pain treatment in the United States. *Pain* 1980;8:85–89.

243. Monga TN, Jaksic T. Acupuncture in phantom limb pain. *Arch Phys Med Rehab* 1981;62:229.

244. Leung CY, Spoerel, WE. Effect of auriculo-acupuncture on pain. *Am J Chin Med* 1074;2:247.

245. Chong-Cheng X. Acupuncture induced phantom limb pain meridian phenomenon in acquired and congenital amputees. *Chin Med J* 1946:99 247–252.

246. Freed S. Acupuncture as therapy of traumatic affective disorders and of phantom limb pain syndrome. *Acupunct Electrother Res* 1989;14(2): 121–129.

247. Tovsa T. Phantom pains of the legs respond to skin magnets of the thorax, Abstracts of ICMART 1997 International Medical Acupuncture Symposium.

248. Ramachandran VS, Rogers-Ranachandran D. Synaesthesia in phantom limb induced with mirrors. *Proc R Soc Lond B Biol Sci* 1996 Apr 22;263 (1369): 377–386.

249. Weinstein S, Sersen EA, Vetter RJ. Phantoms and somatic sensation in cases of congenital aplasia. *Cortex* 1964;1:276–290.

250. Weinstein S, Sersen EA. Phantoms in cases of congenital absence of limbs. *Neurology* 1961;11:905–911.

251. Krane EJ, Heller LB. The prevalence of phantom sensation and pain in pediatric amputees. *J Pain Symptom Manage* 1995;10:21–29.

252. Simmel ML. The Absence of phantom for congenitally missing limb. *Am J Psychiatry* 1961;74:467–470.

253. Smith J, Thompson JM. Phantom limb pain and chemotherapy in pediatric amputees. *Mayo Clin Proc* 70:1995.

254. *See* reference 252.

255. Price DB. Phantom limb phenomenon after reattachment or cross-transfer-three patients histories. *Psychosomatics* 1998 Jul-Aug;39(4), 384–387.

256. Shukla G, Saitu SC, Gurta DK. A psychiatric study of amputees. *Br J Psychiatry* 1982;141:50–53.

257. Sherman, R.A.: Published treatments of phantom limb pain. *Am J Phys Med* 1980;59:232.

258. Bach S, Noreng MF, Tjellden NU. Phantom limb pain in amputees during the first 12 months following limb amputation after preoperative lumbar epidural blockade. *Pain* 1998;33:297–301.

259. Fisher A, Meller Y. Continuous post operative regional analgesia by nerve sheath block for amputation surgery: A pilot study. *Anesth Analg* 1991;72:300–303.

260. Malawer MM, Buch R. post operative infusional continuous regional analgesia: a technique for relief of post-operative pain following major extremity surgery. *Clin Orthop* 1991;266:227–237.

261. Ovechkin AM, Gnezdilov AV, Arlazarova NM, Savin IA, Fedorova EV, Khmelkova El. [Preventive analgesia: true of preventing the post-operative pain syndrome] Preduprezhdaiushchaia analgesiia: realnaia vozmozhnost profilaktiki posleoperatsionnogo bolevogo sindroma. *Anesteziologiia Reanimatologiia* 1996 Jul-Aug;(4):35–39.

262. Nikolajson L, Ilkjaer S, Kroner K, Christensen JH, Jensen TS. The influence of preamputation pain on post amputation stump and phantom pain. *Pain* 1997 Sept;72(3): 393–405.

263. Nikolajsen L, Ilkjaer S, Christensen JH, Kroner K, Jensen TS. Randomized trial of epidural bupivacaine and morphine in prevention of stump and phantom pain in lower-limb amputations. *Lancet* 1997 Nov 3;350(9088): 1353–1357, Nov 8.

264. Woolf CJ, Chong Mun-Seng. Preemptive analgesia-treating post operative pain by preventing the establishment of central sensitization. *Anesth Analg* 1993;77:362–379.

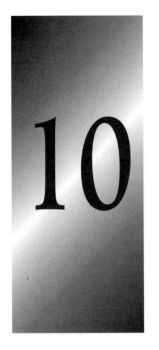

Evaluation of the Adolescent and Adult with Upper Extremity Amputation

Robert H. Meier, III, MD

The history of a person who sustains an arm amputation is paramount to the development of a relevant and comprehensive rehabilitation treatment plan. At the completion of obtaining the history, the treatment team should have a comprehensive picture of the individual. Assessing the individual's life experience prior to the amputation, their experience of becoming an arm amputee, and their hopes and desires for the future are cardinal aspects of the history-taking process.

The history of the events that led to arm amputation is important to describe since trauma is the most common cause of arm amputation. The nature of the trauma can lead to the most appropriate choice of surgical reconstruction and may indicate the type of damage caused to the skin, bones, nerves, blood vessels, and other tissues. Whether the damage was caused by a crush injury, a traction injury, a degloving injury, or blunt trauma may lead to the most appropriate surgery, including attempts to salvage the arm versus primary amputation.

In addition, associated injuries often accompany trauma severe enough to result in an amputation. These injuries may affect the head, spine, brachial plexus, thorax, and the opposite arm. The involvement of other structures essential for upper extremity function will often affect the rehabilitation goals and treatment plan.

An important essential in the history is a statement regarding the presence or absence of pain and a detailed description of any pain that is present. A differentiation should be made whether the pain is located in the residual limb or represents phantom sensation or phantom pain. Which factors improve or intensify the pain are important to include in the history. A current listing of medications, including their doses and indications for use, is important, especially if pain, an altered sleep pattern, depression, or anxiety are present. The dominant extremity should be identified so that the necessity for change-of-dominance training can be determined.

The pre-injury lifestyle and level of functional activity should be recorded. The education level of the amputee and her previous vocational history is essential in planning her rehabilitation program. A listing of her avocational interests is also important. Those things that were most relevant to this individual will assist in focusing the rehabilitation program to restore these relevant life functions as quickly as possible.

It is important to ask questions regarding sleep, appetite, and weight patterns. These are important aspects in determining the emotional adaptive process and the possible signs of anxiety, depression, or a post-traumatic stress disorder (PTSD). The presence of a good sleep pattern may indicate that the adaptive process is going well and that there is probably no problem with significant pain, anxiety, depression, or PTSD.

Questions regarding the nuclear family, marital status, and the presence or absence of a supportive group of important persons are relevant to the psychosocial dynamics that affect the amputee.

It is critical to determine the amputee's level of information regarding a prosthesis, her functional expectations regarding a prosthesis, and her understanding of the rehabilitation process. It is common for the new upper extremity amputee to have received negative information regarding the potential use of an arm prosthesis before being evaluated by the rehabilitation team.

All this information must be gathered to develop the most appropriate rehabilitation treatment plan. Having obtained this information at the beginning of the rehabilitation process, the treatment program developed can most appropriately address the individual amputee's needs. In addition, this comprehensive account of the individual will indicate what further education is essential to restore the locus of control and provide for a more individualized rehabilitation program.

This extensive history will lay the foundation for building a plan that will most likely result in the ideal level of function and emotional adaptation for the amputee (Figure 10-1).

PAST MEDICAL HISTORY

The presence of prior significant illness should be determined and any provision for continuing care of these issues incorporated as a part of the rehabilitation plan. Prior surgeries, especially involving the upper extremities, may affect the expected functional outcome. A list of medications that are currently being taken and others

that have been utilized for pain management should be obtained and recorded. Obviously, any allergies should be noted.

A smoking history should be taken, since there is a known association between the use of nicotine and chronic pain. The use of alcohol and other substances should also be listed, since their use may affect the amputee's response to rehabilitation. The use and response to marijuana should be recorded in considering the treatment of the amputee's pain.

REVIEW OF SYSTEMS

A comprehensive review of systems should be conducted, since the presence of other significant pathology provides a better understanding of comorbid factors that may influence the rehabilitation program and its outcomes. In addition, it is important to identify other symptoms that may require further work-up and treatment during this rehabilitation phase.

PSYCHOSOCIAL

The most essential portion of the history is the amputee's emotional adaptation to the loss of her arm. It has been suggested that the loss of an extremity is similar to losing a beloved family member. Attempting to understand the amputee's emotions and her adaptive process is crucial to the development of an appropriate rehabilitation treatment plan. (See Chapter 6) Some believe that the emotional adaptive process corresponds to Kuebler-Ross' staging of the grief process following death and dying (1). Is important to assess whether the amputee feels she has regained some control of her life following the amputation.

VOCATIONAL/AVOCATIONAL

The type of work performed prior to the amputation and the job title should be obtained. Whether the individual has yet to return to work, and her plans for future work, should be recorded. Her expectation of or need to return to work should also be ascertained. The educational level of the person with the amputation also provides an idea of what potential vocations could be realistic for future planning.

The activities that the amputee enjoyed prior to the amputation should be listed, and whether any of these activities have been tried or successfully accomplished since the amputation should be stated.

FUNCTIONAL AND ACTIVITY LEVEL

This is an opportunity to determine which activities of daily living (ADLs) the person is currently performing

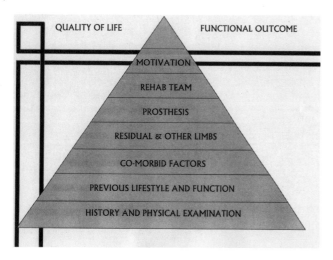

FIGURE 10-1

Pyramid schema of components for successful amputee outcomes and quality of life.

or having difficulty in achieving. This is also an opportunity to chronicle a typical 24-hour day for the individual. The amount or type of activity performed following the amputation should be compared to that performed prior to the amputation. This list should include a wide variety of ADLs, routine indoor and outdoor household tasks, and vocational and avocational activities. This listing of functions will serve as the baseline for future outcome measures and can be used to demonstrate functional improvement during the rehabilitation process.

APPETITE/SLEEP

Disturbances in appetite and sleep patterns are relevant to the amputee's sense of well-being and her emotional adaptation to the limb loss. An insufficient or irregular sleep pattern may also contribute to the quantity of pain experienced. The longest period of uninterrupted sleep should be noted, and the total hours of sleep per night should be quantitated.

PHYSICAL EXAMINATION

Remaining Arm

A long-taught tenet of physical diagnosis states that the normal segments of the body should be evaluated before the abnormal segments are examined. This is important in the evaluation of a person with a unilateral amputation. The "normal" remaining extremity should be examined first to determine any evidence of pathology. This arm will assume the majority of functional demand and be placed under greater use, even if the amputated arm is fitted with a prosthesis.

The amount of scapular abduction (protraction) and forward flexion at the glenohumeral joints of both arms is important to obtain maximum cable excursion for body-powered prosthetic use.

Amputated Extremity

The length of the residual bone, the quality of the soft tissue coverage, and the presence of pain in the amputated limb are three of the most important determinants of prosthetic prescription and of functional outcome with the prosthesis. It is important to measure and record the length from a bony landmark to the end of the bone and to the end of the soft tissues. These measurements determine the length of the lever arm that will be present to utilize the prosthesis. Measuring the glenohumeral and the scapulothoracic ranges of motion separately is important for the understanding of any shoulder pathology and the biomechanics that can be

anticipated for functional prosthetic use (2). The amount of glenohumeral motion will help assess the envelope of motion through which the prosthesis can be used. The scapulothoracic motion will determine the amount of cable excursion that can be generated from one or both sides of the thorax (3). Four inches of cable excursion will provide for the maximum opening of a terminal device and elbow flexion for the body-powered transhumeral prosthesis (4). If the elbow remains, the amount of motion and muscle strength at the elbow is important to quantify and record. Flexion, extension, pronation, and supination should be evaluated.

A description of the scar, its placement, any sensitivity, and the maturity of its healing process should be recorded. The mobility of the scar and the soft tissues over the bone should also be recorded. Good scar mobility decreases the amount of shear that occurs at the stump–socket interface when wearing and using the arm prosthesis. The presence of a neuroma in the scar or in the residual arm, whether this neuroma is painful or not, should be assessed. A neuroma can be the size of a small fishing weight up to the size of a walnut. Palpation of the neuroma will often reproduce pain in the distribution of the peripheral nerve that is involved in the neuroma process.

A description of the end of the residual arm bone is also relevant, since sharp edges, prominent bone edges with little overlying soft tissue coverage, and the presence of new bone formation may make comfortable prosthetic fitting difficult. New bone formation in the soft tissues (heteroptopic bone formation or myositis ossificans) may occur in the presence of trauma, burns, or central nervous system injury. The presence of these bone problems may make stump revision necessary prior to any attempt at prosthetic fitting.

Range of motion measurements must be obtained so that the most appropriate prosthetic prescription is rendered and any limitations of motion that can affect the anticipated prosthetic function are recorded (5). The two most important arm motions are scapular abduction (protraction) that generates scapulothoracic motion and glenohumeral flexion. Scapulothoracic motion must be measured separately from the amount of glenohumeral motion. To separate these motions, the scapula should be blocked by the examiner from any motion. These are essential motions in the use of any type of prosthetic arm. For every 2 degrees of glenohumeral motion, there is 1 degree of scapulothoracic motion (Figure 10-2). In addition, all other arm range of motion at the shoulder should be measured, since they may help substitute for other lost range of motion. At the shoulder, these include flexion, extension, abduction, adduction, internal rotation, and external rotation (Figures 10-3, 10-4, and 10-5).

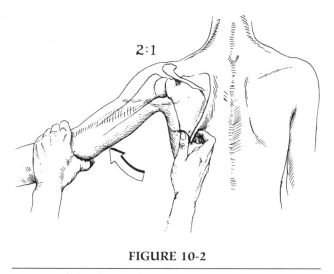

FIGURE 10-2

Ratio of glenohumeral versus scapulothoracic motion.

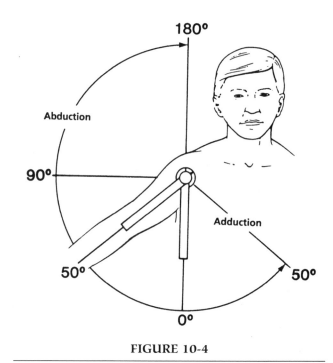

FIGURE 10-4

Shoulder range of motion for abduction and adduction.

A careful testing of individual arm muscles should be performed to determine the strength of each major muscle (6–8). For the transhumeral amputee, the muscles that produce flexion and abduction are most important for body-powered prosthetic activation. In addition, to activate the alternating internal elbow lock, a combination of shoulder extension, abduction, and depression are necessary. The examiner must measure the strength of the primary and secondary scapular movers. This should include the trapezius, serratus anterior, and pectoralis major for scapular stability on the thorax. In addition, the latissimus dorsi assists in downward rota-

tion of the scapula (Figure 10-6). Protraction of the scapula is produced by contraction of the serratus anterior, pectoralis major, and pectoralis minor muscles (Figure 10-7). This motion of scapular protraction on both sides provides cable excursion for elbow flexion and terminal device opening in the body-powered prosthetic design. Forward flexion of the humerus is produced by

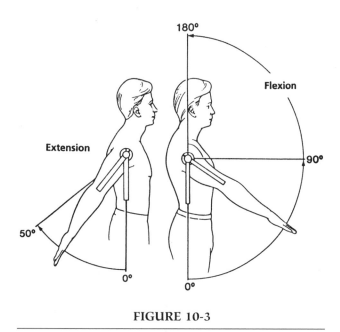

FIGURE 10-3

Shoulder range of motion for flexion and extension.

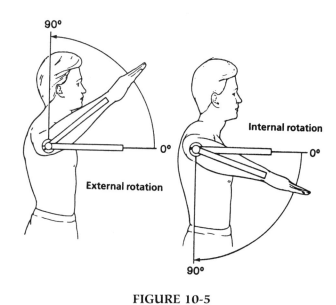

FIGURE 10-5

Shoulder range of motion for external and internal rotation.

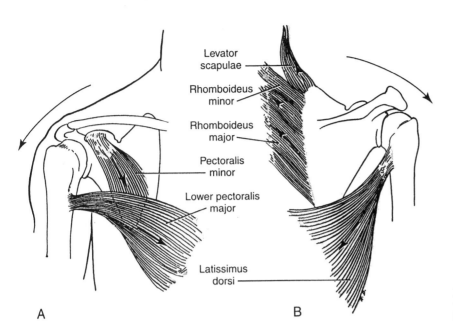

Levator
scapulae

Rhomboideus
minor

Rhomboideus
major

Pectoralis
minor

Lower pectoralis
major

Latissimus
dorsi

A   B

FIGURE 10-6

Muscles producing downward rotation of the scapula.

the deltoid, biceps, and pectoralis major (Figure 10-8). Extension of the arm is produced by the deltoid, teres major latissimus dorsi, long head of the triceps, and pectoralis major (Figure 10-9). Abduction of the humerus is produced by the deltoid and the supraspinatus muscles (Figure 10-10). The presence of triceps, latissimus dorsi, lateral deltoid, and posterior deltoid activity are important for the compound prosthetic elbow lock activating motions of down, back, and out when using a body-powered, alternating locking elbow.

In the transradial amputee, the essential motions that remain should be elbow flexion and extension, and the forearm may have residual pronation and supination (Figures 10-11 and 10-12). In addition to the above shoulder muscles, in the transradial amputee, the elbow flexors (Figure 10-13), including the biceps, the brachioradialis, and the wrist flexors provide forearm life. The triceps produces elbow extension power. In the transradial amputee, the presence of residual wrist flexors and extensors as they cross the elbow maybe important for myoelectric control.

Sensory testing should be performed, keeping in mind both the peripheral nerve sensory pattern and the dermatomal pattern maps (9) (Figures 10-14 and

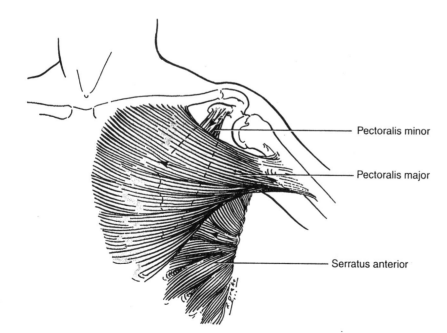

Pectoralis minor

Pectoralis major

Serratus anterior

FIGURE 10-7

Muscles producing protraction of the scapula.

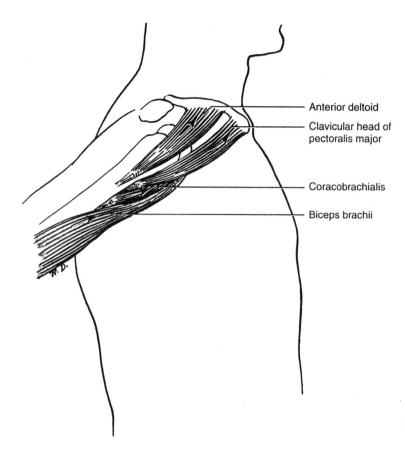

Anterior deltoid

Clavicular head of
pectoralis major

Coracobrachialis

Biceps brachii

FIGURE 10-8

Muscles producing flexion of the arm.

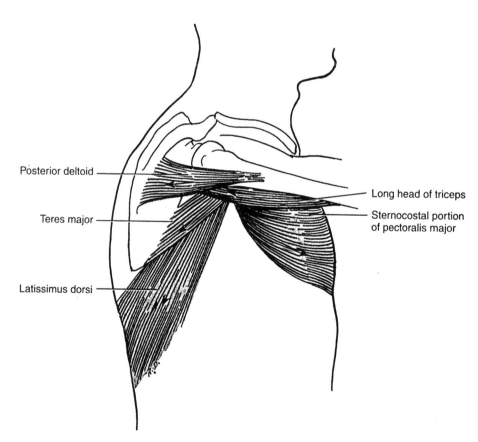

Posterior deltoid

Long head of triceps

Sternocostal portion
of pectoralis major

Teres major

Latissimus dorsi

FIGURE 10-9

Muscles producing extension of
the arm.

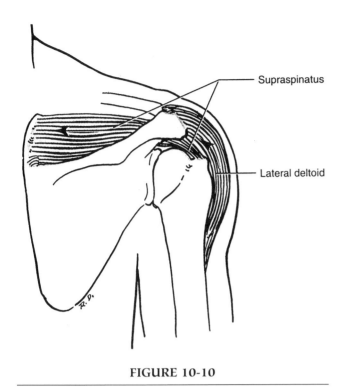

FIGURE 10-10

Muscles producing abduction of the arm.

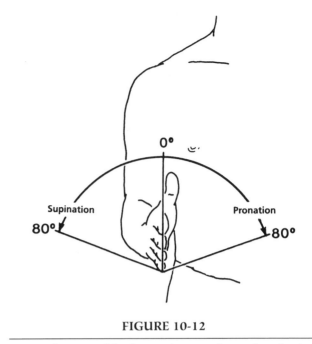

FIGURE 10-12

Range of motion of the forearm in pronation and supination.

10-15). This is a point in the examination where the presence of a brachial plexus or a peripheral nerve injury should be ascertained. Often, these injuries have been overlooked during the acute post-injury period but can now be completely evaluated since the focus is not just on salvaging the person's life or arm.

As this examination is being performed, keep in mind the peripheral neural connections represented by the sensory, motor, and reflex testing. The examiner should always mentally trace the connections between the muscle or dermatome being examined to the peripheral nerve

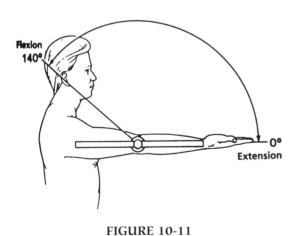

FIGURE 10-11

Range of motion at the elbow in flexion and extension.

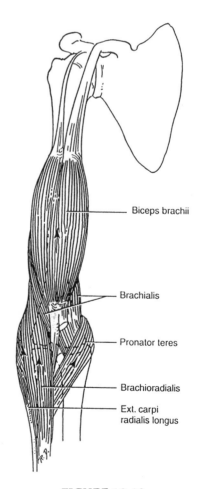

FIGURE 10-13

Flexor muscles of the elbow.

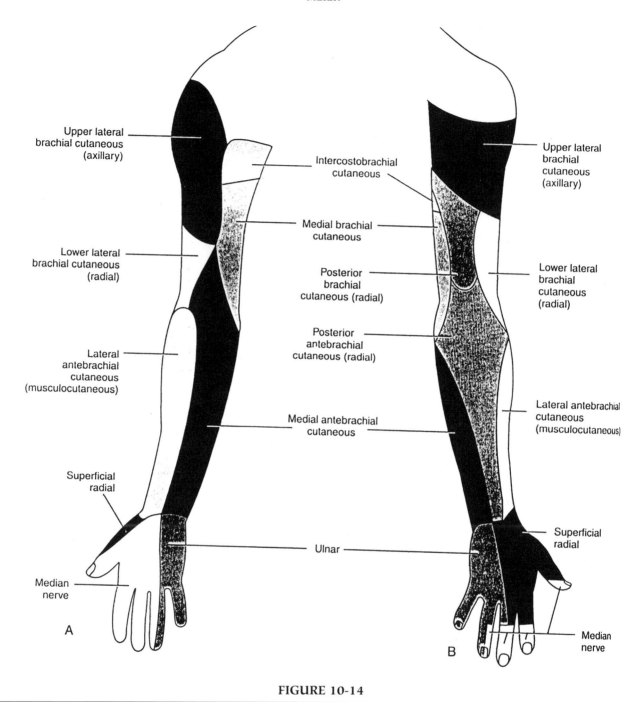

FIGURE 10-14

Peripheral nerve sensory map of the upper extremity.

represented, the region of the brachial plexus from which that nerve arises, and the spinal nerves represented by that muscle and nerve (8) (Table 10-1, Figure 10-16).

Lower Extremities

In the bilateral arm amputee, it is important to examine the lower extremities and trunk, especially because it may be desirable to teach the amputee foot skills that

may assist function. The most common foot skills are useful for toileting and for opening doors. The range of motion at the hips, especially flexion and rotation, are most important for achieving maximum foot skills.

Head and Neck

Frequently, the arm amputee will find that using her mouth and teeth will provide an important functional

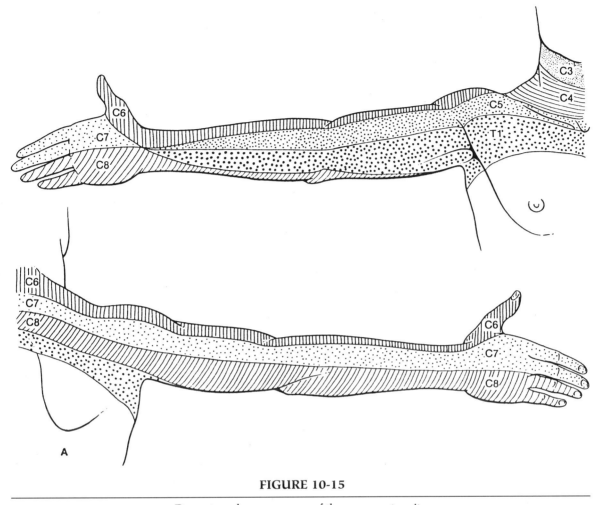

FIGURE 10-15

Dermatomal sensory map of the upper extremity.

assist to the remaining arm. Motion of the cervical spine is important in many amputees. Cervical flexion and rotation are most important for functional placement of the mouth and teeth.

MEDICAL RECORD REVIEW

A thorough review of the post-injury and perioperative records should be included as a part of the history. All dates of surgical intervention should be recorded, as well as a description of the procedures accomplished. A determination of the manner in which the muscles and soft tissues were closed over the bone should be made. An assessment of the quantity of postoperative pain and the manner in which it was controlled should be recorded.

A discussion of the postamputation therapy, both physical and emotional, should be recorded. This assessment should include whether there was change of dominance training, what adaptive equipment was provided, and what exercise program was taught to the amputee. It is also important to ascertain whether any emotional assessment or intervention was provided.

A presentation of the level of function as assessed by the treating therapist should be made. Finally, the source of third-party payment should be included in this part of the record review. In today's health system, differences exist from one payer source to another regarding both rehabilitation service provision and prosthetic sponsorship.

DIAGNOSES

For ease of amputee service provision and health care provider use of the medical record, it is essential to provide proper and complete diagnostic information. This information should include a specified level of arm amputation, the side amputated, the amputation etiology, the date of injury, and the date of amputation (Figure 10-17).

The diagnosis of the type of pain experienced should be placed under the diagnostic listings. Any pres-

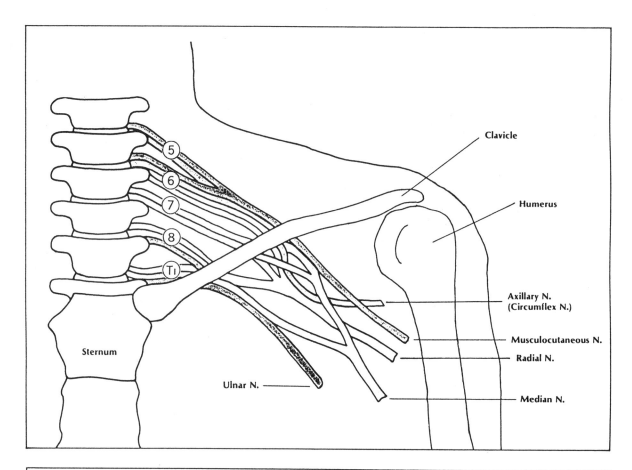

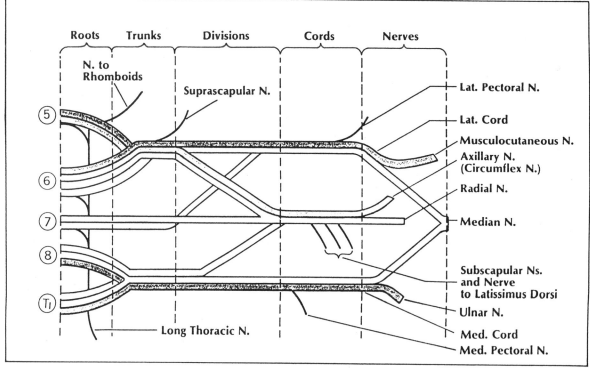

FIGURE 10-16

Schematic of the portions of the brachial plexus.

TABLE 10-1
Muscle and Nerve Chart

MUSCLE	ACTION	NERVE	SEGMENTAL INNERVATION
Sternocleidomastoid	Lateral flexion and rotation of head	Accessory cranial	CN XI
Trapezius	Elevation of the tip of scapula	Accessory cranial	CN XI
Levator scapulae	Elevation of scapula	Nerves to levator scapulae	C3 4
Both rhomboids	Retraction of scapula	Dorsal scapular	C 5
Subclavius	Depression of clavicle	Nerve to subclavius	C 5–6
Teres minor	Lateral rotation of arm	Axillary	C 5–6
Deltoid	Abduction of arm	Axillary	C 5–6
Subscapularis	Medial rotation of arm	Upper subscapular	C 5–6
		Lower subscapular	C 5–6
Teres major	Extension and medial rotation of arm	Lower subscapular	C 5–6
Supraspinatus	Abduction of arm	Suprascapular	C 5–6
Infraspinatus	Lateral rotation of arm	Suprascapular	C 5–6
Serratus anterior	Upward rotation of scapula	Long thoracic	C 5–6–7
Upper pectoralis major	Abduction/flexion of arm	Lateral pectoral	C 5–6–7
Lower pectoralis major	Abduction/extension of arm	Medial pectoral	C 8, T1
Pectoralis minor	Depression of shoulder	Medial pectoral	C 8, T1
Latissimus dorsi	Extension/adduction of arm	Thoracodorsal	C 6–7–8

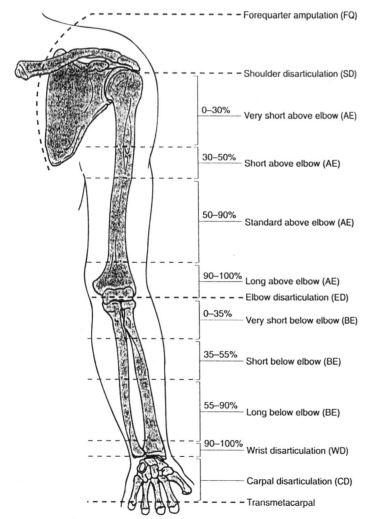

Forequarter amputation (FQ)

Shoulder disarticulation (SD)

0–30% — Very short above elbow (AE)

30–50% — Short above elbow (AE)

50–90% — Standard above elbow (AE)

90–100% — Long above elbow (AE)

Elbow disarticulation (ED)

0–35% — Very short below elbow (BE)

35–55% — Short below elbow (BE)

55–90% — Long below elbow (BE)

90–100% — Wrist disarticulation (WD)

Carpal disarticulation (CD)

Transmetacarpal

FIGURE 10-17

Common levels of amputation in the arm, forearm, and hand.

ence of a mood disorder or of PTSD should be stated here. Other associated injuries should be listed, since they may modify the rehabilitation plan and the eventual outcome. This information is especially important in comparing amputee care outcomes and for third-party payer coverage of the services rendered. This complete information may also be used by government agencies to determine the degree of disability present and the amputee's eligibility for supplemental income and health care sponsorship.

The list of diagnoses for an upper extremity amputee should include, at minimum:

- Specific level and side of amputation
- Etiology of amputation
- Pain and its type
- DSM—emotional disorder (10)
- Associated injuries
- Other comorbid illnesses, either pre-existing or following the amputation

TREATMENT PLAN WITH GOALS

The history and physical examination naturally lead to the development of the initial comprehensive rehabilitation treatment goals and plan. This plan must be directly related to the amputee's perceived needs and goals. Most commonly, this plan is more complete if it contains input from the variety of rehabilitation team members who will be involved in the care of the arm amputee.

From the amputee and the medical record, it should be determined whether a comprehensive rehabilitation treatment plan has previously been developed and what the specific goals and timelines were. In addition, it is important to assess what level of amputee education has been accomplished and what gaps in the amputee's knowledge base exist.

Including the amputee in the development of this plan and using a team conference approach can be the most efficient manner to communicate between the amputee and the treatment team. This direct communication will help to avoid misunderstandings among the several team members and assist in clarifying any areas that may not have clear goals or uniform team agreement.

CONCLUSIONS

A thorough history and physical examination are the basis for developing and implementing the rehabilita-

tion treatment plan for the person with an arm amputation. This evaluation must include much more information than just the history of the amputation and an examination of the amputated arm if it is to meet the needs and desires of the arm amputee. The decision for prosthetic prescription flows from this complete assessment. Only with this type of assessment can any prosthetic prescription be expected to provide the optimal outcomes from the various options of cosmesis, comfort, and function available for the arm amputee. This type of evaluation may also lead to a recommendation to not fit and train in the use of a prosthesis. Instead, the goals may focus on achieving maximum function without the use of a prosthesis. In this manner, the emphasis is placed on the individual who has sustained the arm amputation and not on the prosthesis.

*B*ibliography

1. Jenkins DB, Hollinshead WH. *Functional Anatomy of the Limbs and Back, Eight Edition.* Philadelphia: WB Saunders, 2002.
2. Hoppenfeld S, Hutton R. *Physical Examination of Spine and Extremities.* Saddle Brook, New Jersey: Prentice Hall, 1976.
3. Cocchiarella L, Andersson GBJ. *Guides to the Evaluation of Permanent Impairment, Fifth Edition.* AMA Press, 2000.
4. Kapandji I, Kandel MJ. *Physiology of Joints (Upper Extremity), Fifth Edition.* Edinburgh: Churchill Livingstone, 1982.
5. Kapandji, Honore LH. *Physiology of the Joints: The Trunk and Vertebral Column, Second Edition.* Edinburgh: Churchill Livingstone, 1974.
6. Kandel MJ, Kapandji I. *The Physiology of the Joints: Annotated Diagrams of the Mechanics of the Human Joints, Fifth Edition.* Edinburgh: Churchill Livingstone, 1987.
7. Kendall FP, McCreary EK. *Muscles, Testing, and Function, Fourth Edition.* Philadelphia: Lippincott, Williams & Wilkins, 1993.
8. Tubiana R. *Examination of the Hand and Upper Limb.* Philadelphia: WB Saunders, 1984.
9. Haerer A. *De Jong's The Neurological Examination, Fifth Edition.* Philadelphia: Lippincott, Williams & Wilkins, 1992.
10. Netter FH. *Atlas of Human Anatomy, Third Edition.* Novartis Medical Education, 2003.

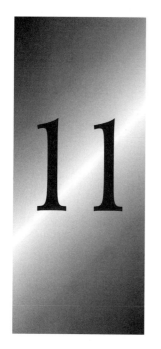

The Prosthetist's Evaluation and Planning Process with the Upper Extremity Amputee

Randell D. Alley, BSC, CP, FAAOP

Evaluation of the Person with an Arm Amputation

A rehabilitative approach that appears to have the most favorable response is one that utilizes an evaluation and planning process that is divided into sections:

1. Interview/practitioner education
2. Physical assessment
3. Patient education
4. Rehabilitation strategy
5. Outcomes assessment (postdelivery assesstment)

The initial stage of the evaluation is an interview, in which the prosthetist attempts to learn all she can about the individual.

It is important to disseminate information to the patient concerning current developments in upper extremity prosthetics. Prior to this, however, establishment of rapport with the patient is a priority.

One of the dilemmas in upper extremity prosthetics is the lack of practitioner experience in the field. The typical prosthetist is given minimal education on the subject in formalized institutions, for various reasons. The instructors have limited time to disseminate their full curriculum, and, they recognize that the vast majority of cases seen will involve lower extremity dysvascular patients. For this reason, the clinician is expected to gain a comprehensive understanding of upper extremity prosthetics in clinical practice. Herein lies the "upper extremity dilemma." Practitioners are given minimal information initially, with the expectation that experience in the field will fortify their knowledge base, yet it is extremely rare that the practitioner is exposed to upper extremity amputation cases. The approximate numbers of upper extremity amputations per year in the United States totals some 10–12,000. These numbers suggest that the average practitioner evaluates between one and two upper extremity prosthetic patients per year, and in many cases, one or two in a career is not uncommon. The upper extremity amputee relies on the evaluating practitioner to provide all the answers, yet in most cases, this practitioner is rarely familiar with even the most basic of upper extremity prosthetic principles. Patients often sense this lack of experience, and this may trigger additional psychological detriments. Indeed, more than half of all upper extremity congenital and traumatic limb-deficient individuals do not wear a prosthesis. One of the more predominant reasons for this involves a bad first experience. This experience is not solely the result of the prosthetic system utilized, but frequently is associated with the initial evaluation. It is, in fact, the author's opinion that many successful outcomes hinge just as significantly on the evaluative method as they do on medical history, education, vocation/avocation, activity level, mechanical aptitude, psychosocial factors, and prosthetic technology.

When evaluating an adolescent or adult upper extremity amputee there exists a certain protocol which, if followed, will result in a patient who is confident, both in the prosthetist's experience and ability, as well as in being able to recognize the most appropriate prosthetic options to maximize his or her rehabilitation potential. The first step is to recognize the specific differences that exist for patients of varying amputation levels and medical history.

One of the most significant aspects of a traumatic upper extremity amputee is the degree of psychological adjustment required to facilitate adaptation and avoid severe psychological distress. Because the majority of all amputations are due to the complications of chronic disease and because most of these amputations can be anticipated, the preoperative period allows the opportunity for psychological preparation of the patient. In addition they write: "Our experience and review of the literature suggest that psychological intervention during the preoperative period is associated with a less complicated postoperative adjustment and grieving experience (1)." This finding underscores one of the most significant challenges facing both the traumatic amputee and the prosthetist. Because the majority of upper extremity limb-deficiencies are traumatic, preoperative preparation is rare. In the absence of the ability to preoperatively prepare the individual, the psychological impact is severe. Clinical and psychological examinations have revealed a high level of aggressiveness, anxiety, and depressive disorders among such patients (2). It is of the utmost importance for the evaluating prosthetist to adjust his or her approach to more effectively deal with these stressors inherent in postoperative cases.

Friedmann writes: "Treating the psychological problems faced by the amputee often has more significance to his life than the quality of the surgery or the nature of his prosthetic device... The disability entailed by amputation... is far more the result of individual and social attitudes than it is with loss of function... It is the loss of ability to relate psychologically, socially, sexually, and vocationally that inhibits amputees most (3)."

Racy describes a four-stage model of the adaptation process to limb loss. The initial stage is the preoperative period, which is lacking in most traumatic upper extremity cases. Experiencing the anxiety associated with one's concerns about body image, the financial impact of medical care, and the ability to maintain personal relationships helps elective amputees prepare for the road ahead. With traumatic amputees, these anxieties are typically experienced post-operatively (4).

BUILDING RAPPORT

Establishing rapport is a priority for the practitioner. The building of rapport is a multifaceted challenge involving comprehensive and current knowledge of, and the ability to effectively disseminate, upper extremity prosthetic principles, terminology, and technology, as well as an ability to perceive the psychological and physical needs of the patient. This perception will lead to situations in which the practitioner can more easily empathize with the upper extremity prosthetic patient's concerns. This empathy will be recognized and most likely appreciated by the patient, thus resulting in improved communication and respect, and possibly leading to a more positive outlook on the road ahead. Psychological intervention during the preoperative period is associated with a less complicated postoperative adjustment and grieving experience. If we apply this finding to the preprosthetic and postprosthetic periods, it can certainly be argued that an improved psychological outcome can be attained with a comprehensive evaluation. It can then further be shown that, with the help of supportive literature, an improved psychological state can lead to an improved sense of well-being and body image, both of which are instrumental to no small degree in prosthetic outcomes.

Practitioner Education by the Amputee

The next phase of the interview allows the patient an opportunity to educate the evaluator concerning past history; medical history (a more comprehensive study of the medical history of these individuals is given in the physician's perspective in chapter 10); previous and current medications; past, present, and future vocational requirements and avocational desires; activity level (prior, current, and anticipated); and extenuating psychosocial factors. During this phase, the prosthetist initially develops an overall sense regarding the essence of the person with the arm amputation. This gathering of data allows the practitioner to piece together the foundation on which the rehabilitation plan will be built.

Physical Evaluation

The obvious physical characteristics of the patient should be noted such as age, height, and weight. These elements may play a role in determining a predisposition toward or away from specific options, but by no means are any a singular determinant of a particular rehabilitation path. The physical evaluation, like the psychological one, is comprised of many discoveries, each of which lends a piece to the puzzle. When taken as a whole, these discoveries assist the prosthetist and other members of the rehabilitation team in to form a successful strategy.

A critical factor that impacts the prosthetic rehabilitation plan is the depth and breadth of the individual's prior or current prosthetic experience. This can range from impressions received from others with amputation to long-term wearing patterns of a particular prosthetic control scheme or socket design established by the patient previous to the current evaluation. When a study is taken comparing the utilization of one option to that of another, many questions should be asked.

What evaluation protocols were used, if any?

What was the psychologic state of the individual (self-esteem, body image, etc.) preoperatively, postoperatively, preprosthetic and postprosthetic?

What interface design was used and how intimate was the fit?

What was the experience of the prosthetist?

What were all the relevant indications and contraindications for the system(s) chosen?

What was the quality of the maintenance and postdelivery assessment programs utilized?

Did the patient have confidence in the practitioner administering care?

Did the patient receive adequate therapy?

Did the patient receive adequate controls training?

Was he or she given a proper description of the capabilities of the system utilized?

Was the individual properly prepared for the weight or the distribution of weight to be encountered?

Was the patient prepared for psychosocial reactions of others to their static (passive) and dynamic (operational) cosmesis while wearing the prosthesis?

What is the climate, and how might this impact results for the various control schemes?

A multitude of variables influence the individual's prosthetic outcomes and it is extremely important to keep them in mind when reviewing the literature assessing comparisons of one type of prosthetic system to another.

Often, an individual will not have a good impression of a particular prosthetic system, although it may be the most appropriate choice. For example, a person may have been fit with a powered system that was improperly designed or unrealistically described during the initial evaluation by an inexperienced prosthetist, thus causing a negative impression of an otherwise excellent option.

Habits developed from long-term usage can have an impact on the individual's ability to properly control a different prosthetic control scheme. For example, if converting a user from cable operation to myoelectric control, the gross body movements utilized to operate the harness and cable system may have been so deeply ingrained that inadvertent generation of electromyographical (EMG) signals may occur when the individual is attempting to operate the powered prosthesis. In this situation, a period of training that reduces or eliminates the degree of gross body movement is required, isolating the intrinsic EMG to volitional activation.

A different situation can occur when a patient has grown accustomed to a particular set of prosthetic parameters, thus hampering their ability to be receptive to new ideas. For example, the individual may have become accustomed to a loose socket fit over the years, either due to wearing prosthetic socks to control volume fluctuations, poor initial design of the socket, weight loss, or fluid redistribution over time. If a more intimate fitting socket is biomechanically advantageous for this individual, it may still be difficult to convince the patient to opt for change. In many cases, a patient's perceived needs can be in direct opposition to a recommended prosthetic intervention that would enable them to realize their maximum rehabilitation potential. Which side wins depends on the individuals involved and the ability of the recommended component or control scheme to present adequate benefits to override patient preference. Prosthetic experience colors an individual's perceptions and often impacts his functional capabilities in many ways. One must weigh the value of theoretic benefits with patient preference and determine the optimal solution.

Nearly every study previously undertaken ignores that these inner perceptions and prior experiences, in addition to a host of other factors, dictate a particular result when regarding outcomes. For this reason, the medical and payer communities are strongly urged to rethink their reliance on studies that have omitted a comprehensive analysis of these variables. The prosthetist must also do his or her part in ensuring that these variables are recognized and dealt with appropriately.

Vocational history, and current and future needs and desires play an important role in piecing together the rehabilitation picture. It has been noted in several studies (and common sense will also tell us) that a fairly small percentage of people with traumatic upper extremity amputations return to their preoperative occupation. For many of these individuals, especially those involved with a vocation that demanded the use of their hands, this is quite a blow not only to their self-esteem but also to their motivation to work at all. The discrepancy in vocational outcomes between those who have lost an arm, especially at a high level, and those who have lost a leg is tremendous. The need for precisely controlled ambulation is typically rarer than the need for fine dexterity at the workplace. Thus, when, regarding vocational requirements, the prosthetist must ascertain the level of realism involved in the goal set of an individual with upper extremity amputation. Levels of expectation must be reasonably set during the evaluation phase to avoid deep disappointment early on in the rehabilitation process. However, it is important to keep in mind that human potentials are never completely defined by the scope of prosthetic systems alone. In many cases, the will of the individual can surprise us with what can be accomplished. It is equally important that the prosthetist does not discourage the patient from learning by personal experience what limits exist. It is our duty merely to describe the operational characteristics of prostheses and to know the general limitations and advantages in each control strategy.

Avocational desires can be just as critical to an individual with upper extremity amputation as vocational requirements. Winchell writes: "Common psychological benefits of recreation include enhanced feelings of well-being, increased self-esteem, improved sleep patterns, better concentration and alertness, less depression and anxiety, decreased stress, reduced dependence on mood-altering drugs, physical and emotional discharge of frustration and anger, and opportunities to interact with others (5)." It is important that the prosthetist regard the level of avocational expectations desired by the patient and that general operational limitations of the intended prosthetic system are discussed. Activity-specific or "adaptive" prostheses are often the best option for individuals who desire to participate in events that demand specialized capabilities and functions. Virtually no limit exists on what can be designed, given enough creativity and patient feedback.

Physical Considerations

It is necessary to categorize and document amputation types. Amputation levels, from partial finger to interscapulothoracic, each require a diverse approach when attempting to determine the most appropriate prosthetic system. A comprehensive description of evaluation techniques specific to each level of amputation is outside the scope of this chapter.

The cause of amputation is not merely important for accurate record keeping, but also plays a key role in the authorization process, which will be discussed later. It is often difficult for patients to talk about the details surrounding their trauma, but knowing the circumstances of injury allows the practitioner to better empathize with, and hence provide better care for, the individual.

The date of injury is extremely crucial in determining the success of the rehabilitation plan. If the patient is fit outside the "golden window" (0 to 90 days postoperatively), studies have shown a significant drop in patient acceptance of a prosthesis. A successful outcome is possible after this period; however, the challenge of overcoming the unilateral patient's propensity for exclusively utilizing the contralateral limb is great.

Patient Education

The education of the patient should follow both the building of rapport and the dissemination of information by the practitioner. This includes but is not limited to information concerning prosthetic history, amputee support groups, amputee demo- and psychographics, prosthetic systems, and developing technology. This allows the patient to gain a better understanding of the foundation underlying the prosthetic rehabilitation process. This understanding leads to an improved ability by both the patient and the prosthetist to identify the optimum prosthetic pathway for superior outcomes. In the Prosthetic and Orthotic Interview, a survey of nineteen organizations belonging to the World Veterans Federation indicates that a major complaint of amputees is "poor dissemination of knowledge to doctors and amputees regarding new prostheses," and "a lack of opportunity for 'input' at the research level (6)."

Prosthetic Options

It is extremely important to both prosthetist and patient that the evaluation consists of a detailed discussion of all available options, together with the inherent advantages and limitations of each option. All too often, a prosthetist simply discusses what he or she feels is the most appropriate prosthetic system, based on the simple observation of physical characteristics or financial status. This approach has several problems. The patient's status may change. The patient may have preconceived notions about what will work best for them based on a variety of past experiences or research. The patient may be able to help others by being a source of accurate information on prosthetic systems.

Finally, a prosthetist's ethical responsibility lies in the unbiased education of the patient. In discussions with prospective payers of prosthetic services, many payers tend to believe the patient will always choose the most expensive option available. Although there are exceptions, most patients and prosthetists alike opt for the system(s) they believe will be the most functional, within the scope of the patient's needs and desires. Ultimately, a successful wearer is the product of matching the appropriate prosthetic system(s) to the physical, psychological, and psychosocial context of the individual.

Prosthetic Language

A discussion of the relevant prosthetic terminology is also very important. If patients are more comfortable with the language of the prosthetist, they will feel more in control of the situation. As has been discussed previously, many traumatic amputees are in a fragile state of mind. In one study, psychiatric manifestations were assessed in seventy-two amputees post-operatively. Nearly two-thirds had psychiatric symptoms in the form of depression, anxiety, crying spells, insomnia, loss of appetite, suicidal ideas, and psychotic behavior (7). Many literary inferences stress the power of language and its effect on self-esteem. Given the fragile psychological state of many recent upper extremity amputees, the avoidance of specific terminology that can trigger a negative body image or self-esteem is imperative. Use of the words "stump" or "nubbins" for example, do not convey the most positive impressions. And, if we agree that self-esteem and body image affect outcomes in some small measure, it stands to reason that a thoughtful approach to the terminology used may bring about a more successful result. In addition, Rogers, MacBride, Whylie, and Freeman state: "there is a complex interplay between physical and emotional factors in the rehabilitative process after amputation of a limb. Although this is recognized by those working in the field of rehabilitation medicine, an overview of the literature indicates that there is comparatively little psychosocial research, education, and innovative programming (8)." It is imperative then, that a prosthetist should attempt to maximize his or her study of relevant literature, as well as establish predefined methods of information gathering and dissemination, to properly set the stage for a successful outcome.

Indications and Contraindications

All relevant factors and their impact on the utilization of the prosthesis must be considered when evaluating the physical characteristics of the individual who has experienced trauma. Whether a patient has undergone unilateral or multilateral amputation, the extent and type of scar tissue, length of lever arm, muscle strength, and range of motion of the affected side are some of the indications and contraindications for particular components or control schemes. Frequently, a characteristic may be an indication or contraindication for several systems. Insufficient limb length (lever arm, weight, and weight distribution issues) can often inhibit or restrict the utilization of any prosthesis.

In many cases, the same characteristic may be a contraindication for multiple systems, yet for different reasons. For example, an individual with residual limb scar tissue may find it painful to operate a conventional prosthesis due to the forces exerted on this area as a result of the gross body movements required (the tension on the cable transfers to the socket and causes an opposite and equal reactionary force within the socket to be generated). This same scar tissue may prevent or distort the transmission of EMG signals to electrodes in a myoelectric prosthesis. Other factors may be more specific and hence more readily understood as to their role in excluding or including a specific control scheme. The desire for active prehension typically excludes the utilization of a passive "non-prehensile" prosthesis or the option of not wearing a prosthesis at all. For example, deficits subsequent to amputation that result in the need for increased grip strength or functional range of motion outside the "frontal envelope" typically preclude or at least negatively affect precision control of a voluntary-opening cable-operated prosthetic system. Severe limitations in the ability to generate sufficient gross body movements whether due to pain or lack of adequate musculature are also considered a contraindication for body-powered prostheses.

The inadequate generation of detectable EMG signals is an obvious contraindication for myoelectric control. However, it is extremely important to note that insufficient and even nondetectable EMG does not automatically preclude the use of a myoelectric system, because effective training can produce a rapid and significant improvement in signal generation. Systems have also recently become much more capable of handling small amplitudes of EMG while subsequently improving shielding capabilities.

In addition to the affected side, contralateral concerns are extremely significant. Tendonitis, decreased hand function, and overuse all demand heightened prosthetic intervention to allay possible future surgical procedures that may be required as a result of these concerns. The prosthetist must evaluate their impact and recommend the appropriate method of control. Finally, some methods of control may inherently lead to future complications. The use of a standard figure eight harness can impinge enough in the axilla to create excessive compression in this region, resulting in tingling of the hand, numbness, and other symptoms that ultimately may progress to nerve entrapment syndrome. The use of a vertically-arrayed dual ring (V.A.D.R.) harness or similar system results in a much more efficient design where harness attachment points are spread along the frontal plane in line with the spinal column and prohibited from translating horizontally under pull. In addition, the axilla angle is widened significantly, greatly reducing axilla pressure for the individual with unilateral limb loss or amelia. An experienced prosthetist learns to look for the tell-tale signs of developing complications, and alters the patient's rehabilitation path to ensure the best possible outcome.

The number of indications and contraindications for each level and severity of amputation is too numerous to list here. It is paramount that the practitioner is well versed in what is appropriate for the varied amputation categories and specific patient requirements.

REHABILITATION PROCESS

Patients often complain of being inadequately involved in their own rehabilitation, with the entire process taking place with minimal input from the end user. For this reason, the details of the rehabilitation plan should be laid out in a clear and concise manner, utilizing terminology that the patient can understand. At this point, the rehabilitation team (including the patient) begins to outline the steps involved in realizing a successful outcome.

Justifications and Authorizations

If a third-party payer is involved, the initial phase of the rehabilitation plan subsequent to a comprehensive evaluation concerns the justification and authorization process. The patient must understand that, for a prosthetic business to remain viable, it must earn a profit. To earn a profit, that same business must be paid for services rendered. As is so often the case, services that are provided before payment is guaranteed frequently are only partially compensated for and may even be denied. Often the business is faced with the agonizing decision to require payment from the patient, to forego future services for this individual, or face continual loss on the patient's behalf, none of which is an ideal situation for either party. To prevent these unfortunate occurrences from happening, a dialog with the patient concerning his or her financial responsibility in such an event, the overall expected cost of the prosthetic system to be utilized, and an annual maintenance estimate is important. In addition, the patient should not be led to assume that authorization is assured. Most at-risk companies require some form of medical or vocational justification before they will even consider a proposal. Because of the previously described psychological state of many individuals with amputation, the danger exists for not only severe disappointment and the possible onset of depression if the "promised" system is denied, but of the complete derailment of the desire to proceed with prosthetic rehabilitation. For this reason, the evaluator

must learn to recognize and prioritize justifiable elements within the rehabilitation plan.

These elements include medical, vocational, avocational, and personal issues. Because electrically powered systems are typically the most expensive option, medical justifications are often mandatory if authorization is to be realized (some indications and contraindications were discussed briefly in the "Indications and Contraindications section"). For other options, vocational, avocational, or personal issues are often all that are needed to justify their value. Prosthetists must familiarize themselves with the numerous reasons why individuals may need to utilize various control schemes, either to help them in their activities of daily living, work, or recreation. It is extremely important that these justifications are discussed with the patient so he understands the relevant factors, and how and why they are significant. Often one may assume an individual is cognizant of the scope of their functional limitations. However, it is difficult enough for an experienced upper extremity prosthetist to foresee all the limitations inherent with amputation. An individual experiencing a recent upper extremity amputation is considerably less aware of what the future holds, whether with or without a prosthesis. Thus, it is paramount that the patient understands how the inclusion or exclusion of a prosthesis, or the utilization of a specific component or control scheme, impacts his rehabilitation. This knowledge will help the patient gain more control of the authorization process and allow him to be his own best advocate. More often than not, a payer will place more merit on the justification coming directly from their client, as opposed to a provider.

An area of justification that would benefit from further discussion concerns "personal issues." Justifying an expensive prosthesis based on this category is a bit more nebulous, but with some measure of care, it can be done. Imagine, for example, that a patient was recently provided with a new prosthesis. The evaluation performed was comprehensive and allowed the rehabilitation team to agree on the best options given the individual's current status at the time. Two months later, the same individual was relocated to a completely different environment due to his occupation or family responsibilities. Because of the new location, the climatic change is severe. Unfortunately, the myoelectric prosthesis, with its intimate fitting socket and stainless steel electrodes, is far too uncomfortable in the extreme cold. Because the EMG signals don't transmit well enough through a prosthetic sock, this patient must endure the temperature of the interface material directly on his skin. This was fine in a warmer climate, but because the material approaches outside ambient air temperature over time, this patient simply cannot tolerate this design given the new situation. This is an example of a problem that doesn't neatly fall into any of the other three types of justifications. However, for this patient, unless something else is provided, it doesn't matter where it falls—a physical requirement is simply not satisfied.

Further defining the prosthetic end of the rehabilitation process is recommended to better prepare the individual for the road ahead. During the initial evaluation, it is important to discuss the tremendous sacrifice in both time and effort required not only from the rehabilitation team, but the individual, in acquiring a prosthesis. It is important to discover early on if a patient is serious about following through with "their end of the bargain." By this, it is implied that patients have a responsibility to themselves, the rehabilitation team, and to the payer (if applicable) to use sound judgment in determining the depth of their desire to utilize a prosthesis. There are certainly no guarantees that the individual won't veer off the intended path as the process progresses for a variety of reasons, not the least of which is the patient's inability to accurately foretell the future. But the initial desire to stay the course should be there. If it is not, then the rehabilitation team should facilitate this motivation in the amputee, or be prepared for the plan to fail. In rare cases, the prosthesis or some other factor can influence the individual to generate this desire serendipitously, but the rehabilitation plan should rarely hinge on this occurrence.

Another reason to discuss the details involved in such procedures as casting and diagnostic analysis, delivery and postdelivery assessment, training, occupational therapy, physician follow-up, and the importance of realistic expectations, is to psychologically "acclimatize" the individual for the trials and tribulations inherent as the prosthetic rehabilitation plan is implemented. Before casting, it is important to warn the patient of the characteristics of plaster wrap (i.e., thermal reaction, adherence to skin and hair during cast removal, and feelings of claustrophobia due to volume containment). During the diagnostic phase, thermoplastics have certain unenviable characteristics such as skin adherence and heat build-up, for example. Psychological issues outlined previously must be dealt with at every turn, even at this early phase in the fitting. To preserve the fragile state of the patient's confidence in his practitioner, it is important to discuss the diagnostic procedure in detail. The significance of this is too often lost on both experienced and inexperienced practitioners alike. A patient may feel that a competent prosthetist should be able to create a perfectly fitting diagnostic interface on the initial attempt, and the adjustments being made to it are a sign of inferior skill. It may be difficult for the patient to remove his limb from the socket

due to the type of plastic being used or the socket design. Donning and doffing effort and the sensations of pressure that are to be expected in the definitive prosthesis should also be discussed in detail.

The difficulties of initial operation inherent in each option should be sufficiently described. If the patient encounters the unexpected, he or she may begin to lose confidence, not only in the prosthetist, but also in the entire rehabilitation strategy. This loss of confidence can defeat a successful outcome. As one can see, at every turn it is paramount to prepare the patient for what may occur. This preparation is a technique used by any experienced negotiator to gain the intended advantage. By addressing as many questions that may arise before they actually do, their negative impact can be reduced or eliminated, thus keeping focus on the issues at hand. In the prosthetist's case, it is crucial to bolster a patient's confidence, positive outlook, and determination to succeed throughout the entire process.

The postdelivery assessment phase is as significant to successful outcomes as the initial evaluation. Because the psychological issues inherent in patient disappointment following prosthetic delivery are extremely hard to overcome, the single most important factor in determining a successful outcome is the degree of separation or divergence between patient expectations and reality. This divergence is almost universally found in individuals with upper extremity amputation prior to prosthetic evaluation, primarily because of the relatively small numbers of individuals experiencing this type of amputation each year.

The law of supply and demand results in relatively few manufacturers, thus generating high component costs and limited technology development. This limited development causes a large discrepancy between the functional capabilities of the human arm and hand and those of an upper extremity prosthesis. Furthermore, due to the small size of the upper extremity prosthetic field, comprehensive media coverage is lacking. Hence, accurate insight into current prosthetic development is not a common characteristic of most individuals, let alone those with upper extremity amputation.

In assessing the progress of the patient during the postdelivery phase, vocational, avocational, and personal issues must all be considered. These aspects must include, but not be limited to an assessment of suspension, wearing time, reliability, durability, and the degree to which the prosthesis satisfies specific requirements. For electric prostheses, what is the electronic efficiency? Is battery life adequate to perform required tasks, or is the ratio between the effort involved to operate the system and battery life acceptable? Is the cosmesis favorable to the patient? Was the weight what the patient expected it to be? What difficulties were experienced, and, just as significant, what goals were realized?

So many questions must be asked at this phase that, in many cases, postdelivery assessment can be as complex as the initial evaluation. It is imperative that as many relevant questions are asked as can be conceptualized before recommending a continuance with the rehabilitation plan or an alternate strategy. Many new horizons may have opened up for the user since the initial delivery of the prosthesis. Much responsibility rests on the prosthetist's shoulders at this point. Throughout the history of both upper and lower prosthetics, postdelivery assessment has been a background player to the delivery phase, to the detriment of many patients desperately seeking solutions to challenges encountered during this crucial period.

OCCUPATIONAL THERAPY

Using occupational therapy (OT), the functional benefits of prosthetic technology should be maximally realized. Delivering a prosthesis to an individual with recent, traumatic upper extremity amputation without functional prosthetic training should be avoided if at all possible. The individual may eventually learn the mechanics of operation, but adequate utilization can be difficult. In most cases, occupational therapists are involved after delivery of the prosthesis. Whereas this is certainly more advantageous than no involvement at all, it is important, if possible, to encourage participation much sooner.

During the initial evaluation, an OT can be an invaluable resource in clarifying issues of functional training unfamiliar to both the prosthetist and the patient. In addition, one of the most significant problems encountered is the lack of cross training among medical professionals of different backgrounds. The deeper the immersion of the therapist in the prosthetic rehabilitation process, the greater his or her knowledge will be. As this knowledge of related fields increases, so too does the ability to provide more comprehensive care in one's own profession.

Certain physicians, burdened with an extensive caseload and the incessant need to research their own specialty, also benefit from a deeper immersion into prosthetics. This rarely occurs, and often not in sufficient detail to allow a broad understanding of the nuances involved in prosthetic utilization. Many studies involving upper extremity prosthetic usage are bereft of useful information or highly biased toward inaccurate,

overly simplified conclusions. Many physicians are forced to rely on these studies to form an overall picture of the efficacy of certain prosthetic options, and are thus predisposed toward an opinion that may be in direct contradiction to an experienced upper extremity prosthetist's recommendation. In addition, because many of the outcomes realized by patients are less than optimal due to an improper evaluation performed by an inexperienced prosthetist, the physician may have little choice but to lay blame with the option chosen, believing that the degree of experience in upper extremity prosthetics is more uniform than it actually is. To counteract this, it is beneficial to not only develop good relationships with local physicians, but also to be present or available during the patient's follow-up visit with the referring physician. This is a unique opportunity to share information in both directions, and it allows the patient additional input to two sources simultaneously. In-servicing is an important method in educating and being educated. It is in this area of cross-specialty education, where the largest degree of improvement is needed.

CONCLUSIONS

Increased knowledge through the sharing of information will ultimately result in a significantly improved climate for all members of the rehabilitation team. It is hoped that the evaluation methods described provide a tool to better substantiate and validate future outcomes and studies concerning individuals with upper extremity amputations. When a standardized and quantifiable set of evaluative protocols is administered, outcome assessment will be much more accurate and helpful in assisting the amputee rehabilitation team in making the most appropriate prosthetic and treatment decisions.

References

1. *J Am Board Fam Pract* 1992 Jan–Feb; 5 1:69–73
2. *Zh Nevropatol Psikhiatr Im S S Korsadova* 1992; 92 2: 74–8
3. Friedmann L. The Psychological Rehabilitation of the Amputee.
4. Racy JC. Psychological aspects of amputation. In: Moore WS, Malone JM, eds. *Lower-extremity amputation.* Philadelphia: W.B. Saunders Co., 1989.
5. Winchell E. *Coping with Limb Loss.*
6. *Prosthet Orthot Int* 1978 Apr; 2 1: 12–4
7. *Shukla GD, Sahu SC, Tripathi RP, Gupta DK Br J Psychiatry* 1982 Jul;141:50–3
8. *Int J Psychiatry Med* 1977–78;8 3:243–255

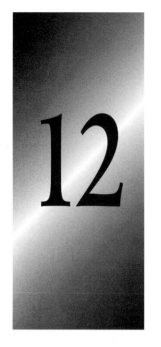

12 Foot Skills and Other Alternatives to Hand-Use

Wendy Stoeker, OTR/L

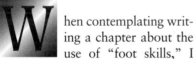hen contemplating writing a chapter about the use of "foot skills," I have realized that it is impossible to separate my views as an occupational therapist and my life experiences as a "congenital bilateral amelic." I was blessed with a supportive, loving, and driven family. I was provided access to the leading prosthetic research and development that was available in the 1960s. I am convinced that I received the best rehabilitation services available, and I know from professional experience that the quality of service for this specific type of disability has evolved into a specialized area of practice for health/medical professionals.

The use of foot skills is definitely a personal choice. I have learned through practical experience that using my feet allows me to enjoy a completely independent life, but other forces play a significant role in my high level of performance. Gravity, leverage, use of my teeth and chin/shoulder area, excellent lower extremity range of motion and highly dexterous toes, my personality and motivation, and my early and almost natural adaptation to foot skills are certainly critical to developing a completely independent lifestyle.

FOOT SKILLS: SOMETIMES OR ALWAYS

Use of foot skills may be essential for all areas of activities of daily living (ADL) or may be used as merely a simple assist or stabilizer. There are numerous examples of people born with portions of their upper extremities missing or who have no arms at all who have developed complete independence in the social, personal, and employment areas of their lives. Reverend Harold Wilke of the United Church of Christ, who was born without arms in the early 1900s, was an example of the attitude he wrote about in his pamphlet, "Using Everything You've Got." Utilizing his feet as the alternative to his hands (coupled with a few commonsense modifications) Rev. Wilke married, had a family, and was able to travel the world independently.

The younger the person is when they acquire a limb loss the better able they are to develop foot skills and other alternative methods of performing the tasks associated with hand function to achieve an independent lifestyle. There are many people who feel that using your feet to eat or perform cooking activities is not an acceptable alternative to use of prosthetics, and that is why there is no single remedy or combination of modifications that can be applied to each person with limb loss. The length of the person's residual limbs directly affects the level of efficiency that a prosthesis can provide. Technological advances continually provide the opportunity for amputees to use prosthetics to achieve independence in ADL. Regardless of the level of independence that the prosthesis provides, foot skills may still be necessary for certain tasks. I have observed the most adept prosthetic users hook their feet around the legs of a chair to move it forward. I frequently wonder how they pull up the sheets and blankets to sleep without the advantage of wearing the prosthesis.

It is possible to achieve dexterity equal to that of fingers and arms. I am not unique in the level of competence that I have accomplished. I can thread a needle, use a sewing machine, light a match or lighter, type over 45 words a minute, shave my legs, and paint my nails (toe nails, of course). I drive a car with no special adaptations but rely on an automatic transmission. I steer with my left foot and brake/accelerate with my right foot. I live alone in a townhouse with strategically placed stools to allow my feet to do their "job." I perform all the household management tasks as well as all of the community access tasks, often sitting down to use my feet and toes and using a laundry basket or bag with a strap to transport objects with my mouth, chin, and shoulder. I am completely independent in *all* of my personal care at home and when traveling across America. My feet have truly provided the skills that hands provide to most people, and I benefit from the sensation of touch that I receive through my toes.

COMPREHENSIVE REHABILITATION PROGRAMS

It is the perspective of occupational therapy as a profession that "developing independence" is the key for individuals with any disability to maximize their unique quality of life. Each individual and her family should be provided with options, resources, training, adaptive equipment/designs, and should be provided with assistance and input from all relevant professionals when considering the use of foot skills as the primary alternative. It is essential that the individual with limb loss is an active participant in the selection of alternative choices for developing independence in his life. Bilateral upper extremity limb loss presents considerations for many common areas of daily life independence: personal care, health, psychological, social, economic, and leisure preferences. Other considerations are equally important when striving for independence: Was the limb loss congenital or acquired? At what age was the limb loss? Physical/medical considerations, length of residual limbs, opportunity for prosthetic fitting, access to a comprehensive rehabilitation program, and personal preference must be considered.

Trying to develop foot skills and various alternative methods to increase functional independence is of utmost importance. People with the motivation and adequate intellect often capitalize on their training and, after returning to their home environments, continue on to develop their own "methods for independence" in all

areas of daily life tasks. In conjunction with prosthetic training, occupational therapy programs for people with bilateral upper extremity limb loss should include development of the fundamental areas of range of motion, strengthening, sensation, balance, mobility, flexibility, and coordination through functional activities for all parts of the body including the neck, back, hips, knees, jaw, and of course, the feet.

An example is that one of the long-term goals would be to improve foot skill function for accessing items from the floor. The short-term goals are to develop strength, range of motion, sensation, and dexterity to pick up items from the floor. Initially, occupational therapists should provide activities to develop the fundamental areas. For example, using toes/feet to pick up pieces of fabric and increasingly larger and heavier items and then transfer them to the prosthesis or a table. With improved proficiency, the therapist should continue to increase difficulty of the activities so that the patient uses his foot to pick up pieces of sponge, 1-inch then 1/2-inch blocks, M&Ms, and rice. Picking up coins would be the ultimate test.

Independent of early intervention following limb loss (regardless of either clinically based or educationallybased therapy services in their younger years), occupational and physical therapy services are an integral part of the rehabilitation process. In order to achieve and maintain an independent lifestyle, these services should be provided at critical stages throughout the lifespan to address the ever-changing physical, economic, and emotional needs at each of life's critical stages. Each person with limb loss will need support and encouragement from her family, and at times the professionals and family members must be insistent and determined to foster the person's decision/commitment to use all of the available resources for maximizing functional independence in every aspect of life.

Physical therapy is essential to promoting independence and addressing muscular, joint, mobility, and balance changes that occur in everyone with bilateral amputations and specifically to those individuals who choose foot skills. When considering the physical problems unique to this population, physical therapists have an expertise in identifying specific areas of the body that incur unusual amounts of stress and strain and then developing programs for aerobic exercise, stretching, strengthening, and so on to enhance each patient's continual physical adjustment to this disability. When providing rehabilitation to people with bilateral upper extremity limb loss, consider this:

Foot Skills + Adaptive Equipment/Techniques + (Prosthetics) = MAXIMUM INDEPENDENCE!!

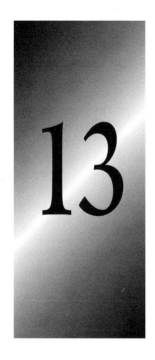

13 Postoperative and Preprosthetic Preparation

Robert H. Meier, MD and Diane J. Atkins, OTR

Ideally, the preprosthetic program should begin no later than when the sutures are removed and the patient is medically stable, generally about 3 weeks following the surgery. It can be helpful to begin some preprosthetic rehabilitation immediately following the amputation surgery. The occupational therapist is the primary person who will be managing and monitoring this program for the upper limb amputee. Nursing is an important adjunct, however, and if the patient is hospitalized, all shifts of the nursing staff should be thoroughly familiar with each of these areas.

PREPROSTHETIC PREPARATION

The objectives of the preprosthetic program are to

- promote residual limb shrinkage and shaping,
- promote residual limb desensitization,
- maintain normal joint range of motion,
- maintain skin mobility,
- increase muscle strength,
- provide instruction in the proper hygiene of the limb,
- maximize self-reliance in the performance of tasks required for daily living,
- determine the electrical potential provided by various muscles (this is known as myoelectric site test-

ing and is necessary if myoelectric prosthetic components are prescribed),
- inform the patient about prosthetic options, and
- explore the patient's goals regarding the future (1).

The postoperative and preprosthetic phase generally begins 2 to 3 weeks after surgery. Healing has essentially occurred by postoperative day 21 (2), and should allow for a vigorous program of prosthetic preparation. Malone et al. (3) have suggested that the first month after upper extremity amputation is the "golden period" during which prosthetic fitting should occur to maximize the level of acceptance and use of the prosthesis.

Promote Residual Limb Shrinkage and Shaping

The shrinking and shaping of the residual limb is accomplished by compression from an elastic bandage, intermittent positive pressure compression, or with a tubular elastic bandage. If using an elastic (Ace®) bandage, it is important that the proper wrapping technique be taught to the patient, family, and nursing staff. The preferred figure-eight wrap is one that is applied with more pressure distally than proximally; wrapping should never be done in a circumferential manner.

The wrapping process begins with the end of the bandage placed diagonally at the distal end of the residual limb. The wrap should encircle the limb from behind and be brought diagonally upward to cross over the end

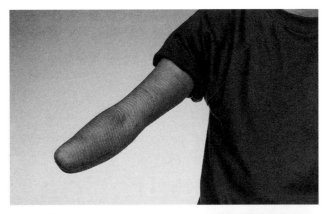

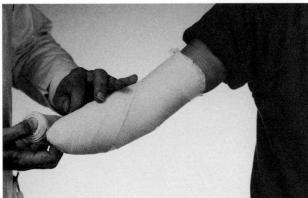

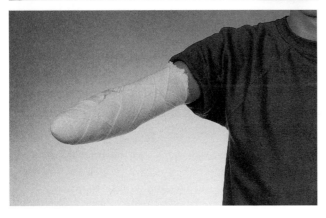

FIGURE 13-1

Wrapping the residual limb is an essential component of the preprosthetic program.

with mild soap and lukewarm water and thoroughly rinsed with clean water. Bandages should not be twisted but laid flat to dry. Washers and dryers decrease their longevity and ruin their elasticity.

The wrap should be worn continuously at all times. Because shaping and shrinking is a dynamic process, the elastic bandage should be reapplied every few hours or more frequently if it slips or bunches. It should always be reapplied every 4 hours while awake. It should be worn all day and all night, except when bathing. A preparatory prosthesis might also be applied early in the shaping process; however, a compression bandage is generally preferred because it affords better monitoring of skin healing and points of pressure. In our experience, elastic compression is superior to the use of a stump shrinker.

Tubigrip or Compressogrip may also be utilized alone, or under the elastic wrap. If used alone, it should be cut twice as long as needed, pulled on to the residual limb, twisted (or sewn at the bottom), and the remaining length should be pulled on as a second layer of compression. If maximal compression is desired, the above technique should be followed by figure-eight elastic bandage wrapping.

Promote Residual Limb Desensitization

Equally important, yet often overlooked, is the desensitization of the residual limb. This process can be helpful in decreasing pain following the amputation surgery. It also better prepares the residual arm for the intimate fit of the prosthetic socket. It can be accomplished with gentle massage and tapping techniques. Desensitization can also be accomplished by vibration, constant touch pressure, or the input of various textures applied to the sensitive areas of the limb. The patient should be encouraged to do these techniques himself. He is aware of his tolerance and can become more "in touch" with his body by practicing this regularly. When healing has occurred, aggressive massage will prevent adhesions from occurring and provide additional sensory input. It should be explained that this will improve the patient's tolerance to the pressure that will be placed on the residual limb by the prosthetic socket.

Maintain Normal Joint Range of Motion

When establishing an effective treatment program, the maintenance of full, active, joint range of motion is essential. Scapular, glenohumeral, elbow, and forearm range of motions are crucial to maintain or obtain to aid in the prosthetic control motions and to maximize the functional potential of the prosthesis.

Forearm range of motion, mainly in pronation and supination, may decrease within 2 to 3 weeks, if this

of the bandage. This figure-eight process should continue with each pattern overlapping the previous one by approximately two-thirds the width of the bandage (Figure 13-1). The wrap should be brought above the next most proximal joint above the level of the amputation for more appropriate suspension of this bandage. The bandage is then secured with tape or special clasps.

No elastic bandage should be used for more than 48 hours without being washed. It should be washed motion is not encouraged. This is especially important for below-elbow residual limbs, longer than 50%, where the remaining forearm motion can be transferred to the prosthetic socket for terminal device positioning. Forearm pronation and supination is a valuable voluntary motion required in virtually all bilateral tasks.

Maintain Skin Mobility

After healing has occurred, aggressive massage will prevent adhesions and provide additional sensory input. Massage should be focused along the healed suture line. Good skin mobility will reduce the shear forces developed at the stump–socket interface and thereby decrease the likelihood of skin breakdown, which may occur with adherent skin, a skin flap, or scarred skin.

Increase Muscle Strength and Endurance

Increasing upper extremity muscle strength can be accomplished in conjunction with a range-of-motion program. Active resistance applied by the therapist, or cuff weights attached to the limb, can be utilized. In addition, it is helpful to use exercise that promotes muscle endurance, not just strength training. This will permit better prolonged prosthetic function during the early prosthetic training phase.

General Full Body Conditioning

During the preprosthetic phase, it can enhance the general quality of well being and improvement for the person with an amputation if they also perform an aerobic conditioning program. Since most arm amputees are previously healthy, young adult men, this conditioning can also hasten the ability to return to work and previous avocational activities.

Provide Instruction in the Proper Hygiene of the Limb

Education in the proper hygiene and care of the residual limb is equally important at this time. The limb should be washed daily with mild soap and warm waster. It should be rinsed thoroughly and patted dry with a towel. This provides additional sensory input into the residual limb as well as allowing the patient to become more familiar with the changes in his body.

Maximize Functional Independence

Another important element in the preprosthetic phase of care is maximizing functional independence. Instruction in change of dominance and teaching one-handed activities is often indicated when working with the unilateral amputee.

The bilateral upper-extremity amputee presents a unique challenge to the amputee team. Before receiving his prostheses, the amputee is often dependent in most activities of daily living. This dependence presents very real anxiety and frustration for these individuals. It is important to express reassurance, support, and realistic optimism to these individuals during this time. Independence for the bilateral amputee can be significantly enhanced by a simple device such as a universal cuff utilized with an adapted utensil, toothbrush, pen, or pencil.

Myoelectric Site Testing

If a myoelectric prosthesis is being considered, the preprosthetic phase should include an assessment of the electromyographic (EMG) signals produced by a muscle. A myotester will gauge the electrical potential generated by various muscles. The electrodes in a prosthetic socket pick up these EMG signals, which are then transmitted to the motor in the prosthesis to produce a desired motion. The discussion here focuses on the most common two-state and three-state control myoelectric systems currently available.

If muscles are difficult to identify for potential myoelectric control sites, it may be more helpful to use a biofeedback machine than the myotester. This equipment can often test multiple muscle sites simultaneously, thus providing direct visual or auditory feedback when a minimal muscle signal is generated.

Two-state control systems activate one action from one muscle site. Two separate muscles are therefore needed to operate a functional prosthesis. A simple contract–relax response activated by a gross muscle movement initiates the electrical potential to operate the motor in one direction. The second muscle site, when contracted, then operates the motor in another direction. In many commercially available prostheses, this principle provides the movement that results in the motions of grasp and release or elbow flexion and extension. An amputee evaluated for this type of system must have two distinct muscle sites, be able to contract and relax each independently from the other, and the muscle sites should be able to be housed comfortably within the prosthetic socket. The Utah Artificial Arm System, which is a two-state system manufactured by Motion Control Inc. for above-elbow amputees, requires the additional ability to co-contract these two muscles simultaneously for unlocking the elbow unit.

The three-state control system uses one muscle site to control two functions. A strong contraction by the muscle causes one function, and a weaker contraction by that same muscle creates a second function. Relaxation of that muscle turns the system off. Use of this type of system requires a more definitive control by the amputee, but it is an excellent system for those with limited muscle sites. This system can also be used to control the movements of several components on one prosthesis by using several, independent muscles. Successful control of this system requires that the amputee be able to differentiate signal levels and be able to change from one level to another instantaneously, without activating intermediate levels (4).

Orientation to Prosthetic Options

The preprosthetic period is an important time to orient the amputee patient and his family to the prosthetic options available to him. The unique differences between body-powered and electric components should be comprehensively described, and examples of each should be shown and demonstrated if possible. Photographs or slides may be reasonable substitutions, but being able to touch and hold the device and understand how it operates is extremely helpful and informative for these individuals. An overview of the advantages and disadvantages of body-powered and electric components should be clearly explained.

Explore Patient's Goals

A careful inventory of the patient's lifestyle, support system, educational background, and future goals should be explored and discussed. The amputee patient is an integral ingredient in the decision-making process of his prosthetic prescription. Involving the patient in decisions that affect his own health care will help to restore a sense of control over his life.

References

1. Atkins DJ. Postoperative and preprosthetic therapy programs. In: Atkins D, Meier R (eds.), *Comprehensive Management of the Upper-Limb Amputee*. New York: Springer-Verlag, 1989, pp. 11–15.
2. Meier R. Amputations and prosthetic fitting. In: Fisher S (ed.), *Comprehensive Rehabilitation of Burns*. Baltimore: Williams & Wilkins, 1984, pp. 267–310.
3. Malone JM, Fleming LL, Roberson JJ, Whitesides TE, Leal JM, Poole JU, Grodin RS. Immediate, early, and late postsurgical management of upper-limb amputation: Conventional, electric and myoelectric prostheses. *J Rehabil Res Dev* 1984; 32(1), 33–41.
4. Spiegel SR. Adult myoelectric upper-limb prosthetic training. In: Atkins D, Meier R (eds.), *Comprehensive Management of the Upper-Limb Amputee*. New York: Springer-Verlag, 1989, pp. 60–71.

14

Functional Skills Training with Body-Powered and Externally Powered Prostheses

Diane J. Atkins, OTR

The impact on a person of the sudden loss of a hand or arm cannot be overstated. The loss of fine, coordinated movements of the hand, tactile sensation, proprioceptive feedback, and aesthetic appearance can only be compensated for to a limited extent by the three types of prostheses that are currently available (1).

Three primary prosthetic options include *1*) a passive, cosmetic arm and hand; *2*) a cable-controlled, body-powered prosthesis; and *3*) an electrically powered prosthesis controlled by myoelectric sensors or specialized switches. In reality, no perfect or ideal replacements take the place of the exquisite mechanisms and function of the human hand (2).

The unusually high rejection rate of upper-extremity prostheses can often be attributed to the following reasons: development of one-handedness, which removes the functional need for the prosthesis; lack of sufficient training or skill in using the prosthesis; poor comfort of the prosthesis; a poorly made prosthesis; the unnatural look or profile of the prosthesis; and the reactions of other people to the prosthesis (3).

Successful outcomes in rehabilitation for the unilateral and bilateral amputee can be attributed to the following reasons:

- Early posttraumatic intervention
- Experienced team approach

- Patient-directed prosthetic training
- Patient education
- Patient monitoring and follow-up

Early posttraumatic intervention and an experienced team approach have been addressed in earlier chapters. The focus of this chapter is to stress the important aspect of prosthetic training. Listening to and acknowledging the patient's psychologic and functional needs is critically important in determining the success or lack of success with prosthetic acceptance and function.

PROSTHETIC TRAINING

Before initiating a program of upper-extremity prosthetic training, one must realistically orient the patient to what the prosthesis can and cannot do. If the individual has an unrealistic expectation about the usefulness of the prosthesis as a replacement arm, he may be dissatisfied with the ultimate functioning of the prosthesis and may reject it altogether. On the other hand, if the expectations of the amputee are more realistic at the beginning of training, then the ultimate acceptance will be based upon the ability of the prosthesis to improve the individual's performance. It is imperative, then, that the therapist be honest and positive about the function of the prosthesis. If she believes in and understands the functional potential of the prosthesis, success can be more realistically achieved.

INITIAL ASSESSMENT

During the therapist's first encounter with the amputee patient in therapy, the following issues must be discussed and documented, if they have not already been accomplished:

- Etiology and onset
- Age
- Dominance
- Other medical problems
- Level of independence
- Range of motion of all joints of residual limb
- Muscle strength of remaining musculature
- Shape and skin integrity of residual limb
- Status of opposite extremity
- Phantom pain or residual limb pain
- Previous rehabilitation experience
- Revisions
- Viable muscle sites (for myoelectric control)
- Previous information regarding prostheses
- Background education and vocational goals
- Goals and expectations regarding the prosthesis
- Home environment and family support

Although this list may appear unreasonably long and too lengthy to document, the assessment will make a significant difference in the therapist's understanding of the individual with whom she is working. The nature of patient–therapist rapport and the subsequent success of therapy will be greatly enhanced if this information is gathered before therapy actually begins.

The time between casting until final fitting of the prosthesis is characterized by eager anticipation and hope that the artificial arm will enable the individual to function as he did prior to his amputation. Unfortunately, the finished prosthesis is often a disappointment for the patient. It is perceived as "artificial looking," heavy, uncomfortable, and awkward to operate. If the patient is appropriately oriented to the realities of the prosthesis and how it looks and operates, he is better prepared to accept the limitations of his prosthesis when it is delivered to him.

INITIAL VISIT

When the upper-extremity amputee visits the occupational therapist for the first time, he will probably be carrying the prosthesis in a bag or sack. It is important to understand this awkwardness and reluctance in putting it on with others "watching." A quiet, nondistracting room with a mirror, plus an atmosphere of acceptance and understanding is preferable.

During the first several visits, the following goals should be addressed:

- Orientation to prosthetic component terminology
- Independence in donning and doffing the prosthesis
- Orientation to a wearing schedule
- Care of the residual limb and prosthesis

Orientation to Prosthetic Component Terminology

Considering that the prosthesis has not become the patient's "arm," it is important that the patient learn to identify the major components of his prosthesis appropriately. Any orientation to identifying such basic aspects as the figure-eight harness, cable, elbow unit or elbow hinge, wrist unit, terminal device, and hook or hand will suffice at this time.

Independence in Donning and Doffing the Prosthesis

It is important that independence is established early in donning and doffing the prosthesis by the "pullover sweater" method. As an alternative, the "coat" method may also be used. Bilateral amputees most often use the "sweater" method.

Orientation to a Prosthetic Wearing Schedule

An orientation to a wearing schedule is extremely important to review during this first visit. Initial wearing periods should be no longer than 15 to 30 minutes, with frequent examination of the skin for excess pressure or poor socket fit. This is particularly important for the amputee with insensate areas and adherent scar tissue. If redness persists for more than 20 minutes after the prosthesis is removed, the patient should return to the prosthetist for socket modifications. If no skin problems are present, the patient can increase wearing periods in 30-minute increments three times a day. By the end of a week, the upper-extremity amputee should be wearing his prosthesis all day.

Care of the Residual Limb and Prosthesis

Following amputation, the skin of the residual limb is subject to irritation and often to further injury and infection. Appropriate care of the skin is therefore a vital part of rehabilitation. The residual limb should be bathed daily, preferably in the evening. It is advisable to not wash the residual limb in the morning, unless a stump sock is worn. The damp skin may swell and stick to the prosthesis and may be irritated by rubbing. The limb should be washed with mild soap and lukewarm water. It should be rinsed thoroughly with clean water. If soap is left to dry on the skin, it may be irritating. After rinsing, the skin should be dried thoroughly using patting motions. Avoid brisk rubbing, which may irritate the skin. Lotions, creams, and moisturizers should not be applied to the limb unless specific orders are given by the physician or therapist.

The socket should be cleaned often, particularly if the individual perspires heavily. In warm weather, the socket may require cleaning at least once or twice daily. The socket should be washed with warm water and mild soap. It should be thoroughly wiped out inside with a cloth dampened in clean warm water. The socket can be left to dry through the night or the inside dried thoroughly with a towel if the patient is going to continue to wear the prosthesis.

If stump socks are worn, several changes may be necessary during warm weather owing to perspiration. If possible, the sock should be washed as soon as it is taken off, before the perspiration dries on it. This will prolong the life of the sock. Mild soap and warm water should be used, followed by a thorough rinse. Allow the sock to dry slowly to avoid shrinkage.

The amputee should be encouraged to inspect his skin daily. If skin disorders develop, the physician should be called promptly. A minor disorder may become disabling if incorrect treatment is used. It will probably be necessary to adjust the prosthesis, and therefore the prosthetist is generally involved at this time as well. Strong disinfectants, such as iodine, should never be used on the skin of the stump (4).

BODY CONTROL MOTIONS

Prior to the upper-extremity amputee practicing prosthetic controls training, several motions need to be reviewed before the prosthesis is actually applied.

- Scapular abduction. Spreading the should blades apart, in combination with humeral flexion, or alone, will provide tension on the figure-eight harness in order to open the terminal device.
- Chest expansion. This motion should be practiced by deeply inhaling, expanding the chest as much as possible, and then relaxing slowly. Chest expansion may be utilized in a variety of ways for the above-elbow, shoulder disarticulation, or forequarter (intrascapulothoracic) amputee. Harnessing this motion with a cross-chest strap is determined by the prosthetic design; in some instances of extensive axillary scarring, it may be used in lieu of the figure-eight harness.

- Shoulder depression, extension, and abduction. This combined movement is necessary to operate the body-powered, internal-locking elbow in the above-elbow amputee. It is advisable to have the amputee practice this motion by cupping one's hand under the residual limb and instructing the patient to press down into the palm. This will simulate the motion required to lock and unlock the elbow in the individual with an above-elbow amputation.
- Humeral flexion. The amputee is instructed to raise his residual limb forward to shoulder level and to push his arm forward, sliding the shoulder blades apart as far as possible. This motion applies pressure on the cable and allows the terminal device to open. Scapular abduction and humeral flexion are the basic motions to review with the below-elbow amputee.
- Elbow flexion/extension. It is critical to encourage the below-elbow amputee to maintain full elbow range of motion. This range will enable him to reach many areas of his body without undue strain or special modifications in the prosthetic design.
- Forearm pronation/supination. In the long below-elbow amputee, it is equally important to maintain as much forearm pronation and supination as possible. This will enable the amputee to position the terminal device where he chooses, without prepositioning the wrist unit. If the amputee has retained more than 50% of his forearm, some degree of forearm pronation and supination is maintained.

PROSTHETIC EVALUATION

Before beginning functional training, it is important to ensure that the prosthesis fits comfortably and that the components function in a satisfactory manner. Ideally, this is accomplished by the occupational therapist and prosthetist working together.

The therapist is encouraged to communicate openly with the prosthetist on a frequent basis not only initially, but also when concerns arise regarding fit or operation.

PROSTHETIC CONTROLS TRAINING

Manual controls are important to review after the prosthesis is applied. One control should be taught at a time and then combined with others:

1. Positioning the terminal device in the wrist unit is accomplished by passive rotation with the sound hand. In the bilateral upper-extremity amputee, a

force against an object in the environment, or between the individual's knees, is necessary to accomplish this positioning.

2. Rotation at the elbow turntable is manually adjusted or controlled by leaning the prosthesis against an object.

3. The friction shoulder joint is manually adjusted with the sound hand or by applying pressure against an object or arm of a chair.

4. If the prosthesis has a wrist flexion unit, this can be manually controlled by applying pressure on the button or, for the bilateral amputee, applying pressure against a stationary object.

Active controls are equally important to review prior to functional training. The upper-extremity amputee is now able to incorporate the body-control motions he learned previously while wearing the prosthesis. It is essential that the harness is adjusted properly before initiating these exercises:

1. In all high proximal levels of limb loss, body-powered elbow flexion/extension is greatly enhanced by a forearm lift assist that responds to scapular abduction or chest expansion. Elbow extension is accomplished by gravity if the elbow unit is unlocked.

2. Elbow lock/unlock is perhaps one of the most difficult tasks to learn in the operation of an above-elbow prosthesis. The pattern of "down, back, and out" is often stated to the amputee to help him repeat the shoulder depression, extension, and abduction pattern. This pattern not only locks but unlocks the elbow in an audible "two-click cycle." Practicing this task should occur in a quiet, nondistracting room where one can hear the clicks without difficulty. This pattern may need to be exaggerated at first, but soon will be barely observable.

3. Before approaching terminal device operations, it is important for the amputee to practice locking and unlocking the elbow in several positions.

4. In the shoulder disarticulation and forequarter amputee, the mechanism to lock and unlock the elbow is often accomplished with a nudge control "button" attached to the thoracic shell. By depressing this button with the chin, one is able to position and lock the elbow where desired.

5. It is important to explain clearly that the elbow must be locked first, in the proper position, before the patient is able to operate the terminal device. As described earlier, biscapular abduction and humeral flexion (as a combined or separate motion) cause the terminal device to open, and relaxing allows it to close (Figure 14-1).

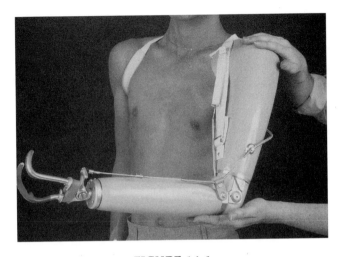

FIGURE 14-1

Terminal device operation.

CONTROLS PRACTICE

A form board is frequently utilized to practice prepositioning as well as tension control of the terminal device (Figure 14-2). Prepositioning involves both manual and active controls to place the prosthesis in the most optimal position for a specific activity. Close attention must be paid to the individual's awkward or compensatory body motions when he approaches an object. Often the amputee will "adjust" his body rather than adjusting or repositioning the elbow and wrist unit positions. A mirror can be effective in assisting the amputee to see the way his body is positioned. It is helpful to instruct the

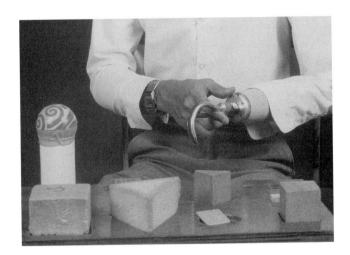

FIGURE 14-2

Form board utilized to practice prepositioning of terminal device.

patient to "think" how his own arm would have been positioned to approach the object. It is often necessary to remind him to maintain an upright posture and to avoid extraneous body movements.

The five motion elements primarily used in hand manipulation are reach, grasp, move, position, and release (5). A form board can be used in training to orient the individual to approach, grasp, and release objects differing in shape, weight, density, and size. Prehension control can be practiced using a sponge or paper cup. The amputee is instructed to maintain constant tension of the terminal device control cable so as not to overly squeeze the object being held. Approach to an object should be such that the stationary finger makes contact with the object and the moveable finger actually "grasps" it. Flat objects can be moved to the edge of the table and then grasped with the terminal device in a horizontal position. Prehension is generally controlled by rubber bands, which can be added as tolerated. Springs may be used as an alternative.

Controls training for the bilateral upper-extremity amputee is an aspect of therapy that may require a longer period to perfect. To learn to separate the controls motion of two prostheses is a complex and coordinated motor process that may need to be practiced frequently. Passing an object back and forth, such as a ruler, may help in reinforcing this pattern.

FUNCTIONAL USE TRAINING

Functional use training is the most difficult and prolonged stage of the prosthetic training process. The success or failure of the individual's acceptance and usage of the prosthesis depends on the motivation of the patient, the comprehensiveness and quality of the tasks and activities practiced, and of critical importance, the experience and enthusiasm of the occupational therapist. The training experience is most effective if the same therapist remains with the patient throughout the entire process.

Use Training for the Unilateral Amputee

It is extremely important to reinforce to the unilateral amputee that his prosthesis will usually play a nondominant functional role. The prosthetic terminal device is most useful for gross prehension activities and to hold and stabilize objects while the sound limb performs fine motor prehension activities. It is unreasonable to expect the prosthesis to assume any more than 30% of the total function of the task in bilateral upper-extremity activities. The sound arm and hand will always be the dominant extremity for all activities performed. The

therapist must be realistic with the patient in viewing the prosthesis as a "helper."

Unilateral patterns of independence occur quickly in the amputee who has lost an arm or hand. It is therefore essential, if possible, to fit the unilateral amputee within 1 to 2 months of the amputation. These individuals definitely show a greater propensity for wearing and successfully using their prostheses. This applies to all amputees fitted with body-powered or electric components (6).

It is appropriate to practice those activities of daily living (ADLs) that are useful and purposeful. Realistic situations should be pursued, so that the individual will automatically use the prosthesis when he encounters the same activity in his daily routine. These activities include:

- Cutting food
- Using scissors
- Dressing activities
- Opening a jar or bottle
- Washing dishes
- Hammering a nail and using tools
- Driving a car

The importance of prepositioning prior to approaching these tasks cannot be overemphasized. The amputee should be instructed to orient the components of the prosthesis in space to a position that resembles that of a normal limb engaged in the same task. As a rule, most difficulties of use are a result of improper positioning.

A valuable and comprehensive guide in orienting the therapist to the specifics of training the amputee is expressed in the *Manual of Upper Extremity Prosthetics* (7). Several of its techniques in training are reviewed in the aforementioned activities.

Cutting Food

It is appropriate to cut food by holding the fork in the hook, with the hook fingers grasping the flat surface of the fork handle and the upper handle of the fork resting on the dorsal surface of the thumb of the hook. The knife is held by the sound hand.

Using Scissors

When using scissors, the material to be cut, such as a sheet of paper, should be placed in the terminal device. The scissors are held by the sound hand. To avoid "flopping," the area to be cut should be as close to the area grasped as possible. The material should be repositioned as cutting angles are changed (Figure 14-3).

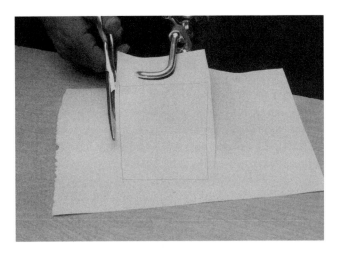

FIGURE 14-3

Scissor-cutting method.

Dressing Activities

Dressing activities, such as fastening trousers, are accomplished by the terminal device holding the waistband or belt loop, while the sound hand tucks in the shirt and fastens the waist hook, snap, or button. The terminal device can "pinch" the fabric at the bottom of the zipper to facilitate zipping with the sound hand. A button hook may be used to assist in buttoning cuffs on the sound side. With the proper prepositioning, the cuff can be buttoned rapidly and reliably. Button hooks are particularly helpful for the above-elbow and shoulder-disarticulation amputee.

Opening a Jar or Bottle

When opening a jar or bottle, the middle of the container is grasped by the terminal device and the sound hand unscrews the lid. All tension should be removed from the cable to assure maximum grasp on the container.

Washing Dishes

To achieve the greatest security of grasp while washing dishes, the dish should be held in the sound hand. Depending on the individual's preference, a dishcloth or sponge is held and manipulated by the terminal device. Submerging the hook in water should be avoided due to a tendency for water and detergents to dissolve the lubricating oils in the hook and wrist units. Periodic cleaning and oiling of the stud threads and bearings may be necessary for the amputee who engages in frequent dishwashing activities. When drying dishes, the sound hand holds the dish while the terminal device grasps the towel.

Hammering a Nail and Using Tools

Hammering nails is accomplished by holding the nail in the hook fingers, rubber-band guard, or special attachment of the #3 and #7 Hosmer-Dorrance work hook. The hook should be pronated to 90 degrees so that the nail is perpendicular to the wood. When correctly positioned, the tip of the nail should just contact the wood. Care and accuracy during the initial stroke results in a greater degree of success.

The amputee may need to be reminded that the prosthesis and terminal device are merely "functional assists" to aid stabilizing. The sound limb, often after changing dominance, becomes the dominant and active extremity.

Driving a Car

Driving a car is an important goal for the individual who has lost an arm. The actual turning of the steering wheel should be done by the sound extremity. If the prosthesis has sufficient function, performance can be improved by using the prosthesis to assist the sound arm in turning the wheel or stabilizing it while the sound arm is involved in another activity. A driving ring is available from most prosthetic suppliers. The fingers of the hook are secured in the ring for turning, but can easily slip out in emergencies.

A list of activities and a rating guide (Figure 14-4), designed by Northwestern University, is a helpful adjunct to the therapy plan in determining which activities are important for the unilateral amputee to accomplish.

Use Training for the Bilateral Amputee

The *Manual of Upper Extremity Prosthetics* from the University of California at Los Angeles (7) is an excellent resource to consult when dealing with the more involved issues of training the bilateral upper-extremity amputee.

Bilateral upper-extremity amputees may be totally dependent upon their prostheses for achieving independence in the following daily activities. Because of this dependence, the following activities are considered essential to review and practice with these individuals:

- Writing
- Dressing
- Eating activities
- Bathing
- Brushing teeth
- Toileting

Single Upper Extremity Amputation – Activities of Daily Living

Name		Age	Sex	Occupation
Type of Amputation		Type of Terminal Device		
Therapist		Date(s) of Test		

RATING GUIDE

0. Impossible
1. Accomplished with much strain or many awkward motions
2. Somewhat labored or few awkward motions
3. Smooth, minimal amount of delays and awkward motions

PERSONAL NEEDS:	0	1	2	3	GENERAL PROCEDURES:	0	1	2	3
Put on shirt					Use key in lock				
Fasten buttons; cuff and front					Open and close window				
Put on belt					Play cards & shuffle				
Put on glove					Wind a clock				
Put on coat					Assemble wall plug				
Lace and tie shoes					HOUSEKEEPING PROCEDURES:				
Tie a tie									
File finger nails					Wash dishes				
Polish finger nails					Dry dishes				
Set hair					Polish silverward				
Clean glasses					Peel vegetable				
Squeeze toothpaste					Cut vegetable				
Put on bra and fasten					Open a can				
Use zipper					Manipulate hot pots				
Hook garters					Sweeping				
Take bill from wallet					Use dust pan				
Light a match					Use vacuum cleaner				
Open pack of cigaretts					Use wet mop				
EATING PROCEDURES:					Use dry mop				
					Set up iron board				
Carry a tray					Iron				
Butter bread					Wash and wring out laundry				
Cut meat					Hang up & take down laundry				
DESK PROCEDURES:					Thread needle				
					Sew on button				
Use dial telephone					USE OF TOOLS:				
Use phone and take notes									
Use pay phone					Layout				
Sharpen pencil					Saw				
Use ruler					Plane				
Use scissors					Sand				
Remove & replace ink cap					Drive screws				
Fill fountain pen					Hammer				
Fold and seal letter					File				
Use card file					Drill				
Use paper clip					Power tools				
Use stapler					Gravel pit				
Wrap a package					CAR PROCEDURES:				
Type									
Write					Drive				
COMMENTS: Band Aid					Change tire				
					Use jack				

FIGURE 14-4

Performance rating of daily activities for the unilateral upper-extremity amputee.

Writing

A pen or pencil is positioned in the same manner, and at the same angle, as a hand would hold a writing instrument (Figure 14-5). In the bilateral upper-extremity amputee, the longer residual limb generally becomes the dominant extremity. The shorter, nondominant extremity is utilized in securing the paper so that it will not slip. Additionally, a forearm leather pad is sometimes added to the volar aspect of the socket to provide an additional source of stability when attempting to hold something flat.

Dressing

Independence in dressing is one of the primary goals for the individual who has lost both arms. Some amputees prefer to wear a T-shirt under the prostheses. If the shirt is straightened out on a flat surface, raised over the head, drawn over the head as the arms are lowered, and then shrugged into place, the task is relatively simple. If stump socks are worn by the amputee, teeth are often used to pull the stump socks tight while the prostheses are put on.

Elastic waistbands, rather than buttons or snaps, are preferred in undershorts and underpants. Socks can be carefully applied by regripping the sock frequently with the terminal device. As an alternative, loops of webbing may be utilized by the individual who tends to poke holes in nylon or silk socks (Figure 14-6). It is strongly recommended that bilateral amputees wear shoes of the loafer, zipper, or Velcro closure type.

Cuffs on long-sleeved shirts should be buttoned prior to putting the shirt on. The nondominant extremity should be inserted into the sleeve first and, by leaning to the dominant side, the amputee can reach behind, insert the prosthesis in the sleeve, and shrug the shirt

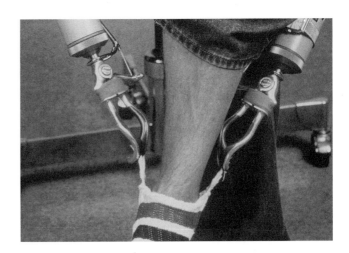

FIGURE 14-6

Loops to assist sock donning.

into place. A simple, useful device that facilitates donning and doffing is a clothing hook mounted on the wall at the appropriate level for the individual. The hook may be of any shape and may be plain, roughened, or covered in rubber tubing (Figure 14-7). A dressing tree may be preferred for the individual with more proximal levels of limb loss. A buttonhook may be used or Velcro mounted behind the button may be a preferred alternative. Many bilateral amputees prefer shirts with short rather than long sleeves, to keep the cuffs from interfering with the thumb of the terminal device.

When donning pants or a skirt, the dominant side should grasp the belt loop or waistband as the amputee inserts the legs into the clothing. This can be accomplished in the sitting or standing position, and the clothing is then drawn up to the waist. The waistband should

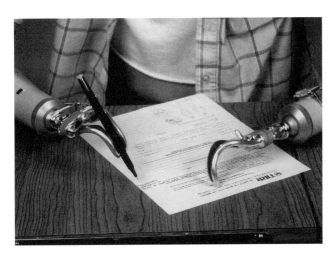

FIGURE 14-5

Position of pen for writing.

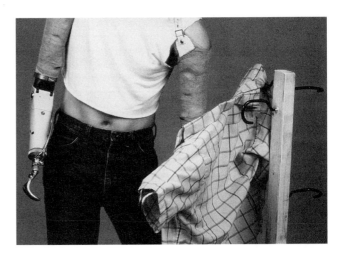

FIGURE 14-7

Dressing tree.

have a hooking clasp or Velcro fastener and should be loose enough around the waist to make fastening easier. An inconspicuous loop or small D-ring may be attached to the zipper tab for easier grasp.

Eating Activities

Prior to attempting to cut meat, the dominant hook is prepositioned at 90 degrees pronation and the assist hook is turned in medially. The dominant hook positions the fork in the assist hook with the tines of the fork facing down. The dominant hook then grasps the knife blade near the handle. It is positioned on the hook finger-thumb hold in the same manner as the fork. The knife cuts the food with a sawing motion and medium force. A serrated blade is preferred.

Drinking from a glass can be accomplished with the dominant terminal device prepositioned in 90 degrees pronation. The glass may be picked up by grasping the rim or encircling it with the fingers of the hook. A cup may be held in the same manner. It is advisable to not fill the cup or glass to the rim, owing to the instability of the container.

It is possible to hold a sandwich in the dominant terminal device with sufficient tension to hold the sandwich without crushing it. A sandwich bag may be used to cover half of the sandwich under the fingers of the hook.

Bathing

Bathing is obviously accomplished with the prosthesis off. A washcloth or small towel may be wrapped around the end of the residual limb. Sewing a strip of elastic in the cloth will prevent it from slipping. A towel can be folded over and sewn to form pockets into which the limbs can be slipped (Figure 14-8).

Brushing Teeth

The cap of a toothpaste tube can be removed by using the teeth and lips while holding the tube between the residual limbs. The toothbrush may be held in the elbow fold, residual limbs at midline, or held in the prosthesis. Head and tongue motion will facilitate proper positioning of the toothbrush in the mouth.

Toileting

Toileting can be accomplished with relative ease if the bilateral below-elbow amputee can manage his clothing. It is preferable for the individual to be trained to have a bowel movement either in the morning before leaving the house or in the evening after returning, rather than during the activities of the day. A wrist flexion unit on the dominant side will assist in the process

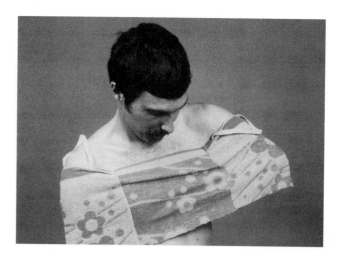

FIGURE 14-8

Adapted towel for bathing.

of wiping after defecation. The toilet paper should be unrolled and folded into a square pad several layers thick. The tissue can be held on the surface of the unit during this process. The center of the pad is pinched by the terminal device and then rotated to approximately 60 degrees supination. The amputee can reach behind the body and place the terminal device and tissue in a position for wiping.

Toileting for the bilateral above-elbow amputee poses a different challenge owing to the limited mobility of the prosthesis behind the body. A combination of dexterity in the use of a prosthesis, plus a high level of foot function in a properly motivated patient, will permit independence at this level. The "seat method" is accomplished by spreading several layers of toilet paper across the toilet seat or on the edge of a bathtub. Moistening the end of the tissue will assist in stabilizing the pad. The amputee sits so the buttocks straddle the seat and by shifting the pelvis from side to side, the wiping action is completed. Several applications may be necessary and considerable practice is required to gain skill and confidence.

The "heel method" is accomplished with the foot resting on the toilet seat and the heel raised. A length of toilet paper is draped over the heel to form several layers as described previously. A forward and backward motion of the pelvis, while squatting on the heel, will bring about a satisfactory wiping action.

Other Activities

Numerous other activities can be attempted by the bilateral upper-extremity amputee. Northwestern University has designed a comprehensive reference list and rating scale (Figure 14-9). Although it is not necessary to

Bilateral Upper Extremity Amputation – Activities of Daily Living

Name		Age	Sex	Occupation
Type of Amputation		Type of Terminal Device		
Therapist		Date(s) of Test		

RATING GUIDE

0. Impossible
1. Accomplished with much strain or many awkward motions
2. Somewhat labored or few awkward motions
3. Smooth, minimal amount of delays and awkward motions

PERSONAL NEEDS:	0	1	2	3	EATING PROCEDURES:	0	1	2	3
Buttoning					Pulling chair from table				
Zippers					Use napkin				
Hooks					Pick up utensils				
Snaps					Drink from glass				
Lacing					Drink from cup				
Tie shoe laces					Eat with a spoon				
Put on socks					Eat with fork				
Put on shoes					Cut meat				
Shorts					Eat soup				
Shirt					Eat sandwich				
Trousers					Eat potato chips				
Tuck shirt in trousers					Butter bread				
Tie necktie					Pass dishes				
Put on belt with buckle					Use salt shaker				
Blow nose					Drink from bottle				
Clean glasses					Pour liquid from pitcher				
Put on watch					Eat ice cream cone				
Wind watch									
Put on topcoat					DESK PROCEDURES:				
Put on hat					Use dial telephone				
Put on overshoes					Use phone and take notes				
Use umbrella					Use pay phone				
Shave					Sharpen pencil				
Shower Lavatory procedures					Use eraser				
Lavatory procedures					Use ruler				
Brush and comb hair					Use scissors				
Set hair					Remove and replace ink cap				
Apply cosmetics					Fill fountain pen				
Squeezing toothpaste					Fold and place in envelope				
Brushing teeth					Open sealed letter				
Put on bra and fasten					Use card file				
Hook garters					Use paper clip				
Hook suspenders					Use stapler				
					Wrap package				
					Unwrap package				
					Turn pages				
					Type				
					Write				

FIGURE 14-9

Performance rating of daily activities for the bilateral upper-extremity amputee.

Bilateral Upper Extremity Amputation - Activities of Daily Living (Con't)									
GENERAL PROCEDURES:	0	1	2	3	HOUSEKEEPING PROCEDURES:	0	1	2	3
Take money from purse					Place dishes on tray				
Take money from trouser					Carry tray				
Pick up change					Pick up objects from floor				
Ring door bell					Operate water faucet				
Use key in lock					Wash dishes				
Turn on lights					Dry dishes				
Use door knobs					Put dishes on shelf				
Turn on faucet					Polish silverware				
Open and close window					Peel vegetable				
Open and close drawers					Cut vegetable				
Use radio & television					Open can				
Play cards					Use egg beater				
Play checkers					Open egg				
Light a match					Mix with spoon				
Light a lighter and smoke					Store in refrigerator				
Wind a clock					Light a stove				
Open and close safety pin					Cook on top of stove				
Open a coke bottle					Cook in oven				
Hook screen door					Manipulate hot pots				
Operate window blind					Sweeping				
Use camera					Use dust pan				
Change record					Dust				
Carry suitcase					Use vacuum cleaner				
USE OF TOOLS:					Use scrub brush on floor				
					Use wet mop				
Layout					Use dry mop				
Saw					Use plug in baseboard				
Plane					Plug in iron				
Drive screws					Set up iron board				
Hammer					Sprinkle clothes				
File					Iron				
Drill					Sort laundry				
Sand					Wash and wring out laundry				
Gravel pit					Hang up & take down laundry				
Power tools					Thread needle				
CAR PROCEDURES:					Sew on button				
					Use pins				
Drive									
Raise hood									
Use jack									
Change tire									

FIGURE 14-9

(continued)

accomplish each activity on this list, the majority of these activities should be reviewed and practiced after determining which needs are of primary importance to the patient.

It has been well documented that bilateral upper-extremity amputees show a strong preference for body-powered rather than electric components (8,9), because of proprioceptive feedback, fewer repairs, and increased fine-motor dexterity skills with a hook versus a myoelectric hand.

The key to effective functional use training is to teach a problem-solving approach with respect to the activity being performed. More advanced bilateral activities should be introduced toward the end of training, to reinforce complex bilateral fine-motor tasks and further refine the motions required to accomplish them. Special assistive devices should be avoided as much as possible. Successful use training is achieved when the amputee uses his prosthesis spontaneously and effectively in all daily activities.

ELECTRIC POWERED PROSTHESES

Electric upper-extremity prostheses have opened a new world of freedom and function for upper extremity amputees. The advent of electronic microminiaturization has allowed the development of prosthetic devices with totally self-contained services of power, motor units, and electrodes (10). Powered prostheses have existed for decades, but not until the 1960s were myoelectrically controlled prostheses clinically introduced. The Otto Bock Company, in Duderstadt, Germany, began this process, as they aimed at developing an electromechanically driven prosthetic hand that would match both the technical and cosmetic demands of a human hand (11).

The clinical use of these devices began in Europe because of government-supported health care systems and a large patient population of congenital (post-thalidomide) amputees. By the late 1970s and early 1980s, North America had an increasing but limited experience with myoelectric prostheses (12). Today, when funding permits, hundreds of myoelectric prostheses are prescribed for children and adults throughout the United States.

The term *myoelectric prosthesis* is often used interchangeably with *electric prosthesis*. A myoelectric prosthesis uses muscle surface electricity to control the prosthetic hand function. The muscle membrane generates an electric potential at the time of contraction. The myoelectric signal is sensed, amplified, and processed by a control unit that powers a motor that drives a terminal device (12). This terminal device is often an electromechanical hand.

Below-Elbow Amputations

A myoelectric prosthesis requires no cables for control, and most below-elbow amputees should not require any straps or harnesses for suspension. Myoelectric prostheses are generally suspended at the condyles of the elbow. The most common condition for which these prostheses are prescribed is a below-elbow amputation, where a natural, functional elbow is retained. Myoelectric controls require minimal physical effort to operate and rarely require adjustment.

The muscle groups in the below-elbow area are used according to their physiologic function—that is, the wrist extensor muscles for hand opening and the wrist flexor muscles for hand closing. Muscular contractions are detected by surface electrodes that are recessed within the wall of the prosthetic socket.

Before prescribing a myoelectric prosthesis, it is critically necessary that the patient is strong enough and able to contract each individual muscle group separately. The surface electric signals are amplified by a miniature electrode and led to the relay system. The relay is responsible for the energy supply to the battery-operated motor in the electric hand. When the alternating contractions of extensor and flexor muscles take place, the direction of the current changes in the electric motor, and the hand opens and closes accordingly. The batteries are energy-storing devices and are rechargeable in a battery charging unit. The unit is plugged in an outlet and generally charged overnight (Figure 14-10).

There are many schools of thought regarding the advantages and disadvantages of myoelectric prostheses. The following list describes some of these points, as

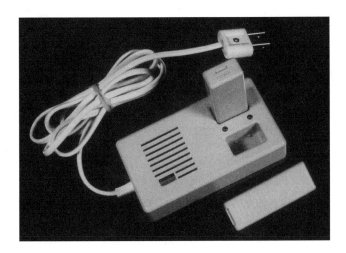

FIGURE 14-10

Battery of myoelectric arm is inserted in battery charger and charged overnight.

opposed to a body-powered, cable-controlled, hook-type terminal devices:

Advantages:

- Improved cosmesis
- Increased grip force (approximately 25 pounds in an adult myoelectric hand)
- Minimal or no harnessing
- Ability to use overhead
- Minimal effort needed to control
- Control more closely corresponds to human physiologic control

Disadvantages:

- Cost of prosthesis
- Frequency of maintenance and repair
- Fragile nature of glove; frequent replacements necessary
- Lack of sensory feedback (a body-powered prosthesis has some sense of proprioceptive feedback)
- Slowness in responsiveness of electric hand
- Increased weight

Although the myoelectric hand is the most commonly prescribed electric terminal device, a specially designed gripping device, or Greifer, is also recommended at times. The Greifer was designed by the Otto Bock Company in Germany and provides a universal working tool that is designed to handle various specialized tasks. It can be used for heavy work in industry or farming and provides for the quick handling and precise manipulation of small objects. Features of the Greifer include a 38-pound grasp, as well as parallel gripping surfaces and a flexion joint for dorsal and volar flexion (Figure 14-11).

Above-Elbow Amputations

For amputation levels above the elbow, the complexity of function and the power level required to accomplish functional movement increases considerably. At the same time, the capability of the patient to operate a prosthesis by harnessing body movement via straps and cables, in the traditional body-power manner, decreases considerably (13). The task of training an above-elbow or shoulder disarticulation amputee how to operate and function with a body-powered prosthesis is significantly more challenging.

Some rehabilitation professionals who work with patients having an upper extremity amputation feel that electric components may be the only appropriate alternative for high-level unilateral or high-level bilateral amputations. Conversely, some rehabilitation pro-

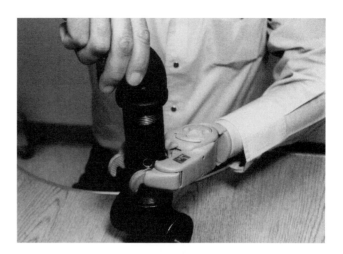

FIGURE 14-11

Myoelectric Greifer is designed as universal working tool with parallel gripping force of up to 38 pounds.

fessionals believe that body-powered prostheses remain the most functional and appropriate type of prosthesis for the majority of patients, despite the level of amputation.

Myoelectric Prosthetic Rehabilitation Program

The purpose of this section is to highlight the following: *1)* preprosthetic training, *2)* muscle-site control training, *3)* the early basics of prosthetic training, and *4)* functional use training. Although many methods are available for activating an electric elbow or hand (e.g., switch, touch, servo, proportional), this section addresses "myo" (muscle contraction) control only, which to date remains the most common method of controlling electric components.

The main focus of this section will be the adult with a unilateral below-elbow amputation. Children with upper extremity limb loss are managed quite differently from adults, and it is beyond the scope of this text to explore rehabilitation techniques in this unique population. Training an individual with bilateral limb loss requires extensive rehabilitation experience and background as well, and it is not recommended for the therapist with little or no previous exposure to rehabilitation of amputation patients. Individuals with bilateral limb loss should be referred to a "center of excellence," where the rehabilitation of persons with amputations is an ongoing specialty area of treatment.

Preprosthetic Therapy Program

An awareness of postoperative and subsequent preprosthetic principles of care is crucial to the successful management of the individual who has sustained traumatic limb loss. The patient has little control over what is happening and must depend upon the health care team to provide the best treatment possible.

The crucial points and treatment goals of a postoperative program include:

- Promote wound healing
- Control incisional and phantom pain
- Maintain joint range of motion (to prevent contractures)
- Explore patient's and family's feelings about change in body
- Obtain adequate financial sponsorship for prosthesis and training (14)

These goals should be addressed by the amputee rehabilitation team, which should include the physician, nurse, occupational or physical therapist, social worker, and patient. Once the sutures are removed, the preprosthetic program can begin. This should include the following goals:

- Residual limb shrinkage and shaping
- Residual limb desensitization
- Maintenance of normal joint range of motion
- Increasing muscle strength
- Instruction in proper hygiene of limb
- Maximizing independence
- Myoelectric site testing and training (if myoelectric prosthesis is prescribed)
- Orientation to prosthetic options
- Exploration of patient goals regarding the future.

The reader is referred to Atkins (15) for additional clarification of these goals if necessary. For the patient receiving a myoelectric prosthesis, this section focuses on a discussion of myoelectric site testing and training.

A myoelectric prosthesis functions by detecting the electromyographic (EMG) signals produced by muscles. A physical examination of the forearm can often detect sufficient wrist extensor and wrist flexor contractions in the below-elbow amputee and sufficient biceps and triceps contraction in the person with an above-elbow amputation. Often however, these signals are weak, and the therapist and prosthetist may require a biofeedback system or myotester (Figure 14-12).

Muscle-Site Control Training

The location of appropriate superficial muscle sites is the most important aspect of the successful operation of a myoelectric prosthesis. The muscle groups selected

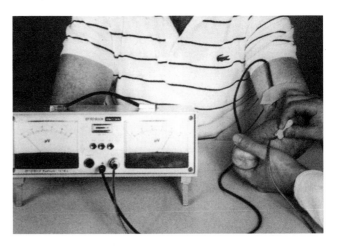

FIGURE 14-12

Otto Bock myotester determines magnitude of muscle contraction.

should approximate normal movements as much as possible. The following muscle groups are generally used during muscle-site selection:

- Persons with below-elbow amputation use wrist extensors and flexors for terminal device (i.e., hand) opening and closing.
- Persons with above-elbow amputation use biceps for elbow flexion and extension and triceps for terminal device opening and closing.
- Persons with shoulder disarticulation and forequarter amputees may use the deltoid, trapezius, latissimus, or pectoralis muscle for control.

It is important to note that the more proximal the level of amputation, the more difficult it becomes for the prosthetist to fit the individual and the therapist to train that individual.

For the patient to understand the desired muscle contraction, the therapist instructs the patient to imitate the desired movement on both sides. The therapist should ask the patient to raise the sound hand at the wrist (wrist extension) and imagine that motion with the phantom hand on the amputated side (Figure 14-13). Often a therapist can palpate the wrist flexors and extensors on the residual limb during this exercise. The patient should be instructed to contract and relax each muscle group separately and on command. For this step, a myoelectric tester is particularly useful since it indicates the magnitude of the EMG signal. Once the maximum response is found, its location should be marked on the skin. This process is often done in the company with a prosthetist, who can select the most appropriate muscle site.

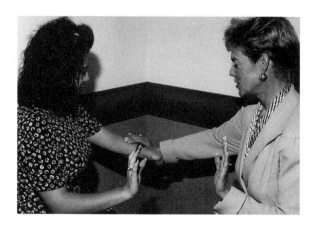

FIGURE 14-13

Therapist instructs patient to imitate desired muscle contraction on both sides.

When measuring surface potentials with the electrodes and a myotester, make certain all the electrodes have good contact with the skin and are aligned along the general direction of the muscle fibers. Moistening the skin slightly with the water may improve the EMG signal by lowering the skin resistance. Begin EMG testing using the most distal portion of the remnant muscles.

The myoelectric tester can be used to train the muscles with both visual and auditory feedback. The goals at this point are to increase muscle strength and to isolate muscle contractions. As confidence and accuracy improve, the visual or auditory feedback should be removed. This task teaches the amputee to internalize the feeling of each control movement. The advantage of creating this internalized awareness of proper muscle control is done so that control and strengthening practice can be continued between treatment sessions without the feedback equipment.

It is essential that the individual with an amputation receive adequate training and practice in initiating these muscle contractions before receiving the myoelectric prosthesis. Anxiety and frustration often accompany the training of an individual learning to use a myoelectric prosthesis. The therapist also needs to recognize muscle fatigue, which is a frequent side effect in this process; time must be given to allow that muscle to relax during the treatment session. The patient's success and effectiveness in using the prosthesis is closely related to the quality of the preprosthetic training.

Early Basics of Myoelectric Prosthetic Training

An extremely important aspect of a myoelectric prosthetic training program is to realistically orient the patient as to what the prosthesis can and cannot do. If the individual has an unrealistic expectation about the usefulness of the myoelectric prosthesis as a replacement arm, he may be dissatisfied with the ultimate functioning of the prosthesis and may reject it altogether. It is imperative that the therapist be honest and positive about the function of the prosthesis. If she believes in and understands the functional potential and limitations of the myoelectric prosthesis, success can be more realistically achieved.

Initial Visits for Myoelectric Orientation

Training with a myoelectric prosthesis should begin as soon as the prosthesis is received, preferably the same day. An excellent resource in the training process of a patient with a myoelectric hand is covered in the text *Comprehensive Management of the Upper Limb Amputee* (16).

During these initial visits, it is important to review orientation to prosthetic terminology, independence in donning and doffing, orientation to a prosthetic wearing schedule, and care of the residual limb and prosthesis.

Orientation to Prosthetic Terminology. Considering that the myoelectric prosthesis is now a "natural extension" of the individual's body, it is particularly important to know the function and names of the major parts such as the electrodes, battery, glove, and electric hand. The initial visit is an appropriate time to introduce the battery charging procedure and the proper use of the battery packs to the patient. Instruction manuals are often included from the manufacturer, and these should be shared as well.

Independence in Donning and Doffing the Prosthesis. Donning the prosthesis should be performed with the electronics in the OFF position to avoid any uncontrollable movements. At times, a residual limb pull sock may be required for donning the prosthesis to accomplish close contact with the limb, particularly for very short residual limbs. The prosthetic arm should be stored in the OFF position, with the batteries removed. The hand should be fully opened for storage to keep the thumb web space stretched.

Orientation to a Prosthetic Wearing Schedule. It is important to review a wearing schedule during the first visit. Initial wearing periods should be no longer than 15 to 30 minutes. This is particularly important if scarring or insensate areas are present on the residual limb. If redness persists for more than 20 minutes in a particular area, the patient should return to the prosthetist for adjustments. If no skin problems exist, the wearing periods can be increased in 30-minute increments three times as day. By the end of the week, full-time wearing should be achieved.

Care of the Residual Limb and Prosthesis. Appropriate care of the skin is vitally important. The residual limb should be washed daily with mild soap and lukewarm water. It should be rinsed thoroughly and dried using patting motions with a towel so as not to irritate sensitive or scar tissue.

The prosthesis may be cleaned using soap and water on a damp cloth. Rubbing alcohol may be used to clean the inside of the socket if an odor develops. The cosmetic gloves stain easily, so special attention should be paid to avoiding ink, newsprint, mustard, grease, and dirt. A glove-cleansing cream can be obtained from the prosthetist that will remove general soil but not stains. The average life of a glove is approximately 6 months. The prosthesis should never be immersed in water, because it will seriously damage the internal electronic components.

Teaching Approach, Grasp, and Release

Simple approach, grasp, and release activities are often accomplished with a form board on which objects of various shapes, sizes, and densities are displayed (Figure 14-14). It is important for the individual first to visualize how the object should be approached and grasped, and then preposition the myoelectric hand. Prepositioning involves placing the terminal device in the optimum position for a specific activity. In approaching a glass, the hand should face in toward the midline to grasp the glass as would a normal hand (Figure 14-15). To approach a glass or cup, the fingers of the hand should

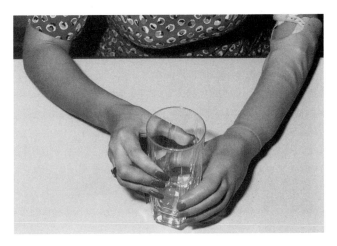

FIGURE 14-15

When approaching a glass, the hand is prepositioned in midline to grasp glass as normal hand.

not be positioned downward, because a normal hand does not approach a glass in this position.

Often the patient adjusts his body, using compensatory body motions, rather than adjusting or prepositioning the hand first. This action is important to avoid because it appears awkward and often becomes a habit. The patient also should make certain the angle of elbow flexion is appropriate if the person has lost the arm above the elbow and uses a body-powered or electric elbow. A mirror can be effective in assisting the patient to see the way the body is positioned and visualize how the sound arm would approach a particular object or activity. It is often necessary to remind the patient to maintain an upright posture and avoid extraneous body movements.

Another important aspect of training an individual to grasp an object is to master the control of the gripping force of the terminal device. This skill involves close visual attention to grade the muscle contraction for a specific result in the myoelectric hand. Styrofoam packaging bubbles work well for developing this skill. The individual must learn how to pick up the styrofoam without crushing it. Too strong a grasp crushes the object being held. Good grasp control through training with styrofoam, cotton balls, or sponges will help develop the control needed to handle paper cups, eggs, potato chips, sandwiches, and even to hold someone's hand. Release is accomplished by visualizing a wrist extension contraction, or hand up or hand open. This response should become quite automatic if good preprosthetic training of the muscles has occurred.

Eventually the effort to perform specific movements will take less cognitive effort; the movements

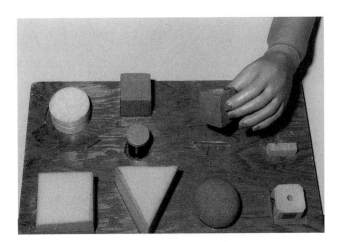

FIGURE 14-14

Form board provides useful tool in practicing approach, grasp, and release of objects of various sizes, shape, and densities.

soon become automatic. Functional use activities can now be introduced into the therapy program.

Activities of Daily Living (ADL)

It is important to keep in mind that the myoelectric prosthesis is used as a functional assist in the majority of bilateral activities. Therefore, most activities of daily living (ADL) will be accomplished with the sound arm and hand. Other than perhaps for practice, it is not appropriate to train a person with a unilateral amputation to eat holding a spoon, write, or brush his teeth using his myoelectric hand. In almost all cases the sound hand becomes the dominant extremity and performs those types of tasks. Occasionally, if the right arm is the dominant arm and is amputated, and the individual is fit with a myoelectric hand in a timely manner, he may prefer to use the myoelectric hand for some of these activities. The critically important component of sensory feedback is often the determining factor in deciding which hand to use. A person with amputation almost always chooses to perform most activities with a hand that has feeling. A myoelectric hand has no sensory feedback.

It is important to review a list of bilateral ADL tasks with the patient to determine which tasks are most important for him to accomplish. Focus on these activities, stressing throughout the activity that the myoelectric hand is used as an assist and stabilizer. The following bilateral activities are good examples to review and practice:

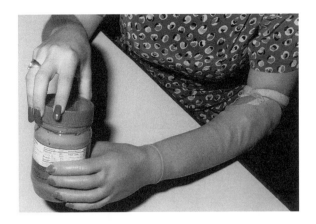

FIGURE 14-16

Opening a jar is accomplished with the myoelectric hand holding the jar and the sound hand turning the lid.

ACTIVITY	MYOELECTRIC HAND	SOUND HAND
1. Cutting meat	Hold fork with prongs facing downward or hold knife as grip strength increases	Hold knife Hold fork
2. Opening a jar (Figure 14-16)	Hold the jar	Turn the lid
3. Opening a tube of toothpaste (Figure 14-17)	Hold the tube	Turn the cap
4. Stirring something in a bowl	Hold the bowl with a strong grip	Hold the mixing spoon or fork
5. Cutting fruit or vegetables	Hold the fruit or vegetable firmly	Hold the knife to cut
6. Using scissors to cut paper	Hold the paper to be cut	Use scissors in normal fashion
7. Buckling a belt	Hold the buckle end of belt to keep stable	Manipulate long end of belt into buckle
8. Zipping a jacket or zipper (Figure 14-18)	Hold "anchor tab"	Manipulate "pull tab" at base and pull upward
9. Applying socks	Hold one side of socks	Hold other side of socks and pull upward
10. Opening an umbrella	Hold base knob of umbrella	Open as normal

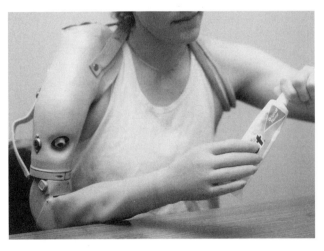

FIGURE 14-17

Opening a tube of toothpaste is accomplished with the myoelectric hand holding the tube and the sound hand turning the cap.

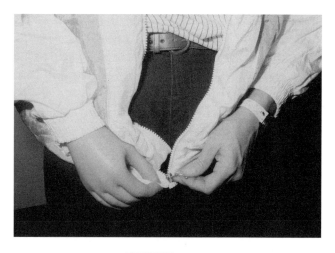

FIGURE 14-18

Zipping a jacket zipper is accomplished by holding the "anchor tab" with the myoelectric hand and pulling the zipper "pull tab" upward with the sound hand.

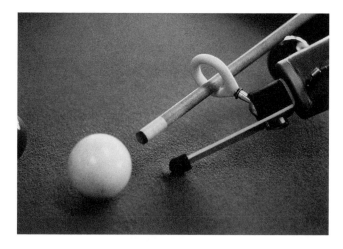

FIGURE 14-19

TRS terminal device for pool.

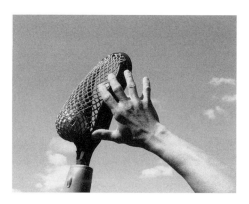

FIGURE 14-20

TRS terminal device for lacrosse.

With practice, these activities and many others will continue to improve and become automatic in their completion. It is extremely important to reinforce and emphasize the fact that bathing, grooming, and hygiene skills involving water must be done without a myoelectric hand because of the damaging effects of water on the electric motor and battery. Additionally, it is important to advise myoelectric users against excess vibration, sand, dirt, and the extremes of heat and cold. These too can seriously impair the electronic components.

Vocational and Leisure Activities

As training proceeds, and a sense of self-acceptance and comfortableness with the amputation is experienced, a therapist should broach the subject of return to work. If possible, the various job requirements can be discussed and then practiced in a simulated step-by-step process. Ideally, an on-site visit could be made by the therapist, and several requirements of the job could be practiced. If changes and adjustments to the work environment are necessary, the therapist could advise in these modifications.

Recreational activities are also critically important to discuss at this time, for these activities contribute not only to physical well-being but also to important psychologic well-being. The terminal devices for recreational activities are not myoelectric. Therapeutic Recreation Systems (TRS) has some excellent terminal device adaptation components that include adaptations for pool (Figure 14-19), lacrosse (Figure 14-20), and soccer (Figure 14-21).

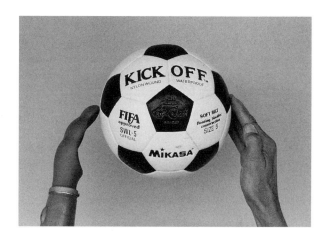

FIGURE 14-21

TRS terminal device for soccer.

Home Instructions

At the conclusion of training, home instructions that include a wearing schedule and care instructions should be reviewed with the patient and the family. A follow-up appointment should also be made at this time, as well as a list of the amputee team members and their telephone numbers, which will enable the patient to contact the appropriate person when problems arise.

CONCLUSIONS

The rehabilitation process of a person with upper limb loss can be a challenging and rewarding process. In the instances of above-elbow, shoulder disarticulation, and bilateral limb loss, significant training and expertise on the part of the therapist is essential.

The potential of the individual with amputation is limitless, and often he is able to accomplish activities one never would have expected. The success of his rehabilitation does not rest solely on the quality of training in the use of a prosthesis. Success is closely intertwined with the quality of his medical management, the quality of the prosthesis, functional training, and the conscientious follow-up of this individual once the rehabilitation phase is complete. Follow-up is critically important and often overlooked. Perhaps the most important aspect of a successful rehabilitation program, however, is the motivation and the desire of the person with an amputation to become more independent. As a team member, this aspect is a pivotal ingredient to cultivate and reinforce. The impact a therapist makes during this important process will remain with the patient for life.

References

1. Millstein S, Heger H, Hunter A. Prosthetic use in adult upper-limb amputees: a comparison of the body-powered and electrically powered prostheses. *Prosthet Orthot Int* 1986; 10:27–34.

2. Meier R. Amputations and prosthetic fitting. In: Fisher S (ed.), *Comprehensive Rehabilitation of Burns.* Baltimore: Williams & Wilkins, 1984, pp. 280.

3. Burrough S, Brook J. Patterns of acceptance and rejection of upper limb prostheses. *Orthot Prosthet* 1985; 39:40–47.

4. Levy W, Barnes G. *Hygienic Problems of the Amputee.* Washington, DC: American Orthotics and Prosthetics Association, 1961, p. 9.

5. Gilad I. Motion pattern analysis for evaluation and design of a prosthetic hook. *Arch Phys Med Rehabil* 1984; 66:399–402.

6. Atkins D. The upper extremity prosthetic prescription: conventional or electric components. *Phys Disabil Spec Inter OT Newslet* 1987; 10:2.

7. Santschi W, Winston M. *Manual of Upper Extremity Prosthetics,* 2 ed. Engineering Artificial Limbs Research Project. Los Angeles: University of California Press, 1958.

8. Trost F. A comparison of conventional and myoelectric below elbow use. *Interclin Inf Bill* 1965; 18:9–16. Spiegel SR:

9. Heger H, Millstein S, Hunter G. Electrically powered prostheses for the adult with an upper limb amputation. *Bone Joint Surg* 1985; 67-B:278–281.

10. Jacobsen SC et al. Development of the Utah artificial arm. *IEEE Trans Biomed Eng* 29(4):249, 1982.

11. Nader M, Ing EH. The artificial substitution of missing hands with myoelectric prostheses. *Clin Orthoped Related Res* 258:9, 1990.

12. Dalsey R et al. Myoelectric prosthetic replacement in the upper extremity amputee. *Orthoped Rev* 18 (6):697, 1989.

13. Scott RN, Parker PA. Myoelectric prostheses: State of the art. *I Med Eng Tech* 12 (4):143, 1988.

14. Meier RH. Amputations and prosthetic fitting. In: Fisher S (ed.), *Comprehensive Rehabilitation of Burns.* Baltimore: Williams & Wilkins, 1984.

15. Atkins DJ. Postoperative and pre-prosthetic therapy programs. In: Atkins DJ, Meier RH (eds.), *Comprehensive Management of the Upper-Limb Amputee.* New York: Springer-Verlag, 1989.

16. Spiegel SR. Adult myoelectric upper-limb prosthetic training. In: Atkins DJ, Meier RH (eds.), *Comprehensive Management of the Upper-Limb Amputee.* New York: Springer-Verlag, 1989.

15 Prosthetic Prescription

Robert H. Meier, III, MD and Alberto Esquenzai, MD

Prosthetic prescription should be accomplished following the completion of the postoperative and the preprosthetic phases of upper extremity amputation rehabilitation, as previously described under the nine phases of amputation rehabilitation (1).

Certain important elements should have been achieved prior to the actual prescription of the arm prosthesis. These elements include stump shaping and shrinking, so that there is some stability of the residual limb soft tissues prior to casting for the first prosthetic socket. Soft tissue stability will provide for a longer period of good prosthetic socket fit before the need arises for modification or recasting for a new socket. This stability of the soft tissues is of particular importance when prescribing a myoelectric device, since an intimate skin–socket fit is essential for electrode activation.

Prosthetic prescription should also occur only after the arm amputee has been educated regarding the types of prosthetic components that are available for his use, and the pros and cons of the variety of prostheses that he could potentially wear and use are discussed. In addition, the process and approximate time period for prosthetic fabrication should be presented prior to prosthetic prescription.

Prior to the actual first prosthetic prescription, an assessment of the arm amputee's anticipated use of the prosthesis should also have been achieved. The actual prosthetic training experience should have been reviewed with the amputee prior to the prescription of the prosthesis.

Before a prosthetic prescription is developed, the funding source of payment for the prosthesis should have been determined and any prescription constraints previously identified. In today's systems of health care reimbursement, not all funding sources will pay for all the possible arm prosthetic components. These prescription limitations most frequently involved passive, custom cosmetic devices and electrically controlled prostheses.

The prosthetic prescription should be developed through input from the rehabilitation team, the patient, and the family, and only after the arm amputee has been presented with the various types of prosthetic arm designs and the possible components that may fulfill his needs. If available, peer demonstration should be implemented. Team and patient concensus should be achieved through this prescription team conference format.

INCLUSION OF THE PATIENT IN THE PRESCRIPTION PROCESS

The development of a prosthetic arm prescription is an inclusive process and should occur once the team has developed an appreciation of the lifestyle and functional capabilities of the person who has sustained the arm amputation. Just examining the residual arm and obtaining a cursory history may give a general ideal of what prosthesis might work best for the amputee. However, this is not an inclusive and comprehensive process, and this type of planning does not provide the amputee with input into the process and include his control of the prescription process. This is an important time to provide some locus of control for the amputee in determining his future appearance and function.

Prior to the actual prescription, the individual should also have had the opportunity to see the proposed components and to touch and feel them. In addition, it can be useful for the new arm amputee to discuss the prosthetic experience of another appropriately matched, successful prosthetic arm user.

MATCHING THE COMPONENTS TO THE INDIVIDUAL

Matching the most appropriate components to the new arm amputee is part of the art of arm prosthetic rehabilitation and generally requires a large amount of arm amputation rehabilitation experience. However, some generalizations can be made to assist the team in prescribing the most appropriate components. Several charts and tables have been developed to assist in indicating the most useful components and prosthetic system designs (Table 15-1 and Table 15-2). These tables are usually based on the relative advantages and disadvantages of prosthetic system and their component attributes.

Those issues found to be most important to upper extremity prosthetic wearing and use are, in descending order of importance, comfort, function, and cosmesis. The prior lifestyle of the individual, including issues of work, play, and family role, are important in the consideration of the arm prosthetic prescription. The issue of cosmesis and the attitude of the arm amputee and his family towards cosmesis must also be determined.

Although this section is mostly concerned with the initial prosthetic prescription, it should be noted that, following the first prescription, it may be determined at follow-up that the prescription should be modified or completely changed. As the arm amputee is trained and becomes more adept at using the initially prescribed device, it may become apparent that other components may provide better function, comfort, or cosmesis than the original prescription.

During the process of the initial prescription, it can be useful to provide some latitude to try a variety of terminal devices (TD) before deciding on the final prescription. The use of a voluntary opening as compared to a

TABLE 15-1
Advantages and Disadvantages of Various Upper Limb Prostheses

TYPE	PROS	CONS
Cosmetic (passive)	Most lightweight Best cosmesis Least harnessing	High cost if custom made Least function Low-cost glove stains easily
Body powered	Moderate cost Moderately lightweight Most durable Highest sensory feedback	Most body movement to operate Most harnessing Least satisfactory appearance
Externally powered (myoelectric and switch control)	Moderate or no harnessing Least body movement to operate Moderate cosmesis More function-proximal levels	Heaviest Most expensive Most maintenance Limited sensory feedback
Hybrid (cable elbow/electric TD)	All-cable excursion to elbow Increased TD pinch	Electric TD weights forearm (harder to lift) Good for elbow disarticulation (or long above elbow)
Hybrid (electric elbow/cable TD)	All-cable excursion to TD Low effort to position TD Low maintenance TD	Least cosmesis Lower pinch force for TD

TD, terminal device.
Modified from Esquenazi A, Leonard JA, Meier RM, et al. 3. Prosthetics. *Arch Phys Med Rehabil.* 1989; 70(Suppl):207.

TABLE 15-2
Comparison of Control Options and Terminal Device Choices

BASIC NEEDS	CONTROL CHOICE		SHAPE CHOICE	
	BODY POWER	MYOELECTRIC	HOOK	HAND
Function				
Fine tip prehension	–	–	X	–
Cylindrical grip (large diameter)	–	–	–	X
Cylindrical grip (small diameter)	–	–	X	–
Flat prehension	–	–	X	–
Hook and pull	–	–	X	–
Pushing/holding down	–	–	–	X
Handling long-handled tools (handle must slide)	–	–	X	–
Ruggedness	X	–	X	–
High grip force	–	X	–	–
Delicate grip force	–	X	–	–
Visibility	–	–	–	X
Cosmesis	–	–	–	X
Comfort				
Low weight	X	–	X	–
Harness comfort	–	X	–	–
Low effort	–	X	–	–
Reliability and convenience	X	–	X	–
Low cost	X	–	–	–

From Sears HH: Evaluation and development of a new hook-type terminal device. PhD Dissertation. University of Utah, 1983.

voluntary closing device is one example. Another example is the use of a voluntary opening hand compared to a voluntary opening hook. In these cases, the amputee can compare the weight of the different devices, their comfort, force generation, and functional use.

BODY POWER VERSUS EXTERNAL POWER

The power generation for an arm prosthetic prescription is quite controversial, and the practice of prosthetic arm prescription in the United States is at variance with the experience in Western Europe and other areas in the world.

The majority of prosthetic arm prescription in the United States today provide a body-powered arm. Externally powered arms have been available since the 1970s in this country, but have not been as widely used as they have been in Western Europe (2). The majority of body-powered arms that have been prescribed also have included a hook terminal device. This practice was largely used in veteran rehabilitation following the Second World War, the Korean Conflict, and the Vietnam War. However, this practice has also been followed in the civilian population of the United States.

In the U.S., the generally held opinion is that the voluntary opening hook terminal device provides more useful function for the prosthetic user than body-powered or electrically powered hands do (3). This is presumed to occur because the visual feedback from the hook is more easily obtained than from either of the hand designs. The surface area of the hook and its fingers is much smaller than the surface area of the hand. Therefore, it is easier to see the object during grasp and release while using a hook. The thinner finger tips in the hook allow for the more precise control of fine objects.

Also, because sensory feedback is not now generally available in an arm prosthesis, the harnessing for the body-powered design is felt to provide better sensory feedback to the arm amputee than the muscle activation used in an externally powered prosthesis.

A comparison vector diagram has been developed by Sears (4), so that the variety of advantages of upper extremity components can be weighed against other features. Figure 15-1 shows the vector diagrams that compare function, cosmesis, reliability, and cost. Figure 15-2 shows the vector favoring myoelectric control for a young student, where cosmesis and grip force are more important than reliability and cost. Figure 15-3 shows a

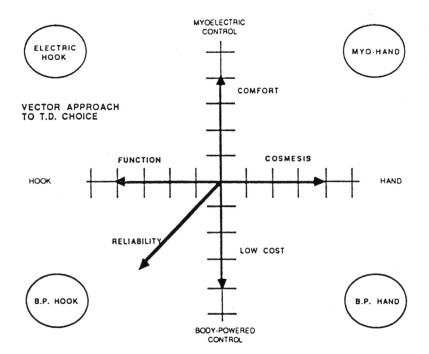

FIGURE 15-1

Vectors comparing function, cosmesis, reliability, and cost for body-powered and myoelectric control.

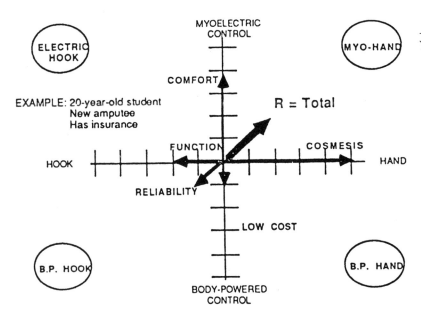

FIGURE 15-2

Young college student with insurance.

more mature laborer who requires reliability and is self funded.

It has long been felt that there is a trade-off between cosmesis and comfort in the prescription of an arm prosthesis (4). The most cosmetic, functional prosthetic prescriptions are heavy and therefore presumed to be less comfortable than the lighter weight body-powered prosthesis with a hook terminal device (TD). This greater weight is not the case when comparing a passive cosmetic arm with a functional body-powered arm using a hook TD. In addition, a passive cosmetic restoration can provide some useful function for the wearer even though it does not provide grasp and release. This function can include steadying an object, keeping paper still, carrying light objects, and pushing an object.

FIGURE 15-3

Mature laborer who is self funded.

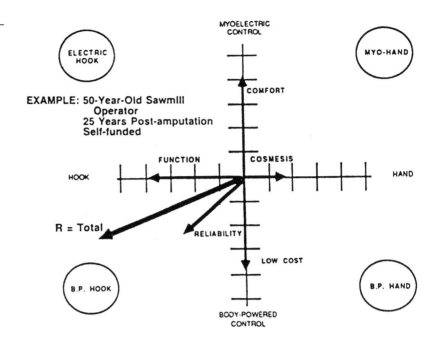

EXAMPLE: 50-Year-Old Sawmill
Operator
25 Years Post-amputation
Self-funded

The durability of a prosthesis is also an important consideration in the prescription process. In general, the body-powered devices are more durable than externally powered designs, and they are also lower in cost. The externally powered devices have a variety of maintenance issues that include battery recharging, inconsistent electrode contact with the skin, fraying wires, microchip board malfunction, and motor malfunction. Some of these items can be repaired by the local prosthetic laboratory, but others may need to be shipped to the manufacturer for repair. The most common issues for repair in the body-powered prosthesis are related to cable attachments disconnecting and battery lifespan. Some improvement has occurred recently with the introduction to the market of rechargeable lithium ion batteries.

The final area of comparison is that of prosthetic cost. If one compares the wholesale cost of components for a transradial amputee using body-powered versus externally powered components, the body-powered prosthesis is about one-fourth the cost of the externally powered design. For the transhumeral amputee, the cost comparison for the body-powered design is one-sixth that of the externally powered counterpart. To date, limited functional outcome and no cost efficacy studies compare these differing designs.

In practical terms, the fitting of an externally powered prosthesis with electrodes requires an intimate socket fit. Usually, a recent arm amputee will continue to have fluctuating soft tissue volumes that will often prevent consistent intimate contact of the electrodes with the surface of the skin. For this reason, it is preferrable that the soft tissues of the residual limb have stabilized before external power with electrodes is fitted. In practical experience, this process often takes from 6 to 12 months from the date of the arm amputation. Considering this difficulty in maintaining consistent electrode contact, it is often the practice to use a body-powered prosthesis at least until these soft tissues have stabilized in volume. Using a body-powered prosthesis first for functional training allows for the body-powered prosthesis to be available for back-up, which can be useful when the person is later fitted with an externally powered prosthesis and the prosthesis needs to be sent in for maintenance. In this manner, the regular prosthetic arm user does not need to go for any period of time without a functioning prosthesis.

In some individual arm amputees, it may be advantageous to mix both body-powered and electrically powered moving arm components. This mixture of design elements is called a *hybrid prosthesis*. If this design is prescribed, special attention should be paid to whether the elbow or the hand is the component that should be electrically powered. In practice, it appears preferable to electrically power the hand to provide greater grasping capability.

COSMETIC PROSTHETIC RESTORATION

Cosmetic restoration has often been overlooked as an important restorative option for the arm amputee, perhaps because of the use of the term "cosmetic." The fact that this type of prosthesis may have useful function, in addition to cosmesis, is often overlooked.

Cosmetic restorations may be either active or passive. In the passive design, the hand terminal device does not have articulated fingers that move. This design may have limited function for use in bimanual activities, where an object must be steadied against the passive side and manipulated with the opposite hand (such as steadying a plate). In addition, a passive cosmetic terminal device can also be of some use in keeping a piece of paper from sliding during writing. The passive cosmetic arm prosthesis may be the lightest and most comfortable design available. It does not generally require harnessing and strapping, which also increases the comfort factors.

The active cosmetic restoration is a cosmetic glove that covers the hand and perhaps the forearm of a prosthesis having a functioning terminal device. This TD could be a hand that has a moving thumb, index, and long finger to provide a three-jaw chuck grasp and release; it may be body or externally powered.

PROSTHETIC FABRICATION PROCESS

Once the prosthetic arm prescription has been developed, the amputee should be educated in the steps of prosthetic fabrication and also receive an approximate time table for the steps of fabrication. The actual delivery date should be estimated so that arrangements for therapy and follow-up visits can be scheduled. This is an appropriate time to discuss what will occur during this rehabilitation phase and the anticipated time suggested for prosthetic training.

CONCLUSIONS

It is essential that the arm amputee understand that prosthetic training is an important component of prosthetic fabrication. Lack of prosthetic training for arm amputees may be one reason for the large percentage of non-use that appears in the American literature. The days when a prosthesis was fabricated and handed to the patient with no further training are hopefully finished. It is the responsibility of the prescribing physician and the prosthetist to assure that arrangements for prosthetic rehabilitation training have been made and that the patient has followed through with the scheduled training in order to achieve optimal wearing and functional use of the prosthesis.

References

1. Esquenazi E, Leonard JA, Meier RH. 3. Prosthetics. *Arch Phys Med Rehabil* 1989; 70(Suppl): 207.
2. Uellendahl JE. Upper extremity myoelectric prosthetics. *Phys Med Rehabil Clin NA* 2000; 11, No. 3: 639–652.
3. Muilenburg AL, LeBlanc MA. Body-powered upper limb components. In: Atkin DA, Meier RH (eds.), *Comprehensive Management of the Upper-Limb Amputee.* New York: Springer-Verlag, 1989.
4. Sears HH. Approaches to prescription of body-powered and myoelectric prostheses. *Phys Med Rehabil Clin NA* 1991; 2.

16 Aesthetic Restorations for the Upper Limb Amputee

Annaliese M. Furlong, CP

Beauty is in the eye of the beholder. Nowhere is this more true than in the cosmetic restoration of the upper limb amputee. While one individual may prefer a device closely resembling the missing limb segment another may favor a lamination with a specific illustration (similar to a tattoo) to symbolize their individuality. Because of the range and diversity of cosmetic options, it is important for the amputee and practitioner to review all restorative options and come to a mutual decision about what best meets the needs of the wearer.

FABRICATION AND MATERIAL OPTIONS FOR PROSTHETIC COVERINGS

Generally, a prosthetic restoration is fashioned to mimic the size, shape, and function of the missing limb segment. The shape, contour, and look of the prosthetic device is usually accomplished by taking measurements and matching the coloration of the contralateral or remaining limb. To some upper limb amputees, the appearance of the outer covering of the prosthesis is as paramount as its function. It was noted by Bowker and Michaels that "Cosmesis should be considered one aspect of function and is probably better termed 'realistic appearance' (1)."

Beasley compared the functional restriction of the individual who chooses to hide the affected hand or limb to that of a forequarter amputee. Although it can be argued that an amputee should have a comfortable body image either with or without the use of a prosthetic device, this does not always occur. For some individuals cosmetic restoration is of paramount importance.

Several options can be applied to a prosthesis to enhance its realistic appearance. These options range from a hard outer covering (lamination) shaped and pigmented to match the patient's skin tone and contour, to a soft, subtle, custom-molded silicone glove replicated from the sound hand and arm and with custom coloration. Several factors can influence the success in integrating a prosthesis with a cosmetic finish. These factors include:

- Desired prosthetic function and design characteristics
- Durability
- Use environment
- Cost
- Length of the residual segment
- Patient lifestyle

The most significant factor affecting the choice of prosthetic finishing is most probably the prosthetic design. Although it may be said that custom silicone allows the highest level of cosmetic realism, it may not optimally serve the individual who is involved in activities that may compromise the integrity of the finish. A passive (nonactivated) prosthesis will not put as much stress on the covering as, for example, a cable driven, body-powered device. This chapter focuses on material qualities as they relate to prosthetic design.

POLYVINAL CHLORIDE

Sometimes referred to as *latex*, the polyvinyl or PVC covering is generally considered one of the more economic choices for prosthetic coverings. These gloves are generally available "off the shelf," with standardized shapes and colors (Figure 16-1). Although the PVC may initially appear the most feasible option, associated costs and wear factors must be considered. Latex is an unstable material that will discolor over time and even more rapidly with increased exposure to ultraviolet rays (sunlight). This can occur within a period of several weeks. Because of this degeneration, latex gloves are best stored and worn out of direct sunlight and are expected to have a life expectancy of 3 to 9 months.

In addition to UV discoloration, latex can harden and become brittle over time. This material can also readily and easily pick up stains and permanent discolorations. Some daily agents that should be avoided include:

- Newspaper print
- Carbon prints
- Fabric dyes
- Food (mustard, juice)
- Shoe polish
- Paint and varnish thinner
- Graphite
- Indelible pencil
- Cigarette smoke

It is recommended that an active user wash the hand at least twice a day using approved cleaning and conditioning agents. The prosthetist can recommend the best cleaning and conditioning agents for the particular glove. Certain nonapproved cleaning agent can actually weaken the material of the glove and or skin.

SILICONE

Silicone has been used in numerous prosthetic applications and contributes to comfort as well as cosmetic affect.

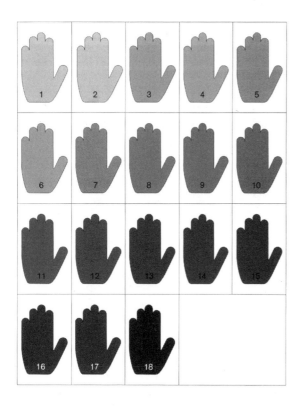

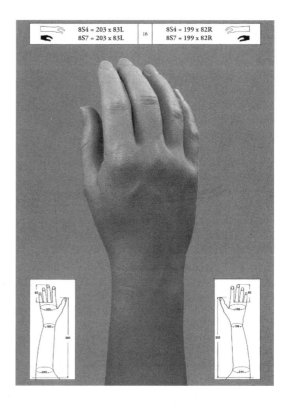

FIGURE 16-1

Otto Bock color selection chart. Courtesy Otto Bock HealthCare GmbH.

Silicone gloves, like PVC, are available in customized and off-the-shelf styles. Silicone off-the-shelf gloves come in a variety of sizes and colors and are made to fit over preformed hand shells (Figure 16-2). Adding color, nails, age spots, hair, freckles, and striations further customizes these gloves. In addition, silicone has an inherent stain-resistant quality and superior durability. Most stains can be readily removed using soap and water.

For individuals who are seeking the optimal in realistic restoration, the custom silicone covering provides the highest level of acceptance (Figure 16-3). Custom gloves are generally fabricated from a mold of the amputee's remaining extremity. Size, color, and shape are duplicated as closely as possible, as dictated by the underlying prosthetic componentry. Although some manufacturers are willing to work long distance with practitioners to design gloves and finishes, others work

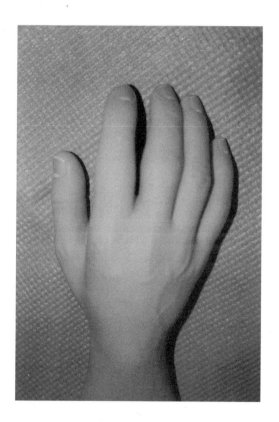

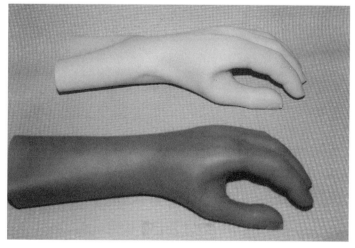

FIGURE 16-2

Realistic glove. Courtesy Otto Bock HealthCare GmbH.

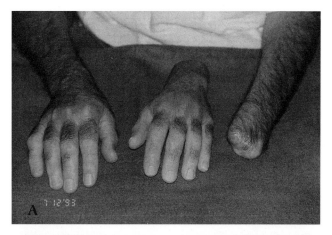

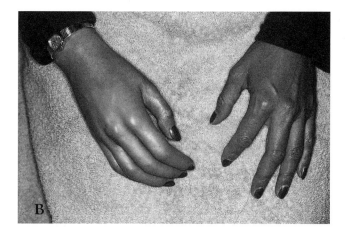

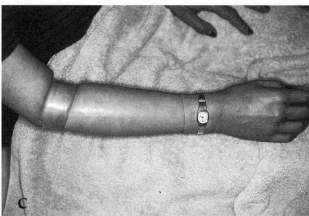

FIGURE 16-3

Custom silicone covering. Courtesy Pillet.

only directly with the patient. Customized silicone gloves also offer enhanced life expectancy (4 to 7 years) and can be repaired if torn. Silicone also offers an inherent improved adhesive quality much superior to latex. This enhanced grip quality allows the patient to manipulate objects that might otherwise slip from their grasp. Hair, nails, and texture can be added to enhance the realism of a cover.

It is imperative for the prosthetist as well as the patient to recognize that skin tone and coloration is dynamic. Changes in temperature or blood flow to the extremity can affect the appearance of the anatomic hand or body segment that is being matched. In addition, seasonal changes can affect appearance. Individuals who seek customized covers generally have a high expectation for the appearance of their prostheses. For an individual who undergoes significant change in skin tone throughout the year, two devices may be warranted, or they may opt for a product that facilitates color change, as is offered by Aesthetic Concerns. The Living Skin product allows skin tone to be altered per seasonal variance. Prior to choosing a manufacturer, it is important consult the patient regarding these various manufacturers and how the product characteristics

best suit the makeup of the particular patient and prosthetic device.

ADDITIONAL OPTIONS

In addition to silicone and PVC cosmetic gloves, skin-like spray-on materials, which only cover the outer portion of the prostheses, are also available (Figure 16-4).

This type of cosmetic covering provides more than just cosmetic restoration; like the prosthetic gloves, prosthetic skin can effectively act as a barrier against dirt and moisture. One distinct advantage that a skin finishing has over lamination is the increased traction provided by the rubberlike finish of the material. Many upper limb amputees find this adhesive quality helpful in stabilizing the objects they are working with.

Cosmetic Options as They Relate to Prosthetic Prescription

The design makeup of a prosthesis, as guided by the prescription, can greatly affect the cosmetic choice. The basic prosthetic designs (for levels above wrist or higher) include:

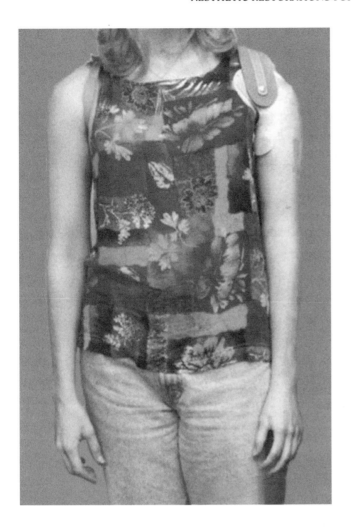

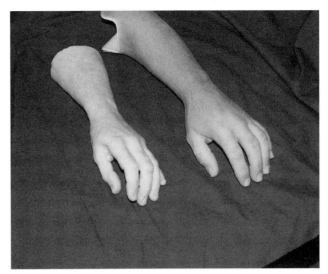

FIGURE 16-4

Spray-on prosthetic covering. Courtesy ARTech Labs.

- Endoskeletal
- Exoskeletal
- Body-powered
- Externally powered (myoelectric, switch, touch pad)
- Passive

Endoskeletal vs. Exoskeletal Prostheses

Endoskeletal and *exoskeletal* refer to the structural component of the prosthesis. By definition, an exoskeletal configuration obtains its structural integrity through its external (or shell-like) makeup and is generally recognized as a hard supportive surface finish. By contrast, endoskeletal refers to an internal base of support. An endoskeletal design usually features a series of tubes that interconnect the components and is covered with a soft foam cover. Several factor affect prosthetic design choice.

The exoskeletal prosthesis has a hardened external cover or lamination. This is by far the most common design for a functional upper extremity prosthetic user. Exoskeletal prostheses are generally hard-pigmented laminate shaped to resemble the missing limb segment (Figure 16-5). As a rule, this option tends to be more durable and able to withstand higher stress and impact. Cosmesis can be enhanced using an off-the-shelf cosmetic glove or a custom silicone forearm and hand.

Endoskeletal prostheses, by contrast, generally provide less functional options but enhanced cosmetic ability. One-piece covers can be applied to provide a continuous cover to the upper arm. The endoskeletal prosthesis uses internal structural components. Along with providing structural integrity, the endoskeletal design also provides a means to attach various components. Generally, this design is composed of a tubular structure to which components (wrist, elbow, shoulder) can be attached to the socket (Figure 16-6). A soft foam encloses the tubing and is shaped to match the residual limb.

The benefits of the endoskeletal design include reduced weight, ease of adjustment, protection from internal components (via the soft cover), and improved cosmetic effect since most of the components are hidden within. Deficiencies include less durability (the cover is

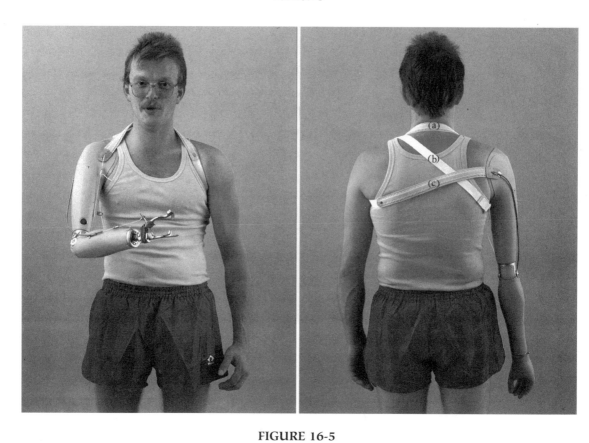

FIGURE 16-5

Cable-controlled prosthetic system. Courtesy Otto Bock HealthCare GmbH.

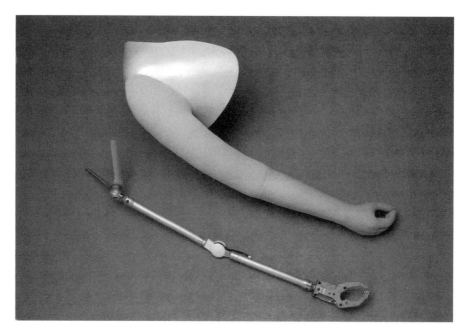

FIGURE 16-6

Endoskeletal prosthetic arm. Courtesy Otto Bock HealthCare GmbH.

more readily torn) and limitation in the type of components that can be adapted. Many of the more heavy-duty components require increased structural support and will not attach to this design.

Body-Powered Design

The body-powered design utilizes cable driven control to translate body motion into function. The need for cable and harnessing limits the choices for cosmetic finish. The cable adds an inherent maintenance factor for any outer covering and tends to be best suited to the exoskeletal finishing. The need for cable can affect the choice of cosmetic finish.

Externally Powered Design

Externally powered or myoelectric designs generally require minimized harnessing and may even be self-suspended. Many users find that the lack of harness and cable enhances the aesthetic component of the prostheses. Just as with the body-powered options, myoelectric prostheses have the option of accepting a hand or hook. These terminal devices can also be interchanged as desired. Externally powered designs will accept any of the covering options of the body-powered prostheses. The position of batteries or other electronic components should be reviewed in relation to cosmetic selection. A cosmetic covering to an externally powered device can also aid in protecting sensitive electronics from exposure to moisture.

Passive Hand

The passive hand is defined by its lack of active grasp function. However, it can function as an assist to the sound arm by providing frictional resistance. Passive hands are available with internal wires that can preposition the fingers. In addition, a higher level of duplication is possible with this design, since moving mechanical components do not need to be accommodated within the finish.

Restoration for Digital Amputation

Digital amputation can present a unique challenge. For some, the deficit is noted as strictly cosmetic. For others, the condition is functional, related to the "hole in the hand" effect. Common complaints associated with digital amputation include increased sensitivity to temperature, lack of soft tissue protection, pain or discomfort associated with manipulation, and a diminished ergonomic positioning, which can lead to overuse syndrome.

Acrylic, latex, PVC, and silicone have all been used in digital recreation, with varying degrees of success. If a portion of the finger segment remains, the prosthetic digit can often be adhered through the use of suction. Suspension becomes more difficult as related to the length of the residual digital segment.

Rigid vs. Articulated

Some prosthetic finger reconstructions offer the option of articulation joints for preposition on the prosthetic segment. Articulation refers to the ability to preposition a segment of the prosthetic restoration similar to that of the anatomic joint. Different options are available. For example, Lifelike Labs uses a wire construct that allows propositioning, whereas Aesthetic Concerns offers a micro-joint positioned within the silicone matrix. It is important to note that the length of the remaining finger segment often dictates the availability of this option.

Thumb Amputations

When it comes to digital prosthetic options, the thumb tends to be slightly more difficult to fit. The main challenge reflects on the complexity of motion that the thumb provides and how this relates to suspension. An amputated thumb represents a 50% loss of function to the hand: opposition, lateral pinch, and abduction can be affected. If a portion of the thumb segment remains, the prosthetic digit can often be adhered through the use of suction (Figure 16-7).

An amputation at the metacarpal–phalangeal joint presents additional challenges in terms of suspension. When there is a well-formed residual thumb segment, the prosthetic restoration can be manufactured to use suction to secure the prostheses in place. However, if there is no such segment to anchor the device to, other options can be employed.

Multiple Digital Amputations

Reconstructing more than one digit may provide challenges similar to that of replacing a missing thumb. Suspension can be achieved by covering more of the hand area or, on occasion, digits can be formed together to enhance adherence and stability (Figure 16-8).

Partial and Total Hand Reconstructions

Partial and total hand prostheses can fall into either the passive or active category. Active prostheses provide dynamic performance augmented by the use of external componentry to provide function. Due to the amount of additional componentry (increased bulk) needed to per-

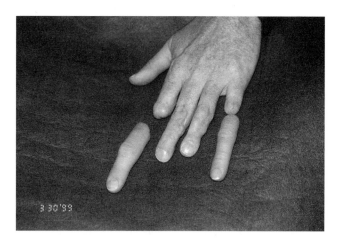

FIGURE 16-7

Thumb prostheses. Courtesy Life Like Labs.

form active tasks, most patients who pursue a "cosmetic restoration" lean toward the passive option.

Passive does not equate to nonfunctional: Many patient find the restored length provided by a digital reconstruction can assist the function of the impaired hand, allow the patient to operate in a more ergonomic fashion, provide protection to the involved segment, and prevent or diminished overuse syndrome.

In contrast, an active hand provides controlled motion. The active prosthetic hand can be subdivided into voluntary open (VO) or voluntary closing (VC) and is usually body powered using cable driven systems. A harness worn against the upper body is connected to a control cable, which in turn provides the designated function. Although any of the aforementioned cosmetic gloves can be utilized in conjunction with the active

hand, cable placement may compromise the overall cosmetic effect.

Arm Amputations

A wide range of prosthetic options is available for the upper limb amputee who is missing the limb at the wrist level or higher. A higher level of amputation dictates the need for additional functional restorative options: This can be viewed as the need for an increased number of components and control mechanisms. These factors should be weighed against the function versus cosmetic factor. In particular, the focus may be on the terminal device, since this is the component most apt to be in view. By definition, the terminal device is that part of the prosthesis that is designed to replace the function of the hand. The terminal device can be fitted as a hand, hook, or other accommodative device.

Passive vs. Active Cable-Driven Hands

A passive hand does not offer an active grasp function. For a patient who has concerns about the weight of the prostheses and is not in need of a functional grip, a passive hand is a viable option. Although by definition prosthetic hands are not heavy, it is important to recognize that the hand is fit to the end of a long lever arm (the prosthetic socket). A good way to demonstrate the functional difference in weight to the patient is to allow them to compare the different hands while holding them away from the body with the shoulder flexed at 90 degrees. Because of this leverage factor, many patient may "notice" the weight of an active hand. No harnessing or control mechanism is necessary with the passive hand.

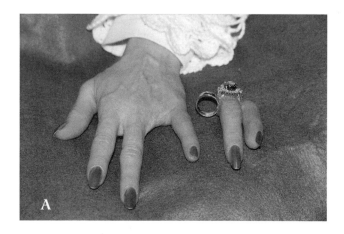

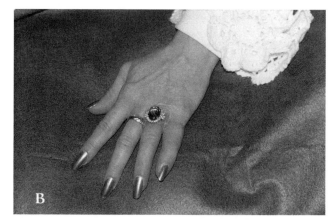

FIGURE 16-8

Multiple-digit restoration. Courtesy Life Like Labs.

REIMBURSEMENT

Getting compensation for a prosthetic device can often be as challenging as getting a good design and fit. Many third-party payers look to the definition of medical necessity to determine if a device is a covered item. When submitting a claim, it is often helpful to provide a clear picture of the various options and variables associated with the proposed prosthetic design. It is important to educate patients, doctors, and payer sources about the functional benefits and drawbacks associated with various prosthetic cosmetics. An expense analyses comparing product life expectancy, functionality, maintenance, and durability can be included with the initial review process to determine long-term costs, and this can often justify higher initial up-front costs. Patient age, lifestyle, compliance, and cost should all be factored into the decision when reviewing these options.

CONCLUSIONS

The aforementioned options are just a few of the restorative alternatives available. However, by no means does review overlook or diminish from the naturalist choice of not wearing a prostheses. Dr. Harlan Hahn suggested "as people become increasingly willing to present their bodies in new and different ways, observers may discover unanticipated aesthetic pleasure in physical characteristics that reflect differences, instead of similarities, between human beings." The choice of cosmetic restoration should be ultimately left to the amputee.

References

1. Michael JW, Bowker JH. *J Prosthetic Orthotics* 1994: 6; 4, 100–107.
2. Fillauer CE, Pritham CH, Fillauer KD. Evaluation and development of the silicone suction socket (3-S) for below knee prostheses. *J Prosthetic Orthotics* 1989: 1; 2, 92–103.
3. Burkhardt A, Weitz J. Oncologic applications for silicone gel sheets in soft tissue contractors. *Am J Occup Ther* 199__: 45; 5, 460–462.
4. Hahn H. *In Motion*, Volume 6. Embodied differences: Achieving a positive identity. Pgs. 30–31.

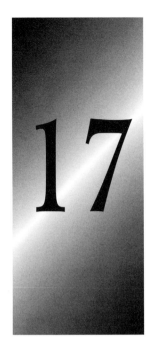

Overview of Body-Powered Upper Extremity Prostheses

Gerald Stark, BSME, CP, FAAOP and Maurice LeBlanc, MSME, CP

Upper extremity prostheses have always been unique in design because of functional and cosmetic issues. Replacing the dexterity and agility of the human hand is not an easy task: The upper extremity prosthesis is expected to not only lock in place when holding an object, but must also provide active movement (i.e., gripping, elbow flexion, etc.). It is also much more visible than lower limb prostheses, making cosmetic concerns particularly relevant. Mechanisms and components to control the prosthesis must be concealed from view. In some cases, function may be sacrificed for more cosmetic alternatives such as a hand for a hook. Movements that activate the prosthesis must also be adjusted to optimize function and minimize the body control movements that activate the prosthesis. Cables and harnesses must be custom fitted to the amputee's form to provide a comfortable, biomechanically efficient, and predictable function.

ARMOR TO ELECTRONICS: A SHORT HISTORY

Armorers were the first to make upper extremity prostheses from hand gauntlets. These early prostheses were used mainly in battle and were of little use during daily activities. The sole functional purpose was to hold a sword or shield and the equally important concealment of any perceived infirmity. The Alt-Ruppin hand (Figure 17-1), circa 1400, is typical of many early active hands that used springs and catches to hold fingers when placed into position. The finger position was then released with a push of a button. In 1812, Peter Ballif, a Berlin dentist, developed a harness and thong system that provided active prehension controlled by shoulder and elbow movement (Figure 17-2). In 1844, Van Peetersen, a Dutchman, controlled elbow flexion in the same way (1).

Although some advances in materials were made, modern prosthetic principles did not evolve until after World War II, as a result of the large number of amputees returning home. The U.S. Army Surgeon General and the U.S. Navy Bureau of Medicine and Surgery initiated an effort to update treatments and componentry methods. The National Academy of Sciences and the National Research Council conducted research largely funded by the Veteran's Administration and the Department of Health, Education, and Welfare. Research in upper limb prosthetics was conducted at the University of Southern California (UCLA) and at Northrup Aircraft. Myoelectric switch control was developed in 1949, but was not refined as a commercial product until the 1980s. Because most of the new research has focused on externally powered prostheses, body-powered

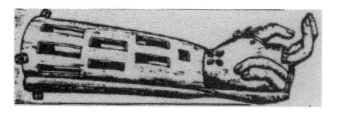

FIGURE 17-1

Alt-Ruppin Hand, circa 1400.

ESTIMATES OF ARM AMPUTEE POPULATION

In contrast to the lower limb, where amputations are relatively common secondary to disease processes such as diabetes, most amputations of the upper limb are primarily due to trauma, congenital deficiency, or tumor. Estimates place the number of arm amputees in the United States at 90,000 with approximately half choosing to wear prostheses (2). The levels of upper-limb amputations are illustrated in Figure 17-3. (3)

Of the 90,000 total arm amputees, approximately 10% are under 21 years of age; 60% are between the ages of 21 and 64 years; and 30% are older than 65 years.

components have not drastically changed in the past few decades due to the low numbers of the upper extremity amputee population and the high cost of manufacturing investment. Most new designs use existing components in combination to enable movements such as wrist or elbow rotation. New materials for cables and harness have been developed that lessen friction and increase general comfort. Many prosthetists are also finding advantages in combining body- and externally powered components to increase proprioception and the separation of controls while decreasing cost and maintenance.

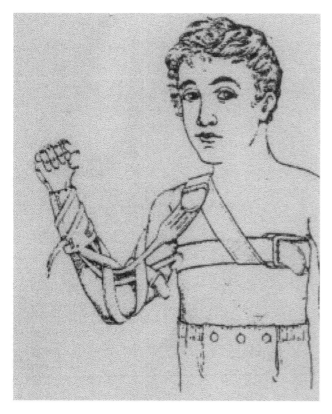

FIGURE 17-2

Ballif harness control system, 1812.

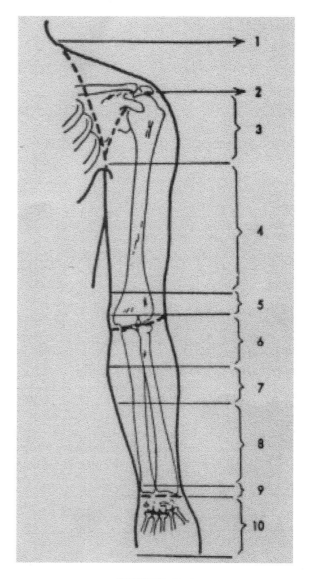

FIGURE 17-3

Levels of upper-limb amputations.

Of the prosthetic wearers (approximately half of the total number of upper extremity amputees), levels of amputation are estimated at shoulder, 5%; above elbow, 23%; elbow, 3%; below elbow, 57%; and Wrist/hand, 12%.

BODY POWER AND EXTERNAL POWER

Many prosthetists and amputees alike engage in a discussion of body-powered prostheses versus externally powered prostheses in the context of high- or low-tech. Both systems exist side by side (and sometimes work together) in the prosthetic armamentarium to address the different needs and goals of the amputee. The real key is weighing the advantages and disadvantages, of both systems to provide the most appropriate technology that will supply the amputee's needs and desires (4).

Body-powered cable systems—similar to bicycle controls—are, although simplistic, nonetheless effective. Cables and harnesses are relatively lightweight, inexpensive, and easy to repair. However, they do require more harnessing than external control systems to activate the prosthesis. Although modern externally powered systems are much more durable than early versions, the repairs still remain fairly expensive when compared to body-powered control. To optimize use, both systems require adjustment and fine-tuning with respect to cabling and harnessing. Unfortunately, many clinicians do not see upper extremity patients regularly to be experienced in componentry or harnessing adjustment. Different functions can be separated using different cable systems, whereas externally controlled prostheses may use a modal switch to alternate between functions using the same input. The use of cable systems to transfer loads to the harness also gives the patient better proprioceptive feedback (ability to determine where the prosthesis is located in space).

The main trade-off for body powered prosthesis is the cosmetic appearance of the device and its dependence on the amputee's physical ability to produce specific body motions to activate prosthetic function. Externally powered prosthesis at the transradial level are especially, cosmetic, since they are self-contained and eliminate harnessing and activation cables. This makes them very acceptable to the new amputee because the prosthesis resembles the anatomic arm, without foreign cables or harnessing. Although a body-powered use has the option of using hooks or mechanical hands, the hands require a lot of effort to use and have far less grip strength than externally powered hands. Cable systems require strength and body movement, whereas external systems minimize body movement requirements by using myoswitches or push/pull switches (5). This makes them useful in cases where strength and excursion are issues, such as with juveniles or high-level amputees.

TERMINAL DEVICES

Terminal Devices (TDs) are so named because they are the most distal component of the prosthesis. Because the TD serves as the primary functional prehensor, it receives more attention with regard to the patient's vocational and recreational needs. Body-powered terminal devices can be separated into four categories: functional mechanical hand, specialized, and passive/cosmetic.

Functional Terminal Devices

The most often used functional TD is the split hook (Figure 17-4). It is popular because it provides lateral gripping and precise manipulation at the tip. The most popular designs are canted to one side to provide better visual feedback and have neoprene lining to grip metal objects. Although only a few types of hooks predominate, more than thirty different hook configurations are available to meet the special needs of the prosthetic client (Figure 17-5).

Most TDs are *voluntary opening*, in that the cable, when pulled, acts to open the device and a rubber band

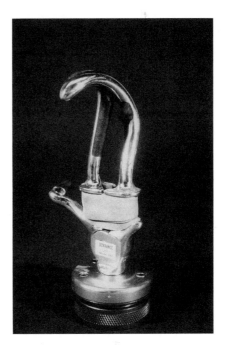

FIGURE 17-4

Hosmer 5XA hook.

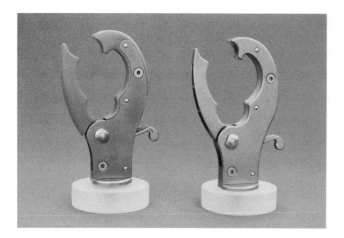

FIGURE 17-5

TRS VC Grip prehensor.

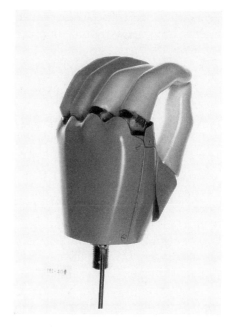

FIGURE 17-6

Dorrance mechanical hand.

or spring provides the closing or grip force. *Voluntary closing* devices, such as the TRS Grip, are also available, in which the cable pull provides the grip force. This has the design advantage of graduated grip force controlled by the patients rather than a passive spring. The control movements are more natural because the hook closes when reaching for an object, but it must be locked closed when carrying objects.

Mechanical Hands

Mechanical hands are used for more cosmetic appeal and to provide an alternative grip pattern (Figure 17.6). Almost all hands (including external power) have a three-jaw chuck or palmer prehension pattern that utilizes the thumb and first two fingers. This grip pattern serves to manipulate small objects at the tip and larger cylindrical objects toward the web of the hand.

Although these mechanisms are more cosmetic, they provide little real functional benefit. The stiff internal spring mechanisms are less efficient and require substantially more effort to open than hook devices. Still, hands are preferred in many instances where cosmetic concerns outweigh pure function. Many prosthetic clients chose to have both hook and hand TDs with a quick disconnect wrist that lets them easily interchange between the two.

Specialized Terminal Devices

Some TDs, designed for singular purposes, resembles tools more than multifunctional implements. Special TDs have been made for golfing, photography, bowling, baseball, swimming, fishing, and a variety of other sports and hobbies. Some systems directly integrate hand tools and kitchen utensils that can be attached to match a certain task. The obvious disadvantage occurs when the proper tool is not available or when the user needs to accomplish other tasks.

Passive or Cosmetic Terminal Devices

Passive terminal devices are primarily hands with bendable or spring loaded fingers that place special emphasis on cosmesis. Most use cosmetic gloves, although other more expensive designs are made to match the coloring and shape of the other limb in detail to the freckles and hair. Although passive and cosmetic TDs have no gripping action, they do provide significant functional value to the unilateral prosthetic user as a holding and positioning aid (Figure 17-7).

PROSTHETIC RECOMMENDATION
BY LEVEL OF AMPUTATION

When assessing each level of upper extremity amputation, it is easy to refer to the componentry from most distal to proximal. The prosthetist will make suggestions for the terminal device, wrist, arm construction, socket, elbow or hinge, shoulder, control system, suspension, and harness. It is important to remember that the more proximal the amputation, the less likely the amputee will wear the prosthesis because of

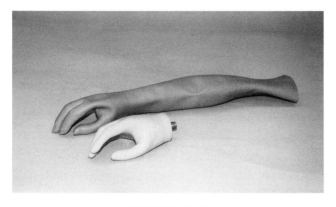

FIGURE 17-7

"Passive" hand and glove.

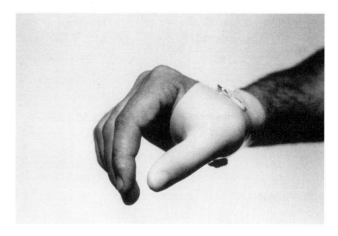

FIGURE 17-8

Opposition post for missing thumb.

increased weight and gadgetry. Long limb lengths present problems in accommodating prosthetic devices. Short limb lengths present problems with suspension and function.

Partial Hand

Partial hand prostheses (Figures 17-8 through 17-11) vary with the functional level of the residual limb. It should be the goal at this level to leave as much of the limb exposed to allow maximum sensation and permit alternate gripping techniques. The prostheses are often simple passive aids rather that active prehensors. The thumb is the most important digit, since it must provide the necessary opposition. If the thumb is amputated, it has been shown that the function of the hand is reduced by 50% (Northwestern University Upper Extremity Manual). A prosthesis for a thumb amputation is usually a passive thumb or opposition post attached to a cuff secured with straps around the wrist. Fingers may be replaced with a simple silicone or rubber prosthesis that is pushed over the remnant with tight fit. If all of the fingers or portions of the hand itself have been amputated, the remaining wrist can still be utilized to provide opposition to a prehension pad that fits below the palmar area. The CAPP Partial Hand, molded as a cuff around the wrist, has three positions and may be swung out of the way. A small body powered hook (a child hook with an infant wrist) or Enabler III [Texas Assistive Devices]) is sometimes used below the palmar area or at the distal end, but involves the enclosing the limb more using a control cable, and a figure-eight harness to activate the prehensor. More active TDs that include external power are not often used because the prosthesis would become noticeably longer than the sound limb.

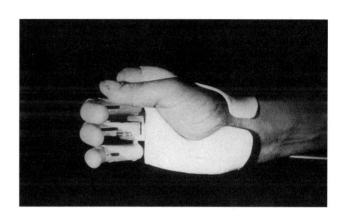

FIGURE 17-9

Partial hand prosthesis for missing fingers.

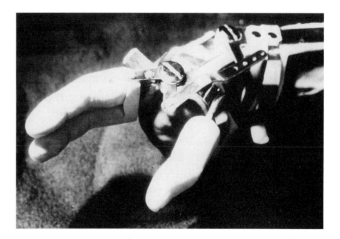

FIGURE 17-10

Wrist-driven partial hand prosthesis for missing fingers and thumb.

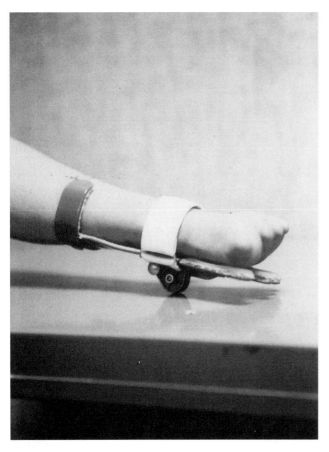

FIGURE 17-11

Opposition post for missing fingers and thumb.

Wrist Disarticulation

The wrist disarticulation prosthesis (Figure 17-12) differs functionally from a partial hand prosthesis in that an active TD of some type is needed in favor of more passive devices. Limb length is still an issue, but componentry is available with low profiles and oval geometries that match the distal end of the limb and minimize the length needed for componentry. Most TDs may be used, provided they are not too long and do not require special wrist configurations. Externally powered system can be used, but do result in some length discrepancy, unless the electronics and battery are placed on the side of the limb, which may increase the overall bulk of the prosthesis. Suspension can be provided over the styloids with a dorsal door or Velcro straps. Pronation and supination restriction must be avoided by using low proximal trimlines that are kept well below the elbow region. The ulnar trimline is frequently left proximal to avoid impingement along the shaft of the ulna when loading or resting on a table. A simple cuff harness may

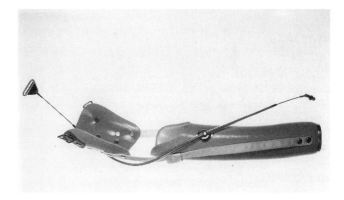

FIGURE 17-12

Wrist disarticulation prosthesis with flexible hinges for forearm rotation.

be used for cable activation only, since suspension may be provided over the wrist styloid processes.

Transradial

The transradial prosthesis (Figures 17-13 and 17-14) offers a greater variety of componentry options. Transradial prostheses may be self-suspending in design or use a harness for more heavy-duty versions. The self-suspending design may be a push-in type for longer limb lengths or a pull-in socket type for shorter limb length. Silicone sleeves that employ a flexible tube rolled tightly onto the arm and attached with a latch or "shuttle pin" are being used more where limb length permits. The self-suspending designs eliminate harnessing for suspension, but supracondylar trimlines eliminate active pronation and supination. For the amputee with 50% or more of the distal forearm remaining, the figure-eight harness with flexible hinges is often used with a triceps pad or humeral cuff as a reaction point above the elbow. Some heavy-duty users may wish to have a shoulder saddle harness that distributes the load over the affected shoulder and lessens axilla pressure. A flexible hinge made of Dacron straps connects a triceps pad to the socket. It is used on longer limb lengths and bilaterals to allow the maximum amount of pronation and supination.

Single axis hinges can be used for heavy-duty wearers. These help unload the forearm and protect it from hyperextension during heavy lifting or torsion. These wearers depend on glenohumeral rotation for activities, since solid hinges eliminate pronation and supination. Special hinges are available for shorter length limbs that may have problems with cubital bunching, range of motion, or loading. The cable system is a Bowden, single control system that employs a

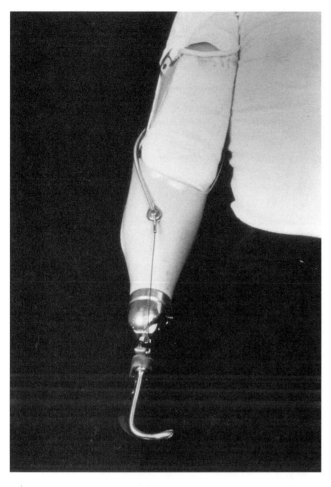

FIGURE 17-13

Transradial (Below-elbow) prosthesis.

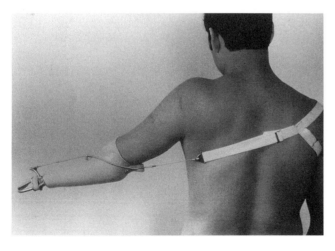

FIGURE 17-14

Transradial prosthesis showing "Figure 9" harness.

cable sliding inside a housing. This permits the same amount of excursion to open the terminal device in any degree of flexion. (See Chapter 18 for more information on external control systems.)

A wide variety of wrists are available to accommodate various needs and goals. The most common, a constant friction wrist, allows passive pronation and supination control. A lock screw is simply tightened against the TD attachment thread. Other wrists allow the user to quickly change TDs and lock rotation by bumping a button or turning a sleeve. Usually the wrists come in three sizes and in round or oval configuration. The oval wrists are used with longer amputations, since this design matches the oval cross section of the residual arm. Various hook and hand terminal devices are available. Frequently, users switch between the two for different tasks, and special wrist and cable modifications may be necessary to activate these differing terminal devices.

Transhumeral

A transhumeral amputation requires an elbow and elbow controls (Figures 17-15 and 17-16). Longer limb amputees prefer to have looser socket designs that allow easy push-in donning. Shorter remnant limbs or designs using external power utilize tighter fitting sockets that may use suction fit. Suction sockets are made smaller than the residuum and are pulled on with a donning sock or sleeve. An air valve is added that lets air out but not in, thus creating the suction fit. The figure-eight harness is the most common harness design used, but it differs slightly from the transradial version. Since full elbow and terminal device operation requires 4-1/2 inches of cable travel (2 inches for teminal device, 2-1/2 inches for elbow), the harness must fit more tightly than a transradial harness. The transhumeral harness should be sewn at its cross point to maximize excursion; this is especially important for short limb lengths. An elastic cross back strap or "Z" control strap may also be needed to keep the harness from riding up the back.

A Northwestern ring is a cross point that uses metal ring. The straps are allowed to move slightly, so that the harness remains flat on the back, which is especially desirable for below-elbow prostheses. The ring harness may not be recommended for short above-elbow prostheses, where the amount of excursion is limited and the movement of the harness may decrease available excursion. To prevent the harness from riding up the back and to increase excursion, double rings may be employed vertically for patients with broad backs or short limb lengths. Additional straps may be needed for shorter limb lengths for suspension and excursion response, but more straps add donning difficulty.

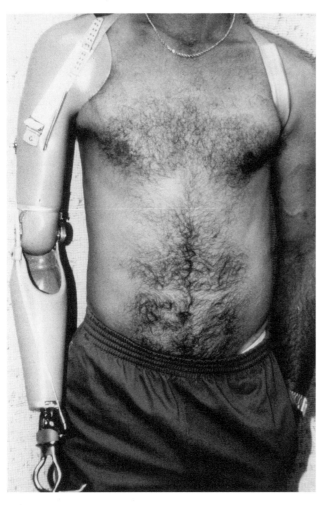

FIGURE 17-15

Transhumeral (Above-elbow) prosthesis.

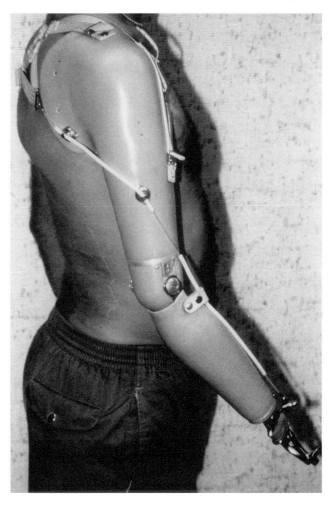

FIGURE 17-16

Transhumeral prosthesis showing dual control cable system.

The lateral suspension strap becomes the main suspensor since the anterior suspension strap is elastic to allow the elbow to lock and unlock in the body-powered arm. The elbow may be a passive friction elbow, mechanical locking, or an externally powered variety. The passive elbow is friction-controlled for positioning, but the mechanical locking elbow is more common. It has a reciprocating lock that locks in eleven positions of elbow flexion. This lock is activated with glenohumeral extension, abduction, and slight depression of the shoulder. The body-powered elbow is flexed with a cable system similar to that used in the transradial system, except that there is a split in the housing. This split cable or fair lead, dual-control system allows a moderate amount of cable shortening to allow the forearm to be flexed at the elbow. The position of the attachments of the cable is crucial for balancing lifting power and excursion requirements.

External springs are also available that aid in the flexion of the elbow by counterbalancing the weight of the forearm. Adjustable friction pads are placed on the turntable above the elbow to allow passive rotation control. It must be adjusted to resist about 6 pounds of force. Other elbows have glenohumeral locking rotation control for activities at the midline. It is important that the elbow be positioned 1-inch lateral from the hip of the amputee and be within 2 inches of the anatomic elbow center for cosmesis and function. The forearm must be constructed of light laminate to allow easy lifting of the forearm and TD. Any wrist may be used, but lighter duty aluminum wrists are most often preferred. Aluminum TDs are often used, rather than mechanical hands because of the greater weight. A small number of heavy-duty users require heavier duty configurations that sacrifice ease of function for durability.

Externally powered arms incorporate hand attachments and use the same electronic hands as those devices used at the transradial level. Their harness differs only because the functionality of the elbow and terminal device is provided by external means.

Elbow Disarticulation

The elbow disarticulation prosthesis (Figure 17-17) differs in that the anatomic elbow center of the amputation is proximal to the distal end of the prosthesis, (that is, the elbow center is lower than the normal side). Special outside locking hinges, usually mounted medially, are used to lock the elbow into place using the same split housing, dual-control cable system as the transhumeral prosthesis. Suspension is provided over the humeral condylar prominences. Often, sockets are con-

structed with a posterior door or spiral groove that allows the socket to be donned by squeezing it over the condyles. If this can be done, all that is required of the harness is elbow and TD activation. Often, however, additional suspension is required through the use of a proximal lateral suspensor to support the weight of the prosthetic arm. The forearm is usually custom made for the prosthesis, since the elbow width dimension is dictated by the anatomic shape and socket thickness. The forearm, made at the same time as the socket, is usually shorter and wider in shape.

Shoulder Disarticulation

Shoulder disarticulation prostheses (Figure 17-18) add a shoulder joint to the componentry list. This may be a passive friction or active locking device or it may be fused to the socket in a monolithic construction. The main purpose of any prosthetic shoulder joint is for donning clothing and positioning for functional activities. A passive device frequently serves this purpose, whereas a locking joint can lock the joint into position for different activities. A monolithic design is built into the socket in a set degree of shoulder flexion. The patient may have to "dress the arm" first, then don the prosthesis next. This is often used for heavy-duty users or children. The emphasis at this level is to keep the prosthesis extremely lightweight.
Figure 17-18.

The more proximal the amputation, the less likely the patient will wear the device, and the reason most amputees at this level reject prostheses because of weight and bulk. Frequently, endoskeletal designs are used with passive elbows and shoulder joints. Externally powered hands are often used, since they can provide superior pinch and easy use in contrast to body-powered systems. (In the past, totally body-controlled systems were often bulky and involved a lot of control and attachment straps.)

Elbows can be used for quick lifting with myoelectric or switch controls. Although heavy, their control involves very little movement and simplifies harnessing. Because this level has so little excursion to be garnered from scapular abduction, special techniques are used to amplify the movement or separate the controls of the harness. A nudge control or paddlelike device that is mounted and activated by the chin of the amputee, can be used to operate the elbow lock independently of lifting the forearm. Excursion amplifiers, which are pulleys that double the amount of cable travel to operate the elbow and terminal device may also be used. A modified harness using "triple control" may be employed; this separates each function to allow a greater range of control. One strap around the tip of the opposite shoulder

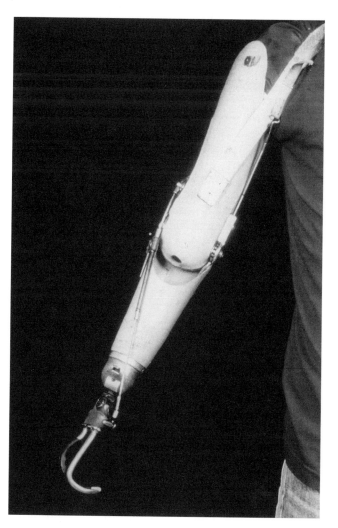

FIGURE 17-17

Elbow disarticulation prosthesis.

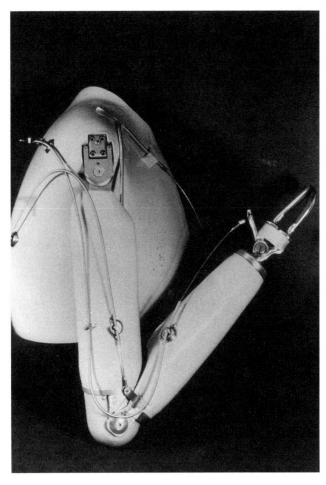

FIGURE 17-18

Shoulder disarticulation prosthesis.

operates the terminal device, another through the axilla moves the elbow, and a nudge control or chest expansion operates the elbow lock (three functions or "triple control"). Many of these techniques have been eliminated with the use of external power, which can deliver more function for those with a limited amount of body movement.

Interscapular Thoracic

Patients who have undergone interscapular thoracic or "forequarter" amputation often have scoliosis in their spine due to the unweighting of their shoulder girdle. The prosthetic goals at this level become more cosmetic and less functional, especially for the unilateral amputee. Many amputees only use a shoulder cap that functions as a cosmetic shirt filler. To bear load for any prosthesis, the coverage of the skin must increase, thus causing a decrease in heat dissipation. For comfort and to improve

heat dissipation from the skin elastic bioelastomers are often used in the attachment devices.

HYBRID PROSTHESES

In many cases of high-level amputation, a passive friction or manual lock elbows is chosen for use with an active TD. The elbow is simply prepositioned and the more functional hand is utilized. With an endoskeletal system, this makes a very lightweight cosmetic system.

Body-Powered Elbow and Externally Powered Hand

One of the more popular hybrid designs is a body-powered elbow and an externally powered hand. The advantages of this system are many: greater pinch force and full opening of the externally powered hand at any position; separation of the controls between the body-powered elbow and externally powered hand means no mode switching is necessary; greater proprioception of the body-powered elbow; less weight and lower cost for the body powered elbow; greater battery efficiency because of fewer components; mechanical simplicity and reduced breakdown; and a combination of controls that reduce the possibility of total failure.

Body-Powered Hand and Externally Powered Elbow

In this hybrid design the heavy elbow design is proximal, so the prosthesis is made to feel lighter. The cable control is dedicated to TD operation and can fully open at any level. Opening the TD requires usually less effort than lifting a longer length forearm. This system works best when a hook is used, and it is limited by the number of rubber bands used for prehension. More prehension is available for a voluntary closing TD, although this combination would be difficult with the body-powered elbow.

NONOPERATIONAL PROSTHESES

Aesthetic prostheses (Figure 17-19 and 17-20) are covered in Chapter 16. Such prostheses typically are referred to as cosmetic or passive prostheses. We include a brief discussion of their use in this chapter because often they are used to provide function even though they are not operational in the sense of being body-powered by a cable.

In the past, upper-limb passive prostheses were considered nonfunctional and for cosmetic purposes only. This distinction is no longer as valid because many "functional prostheses" are becoming more cosmetic, and many "passive prostheses" are used functionally.

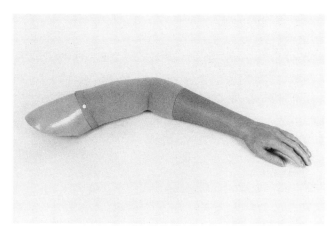

FIGURE 17-19

Transhumeral non-operational prosthesis.

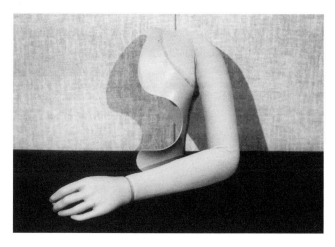

FIGURE 17-20

Interscapular thoracic non-operational prosthesis.

A study done by occupational therapist Carole Fraser in the United Kingdom demonstrated the difference between arm amputees simply wearing passive prostheses versus their actually using them in functional ways (6). She found that "prostheses that might be considered to be worn for purely cosmetic reasons are in fact used functionally when performing everyday tasks." Through analysis of videotapes, she observed that functional users of upper-limb prostheses used active manipulation less than 25% of the time, and cosmetic wearers used their prostheses for nonmanipulative activities as much as the functional users. She also found that arm amputees who chose to wear cosmetic prostheses do not routinely receive training in performing two-handed tasks. Her study suggests that we consider the functional

as well as appearance benefits in using cosmetic prostheses and that amputees be trained in their use.

CONCLUSIONS

Tradeoffs between function and appearance dictate what components are selected for a given amputee's needs. And there are still situations where an amputee may have both a body-powered prosthesis for maximum function and a passive prosthesis for maximum appearance. In general, however, most arm amputees will select one prosthesis for all daily use. Even with one prosthesis, an arm amputee still has the option of interchanging a hook and hand for function and appearance.

Passive prostheses also can be used "functionally" to weight the shoulder of the amputated side to prevent or ameliorate the occurrence of scoliosis due to weight unbalance if no prosthesis is worn. This is usually important at high levels of arm loss.

References

1. American Academy of Orthopaedic Surgeons. *Orthopaedic Applicance Atlas: Vol 2: Artificial Limbs.* Ann Arbor: RT Edwards, 1960, 1–22.
2. LeBlanc MA. Patient population and other estimates of prosthetics and orthotics in the USA. *Orthotics Prosthetics* 1973, 27(3), 38–44.
3. Prosthetic-Orthotic School, University of California at Los Angeles, 1968.
4. American Academy of Orthopaedic Surgeons, *Atlas of Limb Prosthetics*, St. Louis: Mosby, 1981, 95–144.
5. Bray JJ. *Prosthetic Principles—Upper Extremity Amputations, Fabrication and Fitting Principles.* Los Angeles: UCLA, Prosthetics/Orthotics Education Program, Division of Orthopedic Surgery, circa 1974.
6. Fraser CM. An evaluation of the use made of cosmetic and functional prostheses by unilateral upper limb amputees. *Prosthetics Orthotics Intern* 1998;22,216–223.

Additional Reading

Aitken CT. *The Child with an Acquired Amputation.* Washington D.C.: National Academy of Sciences, 1972.

American Academy of Orthopaedic Surgeons. *Atlas of Limb Prosthetics.* St. Louis: Mosby, 1981, 22–132.

Atkins DJ, Heard DCY, Donovan WH. Epidemiciologic overview of individuals with upper-limb loss and their reported research priorities. *J Prosthetic Orthotic* 1996;8, 2–11.

Billock John N. Upper limb prosthetic terminal devices: Hands versus hooks. *Clin Prosthetic Orthotic* 10(2), Spring 1986, 57–65.

Corin JD, Holley TM, Hasler, RA, Ashman RB. Mechanical comparison of terminal devices. *Clin Prosthetic Orthotic* 1987;11, 235–244.

Fletcher MJ, Leonard F. The principles of artificial-hand design. *Artificial Limbs* 1955;2(2).

Kay HW, Newman ID. Amputee survey, 1973–74: Preliminary findings and comparisons. *Orthotic Prosthetic* 1974;28(2), 27–32.

Klopsted PE, Wilson PD. *Human Limbs and Their Substitutes.* New York: Hafner Publishing, 1968.

LeBlanc M, Setoguchi Y, Shaperman J, Carlson L. Mechanical work efficiencies of body-powered prehensors for young children. *J Assoc Children's Prosthetic-Orthotic Clin* 1992;27, 70–75.

Littler JW. On the adaptability of man's hand. *The Hand* 1973, 5(3), 187–191.

Radocy R. Voluntary closing control: A successful new design approach to an old concept. *Clin Prosthetic Orthotic* 10(2), Spring 1986, 82–86.

Santschi WR. *Manual of Upper Extremity Prosthetics,* 2ed. Los Angeles: UCLA, 1958.

Huntington, NY. *Selected Articles from Artificial Limb.* Robert E. Krieger Publishing, 1970.

Setoguchi Y, Rosenfelder R. *The Limb Deficient Child.* Springfield: Charles C Thomas, 1982.

Taylor CL, Schwarz RJ. The anatomy and mechanics of the human hand. *Artificial Limbs* 1955;2(2), 22–35.

Taylor C. The biomechanics of the normal and of the amputated upper extremity. In: Klopsteg P, Wilson P (eds.), *Human Limbs and Their Substitutes.* New York: McGraw-Hill, 1954, 169–221.

Van Lunteren T, Van Lunteren-Gerritsen E. In search of design specifications for arm prostheses, In: Sheridan T, Van Lunteren T (eds), *Perspectives on the Human Controller.* Lawrence Erlbaum, 1997.

Major Manufacturers of Upper-Limb, Body-Powered, Prosthetic Components

Hosmer Dorrance Corporation
P.O. Box 37
Campbell, CA 95008
Tel: 800/827-0070
Fax: 408/379-5263
Internet: www.hosmer.com
Email: hosmer@hosmer.com

Otto Bock Orthopedic Industry
3000 Xenuim Lane North
Minneapolis, MN 55441
Tel: 800-328-4058
Fax: 800-962-2549
Internet: www.ottobockus.com
E-Mail: info@ottobockus.com

TRS, Inc.
2450 Central Ave., Unit D
Boulder, CO 80301
Tel: 303/444-4720, 800/279-1865
Fax: 303/444-5372
Internet: www.oandp.com/commerci/trs/index.htm
E-Mail: trs@oandp.com

Liberty Mutual Research Center
(US representative for Hugh Steeper, Ltd)
71 Frankland Rd.
Hopkinton, MA 01748
Tel: 508/435-9061
Fax 508/435-8369
Internet: www.libertytechnology.com/
E-Mail: twalley.williams@libertymutual.com

Motion Control, Inc.
2401 South 1070 West, Suite B
Salt Lake City, Utah, 84119-1555
Tel: 888/MYO-ARMS, 801/978-2622
Fax: 801/978-0848
Internet: www.utaharm.com/
E-Mail: info@utaharm.com

United States Manufacturing Company
180 North San Gabriel Blvd
Pasadena, California 91107-3488
Post Office Box 5030, Pasadena, California 91117-0030
Tel: 626/796-0477
Fax: 626-440-9533
Internet: www.usmc.com/
E-Mail: usmc@oandp.com

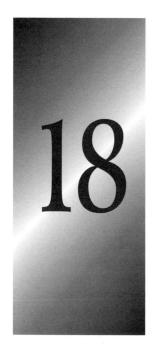

18 Externally Powered Prostheses for the Adult Transradial and Wrist Disarticulation Amputee

John W. Michael, MEd, CPO

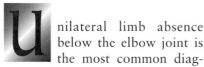nilateral limb absence below the elbow joint is the most common diagnosis encountered in upper limb prosthetic fittings (1). A detailed overview of the prosthetic principles involved in managing this challenge with electrically powered (EP) prostheses can serve as a good foundation for the treatment of more complex and higher level loss. Other chapters deal with the alternatives to such externally powered fittings, and the specifics of other levels and pediatric applications. This chapter focuses exclusively on wrist disarticulation (WD) and transradial (TR) prostheses for adults, which incorporate at least one motorized component.

BIOMECHANICAL LOSS

One of the most universally accepted and clinically useful ways to characterize limb absence is to document the functional losses that have resulted. Although magnitude and specifics vary, and must therefore be determined by individual examination, certain loss patterns are characteristic of these two groups of patients.

The obvious loss, which all upper limb amputees experience to some extent, is that of voluntary grasp and release. The human hand is capable of literally an infinite number of movement patterns, and previous research has established that it is normal to use a variety of specific grasp patterns during activities of daily living (2). Regrettably, even the most sophisticated of available prosthetic terminal devices cannot offer more than a small number of grasp patterns, and none offer direct sensory feedback or the ability to independently control individual finger joints.

The net result is that no prosthetic device can be expected to "replace" what has been lost functionally. At best, a prosthetic terminal device offers only reliable basic grasp and release, so for the person with an intact contralateral upper limb, the prosthesis primarily functions as a "portable vise" to assist the far more useful anatomic hand (3). This is often difficult for the new prosthetic user to believe, based on the expectations that elegant "bionic videos" from the popular media have fostered. The more realistic the amputee's expectations for the prosthetic device, the more likely it will be used successfully long term; thus, the clinic team has a responsibility to gently but firmly correct any bionic fantasies that the patient or their family and friends may be harboring.

Dr. David Simpson has proposed three primary prerequisites for upper limb function (4):

- Proximal stability
- Placement in space
- Grasp and release

This is an excellent conception for prosthetic design. So long as the shoulder and elbow joints are fully functional, proximal stability for these levels is primarily dependent upon the socket design, fitting, and suspension characteristics. These considerations are discussed later in this chapter. As the level of upper limb absence becomes more proximal, a progressively greater restriction occurs in the ability to effortlessly place the limb remnant in space. As a result, the person's "effective work envelope" becomes more constricted as the magnitude of limb loss increases (5).

For example, loss at the wrist joint eliminates the common movements of wrist flexion–extension and radioulnar deviation, thus limiting the ability to preposition the grasping member in space. When the loss is transradial, through the long bones of the forearm, additional losses occur in the ability to pronate–supinate and to support or lift active loads via elbow flexion. The higher the amputation level, the greater these tasks are impaired.

Although modern prosthetic techniques allow the fitting of even residual limbs formerly considered "too short" for active prosthesis use, as a general rule, the shorter the remnant limb segment the more limited the forces the person can comfortably tolerate. As a result, many people with amputation levels in the proximal quartile of the forearm use the prosthesis primarily for light- to moderate-duty activities. Although this is of less significance with unilateral loss, such functional limitations may result in significant disability when there is bilateral upper limb impairment and may justify consideration of special surgical interventions, including limb-lengthening procedures (6).

SOCKET DESIGN PRINCIPLES

Although a detailed discussion of prosthetic socket design criteria is beyond the scope of this chapter, a basic review of the fundamental principles of force distribution and suspension principles can provide a good rationale for the numerous trimline and material variants encountered clinically.

One fundamental tenet of all prosthetic design is to spread the forces over the greatest possible area to reduce the peak pressure per unit area. This reduces the risk of skin trauma, increases amputee comfort, and enhances the user's proprioception of the position of the prosthesis in space. All these benefits are believed to increase the functional use and long-term acceptance of the artificial limb.

Since many functional activities occur at table or desktop level, forearm prostheses must be particularly comfortable and stable in this position. The weight of the terminal device itself, in addition to anything being grasped, creates a force couple, with concentrated pressures at the proximal ulnar surface and distal radial surface inside the socket, as shown in Figure 18-1. For this reason, the preferred trimline along the ulnar surface is near the olecranon or sometimes higher. As a rule of thumb, the shorter the residual limb, and the less stabilizing area remaining below the elbow, the more proximal the trimlines.

The prosthesis must also be stabilized against rotary loads, such as those encountered when turning a door knob or simply holding an object, such as a hammer, with a heavy mass located outside the palmar region. If the residual limb is relatively long, the prosthetist will typically shape the socket to fit very snugly along the contours of the distal half of the radius and ulna, particularly in the region of the interosseous membrane. This "screwdriver fit" helps stabilize the socket against such torque loading.

When less of the forearm remains, and particularly if the remnant is fleshy or obese, it is usually not possible for the socket contours alone to stabilize the socket. In such cases, the trimlines are usually extended up onto the humerus, external hinges are added to a humeral cuff, or both strategies are used. Unfortunately, such proximal stabilization also eliminates any voluntary pronation and supination, and should therefore be avoided to the degree that is prudent.

The prosthesis must also resist axial loading whenever the person is carrying an object such as a briefcase or a bucket. In a self-suspending socket, these forces are carried on the residual limb via either vacuum (suction suspension) or by anatomical (supracondylar) contouring. When a textile harness is used for suspension, the axial loading is distributed across the shoulders and back as well. Many upper limb prostheses use a combi-

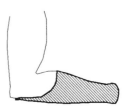

FIGURE 18-1

Typical prosthetic trimlines for wrist disarticulation amputations. Note that the ulnar portion of the WD socket usually terminates just distal to the olecranon to permit maximum loading along the ulnar shaft during lifting activities with the elbow flexed. The WD socket usually terminates well below the epicondyles and cubital fold to permit as much biologic pronation, supination, flexion, and extension movement as possible.

nation of suspensions, for added security and to reduce the unit forces as much as possible.

To allow maximum mobility for placement in space, suspension on the residual limb per se is preferable to avoid crossing the proximal joint. In the case of wrist disarticulation, it is often possible to take advantage of the prominence of the ulnar and radial styloids to suspend the socket. Such suprastyloid suspension is only possible if the styloids are fully developed and have not been surgically altered, so this technique is not always feasible.

Several methods may be used to create a socket that is sufficiently snug just proximal to these bony prominences, including use of a removable panel, a hook and loop strap, or an elastomeric section. When this suspension is tolerable to the amputee and sufficiently secure, the proximal trimlines of the socket can be terminated well below the cubital fold and epicondyles, permitting maximal voluntary elbow flexion–extension and pronation–supination.

When the styloids have been removed, or the amputation level is slightly higher, other suspensions must be used. One of the most popular alternatives is the use of an elastomeric silicone suction sleeve anchored to the distal socket via a shuttle lock arrangement. For myoelectric applications, it is preferable to terminate the silicone sleeve inferior to the selected myosignal sites.

When the residual limb is too short for such a "bikini sleeve" to be successful, some practitioners fenestrate a full length sleeve over the electrode sites or mount the electrodes in the sleeve. Unfortunately, both these strategies decrease the durability of the sleeves and electrode wiring somewhat. So long as the distal socket contours can provide sufficient rotary stability, the trimlines are similar to those noted for suprastyloid suspension.

When the residual limb length is less than about half of the original forearm, the amount of residual voluntary pronation–supination diminishes significantly, and it is not possible for the socket to capture this movement due to the cylindrical cross-section of the forearm at this and higher levels. In this situation, supracondylar suspension via the humeral condyles is commonly used. The shorter the residual limb, the more proximally the trimlines extend onto the humerus, to provide rotary and hyperextension stability in addition to suspension (Figure 18-2).

Unfortunately, supracondylar suspension has two disadvantages: voluntary pronation–supination is eliminated and full elbow flexion is often reduced by 10 to 15 degrees. For the unilateral amputee, these restrictions have limited significance, but any loss of voluntary motion can be critically important in bilateral cases. In

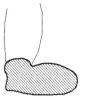

FIGURE 18-2

Supracondylar suspension, typical for shorter transradial amputations, adds stabilizing forces against rotary torque and other loading by extending up onto the humerus, but eliminates voluntary pronation and supination. The more proximal borders also reduce the range of elbow flexion and extension slightly, but this limitation is diminished when flexible materials are used for the socket.

general, supracondylar suspension should be used only when other alternatives are not likely to be effective or when some loss of voluntary prosupination is acceptable to the amputee. The use of flexible socket materials will permit the amputee to forcibly flex the elbow a few more degrees than a rigid socket would allow, thereby reducing the magnitude of this limitation by about half.

Although less common in myoelectric upper limb applications, suspension via rubberlike sleeves that cross the elbow joint is possible in selected cases. Use of suspension straps, such as a figure-eight supracondylar cuff or articulated joints with a humeral cuff, are even more unusual, but have value in special cases. The use of multiple suspension options is increasingly popular, as this increases both patient confidence and comfort when the suspension load is shared by, for example, supracondylar contours in addition to an external rubber sleeve.

Socket materials for upper limb prostheses have evolved in a pattern similar to that seen in lower limb designs: toward increased flexibility and the use of thermoplastic polymers. The advantages of thermoplastic flexible sockets include enhanced comfort, greater range of motion, and superior resistance to perspiration. Laminated thermoset plastics are commonly reserved for the external frame connecting the components to the socket, although laminated sockets are still used frequently.

Making the socket and structural segment of the forearm mechanically independent entities is virtually universal in modern designs utilizing externally powered terminal devices, because the socket is easily removed for component servicing. Such construction also offers the possibility for socket replacement, rather than replacement of the entire prosthesis, in the event of residual limb atrophy.

TERMINAL DEVICES

At this time, all commercial externally powered terminal devices (TDs) use batteries and electric motors for operation, although pneumatic and electrohydraulic designs have been used in the past. Rechargeable batteries, which are incorporated into the prosthesis, power all TDs. If the battery cells are sealed within the prosthesis, the artificial limb must be removed for recharging. Removable batteries that the amputee can interchange are also used in some designs, so a depleted battery may be replaced with a fully charged one without removing the artificial limb. Both battery types have been well accepted clinically.

Nickel-cadmium (Ni-Cd) batteries are the least expensive initially, but their relatively limited capacity and tendency to lose their effectiveness after a few hundred recharges necessitate replacements approximately annually.

Nickel metal hydride (Ni-MH) batteries with significantly more capacity have been introduced, as have lithium ion (Li-Ion) cells. Although more expensive initially, both these technologies are more cost-efficient over the useful life of the prosthesis and are therefore expected to increase in popularity and eventually to displace the NiCad batteries, as has already happened in the cellular phone industry.

All TDs may be conveniently subdivided by their external appearance into those that are handlike, and those that are not. The latter are usually termed "hooks" after the historic TD worn by the Captain in the story of Peter Pan. Hooklike devices are usually intended to be multipurpose tools for use where durability is more important than appearance, such as in the workshop.

One of the most popular "electric hooks" is made by the Otto Bock company and referred to as a "Greifer": German for "gripper." The pointed fingertips facilitate the visual feedback necessary for fine motor tasks and are more durable than the thin plastic gloves that cover electric hands. A thumb wheel allows the user to manually increase or decrease the grip force beyond what the miniature motor can provide, while a small lever permits the user to disengage the drive and passively open the fingers. A unique integrated wrist flexion capability makes precise prepositioning easier.

The Synergetic Prehensor introduced a new grip technology, based on research by Dudley Childress Ph.D. of Northwestern University, using two motors to create the gripping force (7). One motor runs very rapidly and therefore that hook finger opens and closes quickly, making the TD very responsive. A motor that has been geared to provide a great deal of torque closes the second finger very slowly. This provides a powerful, energy-efficient gripping force. The lightweight, hollow

fingers of this TD are replaceable should significant wear occur.

The Steeper company from Britain makes an electric TD they term the "Gripper." This is one of the lightest available alternatives and, like the Synergetic Prehensor, uses dual fast/slow motors to enhance prehension. Figure 18-3 illustrates the three "electric hooks" discussed.

Motion Control in Utah recently released a unique Electric Terminal Device [ETD] designed to be highly water-resistant (shown in Figure 18-4). Like their electric hands, the ETD incorporates a manual quick release lever and an optional integrated flexion wrist that locks in multiple positions.

Several EP adult hands are currently available in the United States from manufacturers in England, Germany, Sweden, and France. They are made in several sizes appropriate for teens and for adults of small and medium stature. All present devices offer palmar prehension, in which the tips of the thumb, index, and middle fingers meet. This is also referred to as "three-jaw chuck" grasp due to the resemblance of the device to the mechanism used in electric drills to grip the bits securely.

Small differences distinguish one adult EP hand from another. The German (Otto Bock) design uses an endoskeletal aluminum inner mechanism covered by a flexible hand shell and then a protective outer glove with a handlike appearance. Some other electric hands have an exoskeletal design, with the glove covering the hard-shelled hand mechanism directly. Control differences are discussed later in this chapter.

Rehabilitation specialists should be aware that it is quite feasible to interchange EP TDs with one another, even if they are from differing manufacturers, and this is often necessary to allow the amputee to perform a full range of activities. The provision of an EP hand and EP hooklike device is the most common example, with the electric hook used typically for workshop and garden activities when the glove covering the hand is likely to be soiled or damaged.

Adapters are also available that allow the use of passive or body-powered (BP) TDs on prostheses that normally utilize EP components (Figure 18-5). For example, the amputee might prefer to use a passive sports mitt for recreational basketball games, reserving the electric hand for work and social occasions where its grasp and release functions are more useful.

WRIST UNITS

A number of wrist units are specifically designed for use with EP TDs. Virtually all offer passive pronation–supination that is resisted by an adjustable friction mechanism or a ratcheting system. The terminal device is preposi-

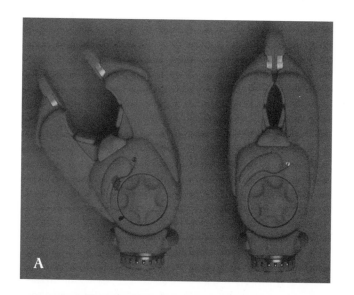

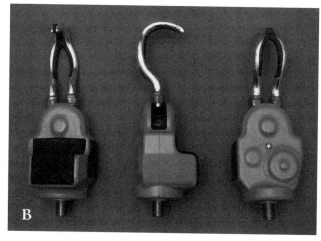

FIGURE 18-3

Some amputees accept the mechanical appearance of various electric hook devices in return for the increased durability and tip prehension they offer, as compared to electric hands. Since they easily interchange with electric hands, many patients use both devices according to the activity being performed. From left to right, the Otto Bock Greifer, Hosmer Synergetic Prehensor, and Steeper Gripper. (**A** Courtesy Otto Bock Orthopedic Industries, Inc. **B** Courtesy Prosthetics Research Laboratory. (Northwestern University/VA Chicago Health Care System. **C** Courtesy Liberty Technologies.)

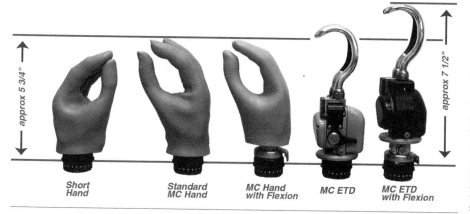

Relative TD Sizes

Short Hand

Standard MC Hand

MC Hand with Flexion

MC ETD

MC ETD with Flexion

approx 5 3/4"

approx 7 1/2"

FIGURE 18-4

The overall length of electronic terminal devices varies significantly, as shown in this illustration, and must be considered when fitting longer residual limbs to avoid a discrepancy with the sound side. Incorporation of a more complex wrist mechanism generally increases the overall length of the TD assembly. The Motion Control hand with integrated wrist flexion shown here is noteworthy because it adds no more length than their standard electric hand. (Courtesy of Motion Control, a subsidiary of Fillauer, Inc.)

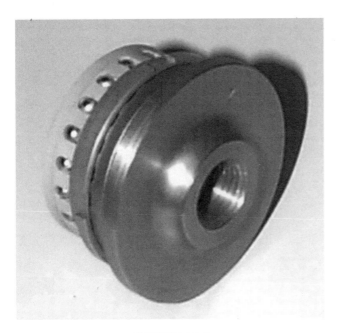

FIGURE 18-5

An adapter that allows the amputee to interchange a myoelectrically controlled and body powered terminal device. (Courtesy Otto Bock Orthopedic Industry, Inc.)

tioned using the contralateral hand or by grasping a fixed object and forcibly rotating the prosthesis. The exception is that, to minimize the length of this component in the case of disarticulation, the wrist unit often lacks rotational capabilities. (Fortunately, anatomic prosupination can usually be captured by the socket design and used for voluntary prepositioning of the terminal device in WD cases.)

The provision of a wrist with a quick disconnect feature is typical, both to facilitate the interchange of TDs and to expedite troubleshooting and repairs. Once again, this feature is often eliminated in wrist disarticulation cases to minimize the component length protruding beyond the end of the residual limb.

Wrist units with powered pronation and supination are available. Although most commonly combined with an EP TD, these wrists can also be used with BP or passive TDs as well. Space constraints prohibit the use of powered wrists with longer residual limbs, but this is not a clinical problem in most cases, as the residual voluntary pronation and supination in the forearm can be used to preposition the terminal device quickly and easily.

For mid-length and higher amputation levels, little or no voluntary prosupination control remains. In this circumstance, the use of an EP wrist may increase the amputee's ability to actively position the TD for optimal grasp. This is particularly important for people with bilateral upper limb impairments who regularly use the prostheses for eating, toileting, and other self-care tasks.

The potential for increased active positioning must be of sufficient value to justify the added weight, control complexity, and cost of the powered wrist. Some amputees with a very short residual limb, for example, may find the addition of another electric motor at the distal aspect of the prosthesis simply makes the prosthesis feel "too heavy," whereas those with a slightly longer residuum may find the added mass insignificant.

Although no absolute indications demand the use of a powered wrist, there is a recent trend toward provision of this component at the time of initial fitting for those amputees who wish to try active prepositioning. The rationale is that the amputee is motivated to master prosthetic technology during the initial fitting, particularly in traumatic cases where bimanual function has been "lost." If fitting with a powered wrist is delayed, the amputee is likely to "work around" this deficit by avoiding activities where active pronation or supination would be useful. Then, not only is their independence reduced from what is potentially possible, but they are more likely to find a powered wrist of limited value, precisely because they unconsciously avoid activities where it could be advantageous.

Conversely, even amputees who receive a powered wrist initially may ultimately decide that it is not sufficiently useful for the tasks they wish to perform. This component can then be deleted from subsequent prescriptions, and even removed from the existing prosthesis if the reduction in weight is desirable.

Wrists that are traditionally considered as "body-powered" components may sometimes be used with EP TDs, although care must be take to route the necessary electrical wires to avoid damaging them. Such special applications are most often utilized in bilateral cases, where even small increases in the "work envelope" of the TD translate into significantly more independent self-care. For example, a flexion wrist that can be locked in multiple positions may be very useful on the dominant side to facilitate midline activities. A number of specialized wrist units can be used with powered terminal devices, including a friction-loaded ball-and-socket wrist from Otto Bock and the Omni Wrist from VASI, which provides free flexion–extension motion under load but returns to a neutral position when the load is removed.

CONTROL SIGNAL SOURCES

The simplest control source for an EP TD is a mechanical switch that is activated by small body movements. Although rarely necessary in the transradial and wrist disarticulation case, switch controls are often used in higher level applications, where the degree of loss or complicating factors, such as severe burn scarring or brachial plexus injuries, preclude the use of electromyographic signals from remnant muscles.

In those rare cases where switch control is needed for a transradial amputee (usually those with extremely short residual limbs), it is generally preferred to mount a microswitch inside the forearm assembly distal to the socket. A very simple elastic figure-nine harness can be used to activate the switch, and only a limited amount of excursion is required for full opening and full closing signals. The Steeper Servo-Hand is uniquely well suited for this application, because the actuator allows the user to control the amount of opening and closing precisely: It is directly proportional to the control cable excursion (Figure 18-6). The full travel of the sliding actuator is 12 millimeters, so pulling it to 6 millimeters will open the hand halfway; 3 millimeters is one quarter opening, and so on.

Virtually all experts now recommend the use of myoelectric controls whenever they are feasible, as this control mode has several advantages over the simpler switch controls. Most importantly, optimized myoelectric controls require zero excursion and very little muscular strength, thus making this the most effortless way to control a transradial or wrist disarticulation prosthesis. In addition, presuming the socket is self-suspending, there is no need for any control harnessing. This makes the prosthesis more comfortable and less encumbering, and it allows the user to operate the prosthesis anywhere within the full scope of their reach (8). In other words, myoelectric control offers the greatest functional work envelope for these levels, allowing the prosthesis to be used overhead, out to the side, and even behind the body—anywhere the user can place it in space.

Finally, the powerful prehension provided by today's electric motors gives the amputee a very strong grip with minimal physical effort, which helps overcome the limitations in finger dexterity and the lack of sensory feedback inherent in all prostheses today. In almost all uncomplicated transradial and wrist disarticulation limb absences, at least one useable myosignal site will exist, even in the case of congenital anomalies. Preprosthetic myosignal strengthening is almost always useful and is highly recommended whenever the strength or control of the signals is anything less than optimal.

It is important for the amputee to develop the ability to control the myoelectric signal precisely, because this will translate into effective grasp and release and long-term use of the prosthesis. Ideally, the amputee should be able to consistently produce a myosignal that varies from a few microvolts to more than 100 microvolts and to generate intermediate levels on command as well. Such a broad range of voluntary signal generation will allow the accurate control of the TD under all circumstances (9).

In addition, the amputee must be able to generate the agonist signal in isolation, without also triggering antagonist activity, and vice versa. It is often necessary for the prosthetist to adjust the potentiometers modulating the agonist and antagonist myosignal signals to overcome less than perfect myosignal isolation, also called *crosstalk*. Increasing the gain of the weaker muscle site or decreasing the gain on the more powerful one will help balance the myosignal signals. Motion Control recently unveiled a microprocessor-controlled circuit called the "ProControl 2" that self-calibrates the gains throughout the day to enhance voluntary control of the TD.

If only one reliable myosignal site is available, a *single site–two function* myoelectric control system may be used. In a typical application, a hard and fast myosignal causes the TD to open, while a gentle and slowly increasing signal causes closing. Fixed speed opening and closing is referred to as *digital control,* because the motor is either running at full speed or off. With practice, many amputees can learn to use this control system effectively. The Otto Bock Sensor Hand is unique in offering multiple control options that are changed by inserting different "coding plugs" into the electronics in the hand. This includes an option for proportional control of both opening and closing from a single muscle site. In this control mode, the speed of opening is directly proportional to the speed with which the myosignal signal is generated. The speed and force

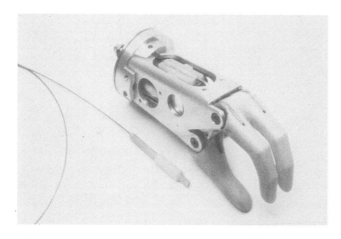

FIGURE 18-6

The Steeper Servo-Hand has a special switch that is connected to a BP control harness. When the amputee's body motion pulls the cylindrical body switch halfway, the hand opens halfway. The amount of hand opening is always directly proportional to the switch travel. (Courtesy Liberty Technology.)

of closing are directly proportional to how rapidly the muscle is relaxed, thus giving the amputee more precise control of the grasping function.

The preferred myoelectric control scheme is to use agonist–antagonist muscles to control opening and closing of the terminal device in a more physiologic manner. For transradial and wrist disarticulation applications, these sites are usually found over the superficial wrist flexor and extensor group in the proximal forearm. The flexor site is typically used to close the electric hand (analogous to finger flexion), while the extensors release the grasp (analogous to finger extension). However, some patients prefer the opposite configuration, so both alternatives must be evaluated with each amputee.

As noted previously, digital or *threshold control* means that the TD opens and closes at a constant speed. Much like the switches that open and close the electric windows in an automobile, this basic control can be quite sufficient for gross grasp and release tasks. With practice, amputees who use threshold myoelectric controls become very adept at controlling the amount of pinch force by limiting the length of time the myosignal signal is generated. To continue the analogy, so long as the closing signal to an electric car window is present it will "squeeze" a trapped finger harder and harder until the motor finally stalls. Control of a digital or threshold TD is quite similar.

General consensus supports that *proportional myoelectric control* is preferable, and some studies also support this notion (10). Particularly for those amputees who use the prosthesis daily, the increased precision in grip strength and the ability to vary the speed of movement of the fingers offers an advantage. Proportional control is initially somewhat more costly to provide than basic digital control but has proved to be similar in reliability.

Despite several decades of research demonstrations (11,12), no commercially available sensory feedback mechanism is currently available for prosthetic terminal devices. As a result, the amputee uses other sensory cues, including visual tracking, to compensate for the lack of direct sensation of the object being gripped. For example, as an object is gripped more and more firmly, the motor change slows down and the frequency of vibrations diminishes. These vibrations are transmitted up the prosthetic forearm to the socket, where the amputee can feel them on the skin of the residual limb. With practice, this indirect sensory feedback provides an excellent cue as to the grip force the TD is generating. Such *extended physiological proprioception* (13) is similar to the effect when you touch paper with a pencil: You can determine easily if you are pressing gently or firmly, even though the pencil itself has no sensory receptors.

The Otto Bock SensorHand is the first prosthetic device to offer a "cybernetic grasp feature" to partially compensate for the lack of direct sensation. An onboard computer monitors force sensors in the thumb tip and fingers. These sensors determine if an object is about to slip from the hand, and automatically and instantly increases the grip strength slightly. This "auto-grasp" feature will sequentially increase the grip force up to 10%, if necessary. When grasping fragile objects, the amputee will generate a slight myosignal, and the hand initially closes with limited pinch force. Because the auto-grasp increases the pinch force no more than 10% beyond the initial grip strength, the object is not crushed. In addition, the amputee can give a very slight extension myosignal signal at any time and the auto-grasp feature will stop immediately. The auto-grasp feature re-engages automatically the next time the hand is opened and then closed.

When an electric wrist is provided in addition to an electric TD, it can be controlled in several ways. In the simplest configuration, a rocker switch can be mounted on the inner side of the prosthetic forearm and simply pressed against the side of the thorax to directly control pronation or supination of the TD. Or, a button switch can be mounted in the same location to serve as a mode selector (Figure 18-7). In this design, the myosignal sites normally cause the TD to open and close, but when the switch is triggered, the myosignal sites now cause the electric wrist to rotate one way or

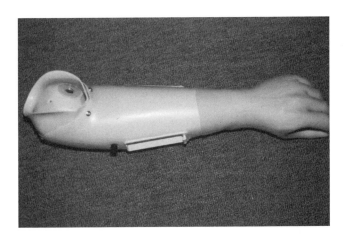

FIGURE 18-7

Transradial prosthesis with a small button switch on the medial aspect. The amputee presses this "mode switch" against the side of the torso to transfer myoelectric control to and from the powered wrist unit to the electric hand. When the user has sufficient myosignal signal control, this mode switching can be done electronically, eliminating the need for an external switch.

the other. Triggering the switch once again causes the myosignal signals to revert to TD control again.

In most TR and WD cases, there is no need for an additional switch if the amputee can learn to change from wrist to hand control by varying the myosignal. Various signal characteristics can been used for such myosignal-triggered mode selection; selection of the optimal method is part of the prosthetic fitting process. The most common method in transradial and wrist disarticulation applications is the use of co-contraction of the agonist–antagonist muscles. Terminal device opening and closing is normally controlled by the two myosignal sites, and may be either speed-proportional or constant speed. An amputee wishing to control the wrist must simultaneously generate comparable signals from both myosignal sites and then relax immediately. This changes the mode to "wrist control." Now myosignals from the two muscle sites will cause the wrist to rotate one direction or the other. An additional co-contract signal and immediate relaxation will return control to the TD mode. This can be termed a *two site–four function* myoelectric control method.

In a similar configuration termed "auto-revert," control automatically returns to the TD whenever the wrist is held stationary for about one second. This avoids the need for two co-contract signals, so the sequence becomes co-contract and relax—rotate wrist to desired location—and pause briefly to initiate TD control again.

HYBRID DESIGNS

Thousands of combinations of externally powered and body powered components are possible. These can be effective clinically, based on the individual needs of each amputee. Two basic approaches should be mentioned to remind the clinic team to consider such hybrid control schemes whenever appropriate. The first is to combine an EP TD with a wrist that can be passively or actively flexed and extended. This is most commonly done to permit bilaterally involved amputees to perform activities of daily living near the midline of the body.

The second option is to use an EP wrist rotator with a BP TD. Particularly when the residual limb is relatively short, the ability to actively preposition the terminal device in pronation or supination is enhanced by this combination of components. Although this is of critical importance in the case of bilateral upper limb impairment, it has also proved to be useful for unilateral applications.

OUTCOMES

The human hand is an incredibly complex structure that performs multiple social, sexual, and self-care functions. Presently available prosthetic replacements restore only a fraction of the functions that have been lost. Even the most technologically advanced designs offer only insensate grasp and release.

This has two important ramifications in the rehabilitation of the upper limb amputee. First, it is not only appropriate but also often critical that more than one TD be provided for the amputee to achieve his full rehabilitation potential (14). For example, a flexible passive mitt is well suited for sports activities such as basketball. A rugged body-powered hook may be perfect for changing the brake discs on an automobile, while an externally powered hand offering a humanoid appearance and powerful grasp might be the optimal choice for office tasks.

Second, it is imperative that the upper limb prosthesis fit securely and comfortably, offering some practical improvement in the wearer's quality of life. If the fit or function is compromised, the long-term result is predictable: rejection of the prosthesis. In fact, present statistics suggest that even in experienced, specialty clinics, the long-term wearing rate for upper limb prostheses averages about 60 per cent overall (15), although the acceptance rate for powered arms at the TR/WD levels is usually somewhat higher (16). The higher the level of loss, the greater the rate of rejection—in part because present technology offers the higher-level amputee only a limited ability to place the terminal device in space. Many amputees find a prosthesis quite useful in the first year or more following a traumatic loss but then gradually find ways to adapt their environment to reduce the need for an artificial limb. This "outgrowing" of the need for a prosthetic device should be encouraged as a very positive long-term rehabilitation outcome.

To offer the amputee the best possible chance for long-term success with an upper limb prosthesis, it is important to provide both rehabilitation and the device as soon as possible after the loss has occurred. Although the literature is not conclusive, some evidence indicates that the long-term prosthetic wearing rate increases for those people who receive a functioning artificial arm within 30 to 45 days of amputation (17). Long delays in rehabilitation—whether due to bureaucratic tangles or other factors—essentially force the amputee to become "one-handed" and "forget about" bimanual activities. If the amputee voluntarily chooses life without a prosthesis, this choice is a positive one and should be supported. But, it is clearly detrimental to delay prosthetic fitting any longer than absolutely necessary for those who wish to adapt to this technology.

A clear distinction exists between using a prosthesis unilaterally, and bilateral applications. For the unilateral amputee, the prosthesis is a "portable vise," which is typically used to stabilize objects for fine manipulation by the surviving hand. Gross grasp and release, and gross placement in space are sufficient for this application, and such functions are available from a wide variety of prosthetic components. It is also quite feasible to perform most activities of daily living with one arm, so independence training without a prosthesis is often useful.

Many, but not all, bilateral amputees find it difficult to maintain full independence without the use of at least one prosthetic device. For the bilateral amputee, the prosthesis is a "survival tool" for eating, toileting, dressing, and other daily living tasks.

Particularly in the case of bilateral transradial/wrist disarticulation loss, prosthetic fitting is often successful. From necessity, many amputees with low-level bilateral loss become remarkably adept users. [This is not necessarily true for higher-level losses or for children born with limb absences. Many in these groups do best with nonprosthetic independence training (18).]

Reliability and durability are of prime importance for bilateral users, so the use of BP components and TDs should be considered. But, EP components have also been used with good long-term success for TR/WD bilaterals. Some clinicians prefer to provide the bilateral one EP arm and one BP arm, thus offering the amputee "the best of both worlds." Others have been equally successful with bilateral EP or hybrid systems. One predominant trend is to offer the bilateral user two differing TDs so that multiple grasping configurations are readily available (Figure 18-8).

CONCLUSIONS

In North America, the most commonly encountered upper limb absences are at the WD and TR levels. In many ways, these levels are ideally suited for prosthetic fitting and, for this reason, the long-term wearing rate approaches 80% in some clinics. The presence of two independent myosignal sites makes myoelectrically controlled externally powered technology technically feasible for most of these amputees. Although the bilateral upper limb amputee makes very high demands on his prostheses, making the rugged and mechanically simple body powered terminal devices therefore quite useful, good success has also been reported worldwide in fitting many of these individuals with artificial arms incorporating externally powered elements.

The control options, terminal device choices, and socket/suspension variants must be individualized for each amputee in accordance with their personal goals and functional capabilities. Although higher level

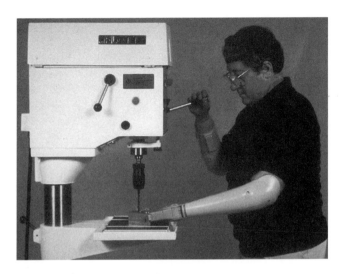

FIGURE 18-8

This bilateral TR/WD amputee uses a powered hook on one side and a powered hand on the other. This combination of TDs offers a variety of grip options necessary for daily tasks. Unilateral amputees may use interchangeable hooks and hands for similar reasons. (Courtesy Otto Bock Orthopedic Industry, Inc.)

amputation places additional demands on both prosthetic design and the amputee operator, most basic principles for component and control selections reviewed for the WD/TR in this chapter remain applicable even in more challenging applications. Strict attention to details—in prescription, fitting, training, and follow-up—is critical to foster the long-term use of upper limb prostheses.

References

1. Atkins DJ, Heard DCY, Donovan WH. Epidemiologic overview of individuals with upper-limb loss and their reported research priorities. *J Prosthet Orthot* 1996; 8:2–11.
2. Murphy EF. Manipulators and upper-extremity prosthetics. *Bull Prosthet Res* 1964; 10(2):107–117.
3. Fletcher MJ, Leonard F. The principles of artificial hand design. *Artificial Limbs* 1955; 2(2):78–94.
4. Simpson DC. The hand/arm system. In *Principles of Prosthetic Practice*. London: E Arnold, 1970. Pp 337–342.
5. Uellendahll KE, Heckathorne C, Wu Y, et al. Prosthetic arm design and simulation system (PADSS) for assessing alternative fittings of upper-limb prostheses. *Capabilities* 1995; 4(3):1–2.
6. Stricker SJ. Illizarov lenghtening of a post-traumatic below elbow amputation: a case report. *Clin Orthop* 1994; 306:124–127.
7. Childress DS. A new synergetic hand prototype. *Capabilities* 1992; 2(2):1.

8. Childress DS, Billock JN. Self-containment and self-suspension of externally powered prostheses for the forearm. *Bull Prosthet Res* 1970; 10(14):4–21.

9. Billock JS. Personal communication. 1999.

10. Sears Hh, Shaperman J. Proportional myoelectric hand control: an evaluation. *Am J Phys Med Rehabil* 1991; 70:21–28.

11. Clippinger FW, Avery R, Titus BR. A sensory feedback system for an upper-limb amputation prosthesis. *Bull Prosthet Res* 1974; 10(22):247–258.

12. Scott RH, Brittain RH, Caldwell PR. Sensory feedback system compatible with myoelectric control. *Med BiolEng Comput* 1980; 18:65–69.

13. Gow D. Control of upper limb prostheses—the Edinburgh philosophy. *Eng Med* 1988; 17:82.

14. Sears HH. Approaches to prescription of body powered and myoelectric prostheses. *Phys Med Rehabil Clin North Am* 1991; 2:361–371.

15. Wright TW, Hagan AD, Wood MB. Prosthetic usage in upper extremity amputations. *J Hand Surg* 1995; 20A:619–622.

16. Datta D, Kingston J, Ronald J. Myoelectric prostheses for below-elbow amputees: The Trent experience. *Int Disabil Stud* 1989; 11:167–170.

17. Malone JM, Childers SJ, Underwood J et al. Immediate postsurgical management of upper extremity amputation: Conventional, electric and myoelectric prosthesis. *Orthot Prosthet* 1981; 35:2, 1–9.

18. Edelstein JH. Special considerations—rehabilitation without prostheses: Functional skills training. In: Bowler JH and Michael JW (eds.), *Atlas of Limb Prosthetics, Second Edition.* St. Louis: Mosby, 1992. Pp 721–728.

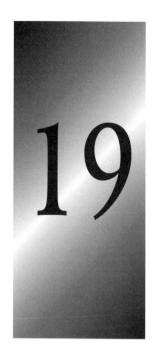

19 External-Power for the Transhumeral Amputee

Harold H. Sears, PhD

A few short decades ago, an electric prosthesis for the transhumeral or higher level amputee would have been considered purely experimental. Today, we can reasonably suggest that every such patient be at least considered for an electric prosthesis. Although there may be those who are simply not candidates, as when reimbursement is impossible or skilled prosthetic care is not available, electric prostheses have something to offer nearly every upper-limb amputee. We might qualify this statement only to say that electric prostheses are often used in addition to another prosthesis, such as a rugged body-powered work/sports arm, or a lightweight cosmetic arm, given the wide variety of activities in which one individual may engage.

In this chapter we summarize the critical advantages and disadvantages of electric prostheses and describe the components available for electric hand, elbow, and wrist. The clinical approaches available to fit transhumeral, elbow disarticulation, and the high-level patient are also described, along with recommendations for some of the key elements for success in fitting electric prostheses.

Specifically, an electric prosthesis offers the transhumeral (or higher level) amputee the following advantages:

- Increased comfort, by eliminating traditional control cables for some or all functions of the prosthesis. The control cables of a body-powered prosthesis can be extremely uncomfortable for many higher-level amputees, sometimes causing a painful nerve entrapment syndrome (1). Cables may also restrict the full range of motion of the shoulder and limit the functional work envelope within which the prosthesis may be used. The elimination of control cables may in fact allow many high-level amputees, or those with brachial plexus injuries, to wear a prosthesis when they would not be candidates otherwise.
- Higher pinch force and the secure grip of electric hands and special-purpose grippers now allow much higher pinch force [usually 22 lb (10 kg)] than traditional hooks or hands provide. This allows a successful combination of a cosmetic hand shape with a high level of function. The body-powered hook is no longer the only functional choice—in fact, the electric hand is even more functional for many activities requiring high pinch force, gripping cylindrical shapes, or the more cosmetic shape of a hand (2).

HANDS (TERMINAL DEVICES)

The most functional element of an arm prosthesis is the hand, or terminal device (TD). Just as the more

199

proximal joints of the natural arm position the hand for prehension or the application of force, the major role of the wrist, elbow, and shoulder joints of the high-level prosthesis is to position the TD to perform tasks.

High pinch force is available in the hand components used with transhumeral and higher level prostheses. But like most prosthetic components, all features come with some trade-offs. Hands featuring 20 lb (10 kg) pinch force are used very widely, but are only available in adult sizes. They are also the heaviest of the available TDs. Combined with a cosmetic/protective cover, the weight of these stronger hands might be 1 lb to 1 1/4 lb (450gm–550gm). This weight can be tolerable for adult males, and many females, but becomes more of a disadvantage for the high-level amputee due to the concentration of weight at the end of the forearm. Modern fitting techniques allow for a much more comfortable fit than ever before, but assessing the weight tolerance of the patient is still an essential element for an appropriate prescription. Lower weight hands are available in the adult sizes, but require a compromise in the pinch force. For instance, a lightweight hand weighing 7.5 oz (215 gm) is available, but produces only about one-half the pinch force of the high-strength hands (3).

This may be an acceptable trade-off between weight and pinch force for those clients whose highest priority is low weight.

The variety of electric hands includes a hand with built-in flexion and extension (a simple locking device allows the wearer to reposition the hand to 30 degrees of flexion or extension and lock the position). This allows much better positioning of the hand at the midline of the wearer's body for dressing, etc., as well as for a wide variety of tasks. (See Figure 19.1.)

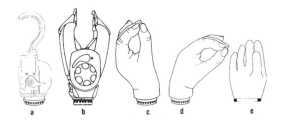

FIGURE 19-2

A variety of interchangeable electric terminal devices (TDs) is available. One type of electric hand (c & d) even allows flexion and extension (to 30 degrees). A body-powered TD can also be interchanged (see Figure 19-10). A "short" hand for up to transcarpal lengths is also shown (e). Many active prosthesis wearers use several TDs for various types of tasks (4).

Shorter versions of the electric hand are also available for wrist disarticulation and transcarpal levels. These versions are significantly shorter and lighter than the standard hand length (by nearly 2 inches [5 cm]). One version is shown in Figure 19-2. These shorter hands (made by at least two manufacturers) offer speed and grip force equivalent to the full-size versions, but do sacrifice the quick disconnect feature to save space; thus, the hand is not interchangeable with work TDs.

COSMETIC/PROTECTIVE COVERS

High-quality cosmetic/protective covers are available from several different manufacturers, in a wide range of cost and appearance. Cosmetic protective covers are available that are indistinguishable from a natural hand at first glance. Although the higher-quality covers are more costly, the important fact to keep in mind is that excellent natural-looking covers are available for electric prostheses, and modern covers can withstand the high pinch forces exerted by modern electric hands. Lifetimes will vary from 6 months to several years, depending on quality.

WORK-TYPE TDS

Given the expense and inconvenience of replacing cosmetic covers, a "Work Hand" is chosen as an alternative terminal device for nearly any prosthesis wearer doing rugged tasks for work or hobbies. Figure 19-2 shows the variety of available work-type TDs. Some are more lightweight, and may be more appropriate for high-level prostheses than others.

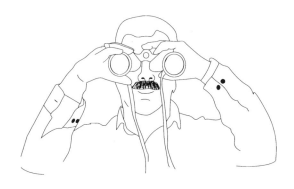

FIGURE 19-1

Electric hands with flexion and extension in the wrist now allow more functional positioning of the hand and the performance of tasks in a more natural manner.

WRIST ROTATION AND OTHER WRIST OPTIONS

Electric wrist rotation (Figures 19-3 and 19-4) is frequently utilized in transhumeral or higher-level prostheses. A number of different TDs can be used with the electric wrist, and either switch control or myoelectric control is available.

The advantages of adding this important degree of freedom have been demonstrated clinically with both unilateral and bilateral amputees. A recently published survey of electric wrist wearers demonstrated that the sound hand is freed from the burden of repositioning the hand by using an easily positioned electric wrist (5). The prosthesis is then used more naturally in the performance of two-handed activities. Cocontraction switching is typically used to transfer the dual-muscle control between hand and wrist. After using the electric prosupination function, the wearer then transfers control back to the hand, to open or close.

In transhumeral cases especially, the use of the electric wrist has become easier and more commonplace since the introduction of simple push and pull switches in the harness or socket. By bumping the switch with a slight abduction of the humerus, the wearer can toggle the proportional myoelectric control between the hand and the wrist.

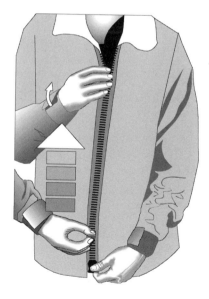

FIGURE 19-3

Use of the electric wrist rotator was formerly considered to be advantageous to bilateral amputees only. However, the unilateral amputee can also easily reposition the TD with the electric wrist, without the sound hand. This allows two-handed activities to be performed more naturally, and more quickly. (Courtesy Journal of Prosthetics and Orthotics.)

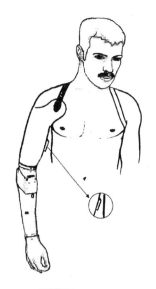

FIGURE 19-4

Electric wrist rotation is utilized much more frequently and successfully now by electric elbow wearers using push and pull switches. In the push version of the switch, as applied to transhumeral cases, the wearer simply bumps the switch, toggling the myoelectric control from the hand to the wrist. Bumping the switch again causes the wrist to turn off, and the control returns to the hand. The pull version of the switch is used more frequently in prostheses for shoulder amputees, since high level amputees can more easily actuate a switch by chest expansion.

ELECTRIC ELBOWS

The current electric elbows (Figure 19-5) must be thought of as the second generation of myoelectric technology, because they are much improved over previous versions. The proportional control of both elbow and hand are available, as well as the aforementioned electric wrist rotation option. Battery systems feature the newer nickel metal hydride high capacity cells, which can last for several days of use, and can recharge in about two hours.

CONSIDERATION FOR PRESCRIPTION OF ELECTRIC ELBOW PROSTHESES

The size and length of the remaining limb, and the weight of the chosen prosthesis are two important factors in any prosthetic prescription.

Size and Amputation Length

Size restrictions may be thought of rather simply: If the amputation level is 2 inches short of elbow disarticulation, an electric elbow can be utilized. At this maximum amputation length, although the humeral length may be longer than the sound-side humerus,

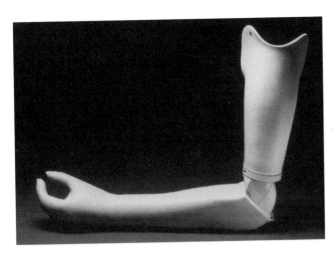

FIGURE 19-5

The Utah Arm 2, a complete electric elbow, hand, and wrist system. All degrees of freedom may be controlled myoelectrically or by ServoPro control. Component weight is 3.3 lb maximum, but the entire prosthesis is usually 4 to 6 lb depending on the socket weight and additional hardware, such as shoulder joints, etc.

the hand positions will be equal, and the overall arm lengths can usually be matched (Figure 19-6). For amputations longer than this length, a hybrid prosthesis would be considered, perhaps a body-powered arm for elbow disarticulation, with an electric hand.

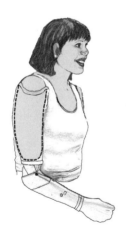

FIGURE 19-6

Maximum transhumeral amputation length. In elective amputations (or if a revision surgery is performed) the ideal length to allow full choice of components is 5 inches (12 cm) short of the elbow disarticulation length. However, the maximum length that allows an electric elbow to be prescribed is 2 inches (5 cm) short of the elbow disarticulation. The position of the hands and forearms can be made equal although the humeral length will be longer than ideal.

Weight

For smaller-sized individuals, weight can be a problem with a complete electric elbow, hand, and wrist system, so weight tolerance is important to evaluate in the prescription of any arm prosthesis. However, fitting techniques have evolved greatly for transhumeral and higher-level amputees so that the weight of electric systems can be suspended with much more stability. Also, if needed, the option of electric wrist rotation may be sacrificed or lighter weight hands may be used.

The smallest electric elbow available is a child to adolescent model for the 8- to 12-year-old range. In adult sizes, the weight of electric elbows varies from 1.5 lb to just over 2 lb (680 kg–900 kg), with the weight of the hand adding approximately 3/4 lb to 1 1/4 lb (340 gm–570 gm). The entire electric prosthesis can weigh between 3 1/2 lb to 4 1/4 lb (1.6 kg–1.9 kg), for transhumeral prostheses. A shoulder disarticulation prosthesis typically weighs 5 to 6 lb (2.3–2.7 kg).

It should be remembered that the effect of prosthesis weight is a very individual matter. For some wearers, a heavier prosthesis is preferable over lighter weight alternatives since the loading on the torso is balanced, thus minimizing spinal curvature and shoulder height imbalance. At the other extreme, some amputees can be hypersensitive to the weight, and cannot tolerate any weight greater than a shell-like cosmetic prosthesis with only passive function. This variable must be carefully evaluated in the prescription process. In lieu of any prior experience wearing a prosthesis, a trial fit may be necessary to realistically evaluate this and other variables (6).

NONMYOELECTRIC CONTROL OPTIONS

As advanced as current myoelectric control systems can be (minimum EMG to control the Utah Arm 2 for instance, is only 10 microvolts), some amputees have very little EMG activity, for example, in the case of severe brachial plexus injuries and some interscapulothorasic (forequarter) amputees. In these cases, proportional control is still available via servo control. Sensors can be of two types: a harness-mounted sensor that detects force or excursion, or touch-pads that sense the pressure at a point inside the socket. When placed anterior and posterior to the acromium, the touch pads replace the usual biceps and triceps signals.

The simplest option, a pull switch, is also available with some elbow components. This option can simplify the fitting and reduce the cost, although at the expense of more natural and easily controlled myoelectric control.

Although the servo control methods may simplify difficult high-level fittings, most clinicians still feel that when adequate muscle control can be developed, myoelectric control is more natural for most patients to operate, and the control of hand function is superior. Such cases should be evaluated carefully, after training for the muscles has been attempted, and a trial fit of both methods may be appropriate.

Simultaneous Elbow and Hand Control

Simultaneous elbow and hand control of the prosthesis is an option with several electric arms. Using the harness-mounted sensor for the elbow control (see Figure 19-7) and myoelectric control (typically from biceps and triceps EMGs) for the hand, the wearer has much more rapid control of the hand than with a system that sequences from elbow to hand upon locking the elbow. The elbow lock is still required to hold significant loads, but for a well-coordinated wearer the system can have a more natural feeling. The advent of microprocessors has allowed the electronic circuitry to be entirely self-contained, with the integrated computers controlling all functions simultaneously.

NONELECTRIC COMPONENTRY

Mechanical or nonelectric componentry is available in several prosthetic configurations.

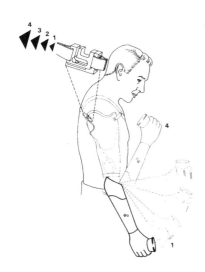

FIGURE 19-7

When myoelectric control is not an option, a force sensor in the harness is used with the ServoPro controller for the Utah Arm 2. Other options include switch control via a simple pull switch mounted in the harness, or touch pads in the socket that can be pushed by the acromium to produce a proportional signal. Simultaneous elbow and hand is also possible using this type of nonmyoelectric control for the elbow and dedicating the myoelectric control to the hand.

Humeral Rotation

Passive humeral rotation is available in several of the electric and body-powered elbow options, with the degree of friction of the rotation joint adjustable by the wearer. As yet, powered rotation is not available, although experimental devices have been reported (3).

Shoulder Flexion/Extension and Abduction/Adduction

New passive joints are available for the shoulder. These joints offer a positive lock for humeral flexion, which is a significant improvement over the purely friction joints formerly available. Friction joints without a lock have a distinct disadvantage, since any flexion or extension at the shoulder cannot be maintained securely because the friction joint too easily displaces from the desired position when the wearer needs to push or pull on objects.

The locking shoulder joint may increase costs somewhat, which is often resisted by payors, but the additional utility that such a joint adds to this highly disabled population is unquestioned and should be pursued aggressively for their benefit.

TRANSHUMERAL AMPUTEES

The choice of an appropriate prosthesis for the transhumeral amputee can be a challenge for even a well-informed clinician. Discussed here are the functions available in current components and current fitting techniques, which both have a tremendous impact on the function that is possible for the amputee.

As mentioned earlier, the electric elbow, wrist, and hand are all available with excellent function for adult-sized amputees. Several "hybrid" combinations of body-powered and electric components may also be reasonable options for some amputees, but require excellent shoulder strength and range of motion.

Electric systems are adopted more widely in the present day, since hand function with proportional systems is not only more functional than the body-powered hand, but also requires less effort than any available body-powered hand. Of course, the elimination of the control cables is a large plus for the fully electric system, giving greater comfort along with the more natural appearance.

The key advantage of choosing electric components at this level of amputation is the freedom from control cables. A lack of cabling translates to more comfort and ease of operation, which can outweigh the higher cost and additional weight of a completely electric system.

Advanced fitting techniques (see Figures 19-8 through 19-11) have also made an enormous contribution to the success of electric prostheses. The range of motion at the shoulder can be increased, the weight of

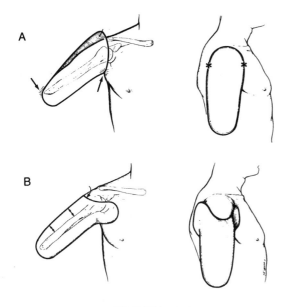

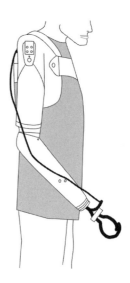

FIGURE 19-10

This hybrid prosthesis is built with an electric elbow and a body-powered hook-type terminal device. The patient's priorities are functional rather than cosmetic. Advantages are: only one body-powered control cable is required (for the TD), and the forearm weight is less than if an electric hand were used. This TD can easily be interchanged with an electric TD via the quick disconnect at the wrist, making the prosthesis fully electric for some occasions.

FIGURE 19-8

The key features of modern transhumeral sockets are the total contact along the entire length of the humerus and the stability in rotation offered by the anterior and posterior stabilizing "wings" of the socket framework. Moving the prosthesis in abduction/adduction is more comfortable and more responsive, and resisting rotation forces (while lifting, pushing, or pulling) is much more comfortable, not being dependent on the harness alone (8). (Courtesy Atlas of Limb Prosthetics.)

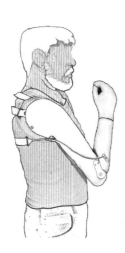

FIGURE 19-9

This hybrid prosthesis features a body-powered locking elbow with myoelectric hand and wrist. The hand is controlled by biceps and triceps EMG signals, connected by cords outside the elbow, or in some cases, connectors internal to the elbow. Two mechanical control cables are still required, however, for elbow flexion and elbow lock, so only patients with very good shoulder range of motion and strength are appropriate for a hybrid of this type.

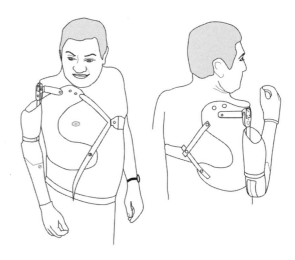

FIGURE 19-11

A modern shoulder disarticulation check socket (or temporary fitting socket), so the usual cosmetic covers are not shown. The electrodes mounted in the flexible interface are comfortably mounted over the appropriate muscle sites, while the stiff frame is anatomically formed around the remnant skeletal features of the clavicle and the scapula. In this design, the shape almost "wedges" onto the remnant shoulder, preventing the socket from shifting on the wearer while in use, while supporting the weight on the scapula and chest. A simple flexion joint is shown. The shoulder joint recommended for the finished prosthesis incorporates a positive lock for humeral flexion.

the prosthesis is suspended more comfortably, and the stability of the prosthesis is increased.

ELBOW DISARTICULATION

The longest length transhumeral cases have the disadvantage of insufficient space in the humeral section of the prosthesis to install either an electric elbow or the internal-locking body-powered components. However, the long humeral length does allow more cable excursion than a high-level patient can generate; thus, the motive for the hybrid prosthesis. Most frequently, the hybrid combination is a myoelectric hand with a body-powered elbow, utilizing outside-locking joints (which unfortunately are accompanied by the greater bulk of the externally mounted joints). In some cases, where the amputation length is no more than 2 in (5 cm) short of an elbow disarticulation length, an internal-locking elbow may also be used.

SHOULDER DISARTICULATION AND INTERSCAPULOTHORASIC LEVELS

The advantages of electric prostheses for transhumeral amputees, such as the elimination of control cables and the higher pinch force of the TD, are even more important for the very high level amputee, because of the greater disability suffered. The combined improvements made recently in components and fitting techniques have made significant contributions to function, cosmesis, comfort, and convenience.

The state-of-the-art electric prosthesis for the high-level amputee integrates all the functions we have mentioned: electric flexion/extension, hand open/close, wrist pronation/supination, and the mechanical shoulder joint with a lock for the flexion position. All electric functions are powered by a single battery pack, and control can be myoelectric or servo for all three motorized degrees of freedom, as the wearer sequences from one to the next via a simple pull switch or push switch.

Fitting techniques have evolved far beyond the large shell-type sockets of a decade or more ago, which were hot and unstable. The nomenclature of mini-frame or micro-frame (7,8) has been applied to the most recent designs, as shown in Figure 19-11. By combining the very strong and stiff carbon materials for the socket external frame with the flexible and more comfortable thermoplastic materials for the skin interface, much more comfortable and stable high-level fittings are being performed.

CLINICAL GUIDELINES FOR SUCCESS

The advantages of early fitting of an arm prosthesis are already well documented (10). With modern techniques and materials, a prosthesis may be fitted very early postoperatively, which is ideal. If the appropriate prescription is uncertain, a trial fit is strongly recommended even for early fitting (6). Unfortunately, wound healing, as well as funding issues, can delay the fitting process. The clinic is generally well advised to expedite the fitting process, even if it means using a simpler body-powered prosthesis. However, a powered prosthesis could be justified for early fitting, if the wound healing is incomplete (contraindicating a body-powered cable) or if the psychologic reaction to a hook-type terminal device would be detrimental to the patient.

Training

Fortunately, the need for proper training with electric arm fittings is being recognized by more clinics and individual caregivers. Training for body-powered arm wearers is equally important, but because the costs of an electric prosthesis are higher, training may be emphasized more strongly (Figure 19-12).

Training is important and distinctly different at two stages of the fitting process. First, at the preprosthetic stage, the focus is on muscle strengthening, increasing range of motion, and in parallel, increasing the client's independence without the prosthesis. During and after the prosthetic fitting, the training focus is on acquiring skills for the operation of the prosthesis and working towards specific tasks required for daily life at home, in hobbies, and on the job (11).

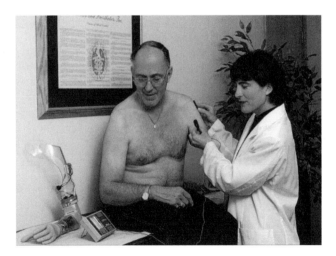

FIGURE 19-12

Training in both muscle strength and everyday usage of the prosthesis is extremely important. Prosthetic utilization is improved because problems in the fit and adjustment can be identified earlier with the aid of the therapist. Also, the wearer can gain confidence in task performance before trying to perform those tasks in the public eye.

For all new prosthesis wearers, training should be thought of as compulsory with the fitting of an arm prosthesis. Two reasons for this that are often overlooked are:

- The patient's frustration with learning to use the prosthesis is lessened greatly if the basic skills can be acquired in a supportive and helpful environment. Arm amputees are much less self-conscious about using their prosthesis if they can develop their abilities before they go out in public.
- Needed adjustments to the prosthesis (to the fit or the controls) are often revealed by the use of the new prosthesis in the therapy setting. The patient alone may not yet have the knowledge to know if adjustment will improve the function, but with the help of a knowledgeable therapist, important feedback is available to the prosthetist to make improvements.

CONCLUSIONS

Improved function, comfort, and appearance in modern electric prostheses are improving the rehabilitation of clients who are motivated to adopt a prosthesis and physically able to wear it.

The presence of the complete rehabilitation team may be more important than ever before. Improved prosthetic rehabilitation requires excellent prosthetic and technical skills, well-timed therapy integrated with the entire process, and informed medical direction. The education of all elements of the rehabilitation team is critical—without any one of these roles, the prosthesis may not make a contribution to the rehabilitation of the amputee.

References

1. Reddy MP. Nerve entrapment syndromes in the upper extremity contralateral to amputation. *Arch Phys Med Rehabil* 1984 (65) 24–26.
2. Sears HH, Shaperman J. Proportional myoelectric hand control: An evaluation. *Amer J Phys Med Rehabil* 1991 (70) 1.
3. Electronic Prosthetic Innovations. O&P *Business News,* 1999 (8) 23.
4. Sears HH. Advances in arm prosthetics. *In Motion* 1999 (9) 3.
5. Sears HH, Shaperman J. Electric wrist rotation in proportional-controlled systems. *J Prosthetic Orthotic* 1998 (10) 4; 92–98.
6. Sears HH. Approaches to prescription of body-powered and myoelectric prostheses. *Phys Med Rehabil Clin NA* 1991 (2) 2:361–371.
7. Migvelez JM, Migvelez MD. The Microframe: The next generation of interface design. *J Prosthetic Orthotic* 2003 (15) 2; 66-71.
8. Andrews JT. In: Bowker JH, Michael JW (eds.) *Atlas of Limb Prosthetics: Surgical, Prosthetic, and Rehabilitation Principles* 2 ed. American Academy of Orthopedic Surgeons, 1992.
9. Sears HH, Andrew JT, Jacobsen SC. In: Meier RH, Atkins DJ (eds.): *Comprehensive Management of the Upper Limb Amputee.* New York: Springer-Verlag, 1989.
10. Malone JM, Fleming LL, Roberson J, et al. Immediate, early, and late post-surgical management of upper-limb amputations. *J Rehabil Res Dev* 1984 (21) 1:33.
11. "Training the Client with an Electric Arm Prosthesis." Video produced by Motion Control Inc., 1986.

*A*dditional Readings

Millstein G, Heger H, Hunter GA. Prosthetic use in upper limb amputees: A comparison of the body powered and electrically powered prostheses. *Prosthetic Orthotic International* 1986, 10: 27–34.

Jacobsen SC, Knutti DF, Johnson RT, Sears HH. Development of the Utah artificial Arm. *IEEE Trans Biomedical Engineering* 1982, BME-29 (4).

Kritter Alfred E. Current concepts review: Myoelectric prostheses. *J Bone Joint Surg* 1985 (67-A) 4: 654–657.

Kohl Sybil J. In: Krvegar DW (ed.) *Emotional Rehabilitation and Physical Trauma and Disability*, 1984.

20 Control of Powered Upper Extremity Prostheses

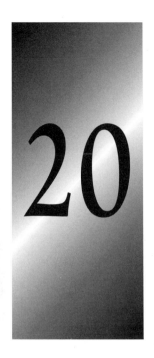

T. Walley Williams, III

This chapter addresses the challenge met by the clinician who wants to prescribe or build a powered prosthesis in today's digital world. During the 1980s, the circuits for controlling hands, wrists, and elbows were analog circuits. Thus, any time a clinical challenge arose that required a new form of control, an entirely new control circuit was needed. The result was that only a small number of circuits had a large enough market to justify development costs. Today analog circuits are giving way to digital circuits that can be reprogrammed on the fly. In some cases, the programming is done by choosing a single configuration plug from a selection shipped with the device. In other cases, much wider choices are available by making selections on a computer screen. This chapter introduces the language and concepts needed to use these new technologies.

THE MEANING OF POWERED

Powered prosthetics usually use a battery mounted on or in the prosthesis. The battery power is delivered to one or more motors by control electronics that are in turn activated by a variety of sensors and transducers. Other power sources have also been used. All of the early work in this field is presented in a single bibliography (1). The thalidomide problem in the 1960s led to a number of gas-powered prostheses. The small gas cylinders are not as convenient as batteries, but gas is still an appealing option because the activators are almost weightless, whereas electric motors are heavy by nature. Recently, the Wilmer Group in the Netherlands has revisited gas power for a child's hand (2). The ultimate success of this effort will probably depend on whether a good interface exists between the electric input devices and controllers available and the gas control logic. In the past, a lack of miniature valves for the proportional control of pneumatic systems existed, but the team in Delft seem to have made significant progress that may again lead to the commercial availability of gas-powered prostheses. However, this chapter discusses only battery-powered prostheses.

MYOELECTRIC CONTROL

The most popular control input for powered prostheses has always been a pair of myoelectric pickups. They are a critical element in the self-suspending transradial socket and permit the elimination of straps and harnesses. Although these pickups are often referred to as electromyographic (EMG), this term should be reserved for the graphic recordings of myoelectric signals, and it will not be used here.

Acquiring the Myoelectric Signal

A myoelectric potential is generated on the skin whenever a single muscle fiber twitches. The typical myosignal used for prosthetic control is the sum of a multitude of individual twitch potentials. This signal is small, typically 5 to 100 microvolts (μ V), and it is overwhelmed by interference signals generated by power lines, machinery, and radio stations. Thus, two constraints are immediately placed on signal acquisition. The signal must be amplified and the interference must be rejected. Both constraints are handled by a preamplifier only or by a preamplifier incorporating additional electronics to smooth the signal and rectify it into a varying direct current (DC) voltage.

The All-In-One Electrode

The typical electrode package is a small plastic box, with three metal electrodes used to acquire the signal and with electronics to convert the signal to a DC voltage. Such electrodes usually have a gain adjustment on the side opposite the metal electrodes. The manufacturer supplies the electrode assembly with additional dummy electrodes and housings, so that the unit can be incorporated into either a laminated or thermoformed socket. Such assemblies accommodate the majority of users. Figure 20-1 shows a typical electrode amplifier assembly.

Use of Separate Metal Electrodes

Some users need the greater sensitivity that can be provided by using larger metal electrodes spaced further apart. However, extra gain can also be incorporated into the controller when the standard all-in-one electrode assemblies are used. A major problem with separate remote electrodes is that each wire connecting the two active electrodes must be shielded until connected to a preamplifier. Along with the reference electrode wire, this adds three rather large cables between the inner and outer sockets. These larger remote electrodes are most often used with higher-level amputations.

Confusion Over Digital and Analog Electrodes

One source of confusion in myoelectric control is the choice of the words used to describe the devices that acquire the muscle signal. The most popular myoelectric pickup is the combination of three metal electrodes with an amplifier and signal conditioner. Although correctly only the three pieces of metal are electrodes, most people refer to the whole device as an electrode. The second source of confusion is the adjective used to describe the electrode assembly. The earliest devices detected whether the myoelectric signal was above or below a threshold. Such a device is a *digital* electrode because it can only output a zero (no voltage) or a one (full battery voltage). In recent years most electrode amplifiers have been made as *analog* electrodes. The output of these devices is an analog voltage that varies with the strength of the myoelectric signal. This is confusing because these analog electrodes are required for the proper functioning of the digital circuits that will control the prostheses of the future.

Digital and Analog Control Circuits

If the variable voltage from an analog electrode is used with a control system for a device such as a hand, how the control system processes the signal determines whether the controller is analog or digital. Analog circuits work by processing and transforming the varying signals themselves. Newer digital circuits convert the varying value of each input to a number that is updated typically a thousand or more times a second. The input values from one or more electrodes, switches, or other inputs are then used by a miniature computer chip to generate motor control instructions. The chips are called *microcontrollers* or *digital signal processors* (DSPs). Such chips can be programmed to work in many different ways, which means that one device, such as an electric hand, can be tried on an amputee with several control strategies until the best is determined.

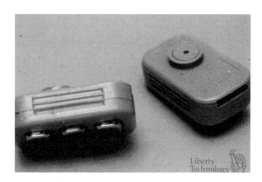

FIGURE 20-1

Two views of one manufacture's electrode assembly. The important elements are the three metal electrodes, the adjustment potentiometer, and the socket for the connecting cable.

Roll-On Sleeves

Many practitioners are now improving the suspension of upper extremity prostheses by using roll-on sleeves. Such sleeves provide almost flawless suction suspension, but they are problematic when electric signals must be passed through them. Several reports in the literature discuss the solution to these problems, but roll-on sleeves will not come into their own until an easy-to-use method is available commercially for incorporating the metal electrodes and cables into an assembly that is reliable enough to last as long as the sleeve itself—about a year. The ideal system will avoid the long shuttle used in transtibial prostheses. Rather it will incorporate a ring around the end of the sleeve that contains the preamplifier electronics, with any needed adjustment potentiometer, along with an alignment and attachment mechanism. Such equipment should appear on the market soon. Figure 20-2 shows a rather cumbersome way to affix wires to a roll-on sleeve.

CONTROL STRATEGIES

A control strategy defines how the inputs from the user are used to control a prosthesis. Typically the microcontroller in a hand or a multidevice controller is programmed at the factory with all the possible strategies that may be needed. This programming is called *firmware*. Later, the person fitting a particular patient selects the best strategy by invoking one or more pieces of the firmware. This selection may be done in any of several ways. Figures 20-3 to 20-6 show some of the microprocessor-based controllers available. These units are so small that they fit almost anywhere in the prosthesis. This small size presents a connection problem, because the connectors are now almost as big as the controllers.

Plugs and Switches for Selecting Strategies

In the least versatile systems, inserting a colored plug chooses from a small number of strategies, usually no

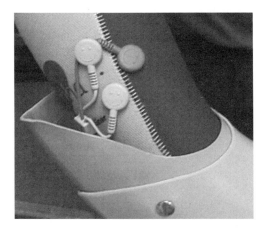

FIGURE 20-2

Remote metal electrodes inside the roll-on sleeve are attached to the preamplifiers by the three snap-on wires of this cable assembly.

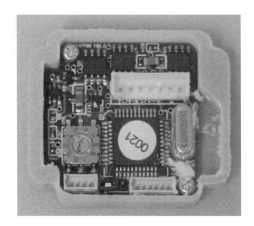

FIGURE 20-3

The miniature switch on this board from a powered gripper measures only 5mm on a side. There are ten possible positions, but less than ten strategies are available.

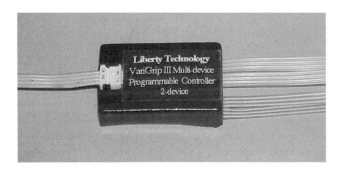

FIGURE 20-4

Controllers are getting smaller. This unit, designed by the author, measures only 27 × 40 × 9.7 mm (1.04 × 1.57 × .38 inches). The outputs on the left control a wrist and a hand. The inputs on the right are from two Otto Bock electrode amplifiers and the computer interface. This controller fits between a wrist rotator and the socket wall of a typical transradial prosthesis.

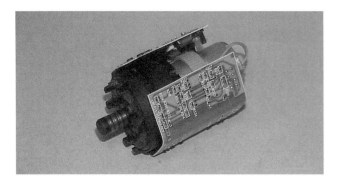

FIGURE 20-5

This controller is shown wrapped around a wrist rotation unit. This configuration can accommodate any residual limb, where there is room for the rotator.

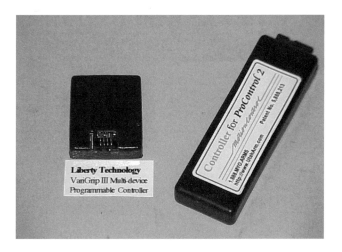

FIGURE 20-6

Two small controllers side by side. Both use a computer interface during patient evaluation and device setup.

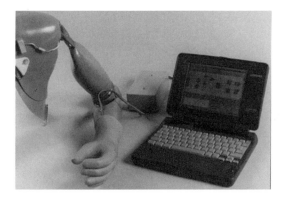

FIGURE 20-7

The elements of a typical system for programming a prosthesis. Information is presented on the computer screen and then downloaded to the prosthesis through an optoisolator and connecting cable. Usually the cable is long enough for the user to operate the prosthesis without pulling the cable. One company makes a controller with a radio link to avoid the cable.

more than eight. Alternatively, the prosthetist or technician will be asked to set the position of a microscopic switch. Figure 20-3 shows such a switch with ten positions. Not all of the positions will select strategies. After a strategy has been selected, there is no possibility for adjustment except for the sensitivity of the myoelectrode amplifiers. This can be a disadvantage when the input signals are too low to boost using the gain control in the electrode. To counter this problem, the Otto Bock company has added duplicate strategies to some of its hands. The extra strategies differ only in having greater input gain. (Of course, this fails when only one muscle is weak.)

Computer-Loaded Strategies

About 20% of the patient population will find that none of the "canned" choices are optimal. When the control circuit can be attached to a computer, more possibilities exist. In particular, a number of adjustments can be made to tune the strategy selected to the user. When a single controller is required to operate three or more devices, virtually every system will use a computer to do the setup and adjustments. Figure 20-7 shows a prosthesis attached to a computer for downloading a program.

Control Strategies Using a Single Input

In many cases, only a single muscle is available for myoelectric control. In addition, there are several other ways for an amputee to generate a single signal with variable strength. The other inputs will be discussed in detail later, but the strategies work the same way.

The Voluntary-Open, Cookie Crusher Strategy

Using this strategy, the hand or gripper opens all the way when the muscle-generated signal crosses a threshold. When the signal ceases, the hand closes automatically until the motor stalls. As it stalls, the current and grip force increase until a battery saver circuit turns it off. The disadvantage of this strategy is that it always closes the hand with its full grip force. This high grip caused the author and inventor of this strategy to call it a *cookie crusher*. The name has become popular, because it helps parents understand what happens. A cookie crusher is usually chosen only for children being fit with a first prosthesis. For the safety of both parent and child, a parental override push button is also provided to open the hand. With modern microprocessor-based circuits, it is so easy to convert a hand to two-muscle control that people sometimes mount a second electrode in the socket to be used when the child is ready.

The Quick-Slow Strategy

Most people can control how quickly they initiate a muscle contraction. With the quick-slow strategy a quick-rise contraction commands the hand to open and a slow-rise commands closure. The Otto Bock company has offered hands using such a circuit for many years. Hand speed is constant, and no adjustments can be made to the quick-slow detector. More recently, digital processing has permitted the expansion of this strategy to include the proportional control of speed and grip once direction has been determined. Furthermore, the thresholds and delay times that make up the quick-slow strategy can be adjusted. With adjustment, many more users can master the quick-slow selection scheme. Figure 20-8 shows a typical computer screen for setting up this strategy. The user is able to watch the signal as it is generated and recorded on a moving strip chart. The user can change the way the signal is generated or the attendant can change the set-up parameters or both.

The UNB Three-State Strategy

This strategy, invented at the University of New Brunswick, is the oldest one-muscle strategy. It is defined by two thresholds. The *off* state is any muscle signal less than the lower threshold. The *open* state is any signal greater than the upper threshold, and the *close* state is any signal strength between the two thresholds. Because speed is not controlled with this strategy, it is rarely used today in its original form. However, microprocessors permit more delays to be introduced when creating a strategy. One company now offers a UNB-style strategy that uses the level of contraction to select direction, followed a few milliseconds later with proportional speed and grip control (3).

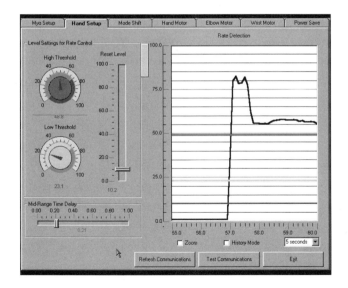

FIGURE 20-8

Screen used to set up one-muscle control of a hand. The photo was made as the strip chart moved from right to left. Three thresholds are shown. The lowest eliminates inadvertent signals. For a slow contraction, the signal must remain between the two upper bands for the 0.2 sec time delay, which it did. The subsequent signal above the third threshold merely controls the speed. For a fast contraction, the signal path would have been almost straight up.

The Alternate Strategy

The alternate strategy was invented by the author for those who have difficulty mastering quick-slow, but who want proportional control. Alternate muscle contractions open and close the hand. Speed and grip are controlled proportionally by the degree of contraction. Because the user may forget what to expect next, the strategy can be set up to default back to either *open next* or *close next* after a settable delay.

The Open-Then-Close Strategy

RSLSteeper has recently redesigned their Powered Gripper. One of the switch-selectable strategies is a variation on the alternate strategy. To open the gripper with one muscle, a strong, momentary signal is generated. The controller automatically opens the gripper all the way. It then redirects the muscle control signal to close the hand proportionally with as much control as with a two-muscle strategy.

Control of Two Devices with One Muscle

Several persons have requested control of both a hand and wrist rotator with a single muscle. Such users are first trained to operate the quick-slow strategy. Then they are taught to make a quick contraction that is held for a settable interval—usually a half second. This action triggers a shift to wrist control, which then uses quick-slow for selecting direction. An important aspect of this strategy is that it can be set up so that if no wrist activity occurs for a settable interval, control reverts to the hand. This auto reversion is often accompanied by a just-audible beep, which may be deleted after the user is trained.

Control Using Two Inputs

Two-muscle myoelectric control is the typical situation that comes to mind when discussing two inputs. Two force sensing resistors (FSRs), such as LTI Touch Pads™, are often used in much the same way, but when the full range of myoelectric possibilities is understood, the use of FSRs becomes a subset as far as control strategies are concerned.

The Simple Myoelectrode Amplifier for Signal Acquisition

Myosignals cannot be used until they have been acquired and processed as individual signals. The simple systems discussed earlier combine the preamplifier with a filter to remove line frequency interference (50 or 60 Hz), a gain stage with an adjustment potentiometer, and a rectifier so that the final output is a DC voltage that typically varies between about .5V to 3.5V. The result is a simple electrode amplifier that will well accommodate about 80% of potential users. The simple electrode is not adequate for a user with weak signals due to scarring, adipose tissue, or partial muscle atrophy or ablation.

Supplementing the Simple Electrode Amplifier

An additional 10% of the patient population can be handled by using the output of a simple electrode amplifier, such as the Otto Bock 13E125, and further processing the signal. Typically, these people need additional signal amplification, and they also require a threshold to remove unwanted interference due to signals generated by motion of the skin with respect to the prosthetic interface or simply due to the inability to fully relax one muscle when the second muscle is being contracted.

The Use of Pure Myoelectric Signal Preamplifiers

The most sophisticated control systems have fully configurable controls that operate directly on the non-rectified myoelectric signal. Such a system can smooth the ripples in the signal more when the signal is weak, less when it is strong, and process the signal in other ways that improve control. In the past, such systems were mainly used by specialists with time to master the many adjustments that are required. Today, these same systems are incorporated into digital processors in the prosthesis that are linked to a computer to guide the prosthetist or technician through the adjustment process.

Fixed Speed Using Two Muscles

Many users wear simple fixed-speed hands. The fixed speed is initiated by contracting the control muscle until the signal strength passes a threshold value. Typically, each of the two input electrodes has its gain adjusted until the user feels that the same effort is required to rise above either threshold. The control circuit decides on direction by noting which signal crosses its threshold first. When the threshold is crossed, the motor runs at a fixed speed to open or close the hand or gripper. The user judges grip force by learning to time how long the muscle is contracted. Users are often so good at this control that they will reject a proportional speed device because it requires them to learn a new way of using their muscles. For many years the electrode amplifier assemblies contained the threshold circuit, and the circuit in the hand simply decided which direction to go. Threshold electrodes are being phased out, so that in the future a patient needing a

new prosthesis with this simple control scheme will require a programmed microprocessor circuit.

Optimal Control of One Device with Two Myosites

Control is usually simple with two strong muscle sites and a fixed speed hand. A simple analog circuit determines which myosignal reaches its threshold first, and this activates the motor in the correct direction. To achieve good proportional control of motor speed is often more difficult. Even after training, the user may not be able to reduce the level of tension in both muscles to zero, or independent muscle control may be difficult. While no control will be optimal for every case, *differential control* has sufficient adjustability to suit a majority of users. When the adjustments are made in the correct order, the system is easy to tailor to the particular user. Only a little additional effort is required to set up a strategy for triggering a shift in control mode when more than one device is to be operated. Figure 20-9 shows how two myoelectric signals are presented on a typical computer screen. All the parameters for setting up the two-muscle control of one device can be adjusted with this screen using the computer mouse. The tabs

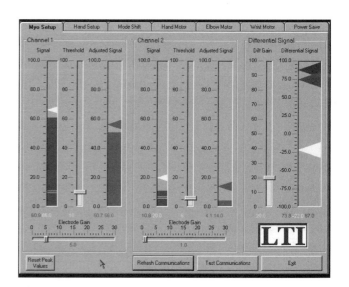

FIGURE 20-9

This screen is typical of those used for setting up a differential motor control system. Each channel has a gain adjustment and a threshold to eliminate signals caused by muscle tremor or electrical noise. The difference between the signals is amplified with the Diff Gain. When channel 1 is greater, the motor goes one way, and when channel 2 is greater it reverses. The arrows in the bar graphs record the maximum signal. These are reset to zero after each attempt by the user to operate the system.

across the top of the screen allow access to other screens for setting the maximum speed of motors and other settings needed when multiple devices are being controlled.

Differential Control with Thresholds

Using two myosites, each muscle will produce a signal with varying strength. With differential control the *difference* between the two signal strengths controls the speed and direction of motion. If the signal from muscle A is larger than that from muscle B, the value A–B will be positive, and the motor will drive in one direction. When A–B is negative, the motor reverses. For values of A–B near zero, the motor cuts out to prevent inadvertent activity. Differential control automatically cancels out any co-contraction, but too much co-contraction will decrease the dynamic range of the signal until proportional control is lost. In these cases, other strategies are better.

Use of Thresholds

Most amputees generate a small amount of myoelectric activity even when their muscles are relaxed. To get rid of this activity, the circuit designer uses a threshold. Signals less than the threshold are ignored. For optimal control, the clinician needs the ability to adjust this relaxation threshold independently for each muscle signal. (This threshold is also called a *noise floor* or a *deadband,* but there are better uses for the latter word, and threshold is at least clear.) With a new patient, thresholds are usually set high. Gradually the user learns to suppress unwanted muscle contraction, and the thresholds are lowered. The clinician should be happy if the user can merely control direction when a myoelectric system is first set up. It is a waste of time to try to optimize all the settings on the first day or even after a single week. No athlete would expect to master a new sport in such a short time, and we should not expect prosthesis users to master a completely new use of their muscles in a short time either. When both direction and speed are controlled with little mental effort, the clinician can proceed to select a mode-shifting scheme if needed.

Using Two Inputs to Also Select the Device Controlled

Although independent inputs are the best way to control more than one device, as amputation levels become more proximal, one runs out of sufficient independent sources of control. One then has to use various methods for shifting control from one device to another. This shifting is usually called *mode shift-*ing. The typical assignment is to control both the hand and wrist with just two myoelectric sites on the forearm. The shift is often triggered by a co-contraction. Digital processors have permitted engineers to invent new ways to select which device is being controlled. Some of these new methods are discussed in the following sections, along with the positive and negative aspects of each.

Co-contraction to Shift Modes

Using older analog circuits, the presence of two signals each exceeding a threshold was easy to detect. This method for mode switching has been in use for two decades. Although it is easy to describe, the method requires the careful adjustment of various gains and thresholds if it is to work reliably. Sometimes the raw myoelectric signals are completely processed through a separate set of threshold circuits, but more often, co-contraction is detected using the two signals after each has had an appropriate gain and relaxation threshold set. Most detectors require both signals to be below these relaxation thresholds before the mode selector is active. When it is active, the direction control system ignores the signals for a settable delay period, while the mode selection system decides whether a co-contraction has occurred. The delay must be kept short or it becomes annoying and interferes with control. Thus, any system starting from a zero reset state is by necessity a rapid co-contraction detector. Such a system will ignore slow co-contractions and is rarely sensitive to an inadvertent shift. The chief difficulty comes with the use of muscles that are not an agonist–antagonist pair in the intact limb. Paired muscles will co-contract together so that the rapid rise is readily detected. In a high-level amputation, muscles are used that do not naturally fire together. For these muscles, another delay is needed to correct for the fact that one of the two muscles almost always fires later than the other.

Alternatively, the detector may simply shift whenever both muscle signals are above set thresholds. This simpler system is more likely to lead to inadvertent mode shifting. The shift may be announced by a beep from the electronics, especially during training. Such a beep is optional on most newer control systems. Co-contraction schemes need frequent attention in the new user. They should be retuned daily, then weekly, and finally monthly, until no further adjustment seems necessary. Figure 20-10 shows the computer screen used to set up a co-contraction method for shifting control from one device to another. This requires a rapid co-contraction of both muscles. For users who cannot master it, a simpler co-contraction scheme is available, but it is more prone to inadvertent mode shifting.

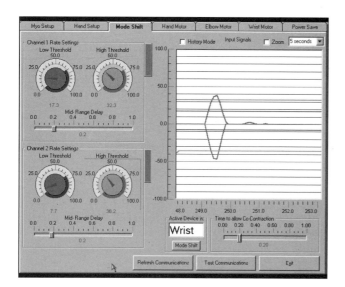

FIGURE 20-10

In the most reliable method of shifting control from one device to another, both the channel 1 signal (from chart center upward) and the channel 2 signal (from chart center downward) must cross both thresholds in the 0.2-second window that begins when either signal crosses the lower threshold.

The First-Muscle-Used Selection Scheme

Clearly, co-contraction schemes take a lot of work to set up correctly, and for some users they are not possible until after an extended period of single-device control has built up the user's abilities. Microprocessors allow the engineer to offer the clinician several new selection schemes that bypass these difficulties. For the first-muscle scheme to work, both signals must reliably descend below their relaxation thresholds. This resets the system, which is easily understood if elbow and hand are used as a control example, with biceps and triceps as the control muscles. Although it is natural for the biceps to flex the elbow and triceps to extend the elbow, it is *not* natural to designate one muscle as the "hand muscle" and the second as the "elbow muscle." Yet, that is exactly how this scheme works. Let the biceps be the "elbow muscle." If the biceps is the first muscle to contract during the zero state, elbow control is initiated. Just enough delay occurs with this first contraction so that the triceps can then be activated if an extension is desired. If flexion is desired, the user simply continues to contract the biceps. In a similar manner, an initial contraction of the triceps will initiate hand control with further activation opening the hand. Since further activation is easier than shifting muscles, triceps should be used to open the hand, because opening is the correct response in almost any emergency. If this concept seems confusing, compare it to the next one, which may be easier for the user to learn.

The Quick-Slow Selection Scheme

This scheme also requires a reliable zero state. The rapid contraction of either muscle selects one device. With hand and elbow, hand would usually be the quick device. A slow, deliberate contraction of either muscle then selects elbow control. Direction is selected by using the correct muscle—biceps for flex or close, and triceps for extend or open.

The Quick-Slow with Co-contraction Scheme

If the user can master a rapid co-contraction, quick-slow can be used to select hand or elbow, while a rapid cocontraction selects wrist rotation.

Returning to the Zero State

People often overshoot when moving a limb, and this is particularly true in myoelectric control, where there is little feedback. Thus it is essential that the user be able to reverse direction without shifting to another device by mistake. A settable delay is provided to enable the user to reverse direction. This delay must be kept short, however, so that the user can quickly shift control to the next device required.

Other Mode Selection Schemes

Many users find co-contraction schemes difficult or impossible. To help these people other triggers may be used for selection. Most often these are single or dual-action switches. (See discussion on Switch Control.)

Simple Switch Activation

Consider the elbow–hand problem. A simple twitch of the shoulder can activate a switch that shifts control from the default device, which is usually the hand to the elbow. The user can hear the switch click and can be confident that control has shifted or, using more recent controllers, a beep can be provided. Although control can be shifted and maintained until another switch activation, it usually takes less mental effort if control reverts to the default device after a delay. A beep may be provided to signal this change, especially if the user chooses to use a long delay before reversion.

Use of a Dual-Action Switch

Because few reliable switches are available to prosthetists, one of the Otto Bock company's dual-action pull switches is often used as a single-action switch to shift between modes. In this case, only the fully pulled state triggers change. For the selection of two nondefault devices, a dual-action switch should be supplemented with a beeper unless the user has acute hearing and can detect the subtle clicks of the microswitches inside the pull switch. The user must know when control shifts. Shift to the first alternate device is announced by a click or beep. The second device is activated by pulling harder than is required to reach the fully pulled position of the switch. A delay must be provided before the first device activates, so that this rapid pull does not activate the wrong device. Using microprocessors and computer setup screens, it is easy to get this delay right for each user, and it is also easy to program beeps, revert-to-default times, and other minor adjustments.

The Switch as a Back-up Trigger

Using microprocessors, it is easy to provide more than one way to trigger a mode shift. The author has used both co-contraction and switch activation on the same user with success. The user was a bilateral amputee, and in some arm positions co-contraction worked well, while in others the switch was best.

SERVO CONTROL OF ONE OR TWO DEVICES

A servomechanism is a closed-loop control. The input can be a position, force, voltage, or any other value. The output likewise can be any of a number of values. The mechanism or circuit compares the *desired* value with the *actual* value and generates a correction signal that operates the motor to change the *actual* value until the two values are within an exceptable difference. Typically, the greater the difference, the more power is delivered to the motor, thus increasing the speed or torque used to make the correction. In prosthetics, the actual value will be elbow flexion angle, wrist rotation angle, percent of hand closure, or some similar value. Usually a potentiometer (or pot) is built into the mechanism to generate this value as a voltage.

Because servo controls are relatively new in prosthetics and because it may be difficult to describe the system, practitioners tend to shy away from this prescription. However, once patients use this system, the advantages are obvious. It is far more intuitive than myoelectric controls because it gives more position feedback to the user.

Prosthetic Servos

To generate the desired value, the author has tried four types of servo input with amputees. The most successful has been the position servo. The input is a linear potentiometer with either 12mm or 25mm (0.5 or 1 inch) of travel that is pulled by a cable made of Spectra™, a lightweight, stiff, strong, and slippery fiber. The cable may be passed through a Bowden sheath so that the pull attachment point can be positioned conveniently. Typically, the cable is aligned across the back as part of a harness system. The line of action should pass over the center of the glenohumeral joint. This location guarantees that the user can accomplish arm forward flexion or abduction of the arm without activating the servo transducer. Forward protraction of the shoulder, however, will pull the cable. With the 12mm transducer pulling the cable, 6mm will half flex the elbow, 9mm will flex it three quarters of full, and so on.

The Set-It-and-Forget-It Strategy

A position servo lets the user employ proprioception to know where the elbow is even in the dark, but considerable mental effort is required to keep the joint under constant surveillance. To reduce mental effort, it is usual to hold the joint in one position for a settable interval, after which the servo circuit "goes to sleep." The user can then relax tension in the cable. The circuit is reactivated by pulling the cable until the potentiometer gives a signal greater than the signal present when the unit went to sleep. For a transhumeral amputee, the use of a position servo to control the elbow will leave a pair of myoelectric signals to independently control another function, such as hand grasp. This is a popular option, especially with previous users of a body-powered elbow.

The Dual-Device Servo

Once a servo has gone to sleep, the signal can be shifted to control a second device. Typically, this is done by reducing the input to zero. If the alternate device is a hand, pulling on the transducer increases the percent-open value until it matches the actual value being generated by the potentiometer in the hand. The hand then opens further. When the transducer is relaxed, the hand closes until it meets resistance, which increases the current going to the motor. The user then has two choices. Holding the transducer lets the hand go to sleep with a light grip. However, by further relaxing the cable pull, the user can let the hand grip increase until it reaches the manufacturer's maximum stall current value, at which point the motor is turned off and the servo circuit goes to sleep.

Keeping the Prosthesis Asleep

It would be easy to shift control back to the elbow by completely relaxing the cable tension, however, this would mean the user could never ignore controlling the prosthesis. Instead, it is better to let relaxation put the controller into "deep sleep." When in deep sleep, a slow pull on the cable reinitiates hand control, while a quick pull shifts control to the elbow. To avoid confusion, a beep can be generated every time control is shifted.

The Pull-Force Servo

If a miniature load cell replaces the linear potentiometer, the servo input becomes the force with which the harness straps are pulled. A pull-force is less intuitive than a position servo, but no actual motion is required, which can be an advantage. Another convenient force servo is one actuated by pushing on a force-sensing resistor (FSR). In prosthetics, the usual FSR is an LTI Touch Pad™. This pad mounts on any flat area 19mm in diameter and is usually pushed by moving the shoulder up or forward against the pad. FSRs do not produce a linear output, but when using digital processors, it is easy to correct for this so that the user feels that the pressure to move the servo all the way is twice as great as that used for going half way. In through-shoulder amputations, a single FSR can be used for servo control of the elbow, while separate FSRs are used for open hand and close hand signals.

The Myoservo

Tension in a single muscle can be used to control an elbow servo. Because myoelectric signals are inherently noisy, the myosignal requires extra filtering for servo use. This slows the response to change slightly, but is not serious.

EXTENDED PHYSIOLOGICAL PROPRIOCEPTION (EPP)

During the flurry of activity that followed the birth of the thalidomide babies in the 1960s, engineer David Simpson coined the phrase *extended physiological proprioception* (EPP). When the concept is applied to the control of a prosthetic joint, EPP requires that the angular speed, position, and torque about the joint be fully coupled to some other body motion so that the user's natural proprioception can be extended to feel the position, velocity, and force of the controlled joint. For instance, protraction and retraction of the shoulder might control elbow position.

Researchers have studied an EPP approach to elbow control and have produced working prototype control systems. EPP has been implemented using standard, available control hardware with both the Boston Elbow and the VASI Elbow for children 8 to 12 years of age. A cable is passed around a pulley that is coaxial with the artificial elbow. The cable must come from above and be tangent to the front of the pulley. It then wraps around the pulley and passes to a fixed point on the forearm. A sensor for measuring the tension in the cable is placed at this attachment point, or it may be placed at the input end of the cable. Typically, the cable is activated by a forward motion of the shoulder. (See the section on harnessing shoulder motion.) This scheme should be called unidirectional EPP or pseudo EPP because there is no way to push a cable. It gives the user complete feedback when using the elbow joint to lift the hand and forearm with or without any added weight.

BETTER PROSTHETIC CONTROL TECHNOLOGIES IN THE NEAR FUTURE

Human beings come hard-wired with a superb control system that starts with supervisory control in the brain and central nervous system. Most people can close their eyes and touch the tips of their fingers together with an accuracy of a few millimeters. If all this is true, why do we ignore most of it when we design prosthetic control systems? The answer is simple. In the past, we lacked the computational ability to collect the information needed for a more natural control system. Further, because only inadequate controls existed, designers made little effort to provide prostheses with multiple joints. This situation should change rapidly in the next 10 years.

Consider myoelectric control: Its great appeal is that it uses sensors external to the skin, and it enables one to harness the muscles that otherwise remain unused after an amputation. For the transradial amputee, it eliminates use of a harness. Offsetting these advantages is the fact that myoelectric control gives no sensory feedback. Experiments to improve on this situation suggest that several new approaches will come to fruition in the near future.

Microcineplasty

In a cineplasty operation, a tunnel of skin is created and internal muscle and tendon structures are altered so that a muscle can be used to move an attachment passing through the tunnel. The biceps cineplasty was popular during and after World War II and is still in use. However, the operation is substantial and the tunnel must be carefully maintained throughout the rest of the user's life. More recently, Dudley Childress and his colleagues at Northwestern University have proposed the microcineplasty, a much less extensive procedure because the purpose of the cineplasty is only to produce motion with relatively little force—the power is provided by use of EPP control circuitry. The electronics are available now and are no longer an obstacle to development. For instance, the author has a circuit that can control four or five motors. All motors cannot be operated simultaneously, but two pairs can. The controller consists of two flat packs with a total volume of less than 1 cubic inch. This technology should improve the lot of the transradial amputee in the near future.

Natural Myoelectric Control

Consider a unilateral transradial amputee. The subject is asked to move the remaining hand and wrist while simultaneously moving the phantom hand. Myoelectric data is collected from multiple sites. After a few sessions of data collection and much number-crunching on a computer, a simple computer algorithm is generated. The subject then uses this algorithm to generate data while moving the phantom limb. This research is well on its way to being a commercial product and is the work of Kristin Farry and colleagues at Intelligenta in Houston, TX. Using a "natural" myocontroller, an amputee will use the hard-wired control system present at birth to control multiple functions simultaneously. Natural control has as its chief advantage over microcineplasty in that no invasive procedures are required. It lacks any instantaneous feedback concerning position, velocity, or force, however the author has observed amputees who were able to control hand grasp and two wrist motions simultaneously with this approach. The system used only two forearm electrodes to collect muscle control data. Recently, Kevin Englehart at UNB has reported even better results by increasing the number of electrodes to four.

Increasing the Number of Myosites

Several years ago, Todd Kuiken, M.D., Ph.D., now of the Rehabilitation Institute of Chicago, observed that in a transhumeral amputee, large muscles remain in the upper arm with little to do except to provide two myosignals (4). At the same time the upper arm contains the remnants of the nerve trunks that previously controlled all of the hand and forearm muscles. He set out to study the possibility of reassigning portions of the biceps and triceps to forearm nerves. Feasibility studies in animals have been successful, and this work is expected to lead to an increased ability for myoelectric control by higher-level amputees within five years. Tremendous challenges must be overcome. For instance, will the neurosurgeon be able to identify useful function in the operating room with the assistance of the patient? Even with the most fortuitous selection of nerve bundles for reenervating parts of these muscles, the techniques

of Farry and Engelhart will probably be needed to recover useful data for natural control using these new multifunctional muscles.

MOTION AROUND THE SHOULDER AND PROSTHETIC CONTROL

A general rule of prosthetic control is that one should avoid using any muscle or motion that is still performing its natural function in a useful way. This precludes most use of shoulder area motion with a transhumeral amputee, because these muscles are still in use for positioning the upper arm. This rule, however, conflicts with the rule that says that as many functions as possible should be independently controlled.

Shoulder Motion Benefits to the Transhumeral Amputee

Using a conventional cable-operated transhumeral prosthesis, protraction of the shoulder assists abduction and forward flexion of the upper arm in producing the 5 inches (125mm) of excursion needed to operate the prosthesis. Using an electric prosthesis, this assist is not needed. In fact, one advantage of an electric transhumeral prosthesis is that it permits operation using any degree of forward flexion or abduction. The disadvantage of the typical electric transhumeral setup is that one pair of myoelectric signals from biceps and triceps is asked to control multiple functions. This sequential control is slow and unnatural. Most amputees can learn to give up their normal use of protraction and retraction of the shoulder when it will give them independent control of additional functions. Protraction is often harnessed to provide switch, servo, or EPP control of a single function; retraction is usually reserved for switch activation.

Isolation of Protraction and Retraction in the Transhumeral Amputee

Figure 20-11 shows a typical modern transhumeral socket. Note the stabilizing wings that prevent unwanted internal and external rotation. To isolate shoulder protraction and retraction, all harness attachments must be made at two specific points on these wings—the centers of rotation in abduction. These points are typically isolated during the fitting of a clear plastic check socket. The procedure is simple. First, you guess the location of the center of rotation. Place a dot of tape here. When the amputee is asked to abduct, the dot will typically move through a circular arc. Move the dot to the center of the arc and repeat the motion. When the dot no longer moves, the center of rotation has been

A

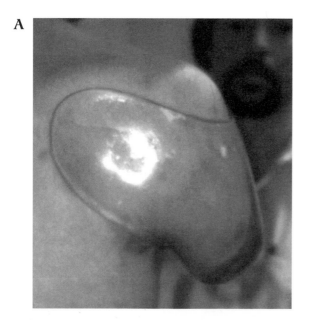

B

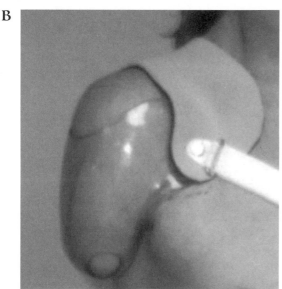

FIGURE 20-11

In the top view, the posterior wing can be seen to lie flat against the spline of the scapula. In the lower view, a neoprene band has been added across the top to aid in suspension. Both it and the chest strap are attached at a point close to the center of rotation in abduction.

located. It helps if the observer is several meters away to avoid parallax. The procedure is repeated in front. These points should be used to provide low friction "hinges" for attaching all subsequent harnessing. Electric prostheses are heavy, so a broad band of stretch neoprene is usually passed over the top of the shoulder, while straps to the contralateral side are independently

attached to the two hinge points. For good control, these straps must not slide on the contralateral side. Both the anterior and posterior straps are made of elastic, with a nonstretch cord or cable attached near the sound side. Ideally, the cord passes inside the elastic strap. (The Otto Bock company offers such a strap with convenient terminations) This cable must pass over the attachment point on the posterior wing. Thereafter, a pulley or sheath is used to route it to the switch or other transducer. The stiffness of the elastic across the back is an important variable. It should be sufficiently resistant so that the user can feel the increase in tension as the shoulder is protracted. A little slack is left in the cables that run to the switches, linear transducers, or force sensors. Switches usually require only 6mm of travel and linear transducers 12mm or 25mm. Friction must be avoided, because the switches and transducers have relatively weak return springs. The author prefers to replace the plastic-covered steel cables provided by most manufacturers with ultraslippery braided cords made of Spectra™. Only special knots may be used with Spectra™, because most familiar knots will simply not hold with this remarkable material. A Spectra™ line of a given diameter will be lighter than nylon, stronger and more stretch-resistant than steel, and almost as friction free as Teflon™.

Shoulder Motion and the Through-Shoulder Amputee

In 1994, the author did a series of experiments to clarify what happens as the shoulder is moved with respect to the spine and rib cage. Although the experiments yielded quantitative data, they were only illustrative because a single subject was studied. The subject was a typical fiftieth percentile man, so the numbers can be scaled to adjust for larger or smaller persons. The critical anatomical fact that links all studies of shoulder motion is the fixation of the clavicle with respect to the sternum. The sternoclavicular joint acts as a center of rotation for any motion of the acromion, which is affixed to the other end of the clavicle. This anatomy generates a constraint. The tip of the acromion can only move on the surface of a sphere with the sternoclavicular joint as the center of rotation.

Quantitative Motion of the Acromion

The experiment was simple. A metal frame similar to that shown in Figure 20-15 (see page 220) was used to provide a reference, rigidly located with respect to the spinal column and rib cage. A cylindrical sheet of translucent plastic was then attached to the frame and a bright spot was marked on the skin at the tip of the acromion. The

BACK

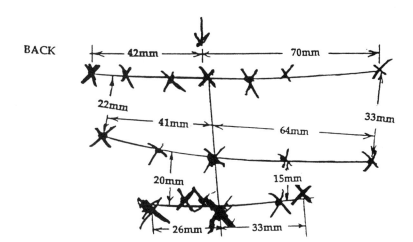

FRONT   **FIGURE 20-12**

Original data on motion of the acromion, showing three "best-fit" horizontal lines and one vertical. The center horizontal line shows the motion of the acromion when the shoulder is relaxed with respect to elevation. The vertical line is neutral with respect to front-back motion. Distances in millimeters have been superposed.

subject then moved the tip forward and back while relaxed with respect to elevation and depression. This created the neutral "horizontal line." In a similar manner, a neutral vertical line was created, and the fullest extent of motion was recorded. Figure 20-12 shows a cleaned-up version of the original recording with the cylinder flattened out. What is immediately apparent is that the tip of the acromion makes a considerable front-to-back excursion as well as up and down. Since the percentage of the sphere of contact that is covered is rather small, one can look at the plot as if dealing with X-Y coordinates on a plane. Thus, motion of the shoulder can cause the tip of the acromion to move independently in two directions roughly orthogonal to one another. Should this motion be used to control positional servos, two joints can easily be controlled independently. However, controlling only two joints with shoulder motion may not be good enough for the amputee, considering how many degrees of freedom have been lost. One more independent control can be added if a pair of muscles can be found for use as myoelectric control sites. These should not be muscles that tie the scapula or clavicle to the core anatomy. A suitable pair would be the lower portions of the pectoralis and teres major. Since the exact anatomy is often uncertain after surgery, the candidate's muscles must first be located and tested as possible myocontrol sites, then verified that they can be fired independently of the position of the acromion or how strongly it is pushing in any direction. If shoulder motion is to be used for control, the proposed myosites must maintain good electrical contact wherever the shoulder is located. A well-designed frame socket can accomplish this.

A Frame to Permit Shoulder Motion and Myoelectric Control

The primary support for a prosthetic arm prosthesis must be a well-designed frame socket. The typical

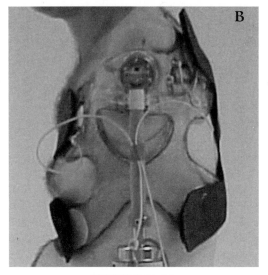

FIGURE 20-13

Two views of a frame socket optimized for myoelectric control. Although the frame seems too low to resist sliding downward when viewed from the front, the side view shows how the posterior wing rises high up the back. This wing and the chest wall form a wedge with an angle of almost 45° that keeps the frame from slipping and holds the electrodes in intimate contact.

shoulder socket for myoelectric control is shown in Figure 20-13. It will support a prosthetic arm and maintain good contact with a pectoralis myosite at the level of the axilla. Downward thrust is taken up by the wedge angle between the anterior and posterior walls. This socket permits anterior and posterior straps to the contralateral side to capture a small amount of forward or rearward motion. Protraction and retraction, however, will move the entire socket. It is an outstanding socket design, but does not work well when forward-back shoulder motion is used, and it will not do a good job of permitting the up-down motion of the acromion to be captured. Figure 20-15, conversely, shows a frame that leaves the acromion freer to move. This socket precludes the location of a pair of good myosites unless the portion immediately over the clavicle has a gap so that the frame can move down snuggly against the chest and back.

Rigging for Dual-Servo or Dual-Switch Control

The study of shoulder motion also yielded information on how to separate two independent motions. Consider the frame shown in Figure 20-15. A small plastic cap covers the acromion. This cap is the moving element, and the frame socket is the fixed element. In front-back motion, the frame attachment points are located close to the midline as shown. Attach a string to the cap in front and another in back. Move the attachments on the frame up and down until raising and lowering the acromion causes the least shortening of the strings.

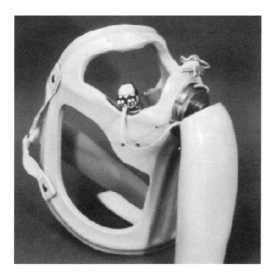

FIGURE 20-14

This frame wraps further around the torso than the previous example. A large opening leaves the acromion free to activate switches, one of which is visible.

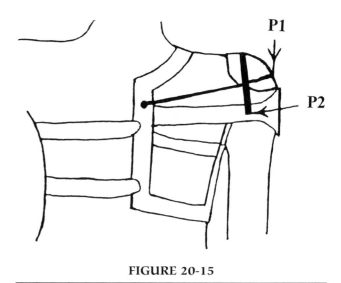

FIGURE 20-15

Posterior view of a frame used to find the optimal locations for "independent" activation cables.

Next, place a piece of string over the plastic cap and pass it down to attachment points on the front and back of the frame. This string should cross the front-back string at approximately right angles. For best results, run this string through a Bowden sheath to permit the friction-free motion of the cable that will activate a switch or servo. Vary the location of the sheath until there is essentially no change in the length of the cord as the shoulder is moved forward and back, and the cord slides inside it. Note that the depression of the shoulder has not been used. A second Bowden sheath across the cap can capture depression. A spring or bungee cord is used to keep this cable in tension until the shoulder is depressed several millimeters. When the spring permits slack in the cable an "unpull" switch can control another function. The author has modified a standard Otto Bock 9X18 pull switch to perform this function.

Touch Control

Multifunction electric control of elbow, wrist, and grasp was first demonstrated as a practical clinical choice by the late William Sauter at the Ontario Crippled Childrens' Centre. His frames were made of aircraft aluminum. Motion of the shoulder activated three dual-action switches, one for each function. Today, the three switches are often replaced by up to five Touch Pad™ force sensing resistors (FSRs). The FSRs are preferred, if sufficient sites are available, because they permit proportional control of speed and grip force. Figure 20-14 shows a typical Sauter frame with switches. Unfortunately the Sauter frame is labor intensive and has fallen out of favor. Instructions for adapting the frame shown in Figure 20-13 and for taking the cast is given in the next section.

Taking a Shoulder Cast for Pads or Switches

This technique requires a rigid cast of the entire shoulder area, almost to the midline. Start by wrapping plastic wrap all the way around the subject as well as across the shoulder. Both the cast and the check socket to follow will need stiffening ribs. Otherwise, when a carbon-fiber-stiffened frame is produced, it will not fit. With your hands on the chest and back, have the amputee move the shoulder both up-down and front-back. Mark a line on the plastic wrap that is protecting the skin to identify the transition from movable anatomy to fixed. Be sure that this transition and all other useful landmarks appear on the positive plaster model. To provide for the free motion of the acromion, you must eliminate a lot of the area that the myoelectric frame uses for suspension. You can replace this by placing your hands on the back and chest wall near the mid line, high but below the clavicle in front. In back, stay both high and medial to minimize the socket shifting when the subject tries to move the acromion through the full range of motion. Mark out two areas, front and back, that have a good wedge angle and are large enough to provide comfortable suspension. These areas will produce the upper wings of a socket similar to that shown in Fig. 20-16. The lower wings can be identical to those shown.

After taking the cast and producing a model, create a bridge above the acromion by adding up to 12mm of a foam rigid enough not to collapse during the thermoforming of the check socket. Cover the top of the acromion and the front and back to full thickness but taper the foam where it approaches the midline and the transition line. At the same time, add plaster on the lateral wall to create room for motion without friction and to mount the attachment ring for the shoulder joint.

Creating a Bridge for Locating Pads or Switches

FSRs must be mounted on a flat surface. Avoid mounting them where the shoulder creates a sliding shear force during the interaction. The five popular locations are straight up, up and forward, up and back, straight forward, and straight back. For either FSR Touch Pads™ or shoulder-activated linear transducers to work well, the socket must leave the shoulder free to move as described above. Few people are making frame sockets for FSR control. Therefore, use the foam technique above or the procedure outlined here the first time you try this:

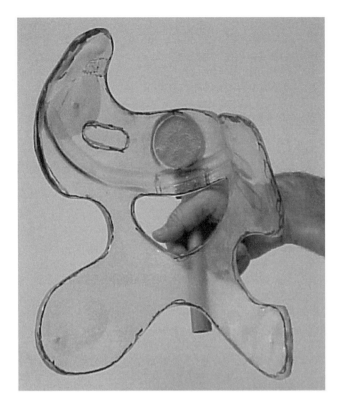

FIGURE 20-16

This myocontrolled socket prevents the forward-back motion of the acromion. To adapt the design for FSR control, you must free up the lateral area and create two suspension areas that are high and near the midline. The lower wings are the same in both designs.

1. First create a rigid frame-style check socket that permits the acromion to move freely. This socket needs a mounting point for the shoulder joint, which is critical, because the full weight of the proposed prosthetic components should be applied during testing and evaluation.
2. If you used the technique described earlier, you will already have a mounting bridge for the FSRs. If you skipped the foam-adding step, you need to create a bridge now. Use a long strip of aluminum with a cross section of about 3 × 35mm. Bend this strip and position it until the amputee can almost touch it when arcing forward and then back while raising the shoulder as far as possible. Rivet or cement it in place when you are sure that it will be over all the bony anatomy that will activate the pads. If you created a plastic bridge in the check socket, you will quickly see where some of the bridge can be cut away.
3. Make several metal disks about 20 to 25mm in diameter. You need one test disk and as many more as you will have control sites.

4. Temporarily tape a test FSR over one disk. Attach it to any device that will report the pressure on the FSR. Typically, the readout will be part of the proposed control system, and the readout itself will be on a computer screen.

5. Take some foam and place a small piece between the metal disk and the bridge. Adjust the thickness of the foam until the amputee can reach straight up and touch the FSR. You want this pad almost as far up as the user can reliably reach. At this time merely note its approximate location.

6. Move the test setup to other points on the bridge. Lots of play at this point will influence where you make your final selection of control points. You are looking for points where bony prominences will reliably activate the FSRs. Posterior points will be the most difficult to find.

7. For your final selection of pressure points, select as many locations as the user can control. Thin amputees will be able to activate more points than those who are well padded. Your final points must survive the process you intend to use to create your definitive socket. To do this, to mix up a little quick-setting cement (body putty works well). Place this between one of the metal disks and the bridge. Have the amputee hold the shoulder comfortably against the pad as the resin hardens.

8. Place the test FSR over each disk in turn and verify that the amputee can generate the full range of control outputs.

9. Fill in the areas between the disks until the disks protrude into "patient space" just a few millimeters. Repeat your tests until the amputee never quite touches the filled in area while moving from disk to disk. When two adjacent disks will control the same device (for example, opening and closing the hand), you may want a continuous smooth surface. The user will then be able to reverse direction easily.

10. Test the resulting locations with the actual prosthetic components. You are particularly interested in how the shifting of weight as the elbow flexes affects the pads controlling elbow motion. Some pad positions will cause jerky motion and may require pad reassignment. If you want to use one of the pads to position the elbow using a force servo, you should locate this pad and test its ability to do its job before selecting any other site.

11. Place the socket with the finished bridge over your original cast. It should now be relatively easy to build up plaster to "cast" the inside surface of the bridge, which will define the inner surface of the definitive bridge in the frame socket.

USING SWITCHES WITH VARIABLE-SPEED CONTROL SYSTEMS

Modern hands, grippers, and elbows are capable of operating at high speeds that make precise positioning impossible. However, since speed is often useful, using a switch to have these devices operate at a single slow speed is also a poor choice. Modern programmable circuits circumvent this limitation in several ways. Three switch control strategies are described here. The input is a dual-action switch with two and sometimes three outputs, depending upon how far the switch is pulled or pushed or which direction a rocker is moved. From a logic point of view, these switches before activation output 0,0 on two lines. When activated, they go through a sequence of 0,1; 1,1; 1,0 or 0,1; 1,0 on the output lines. To make the argument clear, operation of a hand using a pull switch is described with each strategy below.

The Alternate Strategy

When the control is first turned on, the switch will always open the hand slowly when pulled to the first position. Each other position—two or two and three—opens the hand more rapidly. When the switch is released to its unpulled position, the controller reverses direction so that the next pull closes the hand with increasing speed, depending on how far the switch is pulled. Because the user may forget after a few minutes which direction is due to operate next, this strategy often includes a settable revert-to-open time, which might be 2 seconds. Since gripping harder is desirable, a slight delay is built into the response to the first switch position so that the user can set the hand to close next with a quick pull and release.

The Traditional Strategy with Settable Speeds

Using the simplest strategy, the first switch position closes the hand and the second opens it. Before controllers, the speeds were fixed and fast. Using a controller, the two speeds can be independently set to suit the user. Furthermore, a slight delay can be built into the response so that the hand does not grip harder during the time it takes the switch to go through position one on the way to two. If a 1,1 logic position is available between the other two positions, it can be programmed with another speed in either direction. Using this strategy, the user cannot forget what will happen next, but the two speeds are fixed.

The Speed-up Strategy

Here, the first position signals the device to close slowly and the second position to open slowly. As the switch is held in one of the two positions, the speed in that direction increases at a settable rate. In closing, this means that the maximum grip force is also increasing. Releasing the switch momentarily resets the speed to slow. For the open position, dropping momentarily into the closed position will reset the speed. A slight delay is always built into the first or close position. This strategy is not useful for hand control, but it works well to control an elbow.

LINEAR TRANSDUCER OR PROPORTIONAL SWITCH

The linear transducer is a simple variable resistor that can be pulled by a cord or pushed by a phocomelic finger. Typically, this device has a cord that moves 0 to 0.5 inch (0 to 12 mm) or 0 to 1 inch (0 to 25 mm). It can be used to detect almost any relative motion between different parts of the body. Little excursion and little force is required for operation. In fact, a stiffer return spring must often be added to help the user feel when the transducer first engages and to feel how far it has been moved. The linear transducer has been used as a positional servo to control both hands and elbows, but here we consider how it can be used in ways resembling a pull switch, a use in which it lends itself to the operation of several strategies.

The Quick-Slow Strategy

The controller is set up to measure how fast the resistence changes in the first 20% of the pull. Moving quickly through this region will cause the controller to open the hand with a speed proportional to how far out the transducer is pulled. Moving slowly into or through the first 20% will cause the controller to close the hand with a speed proportional to how far out the transducer is pulled. The full range of the transducer is available to control the speed. The transducer in Figure 20-17 is set up to provide quick-slow control of a hand. When the same transducer is activated by protraction of the shoulder, it can operate the positional servo strategy for positioning the Boston Digital Arm. This popular strategy reserves the signals from the biceps and triceps for independent control of the hand.

Two-Position Strategy

Using this strategy, the middle 20% of the range is a dead band with no activation. From 0 to 40% of the

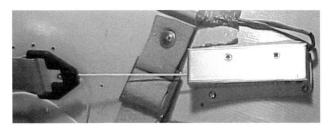

FIGURE 20-17

This linear transducer designed by the author measures 19 × 64 × 10mm (0.75 × 2.5 × 0.37 inches). The cable can be set up to pull 0 to 12 or 0 to 25mm.

pull, the hand closes with increasing speed after a slight delay; from 60 to 100%, it opens with increasing speed. This strategy works well for those who have a good proprioceptive sense for body motion. One can increase the user feedback by using a spring that engages when the transducer reaches the half way point. If the spring is set up to engage at about 70% of full travel, and dead bands are set near 35% and 70%, the transducer space can be divided into three control regions instead of two.

Two-Function Strategy

Adding a spring that engages at about 70% gives the user a way of detecting entrance into a zone that can control a second function, such as elbow flexion. Merely entering into this zone and pulling more or less will control speed but not direction. To control the direction of this extra function, an additional method must be employed. When the transducer output crosses the 70% threshold, the controller waits for a settable small interval long enough for the transducer to reach the 100% level. If 100% is reached, the device will go in one direction proportionally, whereas if 100% is not reached the device will move in the other direction.

FEEDBACK TO THE PROSTHESIS OR USER

The human hand is both a manipulator and a sensor. People use their hands to detect which object they are touching in their pockets and then to control pulling out the right object. Although there is little likelihood that prostheses will ever attain this level of sophistication, much can be done to assist the amputee without increasing mental load.

Autonomous Hand Control

The Otto Bock company offers a semiautonomous Sensor Hand. This hand automatically increases grip force if a held object begins to slip. For a number of years, Peter Kyberd has been working on autonomous hand control. He places several sensors in the artificial hand to detect when a finger or thumb meets resistance. The particular location of the resistance tells the hand which of several grip styles to use. His work will have commercial applicability once manufacturers develop a hand with separate activators for the thumb and the fingers. Also needed are hands where the thumb and finger axes are not parallel; to make full use of this approach, the thumb position should be movable.

Alerting the User

Many of the strategies discussed in this chapter use the same pair of muscles to control several devices. Users need to know which device is in use. Several ways can be used to do this: The controller can be set to revert to the default device so quickly that no confusion ever arises. This is not always practical, so methods have been devised to alert the user. These methods can, in some cases, convey quantitative information as well.

Use of a Beep

Miniature loudspeakers and beepers are widely available for mounting on circuit boards. Simple beepers only emit a single frequency. A miniature speaker can be used to deliver more than one frequency to convey several messages. The author has used beepers both during training and full time. The ability to change frequency is useful. In one case a user could not hear a high frequency beep, but could hear it when the frequency was lowered.

Use of Vibration

A vibrator designed for pagers is the size of a dime. It fits nicely between the inner and outer sockets and imparts a vibration to the entire prosthesis. The frequency can easily be varied. The Motion Control company has a similar way of alerting the user by vibrating the hand motor with a special alternating drive signal.

Varying the Frequency to Convey Information

During the 1970s researchers at MIT and UNB tried various ways to convey grip-force feedback to users. Both mechanical and electrocutaneous feedback were tested. In both cases, varying the frequency worked well to deliver force information, but amplitude changes were accommodated too quickly by the skin to be useful. Now that miniature vibrators are cheap and easy to control with the same microprocessor that runs the prosthesis, we can expect to see many commercial applications of this strategy. (Of course, one can use just two fixed frequencies to alert to two states.)

COMPANIES MAKING CONTROLLERS OR POWERED PROSTHETIC SYSTEMS

Animated Prosthetics, Inc.
Greensboro, NC 27406
(336) 691-9000
www.animatedprosthetics.com

Centri AB
Datavagen 6
S-175 43 Jarfalla, Sweden
+46 8 580 331 65
www.centri.se

Liberating Technologies, Inc.
325 Hopping Brook Rd.
Holliston, MA 01746
(508) 893-6363
www.liberatingtech.com

Motion Control Inc.
2401 S 1070 W Suite B
Salt Lake City, UT 84119
(801) 978-2622
www.utaharm.com

Otto Bock Orthopedic Industry Inc.
3000 Xenium Lane North
Minneapolis, MN 55441
(612) 553-9464
www.ottobockus.com

Variety Ability Systems Inc.
2 Kelvin Ave. Unit 3
Toronto, Ontario M4C 5CB
Canada
www.vasi.on.ca

References

1. Scott RN, Childress DS. *A Bibliography on Myoelectric Control of Prostheses.* Frederickton, NB: Institute of Biomedical Engineering, 1989.
2. Plettenburg DH. *Pneumatically Powered Prostheses: An Inventory.* Delft University of Technology.
3. *Proceedings: UNB Myoelectric Controls.* Frederickton, NB: Institute of Biomedical Engineering, 1980–87, 1989–95, 1997, 1999.
4. Kuiken TA, Stoykov NS, Lowery MM, Taflov A. *Proceedings: International Society for Prosthetics & Orthotics.* Glasgow 2001.

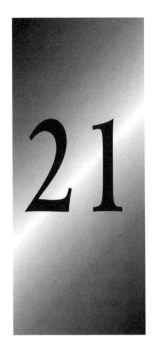

21 Creative Prosthetic Solutions for Bilateral Upper Extremity Amputation

Jack E. Uellendahl, CPO and Craig W. Heckathorne, MSc

The information in this chapter is primarily based on the authors' collective experience serving persons with bilateral arm amputations at the Rehabilitation Institute of Chicago, over a twelve-year period. During that time, we developed several conceptual guidelines for the prosthetic management of these individuals. Our current philosophy has been influenced greatly by the practical input of those served. It has been especially educational to listen to the comments of our clients and to attempt the solutions to basic problems faced in their daily lives as we "fine-tuned" their prosthetic systems over the years. Through the experiences of these clients, we have developed a framework upon which we base our recommendations for prosthetic fitting, knowing what has worked and why. At the same time, problems that have not been solved keep us keen to explore the potential of new components and techniques introduced into prosthetic practice.

The ultimate goal is to provide a replacement for the limbs lost; however, current state-of-the-art is far from that goal. In a hand's exquisite complexity and beauty, nature has provided an instrument that is proficient in accomplishing such divergent tasks as striking with a hammer and playing the piano. The hand is used to express one's self either as a visual accessory to the spoken word or as a subtle, and sometimes more powerful, replacement for words. We greet acquaintances, embrace our loved ones, and hold our babies with our hands and arms. The loss of these emotionally intimate capabilities is profound and, for the most part, still beyond prosthetic restoration. At best, we can provide a variety of tools, including prostheses, that enable the user to better manipulate objects and minimize their dependency on assistance from others for manipulative tasks. The prosthesis as tool is the basic approach taken in this chapter.

ETIOLOGY

The majority of acquired bilateral arm amputations are the result of trauma. These include electrocution, explosions, manufacturing plant mishaps (such as punch press), and farming accidents. A notable cause of bilateral upper limb amputation that is a result of disease is pneumococcemia. We have seen several individuals with multiple limb amputations as a result of this disorder. Over the past dozen years, the Rehabilitation Institute of Chicago has treated more than forty bilateral arm amputees. The majority have had amputations consequent to electrocution.

Children with bilateral limb loss pose special challenges for the rehabilitation team. Congential bilateral limb deficiency is very rare, and the issues regarding prosthetic fitting can be quite different from those of adults. At the more distal levels, (i.e., transradial), they can be successfully fit very similarly to the adult amputee. Indeed, the philosophy for fitting adults outlined herein has merit for children even at higher levels of amputation (Figure 21-1). The problem is that due to their small size and immature cognitive ability at very young ages, children cannot be treated as small adults. With small size comes decreased force and excursion and a lower tolerance for weight. On the positive side, children with congenital limb deficiencies are often much more adaptable than adults having traumatic amputations. They can, with encouragement and tolerance for different approaches, develop great flexibility and skill with their bodies and limbs and achieve remarkable ability (1).

GENERAL PHILOSOPHY FOR FITTING

The basic objective of rehabilitation for the person with bilateral arm amputations is to enable him to become independent in activities of daily living and to promote

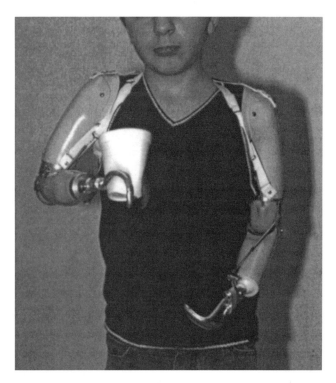

FIGURE 21-1

Bilateral transhumeral child amputee with body-powered prostheses. Note the differences between right and left terminal devices and wrist units, allowing greater manipulative potential.

participation in vocational and avocational pursuits. It is the goal of the prosthetic fitting to restore as much of the lost function as possible without overloading the patient with weight and gadgets. At the higher levels, this poses a significant challenge due to the increased number of prosthetic joints possible and the limited number of control sources. The control system should provide for the simple and reliable function of the various components. It is preferable to employ a dedicated control scheme, where each control source controls only one component. An often used and successful example of this is the unilateral transhumeral prosthesis that uses a body-powered elbow and a myoelectrically controlled prehension device (Figure 21-2). This type of prosthetic system offers straightforward control that is relatively easy to learn and allows the efficient use of the components. It also provides the possibility of coordinated simultaneous control of the elbow and prehensor for more physiologically natural reaching and grasping actions.

Unlike the person with a unilateral arm amputation, the person with bilateral amputations does not have the option of compensating for the inadequacies of a prosthesis through the use of an intact physiologic arm. Therefore, we approach the design of bilateral arm prostheses by considering how diverse prosthetic components might be configured to complement each other's function (and supplement each other's deficiencies) to serve the intentions of the user.

The prosthetist should consider all possible control sources when evaluating the person and then develop a prosthetic design that offers the desired function, the lowest weight, and the most straightforward operation. Control options that provide variable speed are preferable to constant speed options. Control options that provide feedback are favored over those that do not. It is also advisable to use control sources in a natural physiologic fashion when possible; for example, biceps to close a myoelectrically controlled hand or glenohumeral flexion to flex a cable-actuated elbow (2).

In the fitting of bilateral prostheses, it is advantageous to select control arrangements in which the operation of a component on one side does not affect any of the components on the opposite prosthesis. For example, if a client presents with a shoulder disarticulation on one side and a transhumeral amputation on the other, the transhumeral side will generally become the dominant limb. It might then be decided to use body-power for the transhumeral prosthesis to maximize the proprioceptive feedback to the user. In this arrangement, the shoulder disarticulation side will serve as an anchor for the transhumeral control cable, and the shoulder will be protracted to resist displacing forces when the transhumeral prosthesis is actuated. Conse-

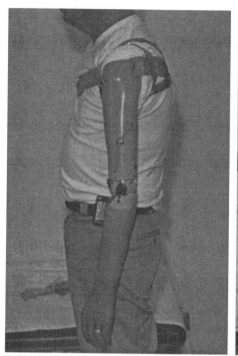

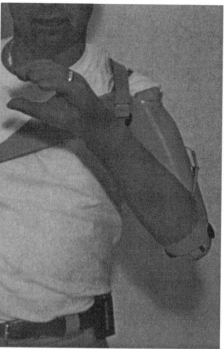

FIGURE 21-2

Dedicated control scheme for the transhumeral prosthesis. Body-powered control of the elbow and myoelectric control of the hand allows simultaneous control of these components.

quently, the shoulder will press into the anterior surface of the shoulder disarticulation socket and associated musculature will contract. In this case, it would be inadvisable to use either a pectoral myoelectric site or an electric push actuator (such as a switch or force transducer) in that region of the socket for control of a component within the shoulder disarticulation prosthesis (Figure 21-3). Faced with the complexity of high-level bilateral fittings, sometimes one seemingly small change in control strategy can cause a chain reaction of control source interaction.

SOCKET/SUSPENSION DESIGN

As with all prosthetic fittings, the socket must fit well to provide a close coupling of the user and the pros-

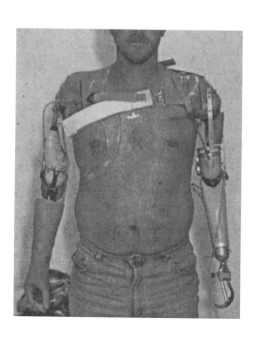

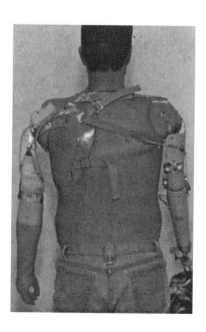

FIGURE 21-3

A hybrid control scheme is utilized for this high-level bilateral. Medial and posterior deltoid muscles control hand operation, thus avoiding inadvertent cross-control.

thesis. Although the socket may not be completely self-suspending, the interface should fit snugly and work with the suspension system to provide a prosthesis that feels firmly connected to the user. A stable prosthesis serves as an extension of the user's body. It should be possible for the user to exert forces through the prosthesis with minimal lost motion; that is, minimal movement of the residual limb within the socket. An intimately coupled prosthesis also provides a stable platform for the attachment of control linkages or transducers, thus enhancing the reliability and efficiency of control actions.

The socket is the foundation of the prosthetic system and any shortcomings will significantly affect the success of the prosthesis. This is true for all types of control systems, body-powered and electric. The socket and suspension system should be designed to allow easy independent donning and doffing whenever possible (Figure 21-4).

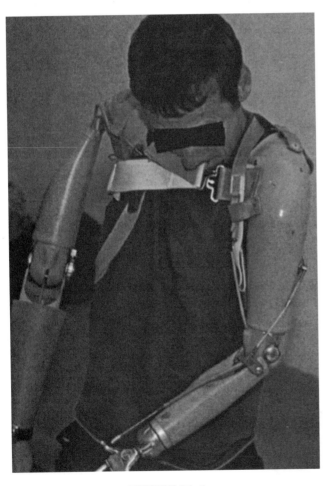

FIGURE 21-4

A high-level bilateral demonstrates independent donning of his shoulder disarticulation/transhumeral prostheses.

CONTROL

Prosthetic components can be divided into two broad classes: mechanical components and electromechanical (or motorized) components. Mechanical components can be controlled either manually or by body movement through a mechanical linkage. Components that are manually controlled are sometimes referred to as passive components. They are positioned by pushing or pulling the component against an external object or, sometimes, against the surface of the body.

Body-powered components are most commonly controlled by a movement of the residual limb relative to the torso. A linkage, generally a plastic or metal cable of fixed length, crosses from an anchor point on the torso to an attachment on the distal part of the prosthetic component. Movement of the residual limb away from the anchor point on the torso forces movement of the distal part of the prosthetic joint toward the anchor point because the length of the cable is fixed. Controlling the positioning and speed of movement of the residual limb directly controls the positioning and speed of movement of the prosthetic component.

The cable actuation of body-powered prostheses provides users with a wealth of proprioceptive feedback through the physiologic joints harnessed to the prosthetic components (3). Users of these devices can readily perceive the position and speed of movement of the prosthetic components. In addition, gravitational and mechanical forces acting on the prosthesis are transferred to the user through the control cable, further enhancing awareness of the prosthetic components. The control cable linking the user's joint position and movement directly to the position and movement of the prosthetic components is the key to the enhanced perception of the prosthesis and associated fine control.

The control of electromechanical components can be done in a variety of ways. One method is to use electrical signals produced by muscles contracting in the residual limb. These signals can be detected at the skin surface and converted electronically into a signal that controls the action of a motorized component. This method is commonly referred to as *myoelectric control.*

Movement of one body part relative to another can also be used to produce an electrical control signal. In its simplest form, the movement can actuate a switch that signals the device to turn on or off. A more sophisticated form converts the movement, by means of an electronic transducer (e.g., a linear variable resistor or linear potentiometer), into a signal that is proportional to the amplitude of the movement. By varying the amplitude of the movement, the user can proportionally vary the response of the prosthetic component, making it move faster or slower or change torque faster or slower.

Proportional electronic control can also be achieved through the application of force with relatively little movement. This is achieved with a type of transducer that is sensitive to applied forces, such as a strain gauge or a force sensitive resistor (FSR).

At present, the control options for electric-powered components do not offer the broad range and extent of proprioceptive feedback available through body-powered prostheses.

Whatever control arrangement is used, it should impose the minimum amount of mental loading on the user. In other words, the control of the prosthesis should not be so complicated as to make it the primary object of the user's attention. Rather, the task the user is attempting to perform should be primary, and the mental effort devoted to the prosthesis should be secondary.

Mental loading can be minimized by using physiologic correlation, isolation of control, and direct control. To establish a physiologic correlation, a control source is chosen that can be intuitively related to the corresponding action of a prosthetic component. The use of muscle contraction to produce a signal to cause gripping by a prehension device is one example. Using shoulder elevation (upward movement of the shoulder) to control the flexion of a prosthetic elbow (upward movement of the forearm) is another example (Figure 21-5).

Isolation of control seeks to avoid the problem of cross-coupling of control actions. Cross-coupling occurs when the control action for one prosthetic component inadvertently influences the action of one or more other components. This is a common problem in the use of bilateral body-powered prostheses, in which the movement to control one prosthesis produces forces that are transferred through the harness to the opposite prosthesis. Hybrid control arrangements that combine body-powered components and electric-powered components can be used to achieve isolation of control (Figure 21-6).

Direct, or dedicated, control (4) assigns separate control sources to each prosthetic component. This method provides the user with immediate access to a component and, sometimes, supports the simultaneous control of two components for the production of coordinated movements. This method generally cannot be fully implemented at higher levels of amputation, when the number of prosthetic joints to be controlled is often greater than the number of control sources (Figure 21-7).

COMPONENTS FOR BILATERAL FITTINGS

Prosthetic components with positioning joints can be divided into friction-type and locking-type. The use of friction joints should generally be avoided for bilateral applications. Friction joints are difficult to keep in proper adjustment. If the force needed to overcome the

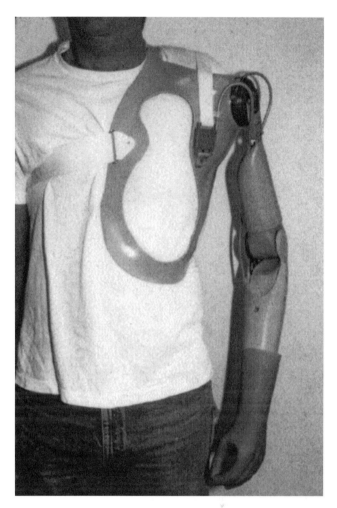

FIGURE 21-5

Use of shoulder elevation for elbow control via a harness pull switch.

friction is set too high, it will be difficult for the user to orient the device as needed. If the force is set too low, the component will not maintain its position against externally applied forces during activities and will slip. Locking joints are preferred for bilateral applications because they can be easily positioned when unlocked yet become a rigid extension of the user's body when locked. Electric-powered components are designed to be self-locking when not powered.

Prehensors

The new bilateral arm amputee will most likely prefer to be fit with prosthetic hands. This is a natural choice, considering that it is reasonable for the amputee to expect that the technology is available to replace the function and appearance of the physiologic hand. However, this is not the case with current technology. If, after

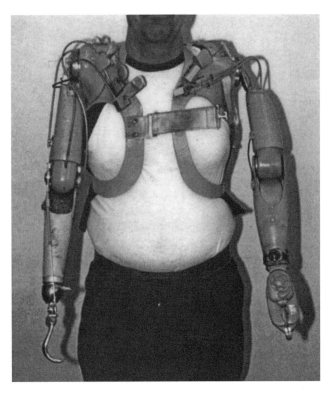

FIGURE 21-6

Isolation of control is achieved for this bilateral shoulder disarticulation amputee by using all body-powered control on the right and all electric control on the left.

a fair presentation of the prosthetic options, and ideally conversations with similar users, it is decided to proceed with hands, then variable speed myoelectrically controlled hands are a good choice. A small minority of clients with transradial amputations have done well with myoelectrically controlled hands.

However, in our experience, relatively few persons with bilateral amputations prefer handlike prehension devices over the long term, even among those who have had the opportunity to use them. Handlike devices are found to be bulky and to obstruct the view of the object being grasped. Most prefer body-powered split hooks on both prostheses or a split hook on one and a utilitarian electric-powered device that is not shaped like a hand on the other. The slender fingers of the split hook allow relatively good visual access to the work area and the objects being handled.

Those who prefer two body-powered split hooks often choose to use two different types of hooks to have greater versatility in the handling of a wide array of objects. This would also be true of persons who use a body-powered split hook and an electric-powered utilitarian device. An electric-powered device also provides prehension forces three to six times the force possible with the number of rubber bands selected by typical split hook users.

Wrists: Rotation

Wrist rotation is essential for the effective orientation of the prehension device. A variety of mechanical wrist rotators are available that use either friction, spring-resisted detents, or locking mechanisms. At the transradial

A 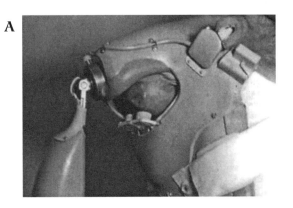   **B**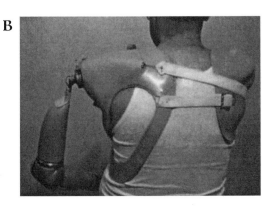

FIGURE 21-7

This bilateral humeral neck amputee is fitted unilaterally, utilizing a combination of body motions to achieve dedicated control of three electrically powered components. **A.** A pair of force sensitive resistors are positioned beneath the mobile humeral segment for variable speed control of the prehensor. The chin nudge–operated rocker switch provides constant speed control of the wrist rotator. The lever situated above the rocker is used to operate the locking shoulder. **B.** A linear actuator is positioned posteriorly using biscapular abduction for variable speed control of the electric elbow.

level, it may be acceptable to use friction- or spring-resisted detent mechanisms. However, at the transhumeral and shoulder disarticulation levels, we have found wrists that can be locked in place to be most effective. If a cable-actuated prehensor is used, the range of wrist rotation will be limited to a maximum between 135 to 180 degrees because of the control cable crossing the joint.

Electric-powered wrist rotation is also possible and can be controlled in a variety of ways, independent of other devices if a separate control source is available or in sequence with other devices if a common control source must be used. In conjunction with an electric prehension device, it is possible to have a rotation range of greater than 360 degrees because no control cable crossing the wrist joint is needed to activate the prehensor (Figure 21-8).

Wrists: Flexion

Almost all persons with bilateral amputations prefer to have at least one wrist flexion unit, and many choose to have wrist flexion incorporated in both prostheses. Flexion is especially helpful for body-centered activities, such as feeding, dressing, oral and facial hygiene, and toileting. All adult-size mechanical flexion units have locking mechanisms. At present, no electric-powered flexion units are available in North America.

Elbows

The selection of the most appropriate elbow should include a careful evaluation of weight, control options, and compatibility with the other components desired. Body-powered elbows are lighter than electric-powered

units, but provide the least amount of live lift. Electric-powered elbows have greater lifting capacity, but are heavier and lack the proprioceptive feedback inherent in the cable control of body-powered elbows.

In our experience, electric-powered elbows are rarely accepted bilaterally. Our most successful applications of electric elbows have been with persons having bilateral shoulder disarticulations who choose to use an electric-powered elbow on one prosthesis and a body-powered elbow on the other. The two elbows complement each other, with the electric-powered one providing greater live lift capacity while the body-powered elbow provides better control in positioning. Persons with bilateral transhumeral prostheses almost exclusively prefer bilateral body-powered elbows as part of the four-function forearm setup (Figure 21-9).

Humeral Rotators

Humeral rotation is generally provided with a friction joint, called a *turntable*, built into the prosthetic elbow.

A

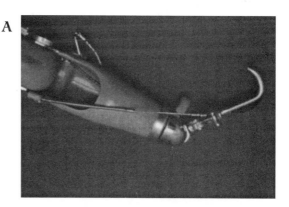

B

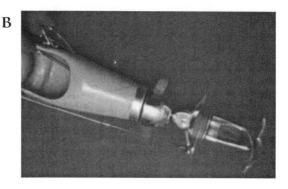

FIGURE 21-9

The four-function forearm setup uses the control cable to **A.** flex the wrist (when unlocked); and **B.** supinate the hook (when unlocked). The same control cable flexes the elbow (when unlocked) and opens the hook (when all other components are locked).

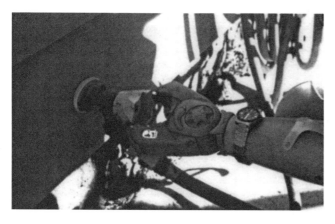

FIGURE 21-8

A bilateral shoulder disarticulation amputee uses the continuous wrist rotation provided by an electric wrist rotation unit to open/close this water spigot.

There are two notable exceptions. The RSL Steeper company offers a locking turntable that is incorporated into their elbow mechanism. However, the lock control cannot be readily adapted to use by a person with bilateral amputations.

Rimjet Corporation offers a locking humeral rotator that is designed for mounting on the proximal plate of a Hosmer Dorrance E-400 elbow, although it is possible to adapt this rotator for other elbows, including electric elbows (5). The lock is operated by a control cable that can be actuated through a control harness or chin-actuated nudge control (Figure 21-10).

Shoulders

Shoulder joints are generally friction controlled and configured with either two separate axes of rotation (flexion/extension and abduction/adduction) or a ball-and-socket configuration. The Liberty-Collier Locking Shoulder Joint (and the MICA Locking Shoulder Joint that preceded it) features a locking flexion/extension joint with friction-type abduction/adduction. The locking mechanism of the Liberty-Collier joint provides free swinging when the joint is not rigidly locked. Free swinging shoulder joints give persons with bilateral

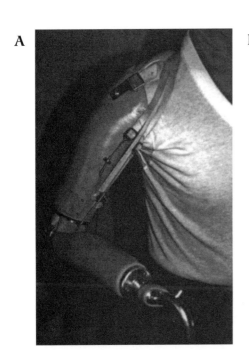

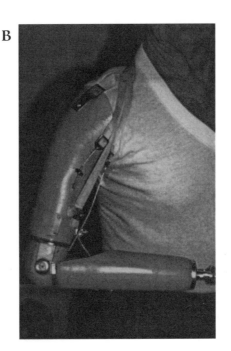

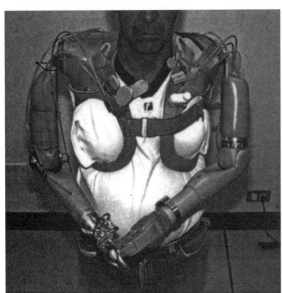

FIGURE 21-10

The positive locking humeral rotation unit **A.** shown in a neutral position and **B.** internally rotated. The humeral rotation lock cable is operated in parallel with the elbow lock. **C.** For the bilateral shoulder disarticulation amputee, locking humeral rotation allows the prehensors to be brought into opposition with each other. Also, the ability to push and pull without loss of humeral rotation position is advantageous.

shoulder disarticulations a more natural appearance and feel when they are walking.

The positioning of the unlocked joint can often be accomplished by simply allowing gravity to orient the arm as the user bends or extends at the waist. Alternatively, the user can push or pull the prosthesis (with very little effort) against an object or ballistically position the arm by swinging the prosthesis forward or backward. When the desired position is achieved, the user locks the joint, and the position of the prosthesis (with respect to the socket) is maintained. The Liberty-Collier Joint locks at 10-degree intervals and is limited to approximately 180 degrees of flexion and 36 degrees of extension to allow for cables crossing the joint (Figure 21-11).

The ease with which the Liberty-Collier Locking Shoulder Joint can be positioned and locked, together with the increased range of positioning of the joint,

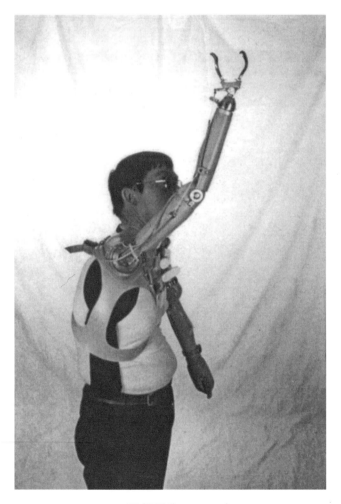

FIGURE 21-11

A bilateral SD amputee demonstrates operation of his prehensor overhead using a locking shoulder joint.

improves the utilization of the total prosthesis. Also, the rigidity of the locked shoulder joint allows the person to use the prosthesis more effectively as an extension of the body, to transmit forces through the structure of the complete prosthesis.

FITTING PRINCIPLES AND CONSIDERATIONS

The bilateral arm amputee presents special difficulties and considerations in prosthetic fitting.

Transradial: Body-powered

The transradial socket should be designed to capture as much residual motion as possible. The obvious range of motion that we are concerned with is elbow flexion, but pronation and supination are also extremely important with bilateral amputations. For the person wearing bilateral transradial body-powered prostheses, the sockets are typically trimmed below the epicondyles and the "screwdriver" shape is accentuated distally whenever there is usable residual pronation/supination. The harness is a standard figure-eight, typically incorporating a ring at the cross point for free movement of the straps, with flexible hinges and triceps pad. Compared with the unilateral figure-eight harness, the bilateral version eliminates the axilla loop, a frequent area for discomfort, and is therefore well tolerated by almost all patients. This type of prosthetic system is easy to don and doff independently (Figure 21-12).

Self-suspending socket designs may be employed in the fitting of a bilateral, as in the case of the person who wishes to switch back and forth between a myoelectrically controlled prosthesis and a body-powered system and have the same "feel" within the sockets of the two prostheses. Socket design for the body-powered arm is essentially the same as for the electric, although one should bear in mind the types of motions and magnitude of forces required for body-powered operation. A socket that works well for a myoelectric fitting might not be as comfortable when the person repeatedly pushes into the distal end when attempting to open the prehension device against the force of seven or eight rubber bands. It should also be pointed out that supracondylar self-suspending sockets block the ability to use residual pronation and supination. The harness for the self-suspending socket need be no more than a figure-nine design although, depending on the level of limb loss on the contralateral side, it may be necessary to provide appropriate anchor points for its harness.

Glenohumeral flexion and biscapular abduction are the body motions used to control the body-powered prosthesis. In the case of the self-suspending socket, it is desirable to attach the cross bar assembly tab to the

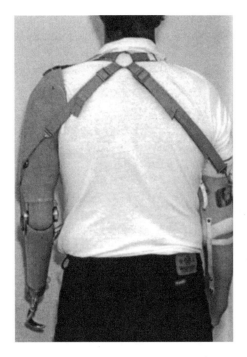

FIGURE 21-12

Bilateral transhumeral/transradial harness for body-powered control.

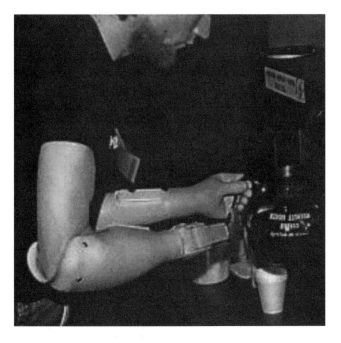

FIGURE 21-13

Bilateral transhumeral amputee using myoelectric prostheses with the Northwestern University socket design.

posterior aspect of the socket, which allows elbow flexion to contribute to terminal device control. Scapular or biscapular abduction is used for tasks near the midline of the body.

Wrist flexion units are certainly indicated for the person with bilateral transradial amputations, and locking wrist rotation units may be employed if length permits for the mechanism.

Transradial: Electric-powered

In the case of the myoelectric transradial prosthesis, it is desirable to provide a self-suspending self-contained prosthesis. The Northwestern University Self-Suspending socket (6) offers the advantages of increased elbow range of motion and easier donning compared with the traditional Muenster design. The socket is donned by pushing in rather than by pulling in. Pulling in is a technique that is to be avoided whenever possible in the case of a bilateral fitting because it makes self-donning difficult. This socket design is favored for all but the short transradial level, in which a higher anterior wall is needed for socket stability. The Northwestern design utilizes a lower anterior wall that allows for good elbow range of motion (Figure 21-13). The three-quarter socket design modification as described by Sauter (7) can be combined with the Northwestern socket. This

modification calls for a cutout to be placed over the olecranon to provide better air circulation in the socket and an improved cosmetic appearance, especially with the elbow in an extended position.

Variable speed myoelectric control is indicated for the bilateral amputee. If length permits, it is often advisable to utilize an electric wrist rotator. Wrist flexion is also desirable.

Transhumeral

Sockets for the transhumeral prosthesis should provide a close coupling of the remnant limb and the prosthesis to maximize the envelope of prosthetic function. Therefore, open shoulder designs (8) are preferred because they allow a relatively free range of motion at the shoulder joint. Another option for socket design is the half-and-half socket, as described by Sauter (9). This socket utilizes a flexible silicone proximal section that is fitted over the shoulder region and is fabricated as an integral part of the socket. The deltoid area is cut out laterally to provide improved flexibility and air circulation within the socket. The socket is rigid from the axilla level distally. This design works particularly well when an all-myoelectric prosthesis is provided, in which case the only function of the harness is to hold the silicone piece in place on the shoulder. Another option, similar to the half-and-half socket, is the flexible shoulder suspension system, in which a strip of Lycra-backed neoprene (or similar material) replaces the silicone "saddle" and is attached to the "wings" of the standard open shoulder socket.

As previously mentioned, body-powered elbows offer functional advantages over electric-powered units when the person has the requisite force and range of motion. A body-powered elbow with a strong counterbalance spring (to reduce the force needed to lift the weight of the forearm and prehension device) should be considered. It has been our experience that when a person with bilateral transhumeral amputations has been provided with myoelectrically controlled and, either concurrently or subsequently, body-powered prostheses, the amputee has, over time, chosen the body-powered system as the preferred option.

The type of body-powered system we use is based on the four-function forearm setup (10), which uses a common control cable to position four different body-powered prosthetic components: split hook, wrist flexion unit, wrist rotation unit, and elbow. The simplicity of the control is both an advantage and disadvantage. It is an advantage because the same physiologic control motion is used to position each of the four components, thus conserving available control sources. The control arrangement, however, is sequential—only one device can be positioned at a time. Therefore, it is not possible to produce coordinated movements involving two or more components. Furthermore, the physiologic control motion—generally glenohumeral flexion at the shoulder for the person with transhumeral amputations—is not well correlated with the action of each component. Glenohumeral flexion is most closely correlated with elbow flexion and wrist flexion, but is not correlated with supination of the wrist or opening of the split hook. The straightforward manner of the control and the presence of proprioceptive feedback appear to outweigh these disadvantages in the experience of our clients.

Therefore, the most successful type of fitting at the bilateral transhumeral levels has been body-powered control including four-function set-ups with or without locking humeral rotation. Usually the only difference between the two prostheses is the terminal device: The dominant side is fitted with a 5XA and the nondominant side with a 555. This affords greater variety in the types of objects that can be manipulated. When body-powered devices are used, it is usually most convenient for the sockets to be worn with a sock (or a tailored short sleeve tee shirt) to allow for easy independent donning and doffing.

Shoulder Disarticulation

The prosthetic interface for the shoulder disarticulation should be designed to spread the loading over as large an area as possible yet cover as little surface area as possible. The large perimeter of the socket will provide a stable foundation for positioning the prehensor in space. This is especially important when electric components are used, because the torque generated can be significant. Any areas of the socket not needed for structural support or for control site location can be cut away. Depending on the preference of the prosthetist, such a "frame" socket can be constructed of either plastic or aluminum. The suspension of the shoulder disarticulation interface can be achieved by using either a simple chest strap or by its attachment to the contralateral prosthesis, depending on the harnessing requirements of that prosthesis.

When fitting the bilateral shoulder disarticulation amputee, it is advisable to start with as simple a prosthetic system as possible. Often only the dominant side is fit initially. Control complexity should be kept to a minimum, starting perhaps with only an activated terminal device and elbow. As the person becomes acquainted with the use of the prosthesis, wrist function can be added, then humeral rotation and a locking shoulder joint. The nondominant prosthesis can be fit once the user has gained confidence in the use of the dominant side. Complexity on the nondominant side can be staged in a similar fashion. In general, the dominant prosthesis of the bilateral pair is configured with all-mechanical, cable-actuated components (similar to the four-function set-up), whereas the nondominant side incorporates either all electric or hybrid componentry (Figure 21-6).

The process of fitting a person with bilateral arm loss at the shoulders can take several months. Most of that time is spent by the person at home developing skills and identifying the problems and functional shortcomings of the prostheses as experienced in normal daily life. These problems should then be reported back to the rehabilitation team and solutions discussed among the members.

Forequarter

Forequarter amputations present significant challenges. Due to the complete absence of residual limb body motions, most control options are eliminated. When only one side presents with a forequarter amputation, that side is used primarily as an anchor point for the control of the longer contralateral side. Our experience with bilateral forequarter amputations is very limited. Individuals who have use of their lower limbs will certainly find foot use most practical. If foot use is not possible due to amputations, paraplegia, or other condition, robotic manipulators may be of value (11).

The most likely control at the forequarter level is a chin-operated nudge control. Force-sensitive resistors arranged under a rocker can provide variable speed control of the prehensor and/or elbow. In cases where the forequarter side is used solely as an anchor for the contralateral side, some clients prefer to have a lightweight passive prosthesis connected to the interface to give a more natural overall appearance (Figure 21-14). In the absence of a full prosthesis, the prosthetic interface should be sculpted with foam to provide shoulder symmetry.

USE OF PROTOTYPE PROSTHESES

In view of the unique presentation of each person and the plethora of possible component combinations, it is our opinion that the ultimate usefulness of the proposed design can only be fully evaluated through the use of a prototype. The prototype prosthesis is an indispensable tool in the development of optimal prosthetic design and component selection. Often patients and payers will not fully appreciate the subtle functional advantages of one system over another. A trial of the proposed components will often allow all parties concerned to jointly

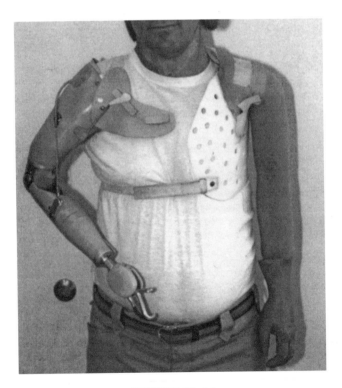

FIGURE 21-14

The passive prosthesis for this forequarter/transhumeral amputee serves as an anchor point for the active prosthesis and provides a more normal appearance.

reach the same conclusions regarding component selection, thus leading to better acceptance and, ultimately, a better outcome.

Critical to the success of this approach is the availability of all component options and the technical ability to mix and match components from different manufacturers. The foundation of the prototype prosthesis is a well-fitted evaluation interface. The components to be evaluated are attached to the interface and adjusted appropriately to allow for a field trial that is fairly representative of function with a finished prosthesis. A prototype might be used for only a few days for the more straightforward fittings, while for the very complex fitting, it might be used for several months. During this time the prototype may undergo dramatic changes in design as various components and controls are evaluated. This process has proved essential in the identification of the most appropriate components and has offered the client a process in which they can have significant input into their prosthetic rehabilitation.

TRAINING

Training of the person with bilateral amputations is often a challenge even for the experienced occupational therapist. The therapist must be well versed in the use, capabilities, and limitations of the prosthetic components employed. It is often helpful, if not necessary, for the therapist and prosthetist to be involved in the initial stages of training to ensure that all parties understand the goals and objectives of the person and the means with which those goals are being addressed. It is useful to periodically come back to the amputee and refocus the goals and objectives. Success can only be achieved when all parties are striving for the same goals.

Training the person with bilateral arm amputations, especially high-level amputations, requires an open mind and the ability to problem solve in creative ways. The occupational therapist should not only focus on prosthetic training but on nonprosthetic function as well. These nonprosthetic options include foot use and other assistive devices. It is sometimes necessary to modify the environment to make it possible for the person to function optimally.

CONCLUSIONS

No one "right" choice exists in the development of a prosthetic system for the person with bilateral arm amputations. However, experience has shown that careful attention to socket fitting, ease of use of the control system, and minimized weight are critical aspects for the successful rehabilitation of these most complicated fittings. Desirable features of an optimal prosthesis are comfort, aesthetics, feedback, variable speed control, and locking joints.

The principles outlined have served as a useful and successfully proven template for the design of bilateral prostheses. However, one should not be constrained by a rigid interpretation of this fitting philosophy, but should consider it a useful starting point. Allowances must be made for situations when physiologic limits, additional disabling conditions, established functional patterns, or the personal preference of the client suggest modification of the general scheme and selection of components and control methods outside the basic approach. Such situations demonstrate the importance of using prototype prostheses and of addressing the unique needs of each individual.

Throughout the design and rehabilitation process, it should be borne in mind that the functional and cosmetic needs of these clients far exceed our present technology. It has been our experience that the most important elements in the success of any particular person are the ability of that person to accept their radically altered circumstances and the motivation to adapt and problem solve as they meet the challenges of their continuing life.

References

1. Uellendahl JE, Heelan JR. Prosthetic management of the upper limb deficient child. In: Alexander M and Molnar G (eds.), _Physical Medicine and Rehabilitation: State of the Art Reviews_, Philadelphia: Hanley & Belfus, 2000; 14(2):232.

2. Childress DS. Control of limb prostheses. In: Bowker J and Michael J (eds.): _Atlas of Limb Prosthetics_. St. Louis: Mosby, 1992, pg. 175–198.

3. Heckathorne CW. Manipulation in unstructured environments: extended physiological proprioception, position control, and arm prostheses. _Proc International Conf Rehabilit Robotics_ 1990, pg. 25–40.

4. Uellendahl JE. Upper extremity myoelectric prosthetics. In: Bussell (ed.), _Physical Medicine and Rehabilitation Clinics of North America, New Developments in Prosthetics and Orthotics_. Philadelphia: Saunders, 2000.

5. Ivko JJ. Independence through humeral rotation in the conventional transhumeral prosthetic design. _J. Prosthetic Orthotic_ 1999; 11(1):20–22.

6. Billock JN. The Northwestern University supracondylar suspension technique for below elbow amputations. _Orthotic Prosthetic_ 1972; 26:16–23.

7. Sauter WF, Naumann S, Milner M. A three-quarter type below-elbow socket for myoelectric prostheses. _Prosthet Orthot Int_ 1986; 10(2): 79–82.

8. McLaurin CA, Sauter WF, Dolan CM, Hartmann GR. Fabrication procedures for the open-shoulder above-elbow socket. _Artif Limbs_ 1969; 13(2):46–54.

9. Bush G. Powered upper extremity prosthetics programme: Above elbow fittings. _Hugh MacMillan Rehabilitation Centre—Rehabilitation Engineering Department Annual Report_, 1990; pg. 35–37.

10. Uellendahl J, Heckathorne C. Prosthetic component control schemes for bilateral above-elbow prostheses. _Proceedings of the Myoelectric Control Symposium, University of New Brunswick_, 1993, pg. 3–5.

11. Weir RF. Robotics and manipulators. In: Olson D and DeRuyter F (eds.), _Clinician's Guide to Assistive Technology_. St Louis: Mosby, 2002; pg. 281–293.

22 Prosthetic Rehabilitation of Glenohumeral Level Deficiencies

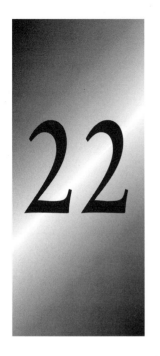

Randall D. Alley, BSc, CP, FAAOP and John M. Miguelez, BSc, CP, FAAOP

Absences at the glenohumeral level (Figure 22-1A,B,C) have long been considered extremely challenging to the rehabilitation team, and successes have been limited. However, using new technologies, techniques, and protocols, prosthetic outcomes have never been more promising. Patients who share the loss of their elbow, wrist, and hand share common functional and psychological requirements. This chapter deals specifically with individuals who have an absence from the humeral neck level to the interscapulothoracic level. Although each level encounters its own challenges, the general rehabilitation plans are similar.

EVALUATION

When evaluating an individual with an upper extremity amputation or congenital amelia, it is important to consider a host of factors, from physical to psychological to social. A comprehensive evaluation of an individual with a high level of limb loss often differs from that of an individual with more distal involvement. This is partly due to the greater physical challenges typically inherent with reduction or absence of sufficient limb length or functional range of motion, and with the limitations of available componentry for more proximal loss (Figure 22-2).

During the physical aspect of the evaluation, tissue condition is of utmost importance (Figure 22-3). At this level, the propensity to use electrically powered components places a demand on the skin-to-socket interface due to the increased weight of the prosthesis on the remaining anatomy and its dynamic distribution as the system is utilized. Many of these high-level cases are secondary to trauma, and epithelial and subsurface layers are often severely damaged. Scar tissue may respond negatively to shear forces, friction, contact pressure, and sensitivity to interface materials, and this must be considered when determining the socket design and control scheme to be utilized. In many cases, due to the need for proper stabilization, weight-bearing, or adequate EMG signal reception, it is necessary for the interface or stabilizing straps to come in contact with damaged areas of the skin. During the evaluation it is important to analyze the anticipated stress to these areas before proceeding. It is also necessary to consider the impact of plaster application and removal in the casting phase, due to the inherent shear, friction, and heat involved in this process.

A second crucial factor to consider during evaluation is the condition of the intrinsic and supportive musculature present. Muscular strength, both in terms of leverage and EMG signal generation for myoelectric control, should be evaluated in addition to muscle and

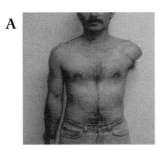
A

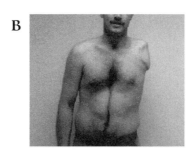
B

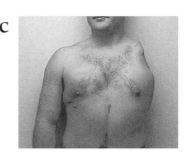
C

FIGURE 22-1

Various levels of glenohumeral deficiency.

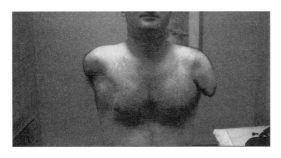

FIGURE 22-2

The bilateral glenohumeral deficiency presents special challenges to the prosthetist.

associated soft tissue range of motion (Figure 22-4). The muscles' ability to function adequately under load or compression plays a role in determining whether there exists sufficient functional range of motion for input devices such as touch pads, switches, force transducers, or linear potentiometers and whether EMG signal generation is adequate for the proper control of myoelectric effectors. In addition, the remaining humerus of an individual with a humeral neck amputation or amelia can be called upon to "assist" in ranging the humeral section or unlocking the shoulder joint, if necessary, thus enlisting the associated musculature. These factors all contribute to the feasibility of the intended system, because they affect interface and frame design, required primary and

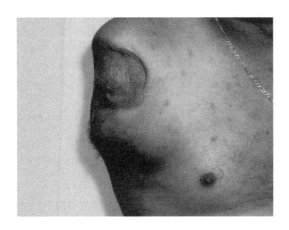

FIGURE 22-3

Tissue condition is an essential component of the prosthetic evaluation.

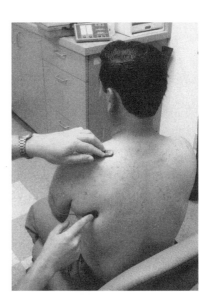

FIGURE 22-4

Evaluating muscle strength and EMG signal potential.

secondary control inputs, (discussed later in this chapter), and useable componentry.

Often ignored or undervalued in the evaluation of individuals with a high-level amputation or amelia is the contribution of the contralateral limb in determining the viability of a prosthetic recommendation (Figure 22-5). Contralateral limb strength, range of motion, grip strength, dexterity, and other physical characteristics play a large part in the person's ability to maximize his potential with the prosthesis. The capacity to don and doff the prosthesis is typically dependent on the contralateral extremity, although systems can be designed to avoid contralateral reliance. If the hand is traumatized by disease, injured, or congenitally affected, not only are donning and doffing issues important, the avoidance of additional stresses placed on it should be a priority. The functional level of the contralateral hand and limb should contribute in determining the appropriate scope of the componentry or control methods.

Lower extremity involvement also affects the prosthetic design (Figure 22-6). The balance and strength of the individual, whether or not assistive devices are used, and the amount of time spent in a wheelchair, for example, all establish guidelines for optimizing functional outcomes. As a case in point, when determining appropriate componentry for individuals utilizing a cane, crutch, or walker, it is important to evaluate the ergonomics of the prehensor and how it will adapt or react to the handle or rail of the assistive device. The materials must be somewhat compatible and not result in a dangerous loss of traction or friction, as would occur with two hard metal surfaces, such as an aluminum hook and aluminum walking bars. The strength of the prosthetic joints—wrists, elbows, and shoulders—must be adequate to withstand the forces incurred during assisted ambulation. To avoid the possibility of injury to the individual and damage to the prosthesis, the durability and compliance of the prosthetic system must be considered in cases where frequent falls may occur.

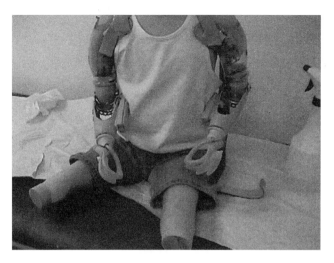

FIGURE 22-6

Lower extremity involvement impacts directly on the upper-level prosthetic design.

A major factor contributing to prosthetic design, and one which should be assessed during the evaluation, is the individual's functional range of motion without the prosthesis. At the glenohumeral disarticulation level and higher, scapular excursion (protraction, retraction, depression, and elevation) can be utilized not only in the generation of mechanical excursion of a control cable, for example, but also for a multitude of switches, touch pads, and other devices that serve as inputs to prosthetic componentry (Figure 22-7). When incorporating gross body movements as secondary control inputs within a myoelectric system, the isolation of these movements is imperative so as not to generate an

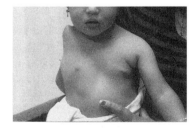

FIGURE 22-5

The contralateral limb plays an important role in rehabilitation success.

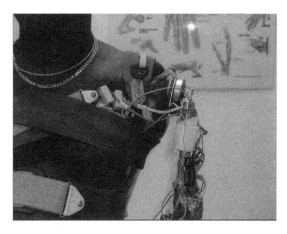

FIGURE 22-7

Range of motion in the shoulder joint can influence prosthetic design, especially in electrically powered units.

excessive activation of the primary muscles used for myoelectric control. If these movements excite a muscle targeted as a myoelectric source above the set threshold, it may cause inadvertent movement of the terminal device or electric elbow. Because of its greater mobility and tactile sensation (in most cases), the remnant humeral neck has additional characteristics that set it apart from the glenohumeral disarticulation and interscapulothoracic levels. The ability to utilize precision spatial positioning for the activation of control inputs should not be ignored. In addition, the direct application of a servo control strap has been utilized successfully in several cases, incorporating the range of motion and kinesthetic acuity of the glenohumeral joint together with the inherent tactile sensitivity to pressure and tension of the external soft tissue (Figure 22-8).

If the individual is currently wearing a prosthesis or has prior prosthetic history, it is imperative that the evaluator determine what the functional range of motion was available and utilized with the previous prosthetic system, or what is present with the current prosthesis. It is important to note that required functional range of motion is a subjective issue. Increased prosthetic mobility may come at the expense of excess weight or a prohibitive complexity of operation. The individual simply may not have the need for the ability provided by a component or feature. An example, unique at this level, occurs during the consideration of which prosthetic shoulder joint (Figure 22-9) to use, if any. The added complexity and mass of a locking shoulder joint over that of a friction design should be weighed against the functional advantage it may provide. In other words, the proposed prosthetic recommendation should achieve an optimum balance between what the user desires and will utilize, and what is realistically appropriate. It is impor-

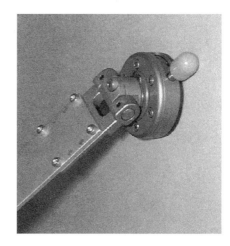

FIGURE 22-9

Locking shoulder joint.

tant to consider, however, that desires and requirements are of a dynamic nature. What the person needs and desires today can certainly change with time or prosthetic experience. It is recommended that the system be biased toward a greater functional potential as the individual gains confidence and a better understanding of prosthetic capabilities. This should not hinder the patient's progression in the early stages of prosthetic rehabilitation. Vocational and avocational requirements may force the utilization of additional features, or focus the prosthesis more narrowly. In any case, the prerequisite functions must be safely and effectively performed with efficiency and reliability.

As discussed previously in the assessment of skin and muscular condition, one must attempt to anticipate the degree of discomfort that may be experienced in utilizing the proposed prosthesis, specifically with volitional movement and weight bearing in mind. If the individual is capable of activating a switch but the discomfort caused by the movement is to such a degree as to impede or discourage this process, then the input protocol should be reassessed in hopes of creating a more favorable outcome (Figure 22-10 and 22-11). It has been often said that if the prosthesis is uncomfortable then it simply will not be worn with adequate frequency, if at all. This is true, yet too often, the practitioner may focus on one aspect of discomfort such as the pressure induced by weight bearing on a specific area, and not take into account the volitional movements required to operate the prosthesis.

One of the dilemmas frustrating both the practitioner and the prosthetic user alike is the difficulty in predicting comfort levels over time. During the evaluation, one should attempt to simulate as closely as possible the pressures to be encountered and the motions

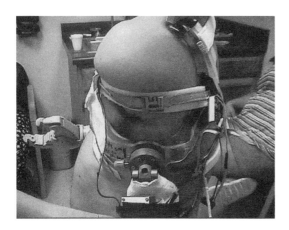

FIGURE 22-8

Force transducer control strap.

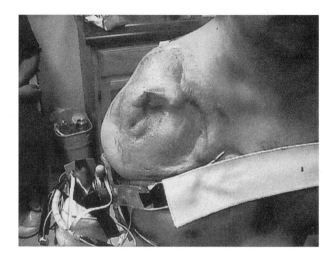

FIGURE 22-10

Prosthetitic interfaces must allow for comfort as well as function.

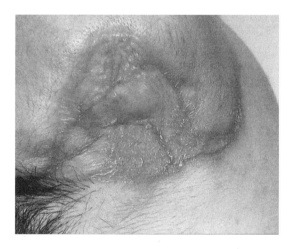

FIGURE 22-11

Tissue condition may preclude the use of intimate skin–prosthesis interface.

acceptance that the user understands and is capable of easily performing the appropriate protocols required for prosthetic operation. In addition, proper care of the prosthesis is imperative, and the system should be designed with the individual's predicted maintenance habits in mind. Comprehensive post-delivery assessments are a critical determinant to long-term success. The level of prosthetic integration is a direct result of the rehabilitation team's ability to respond rapidly to patient concerns, as well as changes in comfort, function, lifestyle, and maintenance issues. A post-delivery assessment must look at each individual matter in addition to their relationship with one another, and this process should be a cornerstone of the rehabilitation plan. It is common for patients to discontinue the use of their prosthesis as a result of inadequate follow-up. Individuals frustrated with excessive down-time, discomfort, or functional and psychological inadequacies present the most significant challenge to long-term prosthetic success. If long-term follow-up is not incorporated properly into the patient's post-prosthetic experience, then the provision of a prosthesis at this level of deficiency should be reevaluated.

THERAPEUTIC CONSIDERATIONS

Therapeutic intervention is a critical factor in determining success at the glenohumeral level of deficiency and above. Although a detailed discussion of proper occupational therapy is outside the scope of this chapter and is discussed elsewhere in this book, therapeutic intervention should consist of three components: preprosthetic, interim, and postprosthetic training.

Preprosthetic therapy should include but is not limited to desensitization techniques, range of motion enhancement, strength training (both of the supporting

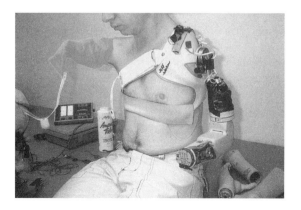

FIGURE 22-12

The ease of donning and doffing is crucial in designing a functional prosthesis.

required of prosthetic usage, recognizing that tolerance may significantly improve or decline with extended prosthetic wear. Once the current spatial requirements have been determined and future usage patterns and comfort levels have been predicted, cognitive ability must be regarded and incorporated into the prosthetic design. Donning and doffing can be a cognitive challenge, especially with supportive and control strapping. Individuals with high levels of amputation or amelia typically require what can be a fairly complex array of control inputs when utilizing either cable-operated or electrical systems (Figure 22-12). It is crucial for patient

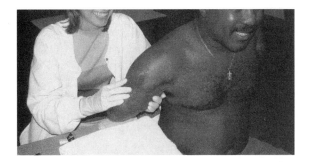

FIGURE 22-13

Range of motion exercises to increase flexibility.

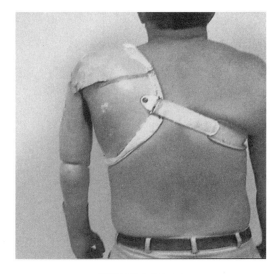

FIGURE 22-14

Bucket or total encapsulation socket.

musculature as well as those muscles involved in direct input to a control device), and wound care if required (Figure 22-13).

Interim therapy involves what is collectively referred to as *controls training*. In addition to maintaining the preprosthetic regimen, the prosthetic user is instructed in the proper operation of the prosthesis. Individuals with unilateral deficiencies receive further instruction in accomplishing tasks restricted to the use of the contralateral hand only. Individuals with bilateral limb deficiencies are instructed in the extended functional use of the feet if applicable.

Consisting of the previous two components, post-prosthetic therapy adds task-specific training, proper care and hygiene of the prosthesis, donning and doffing techniques, and lifestyle integration.

HISTORY OF INTERFACE DESIGN

Typical interface designs for individuals with a high level of limb deficiency can generally be divided into four classes: encapsulation (bucket-style); modified encapsulation; Sauter; and reduced profile (XFrame or Microframe) designs. An understanding of each design's attributes, from both a philosophic as well as a biomechanical perspective, allows a greater appreciation for the current state of prosthetic rehabilitation of the individual with glenohumeral-level limb absence.

Early designs, often referred to as bucket or total encapsulation sockets (Figure 22-14), were of rigid construction and generally covered the entire affected shoulder and torso, often to midline. Devoid of intimate anatomic contouring, this socket relied on excessive skin contact and extensive harnessing. Although this allowed a platform for mounting prosthetic componentry, many wearers complained of the weight of the prosthesis, excess heat, instability, donning and doffing difficulties, and reduced control of terminal devices. In addition, the discomfort this type of design generated due to its exces-

sive vertical loading of skeletal anatomy, poor cosmesis as a result of its extended trim lines, and its range of motion limitations, resulted in reduced wearing times or, in many situations, a discontinuation of prosthetic use all together. These inherent deficiencies were perhaps the principle contributors to the philosophy that still exists in some circles today—that individuals with humeral neck or more proximal amputation levels should not and cannot be fit with a functional prosthesis.

In an attempt to address the limitations of the encapsulation style design, a modified version was developed (Figure 22-15). While continuing to encapsu-

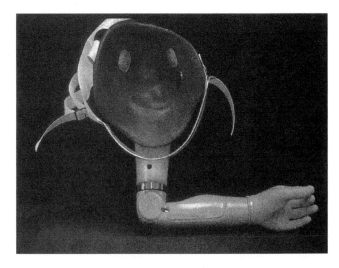

FIGURE 22-15

Modified bucket socket.

late the shoulder girdle, it did not extend to the midline or inferiorly to capture a majority of the torso. This approach, characterized primarily by reduced trim lines, met with partial success in its endeavor to reduce the weight of the prosthesis and heat build-up, and improve range of motion and cosmesis. Although it was an improvement over the previous design, it still did not adequately address its predecessor's limitations. Additionally, due to its greater inherent instability as a result of its reduced profile and continued lack of anatomic contouring, more comprehensive harnessing was required. This often had a negative impact on donning and doffing effort, as well as wearing comfort.

Recognizing that simply modifying the encapsulated socket would not result in a significant improvement, William F. Sauter began to experiment with materials and frame designs not commonly utilized in upper extremity prosthetics (Figures 22-16 and 22-17). Using lightweight aluminum, often used in orthotic management, Sauter molded frames whose trim lines were similar to the previous sockets, with one major difference. The extensive use of "windows" or cutouts significantly reduced heat build-up and overall weight while providing greater stability and reduced donning effort. Although an improvement over previous designs, it continued to generate excessive vertical loading over the acromioclavicular complex, restrict range of motion, and affect cosmesis as a result of its extensive trim line. Because it allowed some mobility of the acromioclavicular complex, this design was primarily used for switch-activated, electrically powered systems. Due to the necessity of maintaining skin-to-electrode contact throughout static and dynamic loading and the increased weight of electronic components, the inherent instability of this socket design limited successful functional outcomes at these levels. Although an

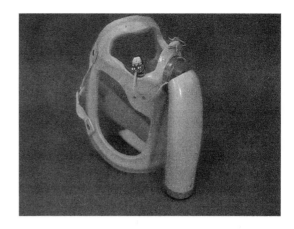

FIGURE 22-17

Sauter socket, front view.

improvement over earlier designs, the Sauter design was not universally adopted due to the high degree of fabrication time and the skill required to create it.

Frustrated by the limitations of the current socket design and platform and its predominantly switch-controlled scheme, the authors recognized the advantages that myoelectric control offered the high-level amputee, principally, an improved functional envelope, increased grip force, variable-rate control of the electronic components, reduced energy expenditure, enhanced cosmesis, and reduced harnessing. By enhancing the stability of the platform, the benefits of myoelectric control could be maximized and thus would alter the perception that high-level amputees could not successfully utilize a functional prosthesis (Figure 22-18). After evaluating current interface designs, it was realized that a better understanding of anatomy would allow for an improved interface. Through cadaver studies and extensive interviews with prosthetic users, eight key areas (critical design criteria) were identified as critical elements for effective interface design:

- Comfort
- Cosmesis
- Stabilization
- Suspension
- Anatomical contouring
- Contralateral/ipsilateral involvement
- Range of motion
- Vocational/avocational/personal

Because comfort is often a key determinant in long-term acceptance and use for high-level amputees, a reduction of interface–skin contact area (footprint), avoidance of shoulder encapsulation, and reduction of interface weight were deemed necessary for improved

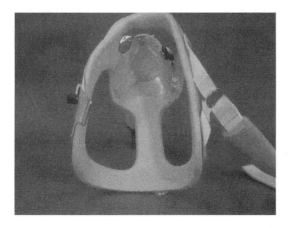

FIGURE 22-16

Sauter socket, side view.

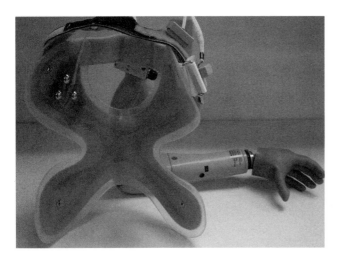

FIGURE 22-18

Alley's XFrame interface.

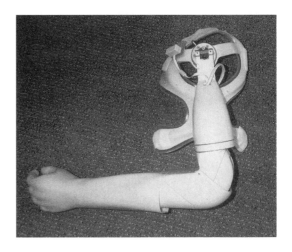

FIGURE 22-19

Reduced profile design with electric elbow and hand with cosmetic glove.

comfort. By incorporating these three factors, the new interface design improves cosmesis and heat dissipation, reduces vertical loading on the acromioclavicular junction, and optimizes the mobility of the shoulder complex by not restricting its range of motion.

Stability in the frame design is achieved in the coronal, sagittal, and transverse planes through soft tissue compression and further anatomic contouring, creating a musculoskeletal "lock" comprised of anterior, posterior, and medial force vectors. This ensures superior vertical loading capabilities (improved suspension and tolerance) and enhanced rotational control. Specifically, this control is achieved by the compression anterior of the proximal aspect of the pectoralis major; posteriorly of the infraspinatus and over the scapular spine; medially of the latissimus dorsi, serratus anterior, and external oblique muscles; and finally, uniformly applied forces to the skeletal substructure. Finally, range of motion should be regarded as having two separate components: translation of gross body movement as it relates to both positioning of the terminal device and the ability to freely range the torso, and the ability to move the shoulder complex to activate a secondary input (Figure 22-19).

This reduced profile interface, often referred to as either XFrame or Microframe (Figure 22-20), capitalizes on its superior stability by capturing gross body movements efficiently, thus resulting in the accurate positioning of the end effector. The specificity of the anatomic contouring facilitates the donning and doffing process by ensuring through its inherent stability, that positioning errors are reduced during application and removal. This feature is critical when designing an interface for individuals with contralateral/ipsilateral involvement, who are further challenged in donning and doffing a prosthesis.

Additionally, because the interface design does not encapsulate the shoulder, the acromioclavicular complex can be positioned independent of the interface. This is useful for activating secondary control inputs (Figure 22-21). Ultimately, all of these attributes maximize the individual's vocational and avocational potential.

The next generation of interface designs will incorporate new materials and techniques that will allow greater comfort and function than ever before. This will result in yet smaller footprints and lighter weight prostheses.

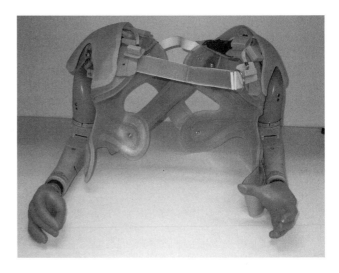

FIGURE 22-20

Reduced profile design for bilateral application.

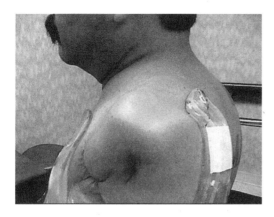

FIGURE 22-21

The Reduced Profile design does not impinge on acromio-clavicular function, thus making secondary control inputs possible.

OPTIONS

At the humeral neck level and higher, although the same prosthetic options are available (with the exception of the prosthetic shoulder joint) as are utilized with lower levels of limb loss, the excursion generated through gross body movement is at a premium. Often solutions that avoid or diminish reliance on these movements are more readily accepted than are those systems that require them to a high degree. The first option to be discussed involves the individual opting to not wear a prosthesis at all. There are a variety of reasons for this, many of which are discussed elsewhere and are outside the scope of this discussion. Focusing more closely on the reasons why a person with a glenohumeral disarticulation or interscapulothoracic amputation chooses not to wear a prosthesis in many cases is a result of the greater disparity between the functional capabilities of the prosthesis and either the contralateral extremity or the limb that was lost. In addition, one of the greatest discrepancies that occurs between human function and prosthetic utility occurs at the shoulder, where the mobility, strength, and precision of the human shoulder joint completely overshadows the capacity of its prosthetic counterpart. Second only to the functional divergence present between the human hand and prosthetic prehensor, this reduced correlation results in a high incidence of prosthetic rejection, as the individual incurring this level of limb loss must deal with significant inequities inherent both at the terminal device and at the proximal joint. Another reason that may induce the decision not to utilize a prosthesis can be financially based. At higher levels, the overall costs of appropriate systems are generally greater than for prostheses of similar design characteristics at more distal levels. This may result in a reduction of insurance authorizations, or require a prohibitive amount of out-of-pocket expense for the intended user.

There exist several advantages and disadvantages for the high-level amputee or amelic patient in choosing not to wear a prosthesis. In most cases, a person is more comfortable due to the absence of prosthetic interaction, whether it be weight, friction, contact pressure, or heat, for example. Tactile sensation is not adversely affected, and the physical range of motion attainable by the individual is not restricted by a socket and frame or harnessing. A lack of prehension is the most obvious disadvantage of not utilizing a prosthesis, but others can be equally detrimental. The overall functional range of motion may be reduced when not wearing a prosthesis, and in rare cases, the lack of volume containment, compression, and tissue or limb stabilization realized without prosthetic use may result in greater discomfort for the individual. Finally, cosmesis may be unfavorably affected in the sense that prosthetic shaping can often provide a higher level of symmetry between the involved and contralateral sides (Figure 22-22).

Often a passive prosthesis is recommended (Figure 22-23). Typically lighter in weight than other prosthetic solutions, this type of system can satisfy cosmetic requirements and cost significantly less (with the exception of silicone designs) than other options. Utilizing embedded wires, passive hands often allow the manual positioning of the fingers, and when utilized with a locking elbow and shoulder joint, provide a limited amount of stabilizing and carrying function. The disadvantages of a passive prosthesis are a lack of active or volitional prehension, a reduced functional envelope, and limited, if any pinch force. The utilization of stabi-

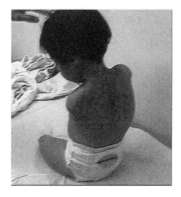

FIGURE 22-22

The decision to prescribe a prosthesis rests on many factors of which human resilience and adaptability is among the greatest.

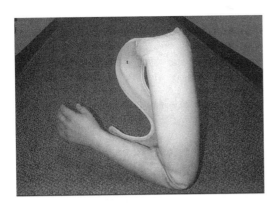

FIGURE 22-23

A passive (non-prehensile) prosthesis.

results in an extremely restrictive and uncomfortable control harness. This can go beyond discomfort and eventually cause nerve entrapment syndrome. As with most cable operated systems, both static and dynamic cosmesis are relatively poor. The presence of cables, external retainers and fasteners, and the like adversely affect static cosmesis, while required gross body movements appear unnatural and serve to degrade dynamic cosmesis. Finally, a poor correlation exists between the neuromuscular recruitment required for the cable operation of componentry and that initially involved either by the contralateral extremity or ipsilaterally prior to amputation. This low correlation often results in a modified development of the neuromuscular system over time, the impact of which is still largely unknown.

The advantages of such a control scheme for individuals with a high level of limb loss are the relatively low initial and maintenance costs, the provision of kinesthetic and biomechanical feedback via the cable and harness, a reduction in weight when compared to electrically powered systems, and finally, the improved environmental resilience of a nonelectrical device.

Several advantages can be gained in utilizing an electrically powered prosthesis that minimally consists of an electric prehensor and elbow for the humeral neck level of limb loss and higher (Figures 22-25 and 22-26). The grip force of the electric prehensor is typically greater than that of its cable-operated counterpart, whereas the functional envelope of an electrically powered prosthesis is often larger due to the reduction

lizing and support straps is often required, which can be uncomfortable.

An entirely cable-operated prosthesis at or proximal to the humeral neck level (Figure 22-24) is characterized by a long list of disadvantages. Inherent in any body-powered system with a voluntary opening prehensor, minimal grip strength can be an issue. In addition, the functional envelope is negatively affected due to the control scheme's reliance on gross body movements and their ability to generate sufficient excursion to adequately manipulate corresponding mechanical effectors. In addition, biomechanical efficiency is paramount, which often

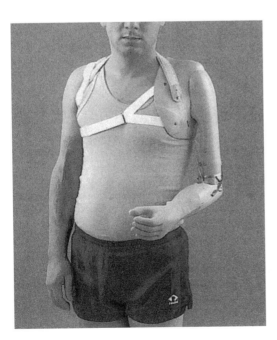

FIGURE 22-24

A cable-operated prosthesis.

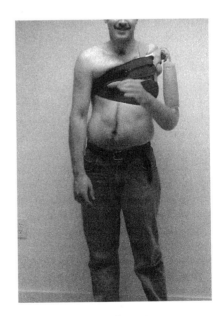

FIGURE 22-25

Electrically operated prosthesis in use.

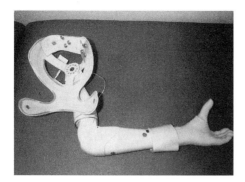

FIGURE 22-26

An electrically powered prosthesis
incorporating the XFrame.

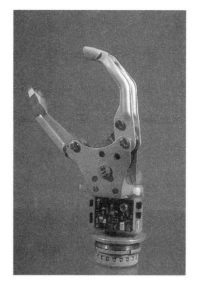

FIGURE 22-27

The Otto Bock Sensor hand.

or omission of the need for gross body movement to yield prosthetic operation. In addition, prosthetic action usually requires minimal energy expenditure, and both static and dynamic cosmesis is frequently superior to that of body-powered systems. There exist a variety of operational formats for primary and secondary control input. If adequate EMG signals can be identified, the most common form of primary control at these higher levels utilizes a myoelectric control scheme. This method usually requires the least amount of energy output by the user and exhibits superior dynamic cosmesis, as little if any detectable external movement is necessary. Other options include the use of a force transducer (generally used in lieu of adequate EMG signals, although not always the case), force sensing resistors (FSRs), and switches. Frequently, some combination of the above is used to satisfy both primary and secondary requirements.

The initial and maintenance costs of an electrically powered prosthesis can be considerable. In addition, the weight and its distribution throughout the prosthesis can be difficult to tolerate for many individuals. The socket and frame must account for this to achieve user acceptance. If properly designed, the negative impact of weight can be minimized or removed as a determining factor. Inherent with most electrically powered systems is the lack of feedback available to the wearer. Although current technology exists to provide information on the level of pinch force being applied or temperature encountered, these features are still in the development stage and have yet to be commercially available. At the time of this writing, several such systems are nearing completion. A clever approach to this lack of feedback has been developed by Otto Bock in the form of a closed-loop configuration inherent in their Sensorhand (Figure 22-27). A sensor in the thumb detects slippage and automatically compensates by increasing pinch force

until slippage is no longer detected. In this case, a lack of pinch force feedback is not as crucial, as the hand increases grip only up to the amount necessary to negate slip. Finally, battery maintenance can be a disadvantage when compared to systems not requiring electrical power; however, with the advent of longer lasting lithium batteries, daily maintenance is not always required.

Incorporating the characteristics of both a cable operated system and an electrically powered one, a *hybrid prosthesis* (Figure 22-28) is configured most commonly as a conventional elbow and electric prehen-

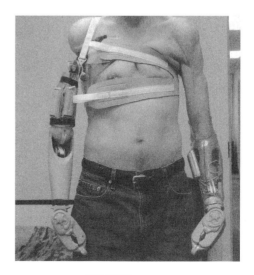

FIGURE 22-28

A hybrid body-powered and electric prosthesis.

sor. The advantages of this configuration are an increased grip strength, increased functional range of motion, reduced weight (relative to a fully powered system), cable feedback, improved elbow flexion velocity (relative to an electric elbow), reduced initial and maintenance costs (as compared to an electric system) and, when balanced against a cable-operated-prosthesis, the hybrid scheme usually requires a less restrictive and less elaborate harness. Finally, a hybrid system allows for the simultaneous operation of both elbow and hand. The disadvantages include the use of a harness for elbow operation and an increased load on the harness with respect to a cable-operated system due to the heavier electric hand. Because of the reduction of available leverage and excursion, a hybrid prosthesis at this level must be considered carefully before proceeding. Although there are successful wearers of hybrid prostheses at considerable levels of limb loss, these individuals are strong and can generate a great deal of gross body movement. However, elbow flexion often suffers, and many users find it hard to flex past 90 degrees.

An adaptive (activity-specific) prosthesis, often generalized as a recreational device, typically possesses a functional advantage over other prostheses for the activity it was intended for. As a result of its specific design, an improved performance of appropriate activities can be expected. Additionally, this specificity often minimizes the required componentry. It should be noted, however, that many activities demand highly customized, complex terminal devices and other components to achieve optimal performance, thus resulting in extensive design and manufacturing costs.

Inherent in its design, the adaptive prosthesis can be of limited value when utilized outside its narrow scope. In addition, authorization can be difficult if it is used specifically for recreation, because avocational pursuits are often regarded by reimbursement agencies as nonessential.

CONCLUSIONS

Historically, it has been argued that the utilization of prostheses at the humeral neck, glenohumeral, and interscapulothoracic levels is generally unsuccessful, with many rehabilitation professionals possessing a strong bias against any form of prosthetic intervention. Although this belief once may have held merit given inadequate assessment methodologies, traditional interface designs and prosthetic componentry, and the insufficient use of occupational and psychological therapy, today, the individual with acquired limb loss or amelia faces a brighter future in which he can expect a much more positive outcome. Possessing greater knowledge and improved techniques, interface designs, and technologies, the rehabilitation team is better equipped than ever before to properly address the challenges encountered at these levels. However, it is simply not enough to selectively incorporate individual tools or techniques; the team that is entrusted to maximize an individual's rehabilitation potential also assumes a great responsibility to comprehensively and appropriately integrate all of the resources outlined in this chapter in the care of their patient.

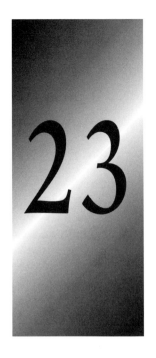

23 Recreation and Sports Adaptations

Robert Radocy, BS, MS and Annaliese Furlong, CP

Recreation and sports activities are integral components of most individual's lives. Recreation and sports pursuits can complement the vocational and family lives of active adults and may have an even greater impact on the quality of the lives of youth, because vocation is not usually a factor. All cultures engage in some type of recreation, play, or sport and these activities have been described or illustrated since mankind established records.

The value of participation in sports, recreation, and play in physical rehabilitation has been well established (1). The profession of therapeutic recreation (recreational therapy) continues to grow, augmenting the more traditional rehabilitation disciplines of physical and occupational therapy. Rebuilding the lives of the sick or disabled using therapeutic recreation techniques can enhance and accelerate the overall rehabilitation process.

"Throughout time, play has been an instinctual way to foster creativity, imagination, and teamwork. Motor skill development, a positive self-image, and confidence are the results of kindling a play spirit... The idea that you can improve fitness through play is unquestionable. Participating in different activities ... moving your limbs through sometimes unfamiliar, though safe ranges of motion ... is what people of all activity levels need to prevent injury..." (2).

In the article "The Power of Play" (2), Chelsea M. Budde discusses the importance of play. "According to developmental experts, interactive play is a critical part of every child's education." Additionally Budde cites M. Anderson: "Children with disabilities need to experience as much play as other children. Children learn cause and effect through play, and problem-solving is a part of everyday life." The complete article provides other insights into how play impacts the lives of disabled children.

Physical disability, including upper limb absence caused by congenital or acquired circumstances can pose additional dimensions to the challenges of therapeutic recreation and sports rehabilitation. In many cases, the loss of a limb requires the advent of a technological aid or aids to allow successful access to the activity. Persons missing a hand or parts of an arm may have sufficient strength, motivation, and talent to be successful in a sport or recreation but they may simply lack the proper tools—the specialized prosthetic accessories or modified sports equipment—to allow them to participate.

Participating in sports and recreation activities for the first time or reaccessing those activities after a traumatic injury involves experimentation and a series of personal choices. Certain individuals will prefer to participate "one-handed," without the use of any special aids. They will accept the challenges of their physical condition and retrain to perform the activity to their own level of satisfaction. That level may be recreational or it may be competitive. Others will seek out technological aids or require prosthetic adaptations or equipment modifications to help achieve the level of performance that they desire. The rehabilitation specialist must take the time to solicit information from the patient/consumer. This data helps make decisions on how to approach sports and recreation pursuits. This process is evolutionary. Overnight success should not be expected or encouraged. Set realistic goals in a stepwise fashion and strive to achieve these goals over a realistic period. No panacea exists when it comes to overcoming the physical access barriers in sports and recreation using technological solutions.

A balance exists in creating "performance" in any sports and recreation activity, when technology is involved. The balance is between physical rehabilitation or physical capability and prosthetic technology and science. The most sophisticated, high performance prosthetic technology or equipment modifications will not create "performance" for an individual who is not physically capable of utilizing it. Range of motion, coordination, and strength, as well as a positive psychological attitude, must exist to achieve high performance using a sophisticated prosthesis or technological aid. Conversely, and as important, the well-conditioned, prepared "disabled" athlete will not be able to perform unless the technology is capable of handling the physical dynamics involved. This concept is very important and should be conveyed by the rehabilitation specialist.

Successful participation in a favorite sport or recreation after an injury that resulted in a loss of a hand or arm can possibly be the "key" to unlocking that individual's overall rehabilitation success. The demand for sports and recreation adaptive technology and specialized equipment modifications continues to increase. This trend has been stimulated by the increased publicity of disabled athletes in the Paralympic Games, as well as the increased profile and popularity of adaptive skiing programs. Specific efforts by the prosthetics and orthotics profession via the Orthotics and Prosthetics Athletics Fund and the personal efforts of recognized amputee athletes like Dennis Oehler, Todd Schaffhauser, Dory Selinger, Diana Golden, and many others have helped fuel this trend. The increased popularity of human interest articles in national publications about the disabled succeeding in a variety of sports and recreation activities has also raised the profile of these efforts and increased general public awareness.

The efforts of a variety of other organizations and associations, like the Amputee Coalition of America and Disabled Sports USA, which advocate for amputees and especially amputee or disabled sports and recreation opportunities, also need to be recognized as contributing to the trend. Refer to the Appendix for a listing of these organizations.

INSURANCE

Insurance issues impact the use of technology when sports and recreation accessibility is involved and may limit the applications, even though the needs exist. Insurance reimbursement itself can be a barrier. Insurance reimbursement has become more difficult for prosthetics in general and is typically nonexistent when specifically applied towards prosthetics or technology for sports and recreation. Alternative resources to finance the expense of specialized prosthetic technology should be considered. Financial assistance from regional, state, or national foundations should be explored (see Appendix), as well as local community resources. Social and community organizations such as Rotary, Kiwanis, ELKS, BPOE, etc. and church associations may rally to help with the fundraising or financing of a particular prosthetic project to benefit a local, disabled youth. In certain cases, a local prosthetic professional will work with patients and families to ease the burden of the costs of such technology by providing some type of credit or structured, extended payment options.

SAFETY

Safety issues can also pose dilemmas and create barriers to the use of prosthetic technology in competitive sports. Rules and regulations that govern and control "play," equipment specifications, apparel, and all the other aspects of sports are written very comprehensively, usually to the detriment of the disabled individual wishing to use an upper limb prosthesis. These rules and regulations will most likely be encountered in high school athletic programs but may affect a youth's participation in competitive middle school and junior high athletics, or community leagues, such as Little League baseball and Pop Warner football. In purely "recreational," leagues, which deemphasize competition, safety is still important but will not be such an obstacle to participation.

High performance prostheses designed with safety in mind are achievable but still may not conform to the strict rules and regulations governing competitive sports and recreation. Special written permission from a governing state athletic association may be required to ensure that specific prosthetic technology will be allowed in competition. Written permission or acceptance is highly recommended, because in almost all instances, the attending referee has total jurisdiction over decisions regarding the topic. Unless a written waiver by a governing authority is available, the disabled player wanting to participate using an upper limb prosthesis may be barred from playing by the referee.

The rules and regulations rarely pertain specifically to prosthetic technology. In most cases, prostheses are prohibited because they are categorized under the rules regarding casts or braces. The National Federation of State High School Association's 1998–99 Rules Book, regarding "Basketball Player's Equipment, Apparel" specifically states:

> The referee shall not permit any player to wear equipment or apparel which, in his/her judgement, is dangerous or confusing to other players or is not appropriate. Examples of illegal items include, but are not limited to:
>
> ART. 1... A guard, cast, or brace made of hard and unyielding leather, plaster, pliable (soft) plastic, metal or any other hard substance—even though covered with soft padding—when worn on the elbow, hand, finger, wrist, or forearm.
>
> NOTE: Each state association may authorize the use of artificial limbs which in its opinion are no more dangerous to players than the corresponding human limb and do not place an opponent at a disadvantage (3).

The intent of such regulations is well meaning, in that it attempts to provide for a safe game environment, but they are written so broadly that they generically prohibit any arm prosthesis without special authorization. Education is key here. The player must enlist the help of the rehabilitation specialist, prosthetist, coach, and parents when attempting to secure a written waiver from the state association. The rules indicate that the state association has the power to allow a prosthesis to be used, but they are going to be heavily influenced by the language of the National Federation's rules. Safety must be demonstrated for other players as well as the prosthetic user. Additionally no advantage can be provided by the prosthetic technology. For example, the surface areas of the anatomic hand and prosthetic device must be equivalent or comparable: A prosthetic device that has noticeably more surface area than the player's corresponding hand could be construed to be an "advantage" and possibly prohibited.

Each state association governing committee will be different. Establish the contact, schedule a meeting to discuss the situation, and try to determine if the committee is willing to discuss an exception and under what circumstances. The assistance of the coach, the prosthetist, and the parents can all be utilized to help develop a solution.

Rules and regulations exist for virtually all competitive athletic activities. They differ slightly from sport to sport, but the general overtone of prohibition exists in all activities. Their fairness may be questionable, but for the time being, they govern high school sports and recreation, and they need to be dealt with professionally.

DESIGN GOALS

The goals required in creating useful prosthetic adaptations for sports and recreation are oriented around duplicating anatomic functions. Sports and recreation are very biomechanically function specific. The biomechanics providing the swing a golf club are quite different from the biomechanics involved in dribbling a basketball, or the biomechanical manipulations of the upper limb while swimming. The factors that must be evaluated include but are not limited to gripping force (prehension), wrist flexion and extension, ulnar and radial deviation, forearm pronation and supination, elbow flexion and extension, humeral flexion, and internal and external shoulder rotation. Prosthetic technology must attempt to duplicate in part or in whole these various biomechanical actions if true bilateral participation in a sport or recreation is to be achieved. In some cases, the equipment itself can be modified to aid in achieving some of these functions. Solutions can be simple and low cost in certain cases and complicated and expensive in others.

Another factor to consider in design is temperature. Temperature can be a significant factor when acceptance or use of a prosthesis is the challenge. It is important to understand temperature extremes and how arm amputees deal with fluctuations of temperature in the prosthetic socket environment.

COLD

One of the chief complaints of amputees who participate in winter sports is intolerance to cold. It is important to recognize that this is due to decreased blood flow to the involved limb. In some instances, an individual may also experience decreased sensation as well, which could leave them at further risk from frostbite. The use of a nylon sheath worn directly against the skin serves to wick moisture away from the residual limb. Wool socks and other interface materials can be used to help keep the residual limb warm. In addition, heating pads and electric socks have also proved successful as means of keeping the arm warm within the socket.

HEAT

Just as the cold weather can adversely affect the comfort of a prosthesis in the winter, heat can cause problems in the summer. The use of a nylon sheath can help provide a cooler stump socket environment by wicking away moisture from the skin. Ventilation holes are another option. Ventilation holes can be added to the prosthesis to assist with air circulation around the stump and result in a more comfortable wearing environment.

POWER OPTIONS

Upper limb prosthetic technology is typically divided into four generic categories regarding function. Passive, body powered, externally powered (myoelectric), and hybrid. The first two categories have been more predominantly used in accessing sports and recreation than the third or fourth, primarily because of the expense, durability, water resistance, and general design attributes associated with externally powered prosthetic technology. Passive and body-powered prostheses are generally less expensive, more durable, inherently water resistant, and are simpler to adapt to sports and recreation accessories than myotechnology. Externally powered prostheses provide the prehension required for most sports and recreation activities but do not provide the wide variety of other biomechanical wrist and forearm functions required.

However, the option of hybrid prostheses exists. The hybrid design combines conventional or cable driven control with external powered components. In some instances, a myoelectric arm can convert to a body-powered design by interchanging the terminal device. This is important to recognize because certain "specific use" terminal devices mentioned later in this chapter can be fit to a myoelectric design. For the patient who does not have the resources for an activity-specific prosthesis, externally powered prosthesis often can be adapted to accept special recreational or therapeutic components.

OTHER FACTORS

Several other major factors affecting and impacting solutions for accessing sports and recreation include the level and complexity of the limb absence. Bilateral limb absence poses a greater dilemma than unilateral, and in general the higher the level of such absence, the more complicated will be the solution if technology is applied. In general, if a dominant limb is lost, it is far easier and more efficient to retrain the remaining limb than to seek a prosthetic solution for a unilateral task. The prosthesis becomes the complement or support for that remaining retrained limb.

Eye dominance is another factor. Eye dominance can complicate the "change over" of handedness, but in most cases eye dominance can be accommodated if a forced change of hand dominance occurs.

Certain sports are more unilaterally performed, while others dictate more two handed, bimanual capability. Bowling is an example where unilateral biomechanics dominate. The best and easiest rehabilitation for the loss of a dominant hand would be to retrain the remaining hand to control the ball, while simultaneously retraining the technique and coordination required to deliver the ball. Canoeing or kayaking however are activities that place a far greater emphasis on bilateral biomechanics and function. It is possible to canoe or kayak one handed, but such a solution is not as effective, powerful, or safe as being able to provide a solution that allows the use of both upper limbs.

The more joints in the limb that require prosthetic duplication, the more complex the solution. At some point for every individual with a high level (transhumeral) arm absence, the trade-off between the complications of prosthetic technology and the level of performance provided are equated. Beyond this point, individuals prefer to operate entirely unilaterally and adjust to the circumstances created. Golf is a good example. Golf is truly a sport that benefits from bilateral involvement. The prosthetic solution for a golfer with a high-level limb absence, however, could be so complicated that it inhibits the player's performance, when compared to that individual's unilateral golf playing capability.

Solutions for the disabled in sports and recreation should always be oriented around the individual's capabilities and desires.

PROSTHETIC SUSPENSION OPTIONS

Conventional prosthetic suspensions utilizing both figure eight and figure nine harnessing can be utilized in sports and recreation, but new technology is available that can enhance performance. Self-suspending prostheses can be improved significantly by building in a cushioned foam liner to protect the olecranon and elbow condyles or by incorporating "roll-on" silicone liner technology. The roll-on liner is a "flexible" inner prosthesis usually equipped with a mechanical fixture that engages or locks down into the rigid, definitive prosthesis. The roll-on provides excellent suspension because it cannot be pulled off. Due to its extensive surface "traction," the liner must be rolled off and on.

Two basic types of roll-on liners exist, the prefabricated and the custom. Fillauer, Inc. was responsible for developing the 3S® custom roll-on technology and Shuttle Lock®. This system is fabricated to fit the exact morphology of the limb using standardized laminating techniques. Prefabricated liners are available from several manufacturers. The liners vary in material, reinforcement, flexibility, and thickness. Considerations for liner selection include evaluating the patient's skin sensitivity, allergies, tolerance to shear forces, limb length and configuration, living climate, and anticipated activity level. Roll-on liners provide excellent suspension and can augment existing suspension technology. Variable suspensions are also possible, which allow for a more traditional type of prosthetic sock wear as well as roll-on compatibility (4).

This type of technology should definitely be considered when a prosthesis is being constructed for sports and recreation. The added suspension is a plus, which can improve control in many activities. Combined with a high strength, carbon fiber reinforced, exterior prosthetic shell, the roll-on liner technology offers performance options to upper limb amputees never before possible.

The remainder of this chapter is an alphabetic exploration of various sports and recreation activities. Examples and solutions are discussed and pictured. Some solutions are one-of-a-kind ideas; others have broader application. In certain instances, the solutions are very custom and individualized, whereas in others commercially manufactured prosthetic accessories or adaptive aids have been developed. The authors hope to provide a comprehensive collection of stimulating ideas and designs that can help provide realistic solutions for those persons missing a hand or arm who are trying to access a favorite sport or recreation.

Archery/Bowhunting

A number of techniques, aids, and apparatus exist to allow a one-handed person or a person with upper limb impairments to shoot a bow and arrow. Prosthetic modifications as well as equipment modifications are presented to illustrate these innovative solutions (Figures 23-1, 23-2, 23-3). Some persons choose to use a prosthesis to hold the bow. Archers with a transhumeral absence, holding a bow with their prosthesis, need to be concerned about "locking" out their mechanical or electromechanical elbow. Archers with a transradial absence will most likely need to increase their arm strength.

Certain prosthetic devices like the Grip 2® can handle a bow with little if any customization. Simple modifications to create a padded gripping area on the bow handle or "riser" can provide for safe and accurate control. In many cases "locking" on to the handle in some manner is preferred. The design needs to allow for the bow to "center" itself in the prosthetic prehensor or

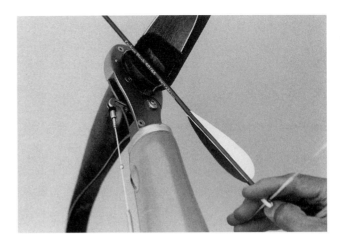

FIGURE 23-1

Grip 3 prehensor application in archery. Courtesy TRS, Inc..

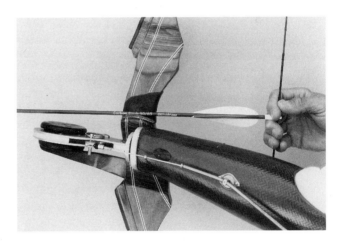

FIGURE 23-2

Custom archery prosthesis and modified bow with extended handle. Courtesy TRS, Inc.

hand so that no torque is induced into the bow. Rigid prosthetic attachments to the bow are also possible but can be more difficult to "tune" to ensure accurate arrow flight. Mouth tabs have been used successfully to hold the string while the bow is pushed away. Other solutions like the Wright Bow Brace® provide a stable, string-holding platform and trigger release for single-handed shooters. Highly impaired persons might consider the use of a cross bow to access archery. Use caution here regarding hunting: only certain states consider a cross bow a legal weapon for their bowhunting seasons.

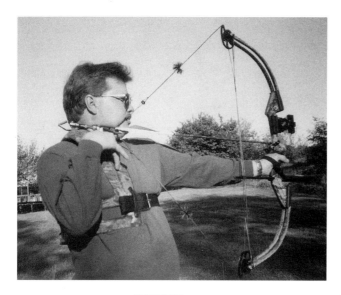

FIGURE 23-3

Wright Bow Brace torso archery adaptation for one-handed archery. Courtesy Mike Chavet.

Archery equipment itself has evolved to make access to the sport easier. New, lighter weight, compact design compound bows, which were designed primarily to open up archery to smaller framed individuals, women, and children, can offer new opportunities for those missing hands or with upper limb limitations as well. These bows are engineered to be easily adjustable for draw weight and arrow length. Most archery pro shops are very accommodating and will gladly help a physically challenged person get involved with this challenging sport.

Two national organizations exist that represent the physically challenged archer/bowhunter, the Physically Challenged Bowhunters of America, Inc. and The United Federation for Disabled Archers. Both these nonprofit, membership organizations provide information, access, and opportunity to persons with physical challenges who wish to shoot a bow and arrow.

Ball Sports

The generic category of ball sports refers to those ball sport activities that require or are enhanced by the use bilateral hand control. Basketball, volleyball, soccer, football, and rugby are good examples. The ball in these activities is controlled by the volar surface of the hand, especially finger and thumb surfaces. Cosmetic (passive) hands have been applied to these activities with minimal success. The design, material, and durability characteristics of cosmetic hands make them a poor choice for these types of activities. Additionally, the protruding

individual fingers and thumb can pose a safety hazard in contact sports.

Prosthetic devices like the Super Sports® and the more recently introduced Free Flex Hands (Figures 23-4, 23-5, 23-6) provide an alternative solution for these activities. These devices were designed to emulate the flexion and extension characteristics of the hand and wrist and duplicate the volar surfaces. They utilize energy-storing materials to provide rebound and strength and have proved to be safe in contact sports.

More exotic custom solutions like the Mills basketball hand (Figure 23-7) challenge prosthetic designers to reach even further in developing highly functional aids for specific sports. The availability of new synthetic

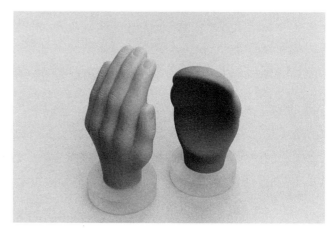

FIGURE 23-4

Free-Flex and Super Sport prosthetic accessories. Courtesy TRS, Inc.

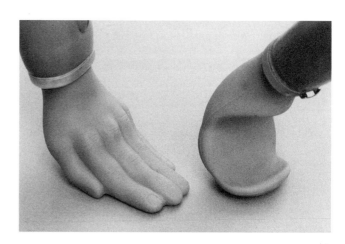

FIGURE 23-5

Free-Flex and Super Sport prosthetic accessories, showing flexibility in action. Courtesy TRS, Inc.

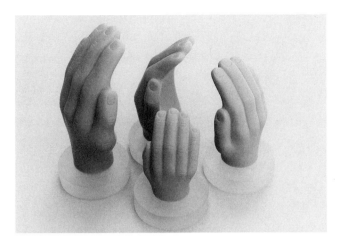

FIGURE 23-6

Various configurations and sizes of the Free–Flex and Super Sport prosthetic hands. Courtesy TRS, Inc.

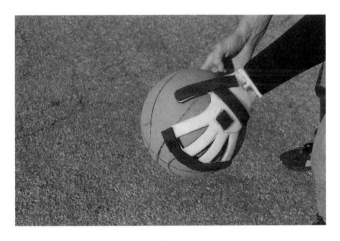

FIGURE 23-7

Mills prototype basketball prosthetic hand. Courtesy TRS, Inc.

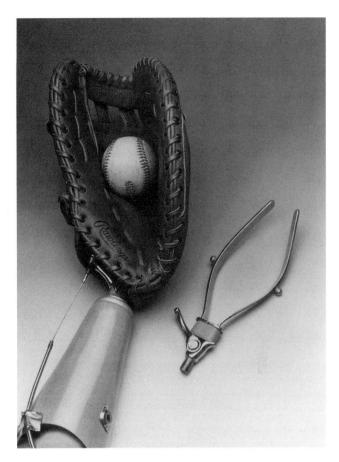

FIGURE 23-8

Baseball glove adapter. Courtesy Hosmer Dorrance Corp.

materials, coupled with the inventive minds of amputees themselves, often create the best solutions.

Baseball/Softball

Baseball and softball are often tackled one-handed: Numerous examples exist of enthusiasts participating or competing single handedly. To a certain extent, one-handed participation has been due to a lack of prosthetic options, not choice. For many years the Hosmer Dorrance Baseball Glove Adapter® (Figure 23-8) provided the only assistance. The Hi-Fly Fielder® and Hi-Fly Jr.® (Figure 23-9) offer newer alternative solutions for catching. These devices allow the user to catch either forehanded or backhanded, thus eliminating the need to pronate. The flexible mesh pocket is bidirectional. Attaching a swivel to the bottom of a bat, as with a Power Swing Ring (Figure 23-9) can duplicate the needed "wrist roll-over" not available in conventional prosthetic wrists. Engaging both arms in the swing adds both power and control. Experiment with cross handed batting or switch hitting to improve the swing and hitting capabilities. Transhumeral amputees may discover that single-handed baseball is much less cumbersome than trying to deal with the weight and mechanics of prosthetic elbows and extra control cables.

Bicycling/Motorcycling

Grasping the handlebars for steering and balance and using the hands for gears, brakes, clutches, and signals are all elements of riding two wheelers, whether body- or externally powered.

Purely one-armed control in bicycling is an option for street riding but probably won't provide enough lat-

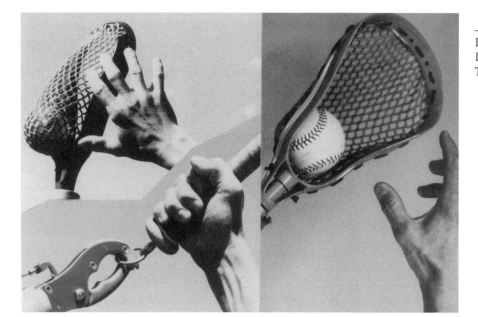

FIGURE 23-9

Hi Fly Fielder, Hi Fly Junior, and Power Swing Ring in action. Courtesy TRS, Inc.

itude for safe mountain biking. Purely one-armed control of motorcycles could prove hazardous, because of the weight, balance, and momentum dynamics that are involved. Trikes or motorcycles equipped with side cars are possible alternatives.

Steering control using an arm prosthesis has proved a viable option in both bicycling and motorcycling. Certain prosthetic prehensors have enough gripping force to adequately control the handlebars; others do not. Voluntary closing devices have been used successfully in this application, and myoelectric hands also perform well. Certain individuals have designed specific, custom handlebar adaptors as an alternative to available prosthetic equipment. Figures 23-10 and 23-11 illustrate two custom modifications. When it comes to convenient shifting and safe braking, bicycle shifting gears can be clustered together on one side of the handlebars, and a single bike brake hand lever can be designed to operate both the front and rear brakes. The Dual Brake Bike Lever illustrated in Figure 23-12 offer this option. Figure 23-13 shows a typical clustered gear set-up along with the dual brake lever system.

On motorcycles, depending upon handedness, the clutch lever can be moved adjacent to the throttle, and the clutch and throttle may be operated simultaneously with one hand. A prosthesis that offers enough gripping function (body-powered or myo) can be used effectively to grasp the handlebars for control and steering. Operating a conventional motorcycle hand brake lever with a prosthesis can prove difficult or compromise safety. Most motorcycles can be modified to operate both front and rear hydraulic disc brakes from a single foot oper-

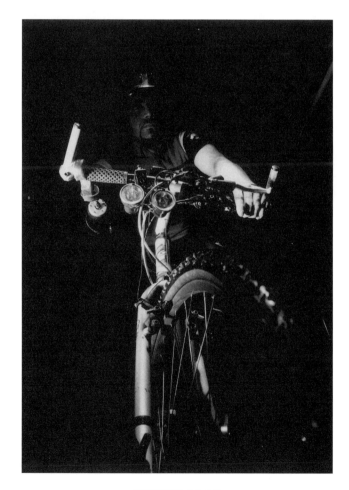

FIGURE 23-10

Custom bicycle adaptation. Courtesy *Active Living Magazine* and Derek Griffith.

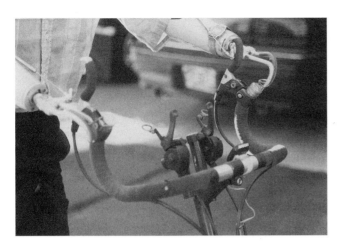

FIGURE 23-11

Custom bicycle adaptation for bilateral amputee. Courtesy NovaCare Inc., Annaliese Furlong.

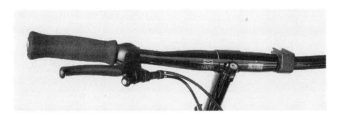

FIGURE 23-12

Dual-brake bicycle lever. Courtesy TRS, Inc.

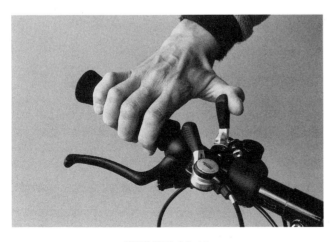

FIGURE 23-13

Mountain bike showing dual bike brake lever and gear cluster. Courtesy TRS, Inc.

ated pedal (Figure 23-14). Motorcycle gears are typically foot shifted, so usually they are not of concern.

Bilateral amputees or persons with a high transhumeral amputation or nonfunctional limb can consider a three-wheeled trike. Figure 23-15 illustrates a bilateral equipped with two split hooks controlling trike handlebars using special steering ring adaptors.

Proper modifications and adjustments to braking systems for both bicycles and motorcycles are extremely important. Consult with certified, trained mechanics to accomplish these types of modifications.

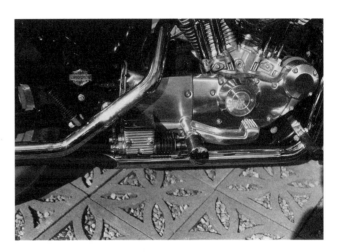

FIGURE 23-14

Custom rear brake foot lever for motorcycle. Courtesy TRS, Inc.

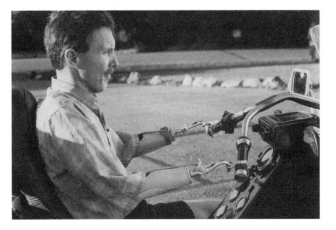

FIGURE 23-15

Custom trike handlebar adaptation for bilateral amputee. Courtesy NovaCare Inc., Annaliese Furlong.

Bowling

Bowling is primarily a single-handed activity. Persons experiencing the loss or impairment of their dominant limb can usually switch dominance and bowl with their opposite hand. Persons not wishing to switch, or those with bilateral involvement, might investigate the Hosmer Dorrance Bowling Ball Adaptor® (Figure 23-16). This device provides a flexible coupling and cable-activated disconnect mechanism to release the ball.

Canoeing/Kayaking/Rowing

The one-handed control of canoe and kayak paddles or boat oars can be cumbersome and impractical, if not dangerous and impossible. Body-powered, voluntary closing prehensors like the Grip® have been successfully used to access these water sports (Figure 23-17). Externally powered hands can provide the prehension necessary, but are more easily damaged and usually cannot tolerate exposure to water. Traditional body-powered split hooks typically cannot provide the power necessary

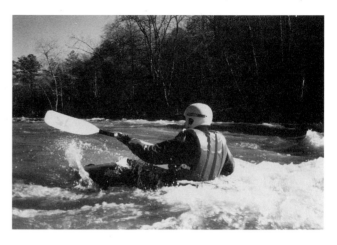

FIGURE 23-17

Grip 3 prehensor in use during whitewater kayaking. Courtesy Dr. Elliot Marcus.

to safely control this type of equipment. Canoe paddles can be easily modified (Figure 23-18) to enhance their control with a prosthesis. Water sports in white water can be dangerous: Never permanently lock a prosthesis onto any canoe or kayak paddle. A paddle can snag up in fast moving water and compromise the boater's safety.

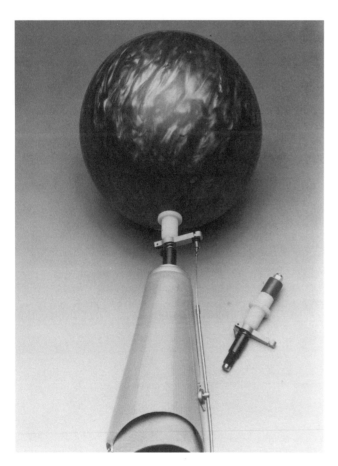

FIGURE 23-16

Bowling ball adapter. Courtesy Hosmer Dorrance Corp.

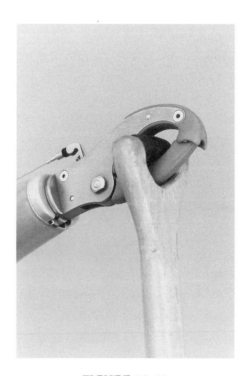

FIGURE 23-18

Canoe handle modification. Courtesy TRS, Inc.

Carpentry

Carpentry is an area that can be deemed an occupation as well as a recreational pursuit. Numerous terminal device attachments are commercially available to promote such activities. Included in this specific group of terminal devices is the Hosmer® #7 Hook and the TRS GRIP 2S® prehensor. Both lend themselves to heavy-duty activity as well as the grasp functions associated with certain tools. However, if the need for a specific terminal device is not deemed practical, a patient can generally utilize most terminal devices to a limited degree (Figure 23-19). Formal training and a review of technique is recommended to promote proper usage and prevent damage to a prosthetic device. For example, a patient should be aware that he is never to use his prosthesis as a hammer or percussion instrument.

Driving/Vehicle Operations/Flying

Driving is often considered a recreation. Handling an automobile, truck, or four-wheel drive equipped with an automatic transmission usually eliminates the need for adaptations for single-handed operation. Most controls can be operated single handedly, although not always conveniently. Manual transmission vehicles typically demand the use of two hands for safe operation. Certain prostheses provide the necessary function with or without additional modifications to the vehicle. Myo-controlled prostheses and modern, voluntary closing prehensors offer a wide range of function to make handling a stick shift or steering wheel convenient and safe. More conventional body-powered prostheses, equipped with a split hook terminal device, usually require the addition of a steering wheel ring or similar aid to ensure safe control over the vehicle.

The selection of adaptive equipment for driving should reflect the need for safety, individual need, and comfort. Some options for upper limb amputees include the driving ring a steering knob, and extensions for turn signal controls. Figures 23-20, 23-21; and 23-22 depict three modifications that enable a prosthesis user to better access auto controls. These devices are mounted right or left according to the handedness and ability of the driver. Bilateral arm amputees can also consider

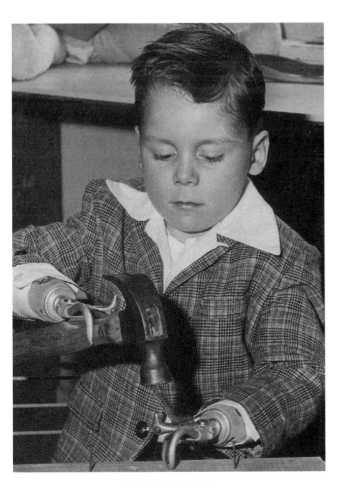

FIGURE 23-19

Child with bilateral involvement using hammer and nail with split hooks. Courtesy NovaCare Inc., Annaliese Furlong.

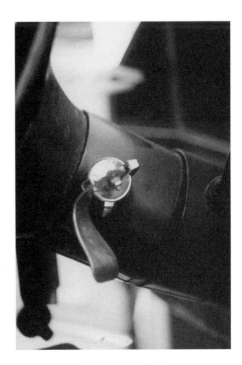

FIGURE 23-20

Ignition switch adapter. Courtesy NovaCare Inc., Annaliese Furlong.

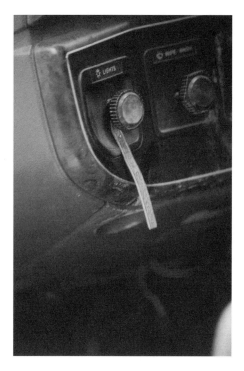

FIGURE 23-21

Light switch adapter. Courtesy NovaCare Inc., Annaliese Furlong.

employing foot activated steering controls along with lever extensions for headlight and turn signal controls.

Flying or piloting a plane requires adaptations similar to those used in driving because the amputee is faced with many of the same types of control and steering oper-

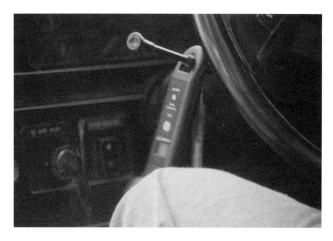

FIGURE 23-22

Turn signal indicator adapter. Courtesy NovaCare Inc., Annaliese Furlong.

ation obstacles. It is important to recognize that there may be certain liabilities associated with adaptive equipment being installed in a vehicle, so consult with the local Department of Motor Vehicles or a rehabilitation specialist. They may be able to provide referrals to vendors and consultants that specialize in vehicular modifications. Additionally, some rehabilitation centers offer specific vehicular driver training to people with varying disabilities. These centers tend to have direct experience with adaptive equipment specialists and can provide the appropriate training to ensure safe vehicle operation. State rehabilitation service agencies are another resource; these agencies are often able to provide resources for training assessment and purchasing assistance for vehicle modification or adaptive equipment.

The Amputee Coalition of America (ACA) (see Resources) can provide a listing of specialized adaptive equipment manufacturers. The local Automobile Association of America (AAA) is another resource.

Firearms

Certain firearms, such as small caliber pistols, can be safely operated with one hand. However, shotguns and long rifles, because of their length and weight, are more difficult to safely control single handedly. When balancing the firearm becomes an issue, specific prosthetic devices have the gripping force and configuration to aid in handling a firearm, whereas others require that the firearm be modified or a special prosthetic adaptive device be designed. Myoelectric hands have been successfully applied to the shooting sports utilizing either rifles or shotguns. Cable-controlled Grip® voluntary closing prehensors have been successfully used for handling pistols and long guns. Traditional split hook technology is a more difficult application because the hook's prehension is usually not capable of stabilizing the gun while firing. Gun accessories like a military strap can aid in the balance and control of a long gun. Oversized rubber grips fitted onto pistol handles provide additional surface area and compliance that can enhance handling with a prosthetic device. Custom modifications and adaptors can be added to the long gun's fore end. Pistol grip style handles or swivel rings attached to a long gun's fore end can provide additional options for safely engaging and controlling a firearm with a prosthesis (5). Any modifications to a firearm should be completed by a certified gunsmith to ensure that the integrity of the firearm and its safety features are not compromised.

Fishing

A variety of options exist for persons wishing to fish. Single-handed fishing can be accomplished utilizing either battery powered, electric fishing reel systems or by fixing the rod onto some type of chest harness or support (10). Voluntary closing prehensors and myo-controlled prosthetic hands or grippers have enough prehension to control fishing reel handles. Typically, the rod is controlled by the anatomic hand and the reel with the prosthesis. The opposite is possible, but most prosthetic wrists do not lend themselves well to the dynamics of casting. The handles of reels can easily be padded or modified to allow for better grasp with a prosthesis. Many fishing reels, both freshwater and saltwater styles, can be purchased either left- or right-handed, so adaptation to an angler's hand absence or dysfunction is easier. The Hosmer Dorrance Ski Hand® has been applied successfully for some lighter duty fishing applications. The hole in this flexible hand, which is designed to receive a ski pole, can be adapted to receive the butt end of a fishing rod as well.

Fly fishing, which requires fine dexterity for handling the line and gear, has been successfully accomplished by the author using a Grip 3® voluntary closing device. The gripping surfaces of this device are made of synthetic rubber, and its quick, natural reflexive action and gripping pressure feedback allow for proper fly line manipulation.

The use of small pliers or surgical hemostats can help any angler hold flies, hooks, lures, and other fishing equipment. Myoelectrically controlled devices are not usually applied to fly fishing, because the angler is typically partially immersed and required to have his hands in the water frequently.

Custom devices are always possible, and the inventiveness of amputees in creating their own solutions is refreshing. However, a device specifically designed for either reeling or rod holding, which completely replaces a standard prehensor or terminal device, has the disadvantage of not being very useful to any other task. A rod-holding prosthesis, for example, might require the angler to change prosthetic devices to bait a hook or net a fish. Both versatility and function are recommended to achieve complete fishing access and success.

Gardening/Agriculture

Numbers from the United State Department of Agriculture (USDA) National Agriculture Statistics Service Records (6) indicate that more than 200,000 individuals per year experience occupational injury that results in lost work time and that 5 percent have permanent impairment. These numbers, compounded by the isolation from support services associated with rural living, catalyzed the development of the AgrAbility Project in 1991. The AgriAbility Project was created to assist physically impaired individuals with education and access to

resources, as well as eliminate barriers to an independent lifestyle. Besides assisting individuals who have experienced amputation, AgriAbility also provides assistance to those suffering from other physical, cognitive, or illness-related impairments. Services include work site evaluation, technical consultation related to equipment modification and work processes, recruitment of community resources, peer support and advocacy, community awareness, evaluation of prophylactic measures to prevent future injury and disability, and networking with other community assistance programs, rehabilitation agencies, and assistive technology centers.

Plowshares, the AgriAbility newsletter, provides technical information on various resources related to the topic. Two articles "Hand controls for agricultural equipment" and "Prosthetic and work-site modifications for farmers with upper extremity amputations" (6) are examples.

Golf

Golf prostheses are probably the most highly evolved of recreational prosthetic adaptations. This is understandable because of golf's popularity and availability to the public. A person's natural handedness and the side of the hand absence or dysfunction dictate different solutions. Two commercially available golf devices, prosthetic the Amputee Golf Grip® and TRS Golf Pro® (Figures 23-23 and 23-24), together are designed to accommodate almost every condition. These devices help create a smooth swing with the power and control required for successful play. Few if any modifications to the clubs are required using these two aids.

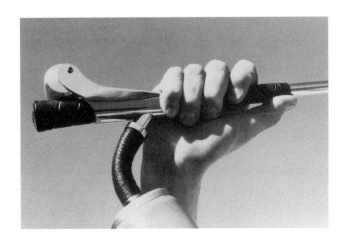

FIGURE 23-23

Golf-Grip golf adaptation for left-hand amputee. Courtesy TRS, Inc.

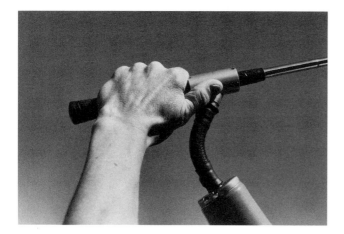

FIGURE 23-24

Golf Pro golf adaptation for right-hand amputee. Courtesy TRS, Inc.

Numerous custom devices have been used as well. Ball and socket joints, custom adaptations into the ends of the clubs, and universal joints have all been applied with limited success to the task of properly controlling a golf club. Most of these custom solutions have certain mechanical inhibitions that limit their application. Golf is a very individual challenge and golfers are very particular about what works for them, so keeping an open mind is helpful in developing an acceptable solution.

Bilateral golfers face even greater challenges. Figure (23-25) shows how one bilateral golfer accessed this game.

Using a prosthesis for golf usually only applies to persons with transradial hand absence. Transhumeral conditions complicate the situation because of the mechanics and the range of motion limitations in the prosthetic elbow. Custom solutions are possible, however. TRS Inc. has worked on special modifications to the Golf Pro® to accommodate above-elbow amputees. In these cases, a short or stubby prosthesis is constructed with no mechanical elbow. The flexion coupling in the Golf Pro® is custom modified to replace the prosthetic elbow entirely and to provide a long flexible coupling and attachment to the golf club's grip.

Single-handed golf is also an option: Reversing the golfer's swing may create options for improved control and power. Over the years, a number of amputees have chosen to tackle golf single handedly and have proved to be competitive.

The National Amputee Golf Association is a nonprofit organization representing amputee and limb-deficient golfers. NAGA coordinates and sponsors tournaments throughout the United States and publishes the *Amputee Golfer* magazine.

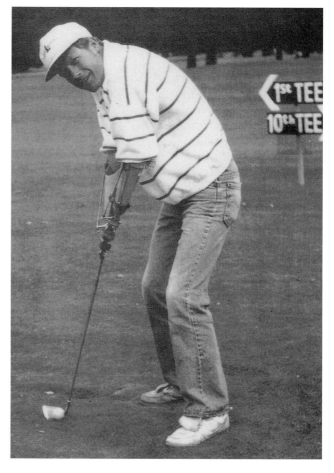

FIGURE 23-25

Bilateral golfer using special adapters. Courtesy NovaCare Inc., Annaliese Furlong.

Hockey (Ice and Street)

Ball and socket adapters designed to connect the end of a hockey stick to a prosthesis have been successful for youngsters wishing to play hockey. The Canadians in particular have used this design to allow their child amputees to compete safely. Adults may need a stronger more versatile adaptation than the simple plastic ball socket design provides.

Two commercially available prosthetic hockey adapters are manufactured. The Slap Shot® hockey device (Figure 23-26) is available in a model for handling the end of the stick and another model to handle the stick's lower shaft. Model preference depends on a person's handedness. Both designs provide for stick control with a prosthesis and are flexible to withstand the forces that can occur playing hockey. Because the design allows for the devices to either flex or bend away, they provide greater safety to the skater during a fall or while

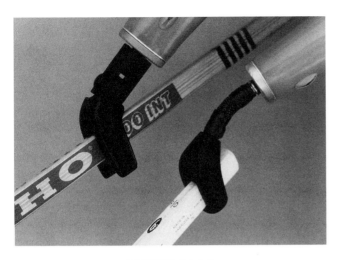

FIGURE 23-26

Slap-Shot prosthetic adapters for hockey. Courtesy TRS, Inc.

being checked into the walls. Both models disconnect easily from the hockey stick.

A variety of custom devices for children have been fabricated, especially in Canada. Over the years a number of these innovative designs have been published in *Champ*.

Horseback Riding/Equestrian Performance

An involvement in equestrian sports can involve more than simply riding. The care of the horse, tack maintenance, and saddling and adjusting harnesses, bridle, and reins can all be involved. A prosthetic device that provides positive prehension and control is most useful. Myoelectrically controlled devices and body-powered, voluntary closing prehensors are most applicable.

A rein bar, which is simply a padded rod attached into the reins, can be installed to aid in control using any prosthesis. A rein bar provides a convenient rigid element to grasp with a prosthesis, an alternative to trying to handle the leather reins themselves.

Mountaineering

Mountaineering can involve rock scrambling, rappeling, and technical and ice climbing. Single-handed mountaineering is a real challenge due to the requirements that rope and equipment handling pose to a climber. Realistically, a prosthesis with a powerful, easily controlled prehensor is necessary. Voluntary closing prehensors like the all metal Grip 2S® have been used in mountaineering. Rugged prosthetic devices such as these can withstand the abuse of the rock and be used for prying, jamming, or

clinging to rock surfaces. Myo-controlled devices should be capable of providing the gripping prehension required for rope handling but probably will not perform well in the other areas described. Rope handling, knot tying, and gear manipulation requires a prosthesis with fine and gross motor function capabilities. Mountaineering enthusiasts should always rely on belaying and other protection and should receive proper training.

Musical Instruments and Instrument Play

Musical instruments, because of their variation in design, require a wide variety of adaptations to be successfully played by the one-handed person or prosthetic user. Some designs are simple, depending upon the musician's particular physical circumstances and the instrument being played. Other situations require complex solutions.

Dr. Rene Baumgartner of Switzerland contributed the following designs (Figures 23-27 and 23-28) that illustrate two solutions, one for guitar and the other for violin. Most prosthetic adaptations for instrument play are semi- or fully customized; however, a couple of exceptions exist to create easier access to certain instruments. TRS Inc. provides a semi-custom fabrication service for creating prosthetic adaptors for guitar, violin, and drums (Figures 23-29, 23-30, and 23-31). A simpler drum stick adaptation for the bilateral amputee is shown in Figure 23-32. The Amend Music Center of Spokane, Washington developed, under a special grant, a unique adapter, that allows a one-handed person to play the saxophone. The Amend Miad® conveniently attaches to any saxophone and provides for a complete range of key operation.

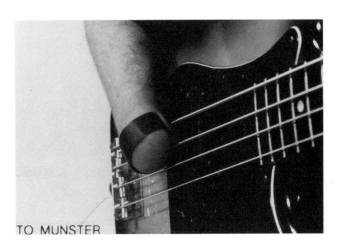

FIGURE 23-27

Guitar modification for transradial amputee. Courtesy Dr. Rene Baumgartner.

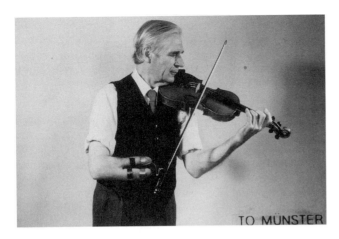

FIGURE 23-28

Violin bow adaptation for Krukenberg arm. Courtesy Dr. Rene Baumgartner.

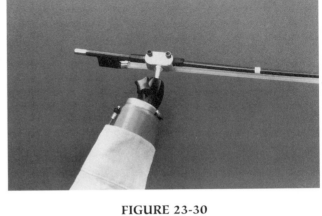

FIGURE 23-30

Violin bow adaptation. Courtesy TRS, Inc.

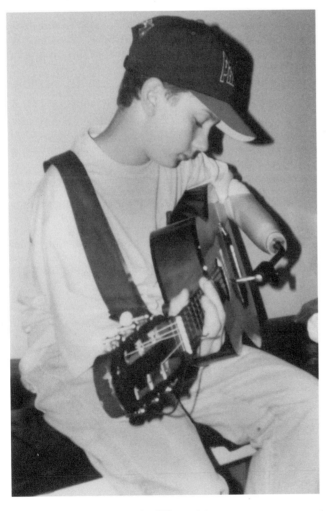

FIGURE 23-29

Guitar prosthetic adaptation. Courtesy TRS, Inc.

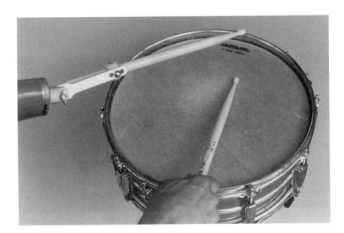

FIGURE 23-31

Prosthetic drum stick adaptation. Courtesy TRS, Inc.

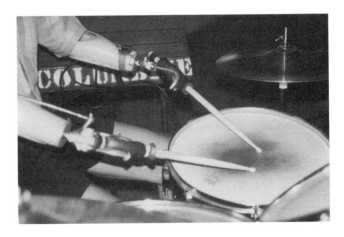

FIGURE 23-32

Simple drum stick adapters for bilateral amputee. Courtesy NovaCare Inc., Annaliese Furlong.

TRS Inc. and the War Amps of Canada are two valuable resources for discovering and exploring ideas about special designs for musical instrument play. Additionally, see references 7 and 8 for specific information about piano playing for children with problem hands.

Penmanship/Writing

Penmanship is an area commonly overlooked for the upper limb amputee. From a functional standpoint, several options exist. For a single amputee who has suffered impairment of the writing hand, the most direct solution is change of dominance. For the bilateral amputee, use of prostheses, or change of function to include foot or mouth skills, are other options.

Although the functional necessity is often addressed, attention to training as related to a neat, legible script is often ignored. A couple of simple tools promoting this task are the alphabetic tracing tablet (available in most school supply stores) and the use of design templates. Both media provide guidance for the motions needed to cultivate the dexterity needed to promote superior penmanship.

Photography

The one-handed control of 35mm format cameras, video, and other types of cameras can be a challenge. A tripod or monopod support can substitute for an absent hand, but these are not necessarily convenient or portable.

Using a prosthesis is very possible and, depending on the camera's shape, no adaptations may be required. Other cameras or specific prosthetic devices may require a specially designed camera adapter. A handle can be attached to any camera via the tripod adapter. The handle can be configured to adapt to any particular prosthetic device. Custom prosthetic adaptations like the Amp-u-pod ® (Figure 23-33) offer other alternatives. This device attaches directly into the prosthesis and allows the camera to be repositioned and locked at almost any angle. For the bilateral arm amputee, these challenges are magnified. See Figure 23-34 for one custom solution that worked well for a photographer with bilateral involvement.

Remote, cable control extensions in various lengths for camera shutters are available in from most professional photographic shops and can add flexibility to handling a camera with a prosthesis.

Pool/Billiards

Pool, billiards, and other similar table top games create the challenge of holding and guiding a cue or stick to

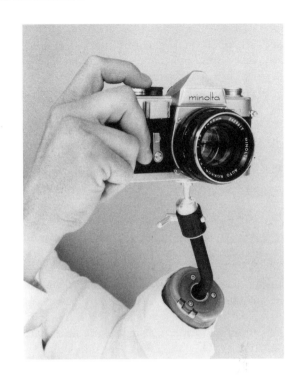

FIGURE 23-33

Amp-V-Pod camera adapter. Courtesy TRS, Inc.

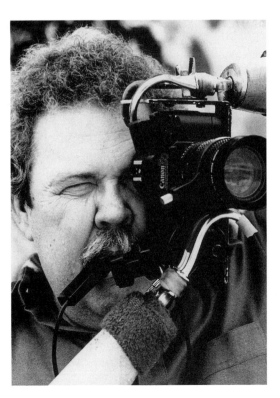

FIGURE 23-34

Camera modification for bilateral amputee. Courtesy NovaCare Inc., Annaliese Furlong.

accurately strike a ball. A wide variety of angles and bridging situations occur that force players to be fairly flexible in their ability to address the ball. Single-handed play is possible using a standard bridge accessory pool stick, but control is not always precise. Persons wearing a prosthesis can cushion or guide the stick on whatever type of terminal device or hand prosthesis they are wearing. Some shot opportunities are usually compromised because of the prosthetic device's configuration or surface materials. A conventional split hook's metal surfaces provide for a smooth stick delivery with some shots, but lack the variable positioning required for all shooting situations. Most prostheses provide the player with a better capability to handle the accessory bridge to provide more shooting versatility.

TRS Inc. manufacturers the Hustler® (Figure 23-35), the only specialized prosthetic device for playing pool and similar games. The Hustler® utilizes a smooth guide ring to control the cue stick and has a lockable angular adjustment mechanism to accommodate an infinite variety of shot situations. The non-slip, padded, monopod, pedestal finger allows the Hustler® to be positioned close into a cluster of balls for "masse" and other more exotic type shot challenges.

Sailing/Boating

Sailing and boating are accessible recreations for persons with hand absence or dysfunction, but the level of boating achievable may be limited by the individual's functional capacity. Prostheses can provide the bilateral control needed for competently handling ropes, pulleys, winches, steering wheels, tillers, and throttles.

Prehensors like TRS Grips® have proved worthy in these activities. Myoelectric prostheses are completely

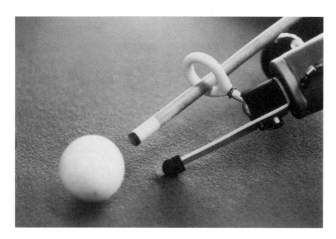

FIGURE 23-35

The Hustler pool stick adapter. Courtesy TRS, Inc.

capable of performing these tasks as long as they are kept dry and free of internal moisture. Conventional split hooks are more limited in their application for these types of activities due to their reduced gripping prehension and configuration.

A saltwater environment can be extremely hard on all types of prostheses, so extra care and maintenance is dictated. Salt is very corrosive to most metal surfaces, so washing prostheses with fresh water after exposure to the saltwater environment is recommended.

Snow Skiing, Nordic and Alpine

These two variations in skiing have certain parallels but are different enough to discuss separately. Alpine or conventional downhill skiing uses the upper body primarily for coordination and balance. The arms and hands control the ski poles, which help maintain balance and, when used properly, help the skier change momentum for quick effective turns. Poles also aid in moving about in lift lines and other situations. Alpine skiers can actually ski very effectively without poles because gravity provides the majority of the force for their propulsion.

Nordic or, cross-country skiers rely a great deal more on the upper limbs. The upper body, torso, arms, and hands control poles that are used for propulsion. A great deal of nordic skiing requires traversing and climbing snow fields. Without the aid of the arms for propulsion, nordic skiing becomes extremely difficult. Armed with this knowledge, it is apparent that a prosthesis could be useful for alpine skiing and is a necessity for balanced nordic skiing. Single-handed skiing is an option for alpine but much less so for nordic skiing.

A prosthesis for skiing will be used much more efficiently by skiers with transradial rather than transhumeral limb absence. A number of custom adaptations over the years have been used to fix the pole to a prosthesis. Split hooks do not have the prehension or configuration to easily hold a pole; however, wrapped with elastic materials, a split hook can be used with moderate success. Two types of commercially available prosthetic accessories exist specifically for snow skiing. Hosmer Dorrance sells the Ski Hand (Figure 23-36). This device is constructed of silicone rubber with an internal reinforcing structure for support. It is available in several sizes. The pole is forced into a hole in the device after the standard pole grip is removed. No cable is used. A twist of the torso, combined with a humeral flexion or thrust, "pendulums" the ski pole forward, due to the Ski Hand's® flexibility. The elastic memory in the device returns the pole to its original position.

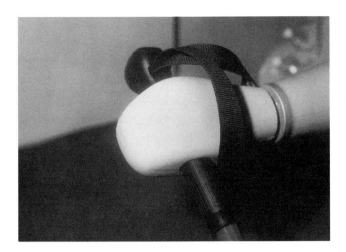

FIGURE 23-36

Hosmer Ski Hand. Courtesy Hosmer Dorrance Corp.

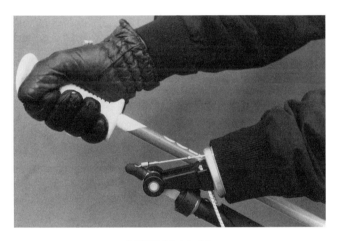

FIGURE 23-37

Ski 2 prosthetic device for alpine and nordic skiing. Courtesy TRS, Inc.

The Ski 2® , built by TRS, Inc. (Figure 23-37), is a cable-powered alternative to the Ski Hand® . The Ski 2® has a quick disconnect pole design not available in the Ski Hand® and pivots either by pendulum or cable force. The standard pole grip is also removed for this application. A shock-absorbing mount within the device absorbs the torsion and shock transferred into the pole during skiing or a fall. The device is also designed to pivot, thus allowing the pole to flex away during a fall. The Ski 2® allows for very quick spontaneous pole plants with a natural, upper body motion. The pole has an adjustable, elastic return system.

Neither device is equipped with a "break away" pole system.

Snow Boarding/ Ski Boarding

Snow boarding (shredding) and ski boarding are two winter sports activities that essentially do not require the use of the hands at all, except for balance and gear adjustments. Snow boarding uses a single board, whereas ski boarding uses two miniature boardlike snow skis, one for each foot.

A safe prosthesis is recommended to prevent against injury during falls. A cosmetic hand with a ski glove will provide some service but a more durable device designed with energy storage such as a Super Sport® or Free Flex® (Figure 23-6) can provide additional function. An externally powered myoelectric hand functions well. A ski glove or mitten can be fitted over such a prosthesis for a more natural look while skiing.

TRS Inc. has experimented with the design of a Winter Sports Hand® (Figure 23-38), for these activities. This passive device, molded using a high-performance polymer rubber, has individual fingers and thumb, fits into a ski glove or mitten, and is designed to be shock absorbent, thus duplicating certain wrist and hand dynamics. This device is not designed to hold a ski pole.

Snowmobiling/ATVs

Positive control and adequate gripping strength are required to pilot these vehicles safely. Most vehicles in these classes have centrifugal clutches, so operating the gas throttle and brakes are the tasks to be mastered. Qualified recreational vehicle mechanics can probably provide some of the best help in modifying these control systems. ATVs have separate brakes for controlling front and rear wheels, much like a motorcycle. Snowmobiles use a lever-style brake similar to a motorcycle.

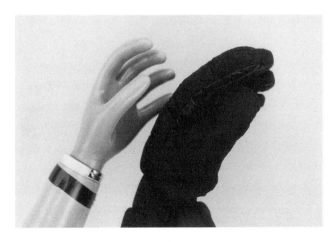

FIGURE 23-38

Prototype Winter Sports Hand. Courtesy TRS, Inc.

Throttles are lever-actuated on the handlebars. Clustering the throttle and brakes on one side provides single-handed control. Refer to the sections on bicycling and motorcycling for additional ideas.

Tennis/Racquet Ball/Squash

A Tennis Service Toss Device® (Figure 23-39), developed by N.D. Kitchen, provides a simple solution for the tennis enthusiast with or without a prosthesis. The tennis ball is controlled within a cup-shaped receptacle attached to the arm or prosthesis. The cupped-ball control device is simply attached to the elastic wrist brace with Velcro. A person with limited hand function could also employ this same concept attached to a glove. Single-handed play, in which the player handles both ball and racquet simultaneously, may be preferred to eliminate the prosthesis altogether. Switching the dominant hand may be required. Racquets are rarely modified to fit onto a prosthesis because of the lack of any truly functional prosthetic wrist suitable for such an activity.

Other alternatives are the Super Sport® or Free Flex® prosthetic accessories. These scoop-shaped hands can provide limited ball handling capabilities, flexible fall protection, and can help prevent injury during contact with a competitor. A cosmetic hand might also be useful but is less durable. Myo hands should also provide adequate function in this type of sport, because myo-controlled prostheses eliminate the cables and harness systems that can restrict movement and inhibit function. A roll-on silicon liner applied to a myo, body-powered, or passive arm prosthesis will improve suspension significantly. An external suspension sleeve made of neoprene, latex, or other elastic material, worn

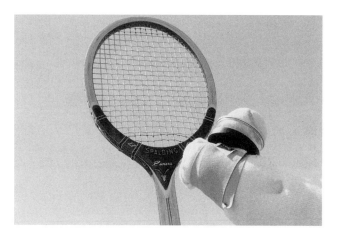

FIGURE 23-39

N.D. Kitchen's Tennis Service Toss Device prototype. Courtesy TRS, Inc.

over the elbow, can also aid prosthetic suspension during rigorous play.

Water Sports

Several factors must be considered when designing a prosthesis that is to be used for water activity.

HARNESSING

Safety is very important. Access to a quick release of the prosthesis is a consideration with many water sports. The ease of donning and doffing the prosthesis can also be a consideration, especially when other sports-related gear may be worn on the torso. A safety release system can sometimes be achieved with the addition of quick release buckles to the front of the prosthetic harness, where they can be more easily accessed in an emergency. Other alternatives include modifying the equipment to allow for rapid, emergency release situations. Testing and dry-land practice are always recommended to ensure that these systems operate properly prior to engaging the actual activity.

SUSPENSION

Suspension can be compromised in a water environment. The prosthesis may work differently under water. Water acts as a lubricant against the skin, and a well-suspended prosthesis might be difficult to control once submerged. Water can seep into the socket and create slippage. Additionally, the body's buoyancy in the water may be different from the prosthesis, thus causing an imbalance. Generally, these conditions can be remedied with the use of some type of suspension sleeve. The sleeve may be made of neoprene (wet suit material) or similar materials and rolled over the socket and up onto the proximal portion of the arm. Another option is a custom, flexible, silicon inner prosthetic sleeve, which interlocks into the rigid, outer, prosthetic shell. Although very functional and stable, this option is expensive. Too much suspension can prove a liability as well. In activities like scuba diving and water skiing, it is important to recognize that it may be necessary to discard the harness and prosthesis in an emergency situation. The quick disconnect harness system already discussed can apply here. Certain materials can be harder to grip or handle when wet, so design the harness and suspension systems accordingly.

A custom cover made of 3-to 5-mm thick neoprene, with nylon fabric on both sides, can function as both a suspension sleeve and also provide flotation for the prosthesis. Prostheses without such a flotation cover will most likely sink once they are discarded in the water. The cover may also provide better buoyancy in saltwater, because the body usually feels lighter than the prosthesis. Experimentation will be required if this buoyancy factor is critical to the activity.

MATERIALS

Certain materials conventionally used to fabricate a prosthesis will not weather well in the water environment. Leather and certain types of foam linings will deteriorate quickly. Synthetic materials that have shown to provide good resistance to water, salt, and UV exposure are recommended to replace the more traditional materials. Polypropylene webbing has been used satisfactorily as a replacement for leather.

MAINTENANCE

Exposure to water, salt, sand, extreme sunlight, and other elements can impact the performance and durability of a prosthesis. Prosthetic equipment should be thoroughly washed, dried, and lubricated as necessary after each use in a water environment to ensure its proper and safe function.

Swimming

Swimming is an excellent source of exercise and therapy for the upper limb amputee. For an individual with a transhumeral or more distal amputation, swimming is therapeutic in improving range of motion and strengthening muscles that otherwise might not be challenged.

The majority of persons with a hand absence swim without a prosthesis and contrary to popular opinion, they don't swim in circles. Custom swimming prostheses are possible using current technology and can provide improved swimming performance. Two-piece prostheses utilizing an inner, roll-on, silicon prosthetic sleeve technology like Fillauer 3S® (1) or ICEROSS® are an excellent choice. A traditional prosthetic suspension can be improved by using a type of flexible suspension sleeve, described in the previous section. A flexible, swimming paddle terminal device like the Freestyle® (Figure 23-40) can provide the necessary displacement for propulsion and simultaneously compensate for the inability of some amputees to pronate and supinate the hand while swimming. A simple flat paddle will suffice if enough arm remains to feather the fin or paddle in the water. Swimming aids can also be attached directly to the arm with straps or elastic banding.

Two other key factors must be considered when developing a swimming prosthesis. First, the overall length of the prosthesis: A swimmer with a short forearm might have difficulty with a full length prosthesis because of the water resistance involved. A stubby prosthesis with a swim paddle may be easier and more efficient to control. A second issue to consider is the design of the fin or paddle: Some swimmers prefer a flat blade

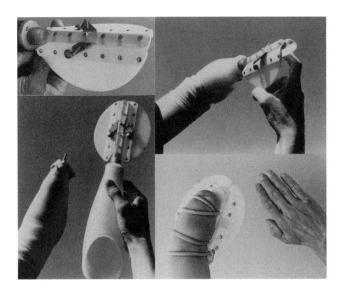

FIGURE 23-40

Freestyle TSD prosthetic swimming device and Freestyle Swim Paddle. Courtesy TRS, Inc.

to a curved or concave shape. The flat paddle planes through the water, whereas a curved or concave design can cause the prosthesis to inadvertently "submarine" as the arm moves forward in the water, as in the Australian crawl stroke. However, the curved design can move water more easily while performing the backstroke. Experimentation and swimmer preference will help develop the best solution.

Water Skiing

This water sport presents special considerations due to the speed, dynamics, and potential danger involved. Single-handed water skiing is possible but extremely stressful and tiring. Using a prosthesis is possible, but extreme care must be given to being able to release the ski rope. A disconnect at the boat is *not* a safe, sole option. The skier must be able to control the rope's release or injury can result. A number of options exist. The rope handle can be modified to accept an end cap that will pull free when the handle is released. This Delgar sling concept has been used successfully. A simple plastic water ski hook can be fabricated to allow for control over a rope handle. The shallow hook releases with a twist of the prosthesis. This hook design should only be used with a supracondylar-style prosthesis, which can be easily doffed. If the hook fails to twist off during a fall, the prosthesis itself will pull off. Covering the prosthesis with a thick layer (5 mm) of neoprene wet suit material will ensure that the discarded prosthesis will float, thus making recovery possible.

Custom water ski devices are also possible. These devices may be designed to snap onto the handle without a release mechanism. The safety release system is then fabricated into the rope. If the skier falls, the action triggers the rope handle section to disconnect from the main rope. Another idea utilizes a terminal device designed to release under a specific load or force. When a fall exceeds this predetermined load, the device breaks free of the handle. This type of design requires a lot of engineering and experimentation to develop and should be approached with caution, due to all the various factors involved.

Windsurfing

Single-handed windsurfing is possible but like water skiing, difficult and tiring. The dynamics of handling the boom, mast, sail, and harness lines can prove overwhelming, especially in heavy wind or rough water. Myo-type prostheses are prohibited because of the real potential for total immersion in the water. Body-powered, voluntary closing prehensors like the Grip 3® have proved functional. Wet suits can restrict cable and harness operation, so prosthetic harnesses and cable systems need to be worn on the outside of tight fitting wet suits to ensure efficiency of operation. Wind surfing requires a powerful grip but also a quick, efficient release of gear. Passive devices have been utilized to a limited extent but lack some of the dynamics required for safe windsurfing in all conditions.

Saltwater environments demand special attention for prosthetic systems, because salt on cables can cause excess friction, much like grit or dirt. Prostheses should be thoroughly washed with soap and fresh water and lubricated as needed after each day's excursion.

Weight Lifting and Conditioning

Weight lifting, training, and conditioning continue to grow in popularity in the general population, and in physically challenged populations. The benefits of strength training for a variety of sports, along with cross-training, can provide measurable performance benefits. Hand amputees and persons with congenital upper limb absence can benefit from weight lifting. Persons missing a hand rarely challenge the affected side of their bodies enough to maintain balanced strength and symmetry. Weight conditioning can reverse the atrophy processes and either build or rebuild muscle. The effects of a therapeutic or recreational weight training program can be better general health, as well as improved muscularity and strength.

A number of custom adaptations have been tried over the years, with varied success, to provide the grasp

and control necessary to handle dumbbells, barbells, and the various handle styles encountered on weight training apparatus. Traditional voluntary opening split hooks have proved of little value. However, voluntary closing devices are useful and specific products like the Grip 2S® (Figure 23-41) can be modified to improve their weight lifting applications even more. A simple locking pin added to the grip device allows for a positive, manually operated locking system to engage dumbbells and other equipment. Using such an aid enables the participant to focus on the specific movement or exercise rather than concentrating on having to maintain prehension via cable tension. Weight lifting performance can also be augmented by the use of a prosthesis that utilizes a roll-on silicone liner. The extra suspension is very beneficial to these types of activities and provides an additional margin of safety when heavy loads are being used. Additionally, a prosthesis that

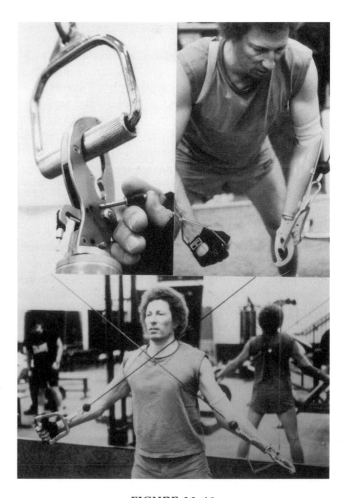

FIGURE 23-41

Grip 25 with locking pin adaptation for weight lifting and other rigorous activities. Courtesy TRS, Inc.

incorporates carbon fiber reinforcement is recommended. TRS Inc. has extensive experience in weight training consultation and the successful application of voluntary closing systems to these activities.

Myoelectric prostheses have enough prehension for most weight lifting activities but the abuse, abrasion, and stress placed on the prosthesis in weight lifting make more conventional body-powered prostheses the popular choice.

CONCLUSIONS

The numerous modifications and adaptations discussed in this chapter are intended to be as comprehensive as possible but reflect only a portion of the potential solutions. A device, technique, or modification that meets the needs of one individual may not be effective for another. In searching out creative solutions, it is advisable to work with a knowledgeable rehabilitation team. It is very important for the patient/consumer to know how experienced a prosthetist is regarding sports and recreation prosthetic design and fabrication and whether a team effort complements that knowledge. Many resources exist and continue to evolve, and information available on the Internet is growing exponentially. Organizations like the Amputee Coalition of America provide information and advocacy for amputees. Publications that include research as well as self-help solutions and resources are becoming readily available; working with a rehabilitation specialist may be the most efficient pathway for accessing these resources and ensuring that the most optimum solution possible is delivered.

References

1. Radocy B. Upper limb prosthetic adaptations for sports and recreation. In: Bowker JH (ed.), *Atlas of Limb Prosthetics,* 2nd ed. Boston: Mosby, 1992.
2. Budde, Chelsea M. The power of play. Amputee Coalition of America. *In Motion;* 7(1), 20.
3. National Federation of State High School Associations. Rule Books. P.O. Box 20626, Kansas City, Missouri, 65195. (816) 464-5400/(816)464-5571.
4. Radocy R, Beiswenger W. A high performance, variable suspension, transradial prosthesis. *J Prosthetics Orthotics* 1995; 7(2), 65–67.
5. Radocy B. Upper extremity prosthetics: Considerations and designs for sports and recreation. *Clin Prosthetics Orthotics* 1987; 11(3), 131–153.
6. Department of Agricultural Engineering. Breaking new ground prosthetic and worksite modifications for farmers with upper extremity amputations. *Plow Shares* #3, Purdue University.
7. Mailhot A. Musical instruments for upper limb amputees. Child Amputee Research Project. University of Michigan Inter Clinic Information Bulletin, Vol. XIII, No. 10, July 1974.
8. Erickson LB. Piano playing as a hobby for children with problem hands. Child Amputee Research Project. University of Michigan Inter Clinic Information Bulletin, Vol. XI, No. 6, March 1972.

Resources

Abilities Unlimited (Keeping Fit booklet), 245 Parkside Dr., Colorado Springs, Colorado. (719) 520-9700.

Access To Recreation. Equipment for the Physically Challenged. (Catalog). Contact: Don Krebs, 8 Sandra Ct., Newbury Park, California 91320. (800) 634-4351, (805) 498-7535, dkrebs@gte.net.

Active Living Magazine, 132 Main Street East, Suite 1, Grimsby, Ontario, Canada L3M 1P1.(905) 309-1639, Fax (905) 309-1640, activeliv@aol.com.

Amend Music Center., Robin Amend, W. 1305 14th, Spokane, Washington, 99204. (509) 456-0376, ramend4034@aol.com.

Amputee Coalition of America (ACA), 900 E. Hill Ave., Ste. 285, Knoxville Tennessee 37915. (423) 524-8772, (888) 267-5669, Fax (423) 525-7917, www.amputee-coalition.org.

Amputee Golfer Magazine, P.O. Box 5801, Coralville, Iowa 52241. (800) 633-6242, NAGAOFFICE@aol.com.

AOPA National Office (Sports Anyone? booklet), 1630 King St., Suite 500, Alexandria, Virginia 22314. (703) 836-7114.

Association of Driver Educators for the Disabled (ADED). P.O. Box 49, Edgerton, Wisconsin 53534. (608) 884-8833.

Department of Veterans Affairs Prosthetic and Sensory Aids Service, Mailing Code 117C, Washington, D.C. 20420. (202) 273-5400, Fax (202) 535-7294.

Disabled Sports/USA (DS/USA), 451 Hungerford Drive, Suite 100, Rockville, Maryland 20850. (301) 217-0960, www.dsusa.org.

Eastern Amputee Golf Association, http://www.eaga.org & Western Amputee Golf Association, www.wagagolf.org.

Handicapped Scuba Association, HSA International, 1104 El Prado, San Clemente, California 92672. Voice/Fax (714) 498-6128 or (949) 498-6128 http://ourworld. compuserve.com/homepages/hsahdq.

Hosmer Dorrance Corp., 561 Division St., Campbell, California 95008. (800) 827-0070, hosmer@hosmer.com.

Little League Challenger Division. A special division for children with disabilities. www.littleleague.org.

National Amputee Golf Association (NAGA). P.O. Box 23285, on-Hudson, New York 10706. (800) 832-8697.

National Amputee Golf Association (NAGA), P.O. Box 23285, Milwaukee, Wisconsin 53223. (800) 633-NAGA, Fax (414) 376-1268, naga@execpc.com.

National Mobility Equipment Dealers Association. (NMEDA). 909 East Skagway Ave., Tampa, Florida 33604. (800) 833-0427, Fax (813) 931-4683.

National Sports Center for the Disabled, P.O. Box 1290, Winter Park, Colorado 80482. (970) 726-1540 www.nscd.org.

NovaCare Inc., Denver, Colorado. Contact Annaliese Furlong, CP. (303) 282-1428. O & P Athletic Fund, 1650 King St., Suite 500, Alexandria, Virginia 22314. (703) 836-7116.

Ossur USA, Inc. (ICEROSS Silicone prosthetic sleeve), 7100 Columbia Gateway Dr., Ste. 120, Columbia, Maryland, 21046. (800)ICE-X727, (410) 290-0130.

Palaestra Magazine of Adapted Physical Education. Palaestra, P.O. Box 508, Macomb, Illinois 61455. (309) 833-1902, www.palaestra.com.

Physically Challenged Bowhunters of America, Inc. (PCBA), RD #1, Box 470, New Alexandria, Pennsylvania 15670. (724) 668-7439.

Toys R Us Toy Guide for Differently Abled Kids, 461 From Rd., 4th Fl., Paramus, New Jersey 07652.(201) 262-7800, www.toysrus.com.

Colorado. (303) 444-4720, Fax (303) 444-5372, (800) 279-1865, www.oandp.com/trs.

United Federation of Disabled Archers, (UFFDA), P.O. Box 50, 20 9th Ave. N.E., Glenwood, Minnesota 56334. (320) 634-3660, bowhunter@wavefront.com.

War Amps Child Amputee Program and CHAMP Newsletter, The War Amputations of Canada, CHAMP Program, 2827 Riverside Dr., Ottawa, Ontario, Canada, K1V OC4. (613) 731-3821, www.waramps.ca.

Wright Archery, P.O. Box 1541, Lethbridge, Alberta, Canada, T1J 4K3. (403) 381-6605, Fax (403) 381-7023.

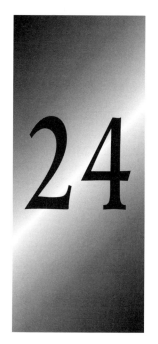

24 Case Studies of Upper Extremity Amputations and Prosthetic Restoration

*James A. Leonard, Jr. MD, Linda Miner, OTR, CHT,
and Mike Hillbom, CP*

CASE 1: PARTIAL HAND AMPUTATION

A 51-year-old man with a history of life-long seizure disorder was involved in a riding lawnmower accident 1 year ago. He sustained amputations of the left thumb at the carpometacarpal joint, distal portion of the middle finger, and tip of the fourth finger. The amputated portion of the fourth finger was successfully reattached. He lives on a farm and reports that he has considerable difficulty with activities of daily living, especially those requiring fine motor coordination and pinch with two hands. He also reports difficulty with his farm chores. His overall health is otherwise good. On examination, there is loss of the left thumb from the carpometacarpal joint distally, and the middle finger is amputated at approximately the level of the proximal interphalangeal (PIP) joint. The range of motion of the wrist and remaining digits of the left hand is normal. Strength is normal and sensation is preserved.

Prosthesis

This man was provided with a self-suspending partial hand prosthesis that utilizes an APRL thumb. He was also provided with a prosthetic restoration for his middle finger for cosmesis. It was recommended that he wear a work glove over the partial hand prosthesis.

Management Issue

Traumatic partial hand amputations are a relatively common occurence. They are usually associated with the digits or parts of a hand being caught, crushed, or cut in some type of machinery whether at work, on the farm, or at home. Loss of function in the injured hand usually results from the loss of prehension. This can be either fine motor, key or the three-jaw chuck-type pinch that occurs with the loss of the thumb, or a more gross grasp that can occur with the loss of fingers other than the thumb. The management issue to be addressed by the rehabilitation team is how to best restore the lost function. In addition to prosthetic treatment, surgical intervention (such as a toe transplant for a thumb amputation) may also be possible.

Teaching Point

For individuals with partial hand amputations, it is necessary to evaluate not only their anatomic loss, but understand how that loss impacts function for their particular life or vocational situation. Individuals with the exact same amputation experience similar cosmetic deficit, but may not experience the same functional deficit. Consider a professional guitar player, a secretary, and a physical therapist who have experienced the amputation of the index finger of the nondominant hand. The functional significance is considerably different for each. Each could be fit with a similar prosthetic finger that would provide excellent cosmesis, but would not satisfy the functional needs of each for their respective occupations. The special functional needs of an individual with a partial hand amputation must be taken into account when considering prosthetic options. For some, cosmesis is the most important consideration when fitting a partial hand prosthesis. For others, it is function. For most, it is the best compromise of these two characteristics (cosmesis and function).

For the case presented, restoration of active prehension was the patient's greatest functional need, but he was also concerned about appearance, hence the desire to also have a prosthesis for the distal middle finger. His prosthesis was fabricated with a thumb from an APRL hand. It would have been easier to fabricate the partial hand prosthesis with a fixed position thumb (an opposition post), but this would have limited the patient's function by restricting the width of objects he could grasp with his left hand. By using the APRL thumb, this man was able to choose which of two positions for the thumb was best suited for the activity he wished to do. This prosthesis provided him with the ability to have fine pinch for small objects and activities such as dressing. He was also able to passively abduct the thumb to grasp the large objects that he commonly encountered around the farm. Initially, he used his middle finger prosthesis and covered both with a work glove to call less attention to his amputations. Eventually, when he became more comfortable being seen in public, he stopped using his finger prosthesis. He continues to use a work glove to cover the thumb prosthesis, not for cosmesis, but to protect the prosthesis.

CASE 2: WRIST DISARTICULATION (WD)

A 25-year-old man working in a metal fabrication plant got his left hand caught and pulled into his machine. He sustained multiple injuries to his left upper extremity including a severe crush of the left hand, multiple lacerations to bone in the arm and forearm, and disruption of the axillary/brachial artery. On the day of injury, he had an arterial repair, suture of his lacerations, and pinning of his crushed hand. A wrist disarticulation was performed ten days later because the hand was not viable. Motor examination demonstrated absent palpable contraction of the biceps and forearm flexor and extensor muscles. Weakness was also present in his deltoid (4) and triceps (3+).

Sensation was intact over the anterior, lateral, and posterior shoulder and anterior arm. No shoulder subluxation was seen. Sensation was markedly diminished on the posterior arm and entire forearm. An EMG 1 month following his injury confirmed the presence of denervation with no voluntary motor unit activity in the left biceps brachii and forearm flexor and extensor muscles. Evidence was apparent of abnormal spontaneous activity and reduced motor unit recruitment in the deltoid; less so than in the triceps. The cervical paraspinal, supraspinatus, and infraspinatus muscles were normal. The diagnostic conclusion following the EMG was that the patient sustained at least severe left musculocutaneous, median, and radial nerve injuries, and these were possibly superimposed on a more proximal brachial plexus injury.

Three weeks following his amputation, the patient was fitted with a preparatory (provisional) body-powered prosthesis. His left upper extremity strength was the same as noted above. His shoulder range of motion was 95 degrees active and 125 degrees passive forward flexion, 90 degrees active and 120 degrees passive abduction, and 35 degrees extension. Elbow range was full passively and passive supination–pronation was limited to half the normal range. The patient also had significant dysesthetic residual limb pain and some phantom limb pain with associated sleep disturbance. This was successfully treated with a low-dose tricyclic antidepressant at bedtime.

Prosthesis

The patient was fitted with a preparatory left wrist disarticulation prosthesis with thermoplastic socket, dual control cable, figure-eight suspension harness, external locking elbow joints with lift assist, full (solid) plastic triceps cuff, quick disconnect wrist unit, cable operated hand, and 5XA terminal device (TD).

Management Issue

This case is not a typical WD. The presentation and management is confounded by the presence of the patient's peripheral nerve injuries and brachial plexus injury. Despite the patient's anatomic presentation as a WD, from a prosthetic function standpoint he presents more as an elbow disarticulation or transhumeral amputation. Would this patient have been better served by a more proximal level of amputation?

Teaching Point

The major management issue typically encountered when prescribing a prosthesis for a wrist disarticulation-level amputation is the selection of componentry and socket design. The long length of the residual limb can limit the choice of wrist and TD selection so that the forearm–hand is not too long for both function and cosmesis. With wrist disarticulation, functional active pronation and supination is preserved (prosthetic range of motion is usually less than the active anatomic range of motion), allowing the prosthetic user to actively position the TD for function "on the fly" without having to preposition it prior to the activity, as he would with more proximal transradial amputations. Some socket designs permit the user to take more advantage of this active range of motion than others.

Typically, a WD amputation would be fitted with a body-powered prosthesis utilizing a single control cable system. To accomodate for the long anatomic length, this patient was fit as a wrist disarticulation-level amputation with the appropriate socket. Initially, the prosthesis had flexible elbow hinges. Rigid external locking elbow joints were subsequently added in place of the typical flexible hinges, because the patient had no active pronation–supination or elbow flexion. The dual control cable system (split housing TD control cable and the elbow lock cable) was selected to facilitate flexion and allowed this patient to position his forearm, lock the elbow, and then operate the TD similar to an elbow disarticulation or transhumeral prosthesis. On this patient's prosthesis, the prosthetist added an elbow lift assist to help accomodate for the weight of the forearm. If needed, two lift assists could be used (attached to both medial and lateral elbow joints) to counterbalance the forearm weight and make cable-assisted elbow flexion easier to accomplish.

Approximately nine months following his injury, this patient began to have some active return of biceps function. One year post injury, the biceps strength is such that the patient no longer requires the use of the elbow lift assist to flex the forearm with the prosthesis and mechanical hand. Triceps strength has also improved, and trace to poor minus function has returned to the proximal forearm flexor muscles. The patient is no longer utilizing the elbow lock. The patient regained sufficient motor recovery to be successfully fitted with a preparatory single-site myoelectrically controlled externally powered prosthesis with shortened friction wrist and hand.

CASE 3: TRANSRADIAL AMPUTATION

A 36-year-old printer whose right hand was caught in an ink press sustained the following injuries: digit amputations, complete degloving of the hand proximal to the wrist, and disruption of the neurovascular bundle. It was determined that salvage of the hand was not possible and an open wrist disarticulation was performed in the emergency department. This was later revised to a long transradial amputation. This man was

fit with a preparatory body-powered prosthesis 2 weeks following his amputation. After 1 week of prosthetic use, the patient was wearing the prosthesis nearly full time and demonstrated excellent control and incorporation of the prosthesis into his activities of daily living. Initial evaluation for a potential myoelectric prosthetic control site was begun 3 weeks post amputation. The patient demonstrated excellent control of both the residual forearm flexors and extensors at this early date, suggesting that he could be a successful user of a myoelectrically controlled externally powered prosthesis. Three and a half months following the amputation, the patient's residual limb volume was felt to be sufficiently stable to permit fitting with a definitive myoelectric prosthesis. Vocational rehabilitation has been complicated by ongoing dyesthetic residual limb pain, phantom limb pain, disordered sleep, and flashbacks of the accident. The pain symptoms were decreased with prosthetic use, pharmacologic treatment, and modality treatment (TENS), but did not show significant improvement until the patient agreed to participate in ongoing psychologic counseling for his flashbacks. He has been unable to return to his former place of employment. He is currently pursuing other types of work. He has recently developed a new symptom of burning pain in his thumb while wearing his myoelectric prosthesis. This was attributed to the presence of a distal median nerve neuroma.

Prostheses

His initial prosthesis was a preparatory right transradial conventional body-powered prosthesis with thermoplastic socket, single control cable, figure-eight suspension harness, flexible elbow hinges, friction wrist unit, 5X hook TD, compression socks, limb socks, rubber bands, and band-applier.

He was subsequently prescribed a definitive right myoelectric prosthesis with self-suspending double wall socket with theromoflex liner and quick disconnect myoelectric wrist unit, Bock electric hand, Greifer, PVC glove, two electrodes, two batteries, and a battery charger. The socket fit of this prosthesis was initially evaluated with a check socket fitting.

Management Issues

Pain and psychologic adjustment issues were the major concerns that the clinic team needed to address with this patient. He demonstrated that he was capable of superb prosthetic function with both his cable-operated and powered prostheses. Prosthetic function was not the issue: He had difficulty resuming his life due to what he initially described as residual limb pain and phantom pain. Many treatments were attempted for his pain, all with limited success. The patient would report that the treatments were helping and his pain was less, but his ability to function in his daily life, as reported by his family and case worker, remained unchanged. After several months working with the team, the patient became comfortable enough to confide in the staff that he was having severe problems with flashbacks of his accident.

The new onset phantom pain in the thumb could be reproduced with the palpation of a 1.5 cm neuroma in the distal volar residual limb. This was diagnosed as a median neuroma from the distribution of the sensory symptoms. Adjustment of the socket fit resolved this problem.

Teaching Points

Three points are illustrated in this case. First, it is preferable that patients undergo prosthetic restoration rapidly following uncomplicated amputation. Fitting a prosthesis within the first few weeks following amputation generally enhances prosthetic use in daily activities and early return to preamputation levels of activity and daily function. Second, neuromas occur commonly but do not generally pose a major problem with upper extremity prosthetic use. If the neuromas are symptomatic with prosthetic wear, although many treatments are available, usually a simple adjustment of socket fit is sufficient to solve the problem. The third and most important point this case illustrates is that of psychologic adjustment following amputation. Although psychologic issues are discussed and intervention offered to all of our patients before or shortly after amputation, as the situation allows, it has been our experience that most patients feel uncomfortable accepting this advice. Treatment team members need to remain alert to the fact that psychologic issues will often present with other somatic symptoms that a patient may find more socially or culturally acceptable. If this point is missed, the team can find itself focused on other issues, such as pain, that may be very time consuming and virtually impossible to resolve until the real issue is identified. In the case of our patient, his cultural heritage played a major role in his initial inability to address the psychologic component of his injury.

CASE 4: ELBOW DISARTICULATION

A 34-year-old man involved in a motor vehicle accident 8 years ago sustained trauma to his left upper extremity resulting in a left elbow disarticulation. He was initially fitted with a body-powered prosthesis with a hook TD, which he did not like because of poor cosmesis. He was eventually fitted with a hybrid prosthesis with a power-operated hand and wrist rotator and cable-operated externally locking elbow joints. This prosthesis is suspended with a shoulder saddle (using a Bowden cable) and chest strap. The patient wears his prosthesis all day. He liked the function that the powered wrist rotator added to his prosthesis, but disliked the weight that it added and has had it removed to lighten his prosthesis. What he dislikes most about his prosthesis is the harness. He finds the harness restricting and irritating, and it causes him to sweat. He came to the clinic requesting a new prosthesis. His current prosthesis is many years old, and the socket is no longer fitting correctly. His shoulder range of motion is full. Strength and sensation are normal. He does have a prominant Tinnel's sign just posterior to the medial epicondyle on his residual limb with dysesthetic sensation radiating to his ulnar sensory distribution in his phantom hand. Skin is intact, without irritation.

Prostheses

The current prosthesis is a definitive left elbow disarticulation prosthesis with single-wall socket with total-contact Thermoflex liner, shoulder saddle and chest strap suspension, dual-control cable body-powered external locking elbow joints, bungee cord forearm lift assist, myoelectric-powered wrist rotator, quick disconnect wrist unit, Bock myoelectric hand, Greifer, two electrodes, and charger.

The proposed new definitive prosthesis will be a left elbow disarticulation prosthesis with single-wall socket using total contact, Thermoflex suction socket liner with cinch strap above the epicondyles, auxiliary supra-acromial detachable gel suspension strap, body-powered external locking elbow joints, bungee cord forearm lift assist, quick disconnect wrist unit, Bock myoelectric hand, Greifer, two electrodes, and charger with an initial check socket fitting.

Management Issues

This man is extremely functional with his current prosthetic design, but he hates the cumbersome suspension harness and wishes to do away with this on his new prosthesis. The bulbous nature of the distal residual limb poses the greatest difficulty to achieving adequate suspension without a suspension harness. The shape does not allow adequate total contact over the entire surface of the residual limb to achieve a suction suspension. One might consider anatomic epicondylar suspension, but clinical evidence exists of an ulnar neuroma in this area that is sensitive and is likely to prevent this type of suspension even if the patient could tolerate the weight of the prosthesis suspended from these bony structures. (Remember he had the wrist unit removed due to the weight.)

Teaching Points

The first point to make is that most prosthetic teams will not manage many amputees with this level of amputation. The bulbous nature of the distal humerus, together with the length make for a difficult prosthetic fit with poor cosmetic appearance. The long length of the residual limb necessitates the use of external elbow joints to maintain level elbow centers and anatomic forearm length with this prosthesis. External elbow joints increase the width of the elbow of the prosthesis over that of the "normal" anatomic elbow. This increased width is a major contributing factor to the poor cosmesis and is the reason to look for other options to provide elbow lift assist other than the use of standard lift assist springs. The use of standard units would only further increase the width of the elbow (the reason for the use of the bungee cord assist in this case). External locking elbow joints are also not as durable as an internal elbow unit (used with transhumeral prostheses). The length of the residual limb also makes this level ideal for the use of a hybrid prosthesis when powered prehension is desired. Practically, this is the only option available, because the length of the residual limb precludes the use of a powered elbow unit. The advent of flexible socket materials, most commonly used in lower extremity prosthetics, does have an application in upper limb prosthetics, especially where the residual limb shape is irregular or skin integrity is marginal or questionable. The use of test socket fitting also allowed the prosthetist to evaluate another suspension option, the feasibility of a vacuum (suction) socket fit utilizing a section of silicone sleeve material at the proximal brim of the socket.

CASE 5: TRANSHUMERAL AMPUTATION

A 37-year-old man sustained an immediate left elbow disarticulation in a conveyor belt accident at work 10 years ago. His amputated arm and forearm were not replanted due to soft tissue injury of the amputated portion of the extremity and contamination of the wound. The wound was left open for several days to ensure no local infection. The amputation was then revised to a mid to long transhumeral amputation and closed. The patient has been a successful prosthetic user since 1 month following his amputation. He was initially fitted with a body-powered prosthesis, which he could operate successfully, but he found limitations using this prosthesis. He had difficulty with what he could pick up with his TD because of the limited pinch force of the TD. He also found he was even more limited in what he could lift when actively flexing the prosthetic elbow. He was not able to generate enough force with the body-powered cable to meet his daily activity needs. Approx-

imately 1 year after his injury, he was fitted with a myoelectrically controlled prosthesis with dual site control, Utah elbow, power wrist rotator, and Bock myoelectric hand. The prosthesis was suspended with a shoulder saddle and chest strap. The patient requested that the rotator be removed to allow shortening of the forearm for equal arm lengths and to reduce the weight of the prosthesis. He next requested that his prosthesis be modified to eliminate the harness, because he found this constricting. He was provided with a suction socket fit and has worn this prosthesis successfully without a harness for many years. He has had difficulty with a cold, dusky purple skin discoloration and breakdown on the distal residual limb requiring frequent prosthetic socket modifications through the years to maintain a good fit. The addition of an air bladder between his outer rigid socket wall and the flexible inner socket, which the patient can adjust as needed, has resolved most fit problems. The patient continues to work full time. He has myofascial symptoms in his left scapular stabilizer and rotator cuff muscles. These symptoms have responded well to myofascial release, stretching, and strengthening, plus the addition of a supra-acromial gel suspension strap. Following treatment of his soft tissue symptoms, he has seen improved active left shoulder range of motion and strength that has resulted in improved prosthetic function.

Prosthesis

The patient was prescribed a definitive left transhumeral myoelectically controlled externally powered prosthesis with laminated outer socket wall with Thermoflex inner suction socket, adjustable air bladder between proximal laminated outer and inner flexible socket to accomodate for volume changes, detachable supra-acromial gel auxillary suspension strap, Utah elbow, myoelectric quick disconnect wrist unit, Greifer, Utah electrode set, two batteries, and battery charger.

Management Issues

Can a transhumeral prosthesis be adequately suspended for function without the use of some form of suspension harness? Is suction suspension adequate for daily activities? Does the use of suction suspension require a change in the conventional wisdom about transhumeral socket design and fit? Are choke syndromes common in upper extremity amputees?

Teaching Points

The use of myoelectrically controlled externally powered components in upper limb prostheses eliminates the need for an attachment point for the control cables on a harness. Thus, the remaining function of the harness is to suspend the prosthesis and hold it securely on the body. Anatomic suspension or self-suspension for externally powered transradial prostheses has long been known and utilized to provide amputees harness-free prosthetic function. The use of a suction suspension socket in conjunction with a myoelectric control system can accomplish the same feat for the transhumeral amputee. The use of flexible thermoplastic materials for the socket interface can make this form of suspension more successful and comfortable. A small one-way suction valve, similar to that used with transfemoral prostheses, is included in the distal socket. In conventional upper limb prosthetic socket design, the socket is not usually designed for total distal contact. Typically, a small gap exists between the distal end of the residual limb and the end of the socket. Such a design in a lower extremity prosthesis would result in a choke syndrome; however, this is not a problem usually encountered in upper extremity amputees. This is true in most cases, except when a suction suspension system is used: To maintain suction there must be total circumferential contact someplace in the prosthetic socket or suction cannot be maintained. To prevent the occurence of a choke, an upper extremity suction socket must have total contact, just as in a lower extremity prosthesis. Unlike lower extremity prostheses, gravity is continually working to pull the upper extremity suction socket away from the distal end of the limb and create a space where a choke can occur. Upper extremity choke syndromes have the same appearance as in the lower extremity (cool, dusky, edematous skin often with ulceration), but may not be initially recognized due to the infrequency of occurence. Choke in the upper limb is treated similarly to that in the lower limb—by restoring total contact. Unlike in the lower extremity, where adding distal padding will often resolve a choke, this approach will not be as successful in the upper limb. The key to eliminating a choke is to ensure that the suspension is adequate. In the case presented, this was accomplished by adding the adjustable air bladder and later the auxillary supra-acromial gel suspension strap. Pigment changes in the skin associated with a choke may be permanent. This patient is able to lift his young child (30 + lbs) using his prosthesis without losing control or his suspension.

CASE 6: SHOULDER DISARTICULATION

A 28-year-old woman sustained an electrical burn injury 6 years ago while at home, with an entrance wound in the right upper extremity and exit wounds through both feet. Her injuries ultimately resulted in a right shoulder disarticulation and bilateral proximal transtibial amputations. She was fitted with a right shoulder disarticulation and bilateral transtibial prostheses. After approximately 1 year of attempting to use her upper extremity prosthesis, she abandoned its use. She continues to use her bilateral lower extremity prostheses. She wears both all day and ambulates without assistive devices. She only uses a wheelchair when she has skin breakdown on her legs and she cannot wear her prostheses. She has been employed in clerical work for the past 5 years. For the past year, she has been waking up at night with "numbness and tingling" in her left thumb, index, and middle fingers. She finds it difficult to use her computer keyboard and mouse at work because her hand cramps up. Examination of her hand demonstrates decreased sensation in the median sensory distribution with some questionable atrophy of the median innervated thenar muscles. Electrodiagnostic testing is positive for a left median mononeuropathy at the wrist with segmental demyelination without evidence of denervation. The findings are consistent with her clinical presentation of carpal tunnel syndrome.

Prostheses

Her definitive right shoulder disarticulation prosthesis included a double-wall socket with foam liner, modified chest strap suspension, body-powered dual-cable control system, nudge control for elbow lock cable, passive four-way shoulder joint, internal locking elbow joint with turntable, friction wrist unit, and 5XA TD.

The bilateral lower extremity prostheses were endoskeletal transtibial prostheses with total-contact patellar tendon-bearing sockets with Pelite foam liners and neoprene sleeve suspensions, lightweight alignable endoskeletal shanks, lightweight multiaxial feet, foam covers, cosmetic underhose, and limb socks.

Management Issues

Did the patient stop using her upper extremity prosthesis because it wasn't the best design for her? Would an externally powered prosthesis have provided her with more function? Has the prosthetic team failed if the amputee rejects a prosthesis? Has the patient's lack of prosthetic use contributed to the development of her carpal tunnel syndrome?

Teaching Points

This case demonstrates a basic principle regarding prosthetic restoration and function. The person with an amputation must derive some benefit from wearing a prosthesis or it will not be worn. The prosthesis must either improve an individual's function or appearance (body image) or it will not be used. The proximal levels of upper extremity amputation require more complex functional prostheses utilizing increasingly complex joint componentry, increased weight, increased heat build-up as body surface area decreases (particularly so in this person with three extremity amputations), and increasingly complex control options for a body-powered prosthesis that are often difficult to master. The prosthesis for this level of amputation often becomes only a passive assistive device, despite the presence of a control system. An externally powered prosthesis with switch control may provide more active function at this level, but does so at the price of increased weight and cost. This patient did not have the insurance coverage or resources to receive an externally powered prosthesis. Externally powered prostheses with sophisticated control systems may lead an amputee to have greater expectations for "normal" or improved extremity function than the prosthesis is able to deliver. Ultimately, the individual must make the final decision to use or not use a prosthesis. If the patient chooses not to use a prosthesis, the prosthetic team should not view this as a failure on their part.

Upper extremity amputees may experience musculoskeletal symptoms. Often these occur in the nonamputated extremity, especially if amputees tend to become predominantly one-handed for ADLs, as has happened in this case. The implications for further loss of function in this patient with only one "sound" extremity can be grave and might require a more agressive therapeutic intervention than would be considered with the degree of carpal tunnel syndrome presenting here. Upper extremity amputees can also experience musculoskeletal symptoms in their amputated limb, particularly in their shoulder girdle musculature (as in Case 5). These symptoms usually respond well to conservative therapies and often result in increased prosthetic use and function.

CASE 7: FOREQUARTER AMPUTATION

A 60-year-old woman underwent a right forequarter amputation at 26 years of age for a giant cell tumor of the right arm. Following healing of her amputation site, she was initially fitted with a functional prosthesis that encorporated a forequarter socket, four-way passive shoulder joint, internal locking elbow joint with turntable and forearm spring lift assist, FM quick disconnect wrist unit, APRL hook, and Dorrance hand. As it was anticipated that she would not wear this prosthesis all day, she was also given a foam rubber shoulder cap to allow her to comfortably wear her clothing when not wearing the prosthesis. She indicated that she was initially able to use the prosthesis to assist with some

activities of daily living and wore the prosthesis regularly mostly for looks until her mid to late forties, while she was working as a nurse. For the past 10 to 15 years she has discarded her prosthesis because it was too heavy. She has continued to use the foam shoulder cap, now disintegrating, to allow the proper fit of her clothing. She returned to clinic after a 20-year absence to have a new foam shoulder cap made. Examination demonstrated a near complete right forequarter amputation. The proximal portion of clavicle remained. The amputation site was well healed, not tender, and without any skin irritation. She was wearing a small remnant of a very old sponge rubber shoulder cap to secure her bra strap.

Prosthesis

A new lightweight ventilated flexible thermoplastic shoulder cap, secured by bra strap or removable chest strap, was prescribed. A lightweight definitive endoskeletal passive shoulder disarticulation prosthesis was also prescribed. The prosthesis had a flexible thermoplastic socket with chest strap suspension, passive four-way shoulder joint, passive manual locking elbow joint, friction wrist unit, foam and nylon cover, passive lightweight hand, and PVC prosthetic glove.

Management Issue

Was it appropriate to provide the patient with a new prosthesis in addition to the shoulder cap, since she clearly indicated that she stopped wearing her previous prosthesis 10 to 15 years earlier and had probably stopped using it for functional activities much earlier?

Teaching Point

Patients with amputations who utilize prostheses need to be seen in follow-up by the prosthetic rehabilitation team at some regular interval. This patient did not return to clinic because she was under the impression that the prosthesis she had been fit with previously was the best available to her. During her initial training with her original prosthesis, the concept of prosthetic function had been emphasized to her. She believed that prosthetic restoration was meant to be primarily functional and, if this were the case, there was not much point in seeking out a new prosthesis. She had learned from experience that the function of a prosthesis for ADLs at her level of amputation was limited. Her prosthesis served her best by providing her with a somewhat normal appearance, minimizing the stares and questions of strangers. When her prosthesis became too heavy to wear, she relied on the use of her shoulder cap to wear her clothing. It was only the advanced state of deterioration of her foam rubber shoulder cap that brought her back to clinic. Significant advances in the materials utilized in prosthetic fabrication permitted the team to provide this patient with a much more comfortable, durable, cooler, and lightweight shoulder cap. The team was also able to show the patient examples of designs of lightweight passive prostheses for her amputation level that provide very acceptable cosmesis. Her new passive SD prosthesis has become her preferred form of prosthetic restoration over the shoulder cap. When considering prosthetic prescription, cosmesis should be given equal consideration along with other prosthetic function.

CASE 8: PARTIAL HAND AND WRIST DISARTICULATIONS

A 49-year-old farmer with insulin dependent diabetes was involved in a farm machinery accident. His hands were caught and pulled into a corn picker. It took approximately an hour to free his hands from the machinery, during which time his hands also sustained severe friction burns from a rotating rubber belt. He underwent multiple surgeries in an attempt to salvage his hands. Due to the severity of his injuries and nonviability, he required an amputation of the right hand at the mid carpus and on the left, amputation of the thumb just proximal to the MP joint and the other four digits at or just distal to the MCP joints. He lacked sufficient soft tissue coverage to close both amputation sites. Bilateral groin flaps were established, and both hands were sutured to the groin for approximately 6 weeks, following which the flaps were taken down and the amputation sites closed. The patient was referred to the upper extremity amputee clinic after successful closure of his amputation sites. Subsequently, he had a web space deepening surgery performed on his left hand to provide him with improved prehension. Following the healing of the amputation sites, the patient was successfully fitted with a right prosthesis and an opposition orthosis for the left hand.

Prosthesis

The right prosthesis was initially a modified preparatory body-powered wrist disarticulation prosthesis with single-wall thermoplastic socket with distal window and removable wall (to accomodate the bulbous shape of the residual limb and to better harness the patient's active pronation and supination), figure-eight harness, flexible elbow hinges, flexion friction wrist unit, and 5X TD. Later he was fitted with a self-suspending (via window and removable distal socket wall) myoelectric prosthesis with Greifer.

Management Issue

What is the appropriate level of amputation for an individual with bilateral upper extremity trauma? When should the prosthetic and rehabilitation teams become involved with the management of patients with upper limb amputations?

Teaching Point

The most salient teaching point associated with this case presentation is the advantage of the early involvement of the rehabilitation and prosthetic teams in the care of patients with upper extremity trauma that might lead to amputation. The surgeons in this case were very diligent and worked hard to provide this patient with the best functional outcome. It was their belief that preserving as much bony length for this patient was imperative, because it was evident that he would lose both of his hands. To this end, they elected to use a groin flap to preserve the proximal row of carpals on the right. The left hand also required a groin flap to close. For 6 weeks, both of this patient's upper extremities were secured to his groin, and he was totally dependent on his family for ADLs. Following take down of his groin flaps, it took another month until his limb was sufficiently healed to be fit with his provisional prosthesis. The preservation of the distal carpal row resulted in a residual limb that was quite bulbous and difficult to fit, as well as a prosthesis that was a bit too long for midline ADLs, even using a wrist flexion unit. The early involvement of the prosthetic team may have helped the surgical team decide that a wrist disarticulation or long transradial amputation would have been just as functional for this patient and could have permitted the primary closure of the amputation site without the need for a groin flap on the right. The patient could have been fitted with a functional right WD or transradial prosthesis within a week or two of his initial injury and provided with some means of ADL independence.

CASE 9: BILATERAL WRIST DISARTICULATIONS

A 20-year-old man sustained severe bilateral crush injuries to both hands in a press while at work. After several surgeries, his hands were determined to be nonviable and bilateral WDs were done. A few areas of delayed healing occurred in his amputation incisions. His pain, secondary to his original trauma and postoperative pain, was managed with Tylox® and Oxycodone®. He also had phantom pain postamputation, which was well managed with gabapentin and amitriptylene. His shoulder, elbow, and forearm supination–pronation range of motion were normal bilaterally. Upper extremity strength and sensation was normal in the remaining upper extremities. Activities of daily living were impaired, with the patient being totally dependent for feeding, dressing, and bathing. He was withdrawn, depressed, and minimally communicative during the period of attempted surgical reconstruction of his hands and following his amputations.

Prosthesis

Approximately 1 week after the completion of his amputations, he was fit with bilateral provisional prostheses. The prostheses utilized synthetic casting material for the sockets, flexible elbow hinges, triceps cuffs, single control cables, friction wrist units, 5XA TDs, and a separate figure-eight suspension harness for each prosthesis.

Management Issue

Loss of this young man's ADL independence and sense of control, with associated reactive depression were the key issues of concern for the rehabilitation team. Discussion centered on the most appropriate approach to provide this man returned control of his environment.

Teaching Point

This man was transferred from the acute care surgical service to the inpatient rehabilitation service. This was done so that ADL, self-care, and depression issues could be dealt with more quickly and intensively than if he were an outpatient. To treat this man as an outpatient would have only prolonged his inability to become independent and in control of his own life and probably would have deepened his depression. He was fitted with his initial prostheses while still an inpatient. He very quickly became quite facile with his prostheses for self-care and ADLs. He used his prostheses many hours each day playing video games with a modified game controller. As he became more functional with his prostheses and required less assistance with ADLs and self-care, he became more interactive and less depressed.

Separate figure-eight suspension harnesses were chosen for his initial provisional prostheses to permit the wearing and use of a single prosthesis (right or left) or both prostheses at the same time. This approach to suspension was used in part because of some concern about the delayed healing of the incision sites on his residual limbs and to facilitate the control of the TDs. For bilateral amputees using body power for both TDs, control is usually linked. To use both TDs for prehension simultaneously, the individual must learn to activate one terminal device while not inadvertently activating the other at the same time. Separate suspension harnessing does not

completely eliminate this problem, but does allow the therapist to have the patient easily remove one prosthesis to concentrate on control training of a single prosthesis. This approach often decreases frustration for the new amputee trying to learn to use the prostheses, results in quicker and more successful prosthetic use, and better initial bilateral prosthetic function. In the case of the patient presented, it also permitted either prosthesis to be quickly removed when it was apparent that the skin was becoming irritated as a result of either too aggressive use or prolonged prosthetic wearing time. The other prosthesis could still be worn and used. The double-harness approach does present some increased difficulty in donning both prostheses and is more bulky than a single harness. As soon as there was no longer a concern about this man's skin integrity and he had demonstrated good independent TD control when wearing both protheses, an integrated single figure-eight harness was fabricated to replace the dual harnesses. It is also possible to design a suspension and control harness system that separates the suspension and control functions of the harness. This harness utilizes bilateral figure-nine axillary loops (or double "O" ring harness) attached to the respective control cables to better separate the control function of the TDs for the two prostheses. This type of design is said to enhance better bilateral prosthetic control and function, but the harnessing system is a bit bulkier and more cumbersome to manage than other harnessing options and, in our estimation, does not completely unlink the TD function of one prosthesis from the other. This case also demonstrates that it is important to fit bilateral amputees as soon as is feasible for ADL and self-care independence. Because the fit of an upper extremity prosthetic socket does not have to provide for weight bearing and is usually not in total contact at the distal end, it is possible to fit a provisional prosthesis very early postamputation even if total wound healing has not occurred. For the bilateral amputee, often the restoration of upper extremity function can be as important as, or more important than, primary wound healing. This does not mean, however, that wound healing, infection, or the condition of the skin can be ignored in favor of function. Common sense should prevail.

CASE 10: BILATERAL TRANSRADIAL AMPUTATIONS

A 31-year-old man with a history of splenectomy as a child developed pneumococcal sepsis as a complication of an aspiration pneumonia. His sepsis progressed to DIC and multisystem organ failure, including ischemia of all four extremities, which necessitated bilateral short transradial and bilateral transtibial amputations with split-thickness skin graft closures of all four limbs. The patient was depressed but cognitively intact. An examination of his extremities demonstrated bilateral short transradial residual limbs of approximately an equal length of 8 to 9 cm from antecubital fossa to distal residual ulna. The split-thickness skin grafts were healed. Elbow extension was –10 degrees full extension bilaterally. Elbow flexion and extension strength was 4 bilaterally. Palpable muscle contractions were present in the residual forearm flexors and extensors on the left and the forearm extensors on the right. There was absence of right forearm flexor muscle mass, presumed to be secondary to previous surgical debridement. His transtibial residual limbs were standard length (proximal third) with split thickness skin grafts having multiple open areas of granulation tissue in the area of the patellar tendons and distal residual limbs bilaterally. Hip range of motion was full bilaterally. He had bilateral knee flexion contractures –30 degrees on the right and – 45 degrees on the left. Quadriceps strength was –3 bilaterally, hip musculature and hamstring strength was 4 bilaterally. EMG demonstrated bilateral femoral mononeuropathies.

Prostheses

The right transradial amputation was fitted with a body-powered prosthesis with single control cable, double-wall socket, figure-eight harness, triceps cuff attached to socket, friction flexion wrist, and 5X hook. The left transradial amputation was fitted with an externally powered myoelectric prosthesis with double-wall self-suspending socket with foam liner, two-site control system, quick disconnect electric wrist, myoelectric hand, and PVC glove. The patient was fitted with bilateral lower extremity prostheses utilizing ischial containment proximal brims, TES belt suspension, external locking knee joints and distal bypass design (little or no contact on the nonhealed distal skin grafts), modular shanks, and lightweight single-axis feet. He was also fitted with custom-molded gel-lined knee pads with exterior soles for limited use in house knee-walking.

Management Issue

What upper limb prosthetic options will provide this patient—or any patient—having bilateral upper extremity amputations with the greatest function? The options include bilateral cable-operated prostheses, bilateral powered prostheses, or one cable and one powered prosthesis.

Teaching Point

This patient was fitted with one cable and one myoelectric prosthesis because it was felt that this approach would result in the most function for this man. The left side was chosen for the myoelectric fitting because of the presence of two good control sites (forearm flexor and extensor muscle groups) to simplify controls training. The goal for the myoelectric prosthesis was to provide this man with significantly greater prehension–grip force together with an increased functional range of prosthetic prehension than a cable-operated prosthesis would provide. The myoelectric prosthesis permitted him to have active prosthetic TD function above the shoulder height, as an example. The goal of the cable-operated prosthesis was increased fine motor dexterity using the 5X hook, improved midline function using the flexion wrist unit, and some sensory feedback via pressure on the residual limb and force on the cable when operating his hook TD. Use of a voluntary closing TD was considered to provide even more sensory feedback, but the patient was not partial to the appearance of the voluntary closing TD.

CASE 11: BILATERAL TRANSHUMERAL AMPUTATIONS

A 52-year-old sustained burns on his upper extremities, face, and trunk 15 years ago when a high-pressure boiler he was repairing at work malfunctioned and exploded. His injuries required bilateral upper extremity mid-length transhumeral amputations. He required skin grafting to his face, trunk, and distal residual limbs to treat his burns. He was right hand dominant prior to his injuries. He has continued to remain right prosthesis dominant since his amputations. He was fitted with his initial set of prostheses 17 days following his injury. The initial prostheses were cable-operated preparatory prostheses. He is currently wearing his third pair of prostheses, which continue to be cable-operated. He is having difficulty fitting in the current prostheses secondary to approximately a 10- to 15-pound weight gain, which he does not anticipate losing. Occasionally, he develops minor skin breakdown on his distal residual limbs. He also has infrequent phantom pain, but not severe enough to request any treatment. On examination, he demonstrated bilateral equal length mid-humeral amputations with mature split-thickness skin grafts on his residual limb. There is no adherence to the underlying bone, and the grafts move freely on the underlying soft tissue. The grafts are not hypertrophic. His active shoulder range of motion is 150 to 160 degrees for flexion, 120 degrees for abduction, and 40 degrees of extension bilaterally. He was unable to get all the way into his prosthetic sockets using only a nylon sheath. Despite his fit problems, he demonstrated excellent bilateral prosthetic control with obvious right side dominance. His prostheses were well worn and in need of replacement.

Prostheses

A prescription was written for new bilateral definitive body-powered prostheses with dual control cable systems, double-wall sockets, single figure-eight harness, internal locking elbow joints with turntable and medially placed lift assists, friction flexion wrist units, and 5XA TDs. His socket fit was to be initially evaluated with bilateral check socket fittings. This prescription duplicated the prostheses the patient was currently wearing.

Management Issue

When is an amputee with weight change likely to experience a change in prosthetic fit? When an established prosthetic user requires a new prosthesis, what is the most appropriate prescription? Do bilateral upper extremity amputees maintain preamputation hand dominance?

Teaching Point

Amputees who use prostheses are likely to experience some change in the fit of their prosthetic socket when the weight gain or loss is 10 or more pounds. Weight loss for conventional body-powered or switch-controlled prosthetic users can usually be accommodated by adding sock ply or padding the socket. For myoelectrically controlled prostheses, the only option to deal with weight loss is to pad the socket, because adding a sock would interfere with electrode contact with the skin, which is necessary for prosthetic function. Weight gain can be managed by reducing sock ply (for those amputees wearing socks with their prostheses) or by heating and stretching the socket to accomodate the increased limb volume. Some materials used in prosthetic design are more amenable to this approach than others. When significant weight change has resulted in a significant increase or decrease in limb volume, the only option to maintain adequate prosthetic function is to fabricate a new socket. A change in volume was one of the factors taken into account in prescribing new prostheses for the case presented. The major reason for prescribing the new prostheses was the significant wear that had occurred.

When developing a prescription for a new prosthesis for an amputee, especially an established user, the prosthetic user's input should be given great consideration. In the case presented, some members of the team thought that the addition of powered components to at least one prosthesis would have provided the patient with enhanced prosthetic function. The patient was very functional and required no assistance from others with his ADLs or vocational or avocational activities when using his prostheses. He was quite satisfied with his current prosthetic prescription and wished no change in the design or components used for his new prostheses, and he made this point well known. It is possible for the prosthetic team to talk a less assertive patient into a "new" or "better" prosthetic design or prescription. Sometimes a change will, in fact, result in improved function for the amputee; more often, it will not, and the team may need to duplicate what the patient previously wore, with regard to prosthetic design, before the patient is satisfied and functioning optimally. When amputees are functioning extremely well with their prostheses, often the best course when prescribing new prostheses is to duplicate what they currently use.

When a person has amputations of both upper extremities and uses bilateral prostheses, one of the prostheses will become dominant for ADL function. If the residual limbs are of equal length, most amputees will maintain the same dominance they had prior to amputation. If the residual limbs are of unequal length, typically the side with the longer residual limb (or more distal amputation level) will become the dominant upper extremity. This is not always the case: some amputees choose to maintain preamputation dominance, even if the dominant side is the more proximal amputation.

CASE 12: BRACHIAL PLEXUS INJURIES

A 47-year-old man was involved in a motorcycle accident and sustained a severe stretch injury to his left brachial plexus. All of the elements of the brachial plexus were involved. Myelography and electrodiagnositic studies suggested that he had involvement of his 5th and 6th cervical roots, distal to the origin of the long thoracic nerve but proximal to the origin of the dorsal scapular nerve, together with root avulsions of the 7th and 8th cervical and 1st thoracic nerve roots. He underwent elective brachial plexus exploration with sural nerve grafting of the proximal 5th and 6th roots to the suprascapular and musculocutaneous nerves. Approximately 18 months after nerve grafting, he had regained some voluntary elbow flexion graded at 1+/2-. He regained no motor function in his supraspinatus or infraspinatus muscle. He had severe wasting of his entire upper extremity, two to three-finger-breadth subluxation of the glenohumeral joint, and no motor function in the upper extremity other than biceps. His trapezius, levator scapuli, and serratus anterior were functioning normally. He had some preserved sensation on the anterolateral proximal half of his arm. The patient had undergone nerve exploration and grafting with the hope that, had he regained sufficient elbow flexion strength, he might be a candidate for transradial amputation and prosthetic restoration to improve his function. When it was apparent that he would not regain sufficient elbow flexion strength to allow him to operate a transradial prosthesis independently, he elected to have a shoulder fusion and transhumeral amputation. Following the healing of his amputation and fusion, this patient had approximately 75 degrees of functional "shoulder flexion" and 65 degrees of "shoulder abduction" using the prosthesis.

Prosthesis

This patient was ultimately fitted with a definitive left transhumeral single-site myoelectrically controlled externally powered prosthesis with double-wall total contact wet fit suction socket, with auxillary supra-acromial gel suspension strap, Utah elbow, myoelectric quick disconnect wrist unit, powered hand, and Griefer. His original suspension had been with a modified shoulder saddle and chest strap harness.

Management Issue

Is amputation and prosthetic restoration too aggressive a rehabilitation approach for someone with a severe brachial plexus injury? Without muscle function, can a person with such an injury attain sufficient prosthetic control to result in useful function and justify prosthetic fitting? What are the surgical considerations to be kept in mind when embarking on this treatment approach? Is this treatment approach appropriate for all patients with complete plexus injuries?

Teaching Point

Amputation and prosthetic restoration is a therapeutic option that should be considered for individuals with severe brachial plexus injuries involving at least the lower trunk (C8, T1) and middle and lower trunk (C7, C8, T1) and resulting in a functionless hand with no demonstrated nerve recovery (after sufficient time for recovery has passed) or the possibility of regaining functional use through reconstruction by muscle transfers or other interventions. It is possible to fit a patient with C7, C8, and T1 root avulsions (or complete middle and lower trunk lesions) with a "prosthosis," which is a hybrid of orthotic and prosthetic technology. The extremity is preserved and an orthotic framework is devised to fit around the paralyzed extremity with an attached cable-operated hook TD attached to the palm of the orthosis. This type of device functions best when the patient has preserved active shoulder function and elbow flexion (i.e., sparing of the upper trunk) to provide some prehension. If elbow flexion is limited, a dual-control cable system, together with elbow lock and lift assist, can be incorporated. For some patients, this approach is an intermediate step to the decision of electing amputation. The level of amputation to be considered for a patient with brachial plexus injury depends on the preserved motor function. If the patient has 3+ or better elbow flexion, together with preserved shoulder function, then transradial amputation and prosthetic restoration is likely to be quite successful. If a patient with plexus injury does not have antigravity elbow flexion, then a transhumeral amputation is the better functional option. If there is preserved good shoulder motion, then the patient will generally be quite successful with the various transhumeral prosthetic options. When there is involvement of the complete plexus (C5 through T1), a transhumeral amputation and prosthetic fitting is not likely to provide the plexus patient with any improved function beyond cosmesis. The lack of voluntary shoulder motion makes it impossible to place the prosthesis, and thus the TD, in space for functional activities. It is possible to provide a patient with a complete plexus injury with voluntary "shoulder motion" to operate a transhumeral prosthesis if there is preserved voluntary motor activity of the trapezius and levator scapuli muscles. This is accomplished by doing a shoulder fusion that results in the transfer of scapular motion to the residual humerus. It is necessary to fuse the humerus to the scapula in a flexed and abducted position (no less than 30 degrees flexion and 30 degrees abduction and no more than 45 degrees flexion and 45 degrees abduction of the humerus) to obtain the best functional and cosmetic results. It has been the experience of our surgical colleagues that the proper humeral–scapular orientation is best accomplished by doing the fusion before doing the transhumeral amputation. Once the fusion heals, the weight of the residual limb (and prosthesis) will cause the scapula to rotate externally so that the arm will come to rest at the side of the trunk. The voluntary contraction of the scapular stabilizers will result in flexion and abduction of the residual limb (and prosthesis), simulating to a limited degree the shoulder motion required to position the prosthesis for use. If sufficient control motion is available, it is possible that the amputee with shoulder fusion may in fact be able to function reasonably well with a body-powered cable-controlled elbow and TD. More often than not, when body power is a considered control option, the function is best utilized in a hybrid prosthesis, with the body-powered cable controlling only the elbow motion. In most cases, the use of externally powered prosthetic components can and does improve the function of the prosthesis for most individuals with transhumeral amputation and shoulder fusion following brachial plexus injury. Most individuals with this procedure typically have limited control motion, which is not sufficient for the motion needed for optimal body-powered prosthetic function. As with all prosthetic decisions, the prescription must be individualized to meet the specific needs of the individual amputee. In the case of our patient, he was able to use his limited biceps function to successfully operate a single-site myoelectric control system. For patients with no available myoelectric control sites, switch control is another option when externally powered components are considered. In our experience, we have had patients who have elected to proceed with shoulder fusion and amputation as quickly as a few months after a complete plexus injury that has no likelihood of recovery or repair, but most wait many years and exhaust all other possible treatment options. Many wait decades before making the decision to proceed with this form of treatment. Often the decision is made after some new traumatic injury to the insensate paralyzed arm, such as unknowingly swinging it through a plate glass window and severely lacerating the arm or accidentally burning the arm or hand on the stove. Often these patients will say that they want to do something because the arm is getting in the way and is "more trouble than it is worth." It takes a great deal of time and effort to counsel these patients regarding this treatment option. As with any other individual who is considering elective amputation—for whatever reason—the team must take care to point out to the patient the realistic functional expectations should she elect this course. Our team has often spent many years discussing the implications of this option with patients before they elect to proceed. With one patient, our discussion went on for 20 years before he decided this was what he wanted to do. Amputation and fusion is an elective procedure and, as with all elective procedures, the pros and cons need to be thoroughly discussed. The process, once embarked upon, requires significant commitment from both the patient and the medical team. This is not a process to rush, and the patient and team should take their time and proceed deliberately and slowly if a successful outcome is to occur.

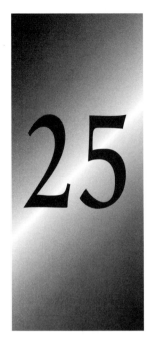

25 Evaluation of a Child with Congenital Upper Extremity Limb Deficiency

Yoshio Setoguchi, MD

hildren with upper extremity limb deficiencies require a multidisciplinary team approach when assessing and developing a rehabilitation program. The team needs to consider both the physical and psychosocial factors or potential problems when prescribing a treatment program.

Children are not "miniature adults." Their needs are different and change constantly. Therefore, the evaluation process must take into account the problems that the limb deficiency will create for the child and his family. The child's needs change with growth and development; therefore, the multidisciplinary team must be composed of professional staff with the knowledge and experience of dealing with children and their needs as they progress through various phases of growth and development. A thorough knowledge of the effects of the stages of growth and development is essential in establishing a treatment program, because these stages affect both functional and prosthetic needs. Physical and cognitive development must also be carefully evaluated as they affect the treatment program.

The team should consist of a physician (either a pediatrician, orthopedic surgeon, or physiatrist with a background in pediatric rehabilitation), a medical social worker, an occupational therapist, a physical therapist, and a prosthetist (Figure 25-1). Each discipline plays a

vital role in the evaluation process and the development of a treatment program.

The challenges in treating the upper extremity limb deficient child lie in the fact that not all patients are candidates for prosthetic fitting. Many of these children have very functional extremities even with partial deficiency and may not require prostheses to improve function. In addition, in upper extremity deficient children, many variables are still not completely understood, and these affect successful prosthetic outcomes. Therefore, the team must assess not only the physical problems but also the developmental status, the growth potential, the family environment, and the psychosocial situation of the family in following through with the treatment program, before developing a treatment plan.

DEMOGRAPHICS

Congenital limb deficiencies of both the upper and lower extremities can be classified into two basic types: transverse and longitudinal (1–4). The transverse deficiencies are those in which the limb is absent across its longitudinal axis (Figure 25-2), such as elbow disarticulations or below-elbow deficiencies, as seen in standard acquired amputations. The longitudinal absences are those in which the deficiencies are present along the axis of the limb, but do not extend across it, such as radial or

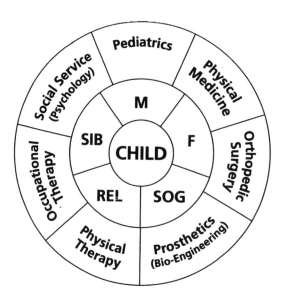

Inner Circle: Treatment to include besides patient, M=Mother, F=Father,
SIB=Siblings, REL=Relatives, and SOB=Grandparents.
Outer Circle: Treatment Team

FIGURE 25-1

Team approach to the treatment of a limb-deficient child.

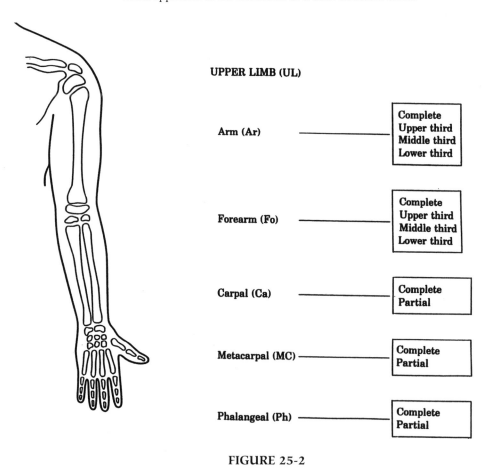

FIGURE 25-2

Transverse limb deficiencies (Congenital amputations).

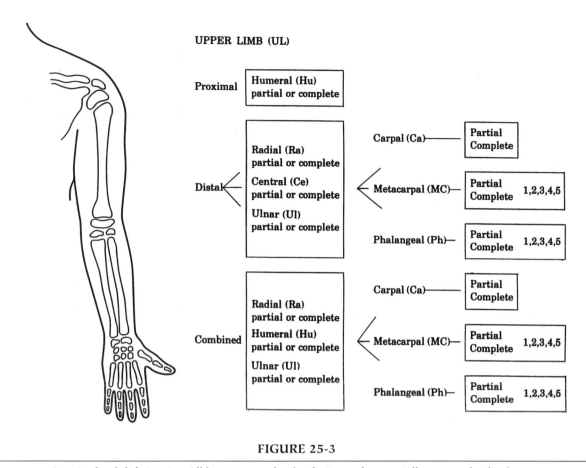

FIGURE 25-3

Longitudinal deficiencies: All bones named to be designated as partially or completely absent.

ulnar deficiencies (Figure 25-3). In some cases a patient may have a combination of the two types of deficiencies. The above classification is based upon the determination of the absent skeletal elements, not on any prosthetic or treatment criteria.

In the congenital limb deficient population, upper extremity absences are more common than lower extremity absences by a ratio of about 60 to 40%. The reason for this difference is unknown: No gender differences predominate in the occurrence of the deficiencies; and no significant racial predominances have been identified.

In most cases, the causes of congenital limb deficiencies are still unknown, and the majority of patients seen with this condition are classified as idiopathic or etiology unknown. These conditions occur sporadically and are believed to be nonhereditary.

Only about 1 to 2% of the cases are due to hereditary or chromosome abnormalities. Generally speaking, the latter group of patients—those with limb deficiencies as part of a chromosome abnormality—are usually not seen in a child amputee clinic except for diagnostic eval-

uation, as they are not candidates for prosthetic and rehabilitation programs.

The hereditary conditions without chromosome abnormality (at least at this time) include quadrilateral partial hands and feet deficiencies; several syndromes involving radial deficiencies, such as Holt-Oram syndrome and TAR absences; and Robert's syndrome with upper extremity phocomelia.

Another group of patients are born with limb deficiencies that can be considered acquired amputations. These patients have limb deficiencies believed to be secondary to constriction or amniotic bands, intrauterine constraints, or intrauterine or postnatal vascular injuries resulting in thromboembolic phenomena.

Congenital constriction bands are the most common cause of amputation in this group. The currently accepted theory is that these amputations and deformities, primarily of the distal extremities, are caused by amniotic bands that constrict the extremities much as a ligature would do and create the amputations. In this author's experience, most cases seen show the involvement of more than one extremity.

ASSOCIATED MEDICAL PROBLEMS

Although uncommon, associated medical problems are sometimes seen with limb deficient children (5). It is important to recognize these syndromes and to develop a treatment program that covers not only the limb deficiency but also the medical problems.

Craniofacial Abnormalities

In the past, several cranial abnormality syndromes were associated with limb deficiencies, primarily involving the hands and feet (6). Recently, these have been consolidated into one group, titled "oro-mandibular limb dysgenesis," because of considerably overlapping symptoms among the various syndromes. Included in this new title are the following syndromes:

- Moebius Syndrome. The craniofacial anomalies classically manifest as paralysis or paresis of the VII and VI cranial nerves, but may also involve other cranial nerves. The clinical features include facial palsy or paresis, ptosis, strabismus or nystagmus, small mouth, tongue hypoplasia, and usually terminal deficiencies involving the hands and feet. Clinical symptoms include lack of facial expression, so that many of these patients are diagnosed as mentally retarded; lack of lateral movement of the eyes resulting in "tunnel vision"; poor feeding; and difficulty in handling oral secretions. Later, patients develop speech problems. Limb defects occur in approximately 50% of cases, with the most common deficiencies being hypoplasia of digits, syndactyly, and clinodactyly, but higher levels of reduction deformities are seen.
- Hypoglossia–Hypodactylia Syndrome. The classic features are small or absent tongue with micrognathia, and distal limb anomalies, such as the absence of the digits. However, the limb anomalies are quite variable (7).
- Hanhart Syndrome. Features include micrognathia but with normal tongue and distal limb deficiencies (8).
- Glosso-Palatine Ankylosis Syndrome. Major features of this condition are the presence of intraoral attachments (frenulae) between tongue and palate and between upper and lower arches. The limb anomalies are primarily distal, but can be quite variable.
- Limb Deficiency–Splenogonadal Fusion Syndrome. The primary feature is that of a cordlike structure connecting the spleen with the gonadal structure on the same side. This condition also presents with abnormalities of the oral structures, particularly the mandible.

- Charlie M. Syndrome. Distinguishing features include hypertelorism, facial paralysis, absent or cone-shaped incisors, cleft palate, and limb reduction deformities primarily involving the hands and feet.

Radial Deficiency Syndrome

Whenever a newborn presents with unilateral or bilateral radial deficiencies, with or without the absence of the thumbs, and with radially clubbed hands and occasionally with involvement of the humeri and elbow joints, the possibility that the child represents one of the following syndromes must be considered:

- Thrombocytopenia Absent Radii (TAR). Patients may present in the newborn period with ecchymosis and petechiae due to thrombocytopenia and absence or hypolasia of the megakaryocytes (9). In addition to the radial deficiencies, these patients may present with other skeletal anomalies.
- Franconi's Pancytopenia. Usually, these patients present with skeletal anomalies at birth, but the hematologic symptoms do not manifest until 5 to 6 years of age and occasionally not until 10 years of age. This condition is felt to be autosomal recessive. Early prenatal and postnatal diagnosis can be made by demonstrating a high frequency diepoxybutane-induced chromosomal breakage in peripheral blood lymphocytes as well as in cultured amniotic fluid cells.
- Holt-Oram or Hand-Heart. This syndrome manifests with radial deficiencies and congenital heart anomalies (10). The most common heart defect is an atrial septal defect, but other heart lesions have been described, such as the tetralogy of Fallot seen in Lewis-Franchischetti syndrome. Associated anomalies include Poland's anomaly, pectus excavatum, and scoliosis. The inheritance pattern is autosomal dominant with variable penetrance.
- VATER Association (also called VACTERL). A group of associated anomalies involving the vertebral bodies (hemivertebrae); anal orifice (usually atresia but may be present as ectopic position); tracheoesophageal fistulae, most commonly the "H" type; renal system; cardiac system; and limbs—usually radial defects (11). Associated problems include intrauterine growth retardation, a single umbilical artery, and abnormal external genitalia.
- Baller-Gerold Syndrome. A relatively rare condition, presenting with radial defects and occasionally phocomelia associated with the premature closure of the coronal cranial sutures.

- Trisomy 18. This anomaly presents with severe multiple congenital anomalies including growth and mental retardations.
- Blackfin-Diamond and AASE Syndromes. Very rare conditions with hemotologic abnormalities presenting as aplastic anemia.

Associated Musculoskeletal Disorders.

Two musculoskeletal disorders are commonly associated with upper limb deficiencies:

- Congenital Constriction Band. In addition to the amputations and soft tissue band deformities described earlier, the disruption of craniofacial structures with facial clefting and deformities of the abdominal wall also occasionally occur (12).
- Poland's Syndrome. This deficit presents with a unilateral absence of the pectoralis minor muscle and the sternal portion of the pectoralis major muscle group and is associated with some type of abnormality of the ipsilateral hand. In girls, breast asymmetry is often seen in puberty and may present as a significant cosmetic problem.

Dermatologic Conditions

Two dermatologic conditions are seen in some cases of upper limb deficiency:

- Ectodermal Dysplasia, Ectrodactyly, and Clefting (EEC). This condition presents with abnormalities of the structures derived from the embryonic estoderm including skin, hair, nails, and lacrimal and sweat glands. Limb deficiencies are usually distal and usually present as clefting of the hands and feet.
- Adams-Oliver Syndrome or Aplasia Cutis Congenita. This condition is rare and its recurrence is felt to be autosomal dominant. Clinical features include the absence of patches of hair (alopecia) in the scalp, with or without cranial involvement, and transverse type skeletal deficits that may involve one or more limbs.

More than 80% of inheritable limb deficiencies are associated with anomalies of structures other than the musculoskeletal system. The upper extremity limb deficiencies are more likely to be associated with syndromes of defect. If viewed from the point of frequency of involvement of other organ systems, the most common nongenetic occurrence is seen in the genitourinary system, the musculoskeletal system, and the respiratory system. In genetic conditions, craniofacial and cardiovascular disorders are more common. Fortunately, these associated medical problems are still quite rare and make up a small portion of the limb-deficient population.

EVALUATION

The development of a rehabilitation program for a child with upper extremity limb deficiency begins with a complete pediatric assessment. This is usually done in the newborn period by the primary care physician. Besides providing the parents with an accurate diagnosis or a future treatment plan, the most important role the physician plays at this point is that of someone who understands their concerns and questions regarding their newborn having a congenital limb deficiency. They need to be reassured that appropriate medical facilities, such as child amputee clinics, are available with staff who have experience in dealing with the limb-deficient child. They need to be told that it is normal for parents of children born with deformities to have feelings of sadness, anger, embarrassment, guilt, and isolation. The primary care physician need not have a thorough background in rehabilitation, but he can provide a foundation for future treatment. The caring manner in which the physician addresses the child and his family can be the basis of a healthy adjustment.

At the initial team evaluation, the team physician is usually the first member to see the patient and family. The manner in which both the child and family are handled is very important. The birth of a child with a birth defect, specifically a limb deficiency, is a very traumatic event for the parents.

The mother usually is the first to sense that there are problems with the child that she has just delivered. Mothers often describe the sudden quietness that comes over the delivery room personnel following the delivery. Often the infant is immediately removed from the delivery room into the neonatal intensive care unit (NICU) without explanations. Mothers have said at our first consultation that they became extremely frightened at that moment, imagining bizarre situations. In fact, some mothers, when allowed to see their baby, have said that "they were relieved that only a single limb was involved." However, others described extreme isolation and even anger at the fact that the child's problems were not immediately discussed with them. They have stated that it is not so much what was said but how it was said that had the biggest impact on them. Often, this initial reaction persists for years to come in the mother's mind.

Once the mother is made aware of the child's condition, the next person to learn about the child's condition is the father. It is usually left to him to notify other family members, including grandparents, relatives, and friends. Often, these responsibilities require so much of the father's energies that he doesn't have time to grieve.

In the initial evaluation, it is important to have the parents discuss their initial reactions and discuss ways for them to verbalize and validate their feelings and the ways in which they have compensated for their feelings.

Some initial questions that the team physician must discuss with the family include:

- Is the condition hereditary? A thorough medical history and physical examination is important. Although the majority of unilateral limb deficiencies seen in the child amputee clinic are sporadic and no etiologic factors are identified, it is essential that syndromes and inheritable conditions be identified. In certain cases, where multiple anomalies are noted, a genetic consultation may be in order.
- If not hereditary, is there a cause for the limb deficiency? Parents may be concerned with medications that the mother may have taken, exposures to environmental toxins, exotic foods that were ingested, and traumatic situations that occurred involving the mother during the pregnancy. Although in most cases the family is told that no etiologic factors are known, this fact alone is reassuring.
- Are there other medical problems? As noted earlier, certain types of limb deficiencies are frequently associated with other medical problems. However, the more common transverse deficiencies usually are not associated with other congenital anomalies. Related to this question is that of concerns regarding the mental and cognitive abilities of these children. Most have normal growth and development. The family is reassured that the patient will have normal developmental milestones and be able to attend regular schools.
- Is one parent responsible for causing the limb deficiency? Usually, when this question is asked, the parents have many unresolved guilt issues and often are looking for someone or something to blame for their child's condition. Cultural and/or ethical issues are often raised. One such example is in the Hispanic population, in which a superstitious belief persists that the child was "marked" by the mother exposing her unborn child to the eclipse, thus putting the responsibility for the condition on the mother. This is a rather heavy burden for the mother, and it is important that these issues be raised and discussed as soon as possible.

To complete the initial pediatric examination, it is important to get an accurate family history, prenatal and birth history, and if the child is older, a good medical history and assessment of the overall growth and developmental history of the child.

To confirm the diagnosis, x rays should be taken of the limb involved. In our clinic, x rays of the sound limb are also usually taken, and by comparison help to illustrate the limb deficiency present.

At the initial evaluation, it is important that the family be seen by the team social worker, or in some cases, by the team psychologist. The psychosocial issues that must be dealt with include:

- Initial reactions at the time of birth and the response of the parents to these reactions. Positive and negative aspects must be explored, as then relates to the family's handling of the child's medical treatment program.
- Reactions of the immediate family and how they have helped or hindered the parents in coping with the condition and treatment goals.
- Past history of family's adjustments to previous stresses. Previous occasions of stress are a good indicator of the parents' abilities to cope with the needs of the limb-deficient child. This knowledge may help the social worker to plan an intervention program and follow-up for the parents.
- What the parents envision as problems in caring for their child. This information is very helpful for the other team members such as the physician, therapist, and prosthetist. Unrealistic goals need to be brought up and clarified as soon as possible. Realistic objectives need to be validated and parents complimented on their abilities to work out their feelings and plan for a healthy future for their limb-deficient child.
- Expectations of the family regarding treatment options. In our clinic, the social worker is usually the last team member to see the patient and her family. This order of interview allows the social worker to ensure that the family understands the treatment options provided. If any questions arise, then these issues are brought up at the team meeting and again discussed with the family.

The occupational or physical therapist plays a vital part in the initial evaluation of the limb-deficient child. The two major responsibilities of the therapist are to assess the child's growth and development and to develop a prosthetically and therapeutically appropriate treatment plan. If the child appears to be delayed in her developmental milestones, the therapist should provide a stimulation program for the parents. In many cases, the child is *not* developmentally delayed: Because of the limb deficiency, the family's overprotectiveness has not allowed the child to progress in a normal fashion with developmental milestones. Encouraging the parents and especially the caregiver to allow the child to be left on the bed or floor to try to manipulate her environment is very important.

The therapist also provides the initial orientation to a prosthetic program. The various prosthetic options, including the various types of terminal devices (in the case of upper extremities absences) must be carefully presented, with a discussion of both the advantages and possible disadvantages of the various fittings or components. Often, the parents are then introduced to other families with children already fitted, or in some cases movies or videos are shown of other children wearing and using the types of prostheses that the child might be fitted with.

The prosthetist also is involved in the orientation program. Here, discussion centers around amplifying the information provided by the therapist. Then, if the family is interested, they are given an overview of the prosthetic fitting process. This latter information will again be provided when the prescription is written, but is offered here to reassure the parents.

Many children seen in our clinic require some surgical intervention prior to prosthetic fitting. A thorough explanation of the benefits of surgical conversion and its impact on future prosthetic fittings is needed. Often, the introduction of another patient with the same condition who has previously undergone the procedure is helpful.

To complete the initial evaluation in those patients with some digits present, before final decisions regarding prosthetic treatment are made, a hand surgery consultation is very helpful. With advances in limb lengthening and toe-transfers, as well as new reconstructive techniques, the family must know all their options before starting on a treatment program.

The first clinic visit can be a very traumatic experience for the family. From the initial contact on the phone when this appointment is made to the family's presentation at the waiting room area, the manner in which the family is received and the atmosphere of the clinic is very important in preparing the family for this initial evaluation. As many clinics point out, the waiting room and the presence of other children with limb deficiencies, many of them wearing prostheses, may be a positive or negative experience for the new family. Ideally, other families can be very helpful, because they can function as a support group; older patients and their parents can be role models in discussing initial reactions as well as prosthetic experiences. Lifelong friendships may be established in the waiting room.

Once the prosthetic treatment program is established and discussed with the family, it is important that the parents have a chance to digest the information and have all their questions answered. It is important that parents have sufficient time to discuss their concerns

between themselves and their families before coming to a decision. Unless the family has already been exposed to prosthetic rehabilitation, parents are not ready to make a decision on the first visit. In our clinic, we often suggest that parents go home without making a decision, so that they can take time to discuss the various issues involved and then make up their minds. However, it is important that the clinic makes a follow-up appointment before the family leaves.

Allow the family sufficient time to discuss the recommended treatment plan and to verbalize to each other their concerns and questions. Even if the family decides against prosthetic fitting, it is important to interview the family a second time to be sure that the information that they have retained is accurate and relative to their child's limb deficiency. It is not unusual that parents confuse what was said with what they heard from friends, acquaintances, or the news media.

Once the family has decided on a prosthetic or therapeutic treatment program, it is important that they commit to the following responsibilities:

- Establishment of a full-time wearing pattern immediately, if possible, after receiving the prosthesis. Often families are allowed to set their own time limits regarding prosthetic wearing, starting with just a few hours a day. Some parents allow the child to dictate the length of wearing time, using the excuse that "she cried and was uncomfortable so they took the prosthesis off for a rest period." This behavior pattern sheds negative light on the value of the prosthesis and often leads to feelings of "nonimportance" regarding the prosthetic program. The same is true for any therapeutic treatment program: Consistency and full time use is the best approach to successful fitting.
- Persual of an ongoing training program. It should not be left to the patient and family to teach the child the functional advantages of a prosthesis. A consistent, ongoing therapy program is essential. Therapy should begin by having the therapist assist the parents in establishing a full-time wearing pattern and thus developing a consistent, spontaneous use pattern that incorporates the prosthesis in all appropriate bimanual activities, especially activities of daily living (ADLs).
- Maintenance of the prosthesis in good fitting and good working order. This means not only having the prosthesis repaired when not functioning, but maintaining a regular evaluation program through the prosthetist to make appropriate adjustments for growth and to make minor repairs so that major functional problems are minimized.

The initial evaluation of the upper extremity limb deficient child typically ends when the first prosthesis is fitted. With standard unilateral partial deficiency, such as B/E, E/D, and A/E deficiencies, the first fitting occurs when the child develops a good sitting balance posture. Some amputee clinics fit the child even before this developmental milestone. However, regardless of when the first fitting occurs, it is important that the team prosthetist and occupational therapist check the prosthesis on the patient to ensure that it meets the prescription recommendations and that the prosthesis is comfortable in all the patient's activities.

A successful rehabilitation program then makes certain that the child continues to gain confidence in her abilities to make maximum use of her residual limb and prosthetic fitting to perform all necessary activities to lead as normal a life as possible.

References

1. Frantz CH and O'Rahilly R. Congenital Limb Deficiencies. *Journal of Bone and Joint Surgery* 1961; 43A:8.
2. Hall CB, Brooks MB and Dennis JF. Congenital Skeletal Deficiencies of the Extremities: Classification and Fundamentals of Treatment. *JAMA* 1962; 181.
3. Burtch RL. The classification of congenital skeletal limb deficiencies, a preliminary report. *Inter-Clinic Information Bulletin* 1963, 3:1.
4. Kruger LM. International Terminology for Classification of Congenital Limb Deficiencies in Amer. Academy of Orthopedic Surgeons, *Atlas of Limb Prosthetics: Surgical and Prosthetic Principles,* CV Mosby Co, 1981, 501–518.
5. Herring JA and Birch JG (ed). *The Child With a Limb Deficiency,* American Academy of Orthopedic Surgeons, 1998.
6. Steigner M, Stewart RE, Setoguchi Y. Combined limb deficiencies and cranial nerve dysfunction: Report of six cases. *Birth Defects* 1975; 11:133–141.
7. Cohen MM Jr, Pantke H, Siris E. Nosologic and genetic considerations in the aglossy-adactyly syndrome. *Birth Defects* 1971, 7:237–240.
8. Wexler MR, Novark BW. Hanhart's Syndrome: Case report. *Plast Reconstr Surg* 1974; 54:99–101.
9. Hall JG, Levin J, Kuhn JP, Oppenheimer EJ, van Berkum KA, McKusick VA. Thrombocytopenia with absent radius (TAR). *Medicine* 1969; 48:411–439.
10. Holt M, Oram S. Familial heart disease with skeletal malformations. *Br. Heart J* 1960; 22:236–242.
11. Quan L, Smith DW. The VATER Association: Vertebral defects, anal-atresia, T-E fistula with esophageal atresia, radial and renal dysplasia: a spectrum of associated defects. *J Pediatrics* 1973; 82:104–107.
12. Jones KL, Smith DW, Hall BD, et. al, A pattern of craniofacial and limb defects secondary to aberrant tissue bands. *J. Pediatrics* 1974; 84:90–95.

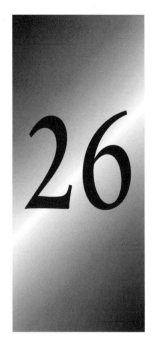

26 Training the Child with a Unilateral Upper-Extremity Prosthesis*

Joanna Grace Patton, OTR/L

The developmental frame of reference and the concept of early prosthetic fitting provide a sound clinical approach to treatment for a child with unilateral upper-extremity limb deficiency or amputation.

The theme of early fitting is cited in the literature and prevalent in past and current practice. In a 1972 literature review, Sypniewski reported the dominant point of view favored early prosthetic fitting for the child with a transverse forearm deficiency (1,2). Then and now clinicians agree on "early fit" (1,2), but do not always agree on the same developmental time frames.

A 1965 study by Brooks and Shaperman reported that children who received a below-elbow prosthesis before age 2 developed better wear and use patterns than children fitted after 2 years of age (1,3). Clinical experience demonstrates that the baby between ages 6 and 18 months adjusts more easily to a consistent prosthetic wearing pattern, whereas the more independent and often negative 2 to 2-1/2-year-old may resist initial fitting. There are always exceptions, and a highly motivated child fitted at an older age still has the potential to develop good prosthetic skills. Nonetheless, school-age children fitted for the first time have already developed alternative methods of performing two-handed activities.

The emergence of the newer electric components for children during the 1970s and 1980s has also influenced the way clinicians and families view the prescription and training process. Proponents of very early myoelectric fitting feel that the first infant passive prosthesis should be fitted as early as 3 to 4 months of age (1,4–6). However, no substantiating data exist to support better wear and use outcomes with this extremely early period of fitting. Future outcome studies, which assess age at first fit as well as prosthetic wear and use patterns for the child with unilateral upper extremity limb loss, may provide objective data and insight into these issues. Nonetheless, the controversy will probably continue for some time.

The Child Amputee Prosthetics Project (CAPP), formerly at UCLA and now at Shriners Hospital for Children—Los Angeles, continues to base treatment on the developmental frame of reference. The first infant passive below-elbow prosthesis is prescribed when the baby sits independently (1,7). The prosthesis is less likely to hinder development, since the baby is no longer rolling. For the

* This chapter is adapted from material presented in the *Atlas of Limb Prosthetics, 2nd Edition*, published by Mosby. Selected information from the chapter by Joanna G. Patton entitled "Developmental Approach to Pediatric Upper-Limb Prosthetic Training" is incorporated into this format.

baby with a short forearm segment, the prosthesis may offer stability when she begins to creep and pull to stand. Through clinical experience, the CAPP team believes that the acquisition of good sitting balance is a reasonable time to fit the first infant passive prosthesis (1,7).

FAMILY, PATIENT, AND TEAM ORIENTATION

Children with limb deficiencies need special medical and technical intervention. They receive the best care in centers that have a multidisciplinary team and the knowledge and experience to provide comprehensive care. The team is usually comprised of a physician, prosthetist, occupational therapist, social worker, psychologist, and other health professionals. The family and patient are also part of the team and certainly the focus of the treatment (7).

The role of the occupational therapist may vary depending on the clinical setting. At CAPP, the therapist is an integral part of the team and monitors the baby's development. She reassures the family that the baby who has a transradial/ulnar deficiency (below the elbow) has the potential for normal development. The baby will achieve all developmental milestones unless other medical or neurologic problems interfere. These factors are usually unrelated to the limb deficiency (1,7).

Along with other team members, the occupational therapist provides information about prosthetic components and realistic expectations of prosthetic function. Later, the therapist will participate in the prescription process, help evaluate the new prosthesis, and conduct the prosthetic and activity of daily living (ADL) training sessions.

Early access to care and support is most critical for parents and families. If possible, parents should be referred to the team soon after the baby's birth. Some individuals are overwhelmed with shock, anger, confusion, and depression; others seem to cope more effectively. All families, however, need an opportunity to discuss their fears, concerns, and feelings about the limb deficiency (1,7,8). Sometimes parents focus on future events and ask questions such as:

- Will my child be able to care for himself?
- Will my child be able to play like other children (ride a bike, swim, etc.)?
- Will my child be able to attend regular school?

It is important for parents to know that the child with a unilateral limb loss has the potential to do all of the above. He needs to be accepted and treated like other children in terms of performing daily tasks, going to regular school, and participating in normal play and recreational activities (1,7,8).

Well-meaning and overprotective relatives and friends sometimes provide misinformation or interfere with the family's decisions concerning treatment. Therefore, to clarify information about the baby, the siblings and extended family members are encouraged to attend the orientation sessions (1,7,8).

Misconceptions about prostheses are commonplace. Therefore, families must have accurate information about the state-of-the-art prostheses and the availability of components at the center where the baby is being treated. Some parents may want the prosthesis solely to complete the missing limb. Others may ask, "Does my child need a prosthesis?" The upper-limb prosthesis does not change the central nervous system nor does it alter the ability to achieve developmental milestones such as creeping, sitting, or walking. With or without a prosthesis, the child with a unilateral limb deficiency will be able to accomplish most, if not all, daily living, recreational, and vocational activities. One of the benefits of the artificial limb is to provide a method to perform two-handed activities at the midline of the body. The prosthesis is an assist to the sound extremity and eliminates the need for substitute grasp patterns (1,7).

Parents must assimilate information provided by the team and ultimately make the decision about prosthetic fitting. If they choose a prosthesis for their child, parents need to establish a consistent wear and use pattern. The child's ability to learn to use the prosthesis skillfully takes place over a period of time. Therefore, the family's time, energy, and commitment to the prosthetic program are essential to produce a positive prosthetic outcome (1,7).

THE INFANT PASSIVE
TRANSRADIAL PROSTHESIS

The infant prosthesis must be as lightweight as possible. At CAPP, the below-elbow prosthesis has a full cuff and an infant chest harness (Figure 26-1) instead of the traditional figure-eight harness (1,7).

A polyvinylchloride (PVC) gauntlet provides some friction for the prosthetic forearm, to prevent the baby from sliding when he creeps on all fours (1,7).

Parents are able to choose the terminal device (TD) for the first prosthesis. The benefits of the CAPP Terminal Device No. 1, the 10X Dorrance hook, and the infant foam-filled Steeper hand are explained. The CAPP TD No. 1 and the hook may be opened manually to place a toy into it. The CAPP TD has a large grasping surface as well as a friction cover (1,7,9). Both features provide a good grip on objects. Passive hands have no ability to hold. However, they do provide a pleasant appearance, which is extremely important for many parents (1).

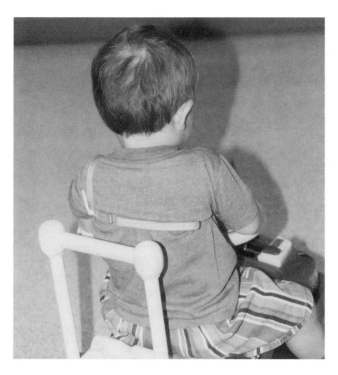

FIGURE 26-1

Prosthesis with infant below-elbow harness.

Evaluation of the New Prosthesis

A checkout or evaluation is completed when the prosthesis is issued to the baby. The components and quality of workmanship must be in accordance with the prescription and the standards of the clinic. An ideal clinical situation allows the prosthetist and therapist to do the evaluation together. Many times, logistics makes this scenario impractical. The occupational therapist will observe the baby during play and evaluate the fit and comfort of the prosthesis. The socket and harness should provide comfort and stability as well as freedom of movement while the baby creeps on all fours, pulls to stand, and clasps large toys. The prosthetist is notified if there are problems in order to make the necessary adjustments (1,7).

Family Instruction

When the prosthesis is given to the baby, the family will need two to three follow-up sessions during the first few weeks. The therapist will provide support and guidance concerning the baby's use of the prosthesis. It is important for the parents and extended family members to understand and comply with the following instructions (1,7):

- Learn to apply and remove the prosthesis.
- Clean the prosthesis and keep it in good working condition.
- Establish a consistent full-time prosthetic wearing pattern for the baby.
- Encourage the baby to include the prosthesis in daily developmental activities.
- Learn to recognize when prosthetic adjustments are needed. Keep recommended appointments with the clinic or local prosthetist (1,7).

It is reasonable for the baby to wear the below-elbow prosthesis during the time he is awake. It should be removed when the baby sleeps, takes a bath, or is ill. Climate changes, especially very hot weather, may vary the wearing pattern. The baby's movements may initially appear awkward or clumsy with the prosthesis. However, within the first few weeks, she will become accustomed to the increased weight and length of the prosthesis and to the decreased tactile sensation to the residual limb (1,7).

Parents should assist the baby if the prosthesis becomes entangled in clothing or furniture. Eventually the baby will incorporate the prosthesis as a stabilizer when she creeps on all fours and pulls to stand (Figure 26-2). By presenting a large ball or stuffed toy, the baby will reach out and learn to clasp with the prosthesis and the sound arm. If the TD can be opened manually, toys, crackers, and cookies may be placed into it. Initially, the 12- to 15-month-old baby will ignore the object or pull it out of the terminal device. As parents repeatedly place toys or food into the TD, the baby becomes aware that it holds an object (1,7). This concept becomes more meaningful between 15 to 18 months of age, when the baby begins to put toys in and out of a container (Figure 26-3). Gesell describes this developmental activity as the container/contained concept (1,10). To make it easier for the toddler to open the TD with the sound hand, a soft spring is placed on the CAPP TD. The manufacturer issues the CAPP TD with a medium spring, but the prosthetist can easily change it to a soft one (1,9).

Readiness Criteria to Activate the TD

Between 18 months and 2 years of age, the child demonstrates developmental changes that help them to learn the operation of the cable system. In her book, Pulaski states that the 18-month-old performs activities by trial and error (1,11). During this period, the child is in constant motion. At 2 years of age, the child shows more purpose and intention in behavior. He has the capacity to follow directions and begins to understand cause and effect (1,11).

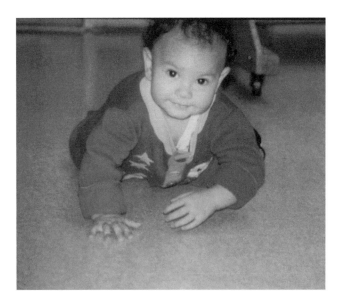

FIGURE 26-2

Baby uses infant passive prosthesis to creep on all fours.

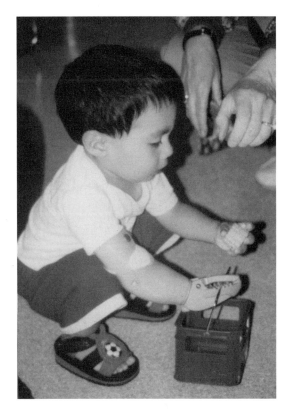

FIGURE 26-3

Child learns about the holding function of the terminal device.

Because treatment at CAPP is based on principles of child development, it is reasonable to capitalize on this period of change in cognitive and motor development by adding the control line or cable to the below-elbow prosthesis (7). Because some 2-year-olds are more cooperative than others, the following readiness criteria are used as indicators of the child's ability to learn to operate the TD. The child must demonstrate all or some of the following criteria (7,1):

- Have a 10-minute attention span and be able to focus on an activity.
- Follow directions that have one or two steps.
- Understand that the TD is able to hold an object. Attempt to open it with the sound hand.
- Show a willingness to be still. Allow the therapist or parent to move the arm with the prosthesis through the control motion.
- Demonstrate an interest in age-appropriate bimanual play activities (1,7).

The behavior of the 2-year-old can sometimes be volatile and unpredictable. The child may initially appear ready for the control line, but then may be uncooperative and negative in the therapy or home setting. Both the therapist and parents must be patient: there is no need to force the child to learn TD operation. Postpone the formal training until the child is more cooperative. During normal play, as the child reaches forward or leans over, tension on the cable or control line will cause the TD to open. Parents should call attention to this inadvertent operation to reinforce the learning process. During the formal training process, the therapist needs to be creative and flexible when using toys that provide for the repetitive opening and closing of the TD (1,7).

Evaluation of the Prosthesis with Active TD

When the control line is added to the existing or new prosthesis, other changes are also made. The infant harness is changed to a figure-eight harness (Figure 26-4). The TDs of choice at CAPP are voluntary opening ones such as the CAPP TD No. 1, a 10X Dorrance hook, or a child-size mechanical hand (1,7).

The mechanical and functional evaluation of the prosthesis is essential for good fit and function. Because children differ from the adult in range of motion and strength, the following items are important for a child's prosthesis (1,7):

- The cross point on the harness is centered and stitched. The cross is in the middle of the back slightly lower than C7, rather than toward the sound side.

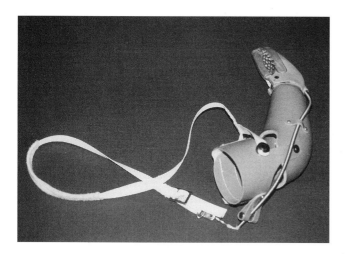

FIGURE 26-4

Below-elbow prosthesis with figure-eight harness and CAPP TD.

- The spring on the CAPP TD is changed to a soft one.
- The 10X hook has 1/4 to 1/2 of a rubber band instead of a full band.
- The cable housing is lined with Teflon to increase efficiency.
- The axilla loop is padded with dacron felt and nylon tricot instead of plastic tubing.
- Extra rubber bands and CAPP TD covers are always provided (1,7).

With busy lives, it is easy for parents to forget to care for the prosthesis. Part of the evaluation and training process is to impress caregivers with the necessity to maintain good personal hygiene for the child and to follow these prosthetic care and maintenance procedures:

- Wash the socket every night with soap and water or alcohol.
- Wash the harness once or twice a week.
- Remove dirt and sand from the inside of the CAPP TD with a brush or air hose.
- Clean the cosmetic glove with alcohol, soap, and water or the manufacturer's cleaner. Alert parents that the cosmetic glove that covers the child-size hard plastic mechanical hand will tear easily during play.
- Adjust the wrist friction with the appropriate tool to prevent inadvertent movement of the TD during use.
- Keep appointments for repairs and harness adjustments (1,7).

Learning the Control Motion to Operate the TD

The young child learns to actively open the TD using the cable system when the therapist and parent repeatedly moves the shoulder (on the side with the prosthesis) through the control motion. The therapist may sit behind or beside the child. The child is given a toy to hold in the sound hand. The therapist places one hand on the child's shoulder and the other hand under the prosthetic forearm to move the shoulder into humeral flexion (Figure 26-5). When the TD opens, the child is told to place the toy inside (1,7). Some children do not like the feel of the pressure created by the axilla loop of the harness. To lessen the pulling sensation, the child usually extends the shoulder. Slack is created in the control line, thus preventing the TD from opening. To minimize frustration, the therapist stabilizes the child's shoulder, assists with the control motion, and helps to place the toy in the TD. To make it easier to open the TD, the control attachment strap may be tightened slightly. With "hands on" assistance from the therapist, the child also needs to learn to return the shoulder to a neutral position to relax tension on the control line. Once the activity is completed, most children pull the object from the TD with the sound hand (1,7,12).

If the child is cooperative, formal training sessions may be conducted two to three times a week until the child is able to independently perform the following:

- Use a refined shoulder flexion motion to open the TD (humeral flexion, not abduction).
- Place an object correctly and securely in the TD.
- Return the shoulder to the neutral position to relax tension on the control line. Hold the object with the sound hand until the TD closes completely.

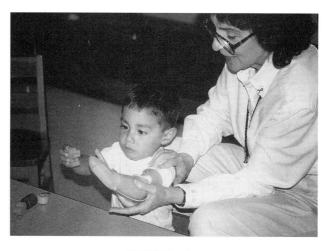

FIGURE 26-5

Child learns the control motion to open the TD.

- Pull the object out of the TD with the sound hand or use the control motion to actively release it.
- Use biscapular abduction to open the TD at the midline of the body. (Some children learn this second control motion without assistance. Others need instruction.)
- Continue to use the prosthesis as a unit to stabilize or clasp large items (1,7).

Parents are instructed in the training procedures to help the child at home. Sometimes parents provide the only training available. Adults should not expect the child to use the prosthesis to stack blocks, grasp items from a table, or eat with a spoon. It is not appropriate for the child to use the prosthesis to perform dominant hand skills; the prosthesis is an assist to the sound hand (1,7,12).

Because children respond to purposeful play and not to drills, the best approach is to use developmentally appropriate toys and games that require the use of two hands. Appropriate, repetitive, fun activities reinforce the learning process for the young child. Some activities include:

- Large wooden or plastic beads with a strong cord or leather lace. (Hold the bead in the TD and the string in the sound hand.)
- Threaded nested toys or small jars with candy or raisins inside. (Hold the jar with the TD. Remove and replace the top or lid with the sound hand.)
- Do-A-Dot Art paint bottles with screw on caps. (Hold the bottle in the TD. Remove the cap with the sound hand.)
- Large felt-tipped markers or pens (1). (Loosen the cap to facilitate removal.)

Functional Use Training

Once the child learns the control motions, the focus of the training process shifts to the acquisition of prosthetic skills. These skills facilitate the use of the prehensile function of the TD and help the child to use the prosthesis more effectively. The young child cannot learn all the skills or assimilate all aspects of training at one time. Stages of training often overlap. Learning takes place along a developmental continuum as the child's cognitive ability and fine motor coordination increase. The following skills are introduced when the child is ready to learn them. These skills are taught in conjunction with bimanual activities that are commensurate with the child's developmental age and interest (1,7):

- Place an object securely in the TD. Reposition the object as needed.
- Refine the size of the TD opening, especially for small or thin items.

- Preposition the TD as required for different activities (Figure 26-6).
- Actively release an object from the TD using the control motion (1,7). (Actively toss the object from the TD into space.)

First, the therapist provides demonstration and verbal instruction to teach skills and to remind the child to include the terminal device. Later, a trial-and-error approach is permitted to encourage the child to do the activity on his own. If he appears awkward when using the prosthesis or cannot complete the task, the therapist intervenes. Children often avoid repositioning an object or prepositioning the TD (1,7). They substitute shoulder motion to place the TD in what they perceive to be a good functional position. The therapist may either correct the child's method of performance or ask him to demonstrate another way to do the activity (1,12). One method is to have the CAPP TD mimic the position of the sound hand (1,9).

The child with a unilateral limb deficiency uses the prosthesis as an assist. The standard training procedure is to pick up the object, place it into the TD, and complete the activity with the sound hand. The child must also learn to reach out with both the prosthesis and sound hand to grasp a stationary object in space (1,7,12). Youngsters learn this skill easily because they play with toys that encourage this two-handed approach. These toys include tricycle, tyke bike, swing, see-saw, doll carriage, shopping cart, wheelbarrow, and Play Doh with rolling pin (1,7).

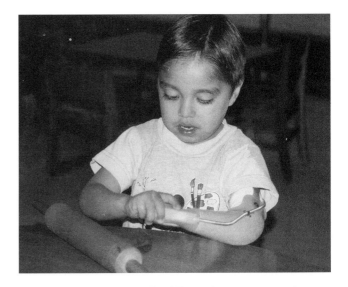

FIGURE 26-6

Child prepositions the CAPP TD.

To encourage the child to motor plan and problem solve new activities, the therapist uses fine motor manipulative toys, arts, and crafts as well as appropriate daily living activities.

The pre-school child may be easily bored with table-top activities. Imaginary play allows the therapist to vary the work space and to provide a more creative environment (Figure 26-7). The following activities provide incentive for the young child to practice skills and develop spontaneity with the prosthesis: tea party, wash dishes with real soap suds (Figure 26-8), dress and undress a doll, wash doll clothes and hang on a line, dress-up play with costumes and make-up, play musical instruments, plant flowers or seeds in a pot, blow bubbles (Figure 26-9), floor play with trains and large Duplo pieces, play baseball with a plastic bat and ball, and outdoor play on playground equipment (1,7).

Formal therapy is no longer necessary by the time the child enters kindergarten. However, before the child goes to school, the therapist needs to review the following skills: don and doff the prosthesis, don and doff a sweater or coat, stabilize clothing to zip a jacket or button a sweater, hold paper and cut with a scissor (Figure 26-10), open glue bottles, open a milk carton or lunch pail, learn to tie shoe laces, and wash hand and prosthesis (1,7).

The school-age child continues to benefit from periodic assistance to learn additional skills. These skills include:

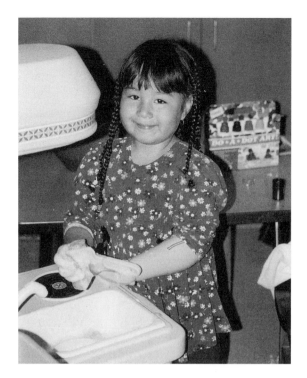

FIGURE 26-8

Creative bimanual activity used in the training process.

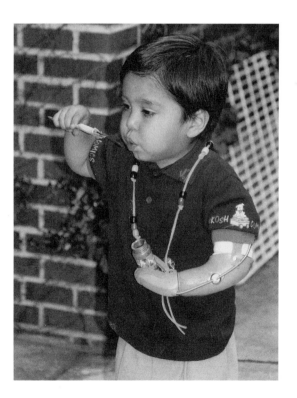

FIGURE 26-9

Blowing bubbles coordinates use of the TD and sound hand.

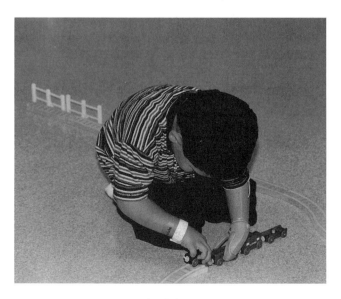

FIGURE 26-7

Floor play activity encourages use of the prosthesis.

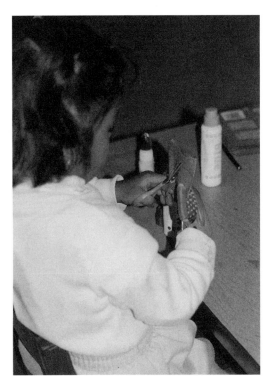

FIGURE 26-10

Child learns to reposition paper in the TD to cut with a scissors.

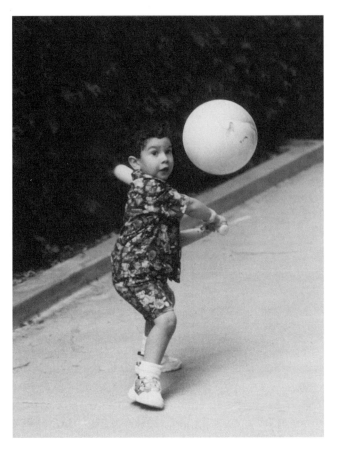

FIGURE 26-11

Child demonstrates skillful and spontaneous use of the prosthesis.

- The ability to actively grasp an object from the floor or table with the TD; needed when the sound hand is occupied.
- The ability to maintain a slight amount of tension on the control line or cable to control pressure grip on the TD; needed to hold a soft object like a sandwich or a fragile object like an egg without smashing it.
- The ability to keep the TD closed when bending or reaching; needed to keep the device closed to tie shoe laces. Child may need to move the harness high on the back to relieve tension on the control line (1).

The goal of prosthetic training is to help the child achieve some degree of skill and spontaneity with the prosthesis (1,12) (Figure 26-11). Formal therapy focuses on practice and repetition to build good habit patterns. However, a child's successful prosthetic experience depends in part on his parents. It is important that parents attend therapy sessions to learn how to assist the child. When their youngster enters school, parents introduce the prosthesis and its function to the teacher. Finally, they must reinforce the daily use

pattern and encourage the child to include the prosthesis in activities at home, at school, and in the community (1,7,12).

Functional Need and Changes to the Prosthesis

Adequate grip force is a common need for individuals who use cable-operated, voluntary-opening TDs. The soft spring on the CAPP TD allows the device to open easily. However, the child is often frustrated with the minimal grip force and inability to hold an object when resistance is applied by the sound hand. As soon as the child has enough strength to pull against the medium spring (Hosmer 71622), it should be used to replace the soft one (Hosmer 71623). A third and stronger spring is available for the older child (1,9,13).

Some parents do not like the appearance of the CAPP TD or Dorrance hook. An alternative is a childs-size mechanical hand. Although the configuration of the hand lends itself to cylindrical objects like a bike handle, there are major disadvantages. The child's size 2-inch and 2 1/4-inch hands from Steeper Ltd. have a minimal grasping surface for small objects, require excessive operating force, and achieve only minimal opening. The 2-inch hand has a weak pinch. The glove frequently prevents complete closure. Therefore, the 2-year-old who wears the hand will be frustrated and unsuccessful in his attempt to learn TD operation (1,13,14). However, some older children are able to perform bimanual tasks with the 2 1/4-inch hand (Figure 26-12).

As the child gets older, interests, functional needs, and skill levels change. At CAPP, some teenagers (especially boys) prefer the versatility of the Dorrance hook. They like the fine tip prehension and the ability to increase grip force by adding rubber bands. Different types of hooks provide a secure grip on tools. The stainless steel hook is durable enough for manual labor (1,13).

The voluntary closing Adept and Grip Prehensors manufactured by Therapeutic Recreation Systems (TRS) provide increased prehension force. These prehensors allow the individual to control the amount of force exerted to do an activity. The Adept devices are made for children and adults. The Grip device is an adult component that is used for heavy-duty tool use and outdoor and recreational activities (1,13,14).

The need for cosmesis increases during the teenage years. A mechanical hand provides some aesthetics, but does not have the same potential for function as the CAPP TD or Dorrance hook. Children frequently complain that the mechanical hand does not hold objects securely. They find it easier to use the prosthesis as a stabilizer rather than rely on the weak prehension force (1,13,14).

A myoelectric hand provides the advantages of excellent pinch force and a pleasing appearance (Figure 26-13). The cable and harness system are eliminated. The hand opens and closes with the patient's arm in any position. However, increased cost and the lack of

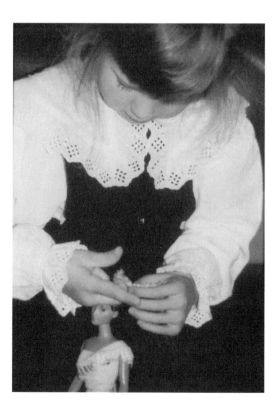

FIGURE 26-12

Child uses 2 1/4-inch Steeper mechanical hand to braid her doll's hair.

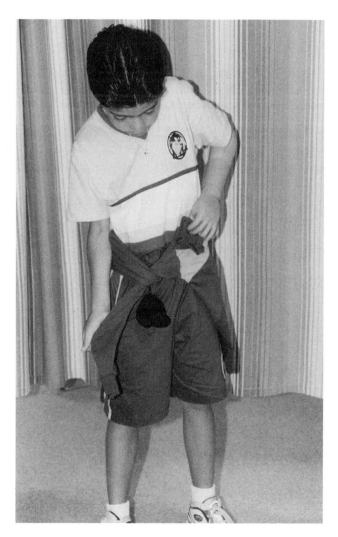

FIGURE 26-13

Myoelectric prosthesis provides good pinch force to tie the jacket.

available funding make it difficult for most children to receive this type of prosthesis (1).

At school or in the community, children may be required to remove the prosthesis for body contact sports. Sometimes, the TD may be perceived as a weapon. TRS manufactures the Super Sport Hand, which has a concave shape and is made of a flexible polymer. This device may be an appropriate alternative for certain sports activities (1).

Expectations of Wear and Use with the Below-Elbow Prosthesis

Based on clinical observation, it appears that many patients who have a transverse deficiency below the elbow continue to wear and use some type of below-elbow prosthesis as adults.

Prosthetic use patterns may vary during different developmental time periods. The pre-school and school-age child participates in many play activities that require the use of two hands.

Arts, crafts, toys, and games used in kindergarten and early elementary school reinforce the use of the prosthesis as practiced in the formal therapy setting.

As the child grows, the unaffected hand increases in strength and fine motor coordination. Some teenagers may rely on the sound hand to perform most tasks and use the prosthesis primarily as a stabilizer. This pattern is reinforced when the TD does not provide the fine prehension or grip force needed for the activity.

Most children and adults who demonstrate good motor planning and good problem solving skills have a better chance to develop excellent use of the prosthesis, which includes using the prehensile function of the TD to perform two-handed tasks and using the prosthesis in a natural and spontaneous manner.

UNILATERAL TRANSVERSE DEFICIENCY AT OR ABOVE THE ELBOW

The baby with a long residual limb at or above the elbow may receive the infant prosthesis when he sits independently. The baby with a short limb may benefit from the prosthetic fitting when she is walking, because the prosthesis may interfere with the ability to move freely. To provide the best possible outcome for the child with high-level limb loss, the team members need to evaluate the level and type of deficiency. Often the length, shape, and strength of the residual limb, as well as the range of shoulder motion, determine whether the child is a candidate for a standard prosthesis. To help the family make a decision about prosthetic fitting, the team provides the following information:

- The baby's functional potential and the developmental time frames for acquiring skills.
- Guidelines to help the baby achieve developmental milestones.
- Realistic expectations concerning the use of a prosthesis (7).

The Infant Prosthesis

The elbow disarticulation and above-elbow prosthesis can be an exoskeletal type with an elbow lock. A pull tab on the lock allows an adult to reposition the forearm. Friction hinges provide an alternative to a locking mechanism; these hinges are less bulky and allow the forearm position to be changed. However, the elbow cannot be locked in one position. Terminal device options are the infant hand or mitt, the CAPP TD, or the 10X hook. The prosthesis needs to be comfortable and secure as the baby moves and plays, therefore, a modified figure-eight harness with a chest strap is used to keep the socket and harness in place (7).

Family Instruction and Expectations for Use

The baby with the long residual limb is expected to wear the prosthesis all the time he is awake. The family is asked to develop a consistent full-time wearing pattern to help him become accustomed to the prosthesis. Parents can encourage the child to reach out and clasp toys with both arms (Figure 26-14) and to lean on the prosthesis for balance. It is important to note that the baby who has an elbow disarticulation or above-elbow prosthesis cannot use the artificial limb to support the weight of the body to creep on all fours. Before the child is able to walk, the preferred method of mobility is to scoot on the buttocks (7).

If the baby has a short, weak limb, he may tolerate the prosthesis for fewer hours per day. This baby cannot reach out to clasp big toys with both arms because the residual limb cannot lift the weight of the prosthesis.

In addition to placing toys and food in the TD and calling attention to the holding function, parents need to reposition the forearm periodically. If the forearm remains in one position, the child may resist learning to lock and unlock the elbow at a later time (7).

Activation of the TD: Single versus Dual-Control Cable System

The criteria to determine readiness to activate the TD have been discussed in the previous section. When the child is ready to learn to operate the TD, a cable is added to the new or existing prosthesis.

A dual control system is the standard control line or cable for an elbow disarticulation or above-elbow pros-

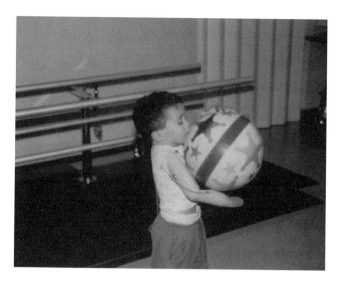

FIGURE 26-14

Child includes the prosthesis to clasp a ball.

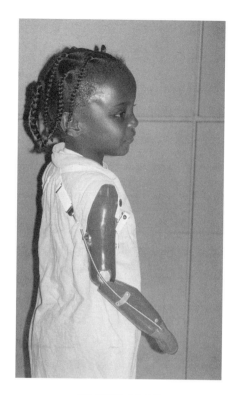

FIGURE 26-15

Elbow disarticulation prosthesis with a single control cable.

thesis. This cable has two functions: The patient performs the control motion (humeral flexion and/or scapular abduction) and the forearm lifts when the elbow is unlocked; the same control motion opens the terminal device when the elbow is locked. With the elbow locked at 90 degrees of flexion for most table-top activities, slack is produced in the cable system. The child does not have the power or range of motion in the shoulder girdle to take up the slack and cannot achieve full opening of the TD (7).

The single-control cable operates only the TD (15) (Figure 26-15). It requires the same amount of range and strength to open the TD with the forearm in any position, therefore, the 2-year-old finds it easier to learn TD operation with the single-control cable and has more success in the training process (7) (Figure 26-16).

The training procedures, which include learning the control motion, acquiring skills, and developing a spontaneous functional use pattern, are similar to procedures described earlier. Once the child has learned to open the TD and begins to use it to perform bimanual activities, he must become aware of how to preposition its components. A child with a limb loss above the elbow has less mobility of the arm when he wears the prosthesis. Therefore, it is necessary to preposition both the elbow and the TD to place the prosthesis in a good functional position to complete a task. Initially, the therapist and parents will preposition components for the child and call attention to the process (7,15).

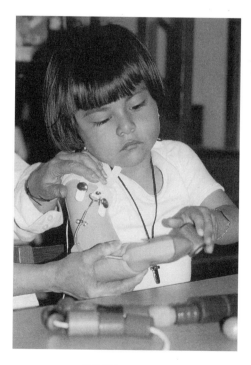

FIGURE 26-16

Child learns to operate the TD. The elbow disarticulation prosthesis has a single control cable.

Developmental Readiness Criteria to Learn Forearm Lift and Elbow Lock and Unlock

In a study that describes how young children learn to use an above-elbow prosthesis, Shaperman states that most 3-year-olds are aware that the forearm position can be changed (15). To show the child how and when to change the position of the forearm, the therapist does the following:

- Demonstrates how to pull the tab or billet on the elbow cable to lock and unlock (7,15). (This cable system exits the locking mechanism of the elbow joint and is separate from the single- or dual-control cable.)
- Varies the child's position in the play environment (7,15) (the child performs bimanual activities sitting on the floor, standing, or sitting at a table.)

Through observation and imitation, the child learns to unlock the elbow. The child then supports the prosthesis on a table or on her knee to maintain the desired position before relocking (Figure 26-17).

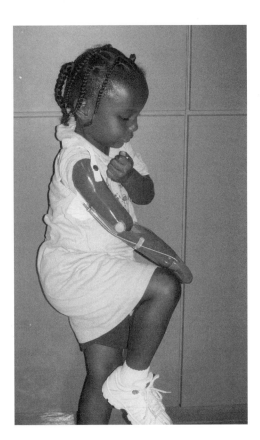

FIGURE 26-17

Child supports prosthesis on her knee while manually locking the elbow.

Shaperman states that children between 4 and 4 1/2 years of age are able to learn to actively lift the forearm and lock and unlock the elbow using the appropriate cable systems (15). She describes the developmental criteria that determine when the child is ready to learn these skills (15).

Clinical practice at CAPP suggests that children between 4 1/2 and 5 1/2 years of age appear to meet these readiness criteria more easily than the younger child:

- Child is able to effectively operate and use the TD.
- Child is able to see a purpose for and has a need to position the forearm.
- Child is able to manually operate the elbow lock tab or billet and tries to position the forearm.
- Child is able to follow verbal instructions and perform some drill activity. Because the elbow lock is a positioning component, practice and repetition are required to learn the control motion sequence.
- Child has sufficient range of motion, strength, and coordination to operate the dual-control cable system and the elbow lock system. The child must be able to flex the forearm to 90 degrees and then take up the additional cable slack to achieve full TD opening.
- The child must be able to utilize a medium spring on the CAPP TD or at least one rubber band on the hook to achieve separation of controls. Without sufficient loading, the TD will begin to open when the child uses the dual-control cable to lift the forearm (15).

Changes to the Prosthesis

The dual-control cable replaces the single-control cable on the prosthesis (Figure 26-18). The elbow lock tab or billet is attached to the harness, and a front suspensor replaces the front support strap. A flexion stop is used to prevent the forearm from hitting the child in the face while he learns to control forearm lift. The TD spring tension or rubber loading is increased as previously described (15).

Teaching the Controls

Forearm Lift

It is appropriate to teach elbow lift first because the child already uses the same control motion to open the TD. The therapist unlocks the elbow. He then demonstrates the control motion (humeral flexion) to show the child that the forearm lifts. Most children learn this operation quickly. However, they do need practice to regulate the degree and speed of forearm lift (15). The

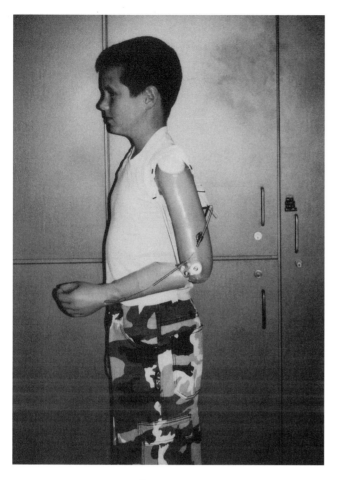

FIGURE 26-18

Elbow disarticulation prosthesis with a dual-control cable system.

flexion stop can be removed once the child is proficient in controlling this motion (15).

Sometimes the child who has a short, weak limb uses body swing to move his humerus. Without this momentum, he cannot move the cable system to achieve forearm flexion (15). The prosthetist can make changes to increase the mechanical advantage. He can adjust the harness to improve socket stability or reposition the lift loop that guides the dual-control cable. If the lift loop is close to the elbow center, greater force is required to flex the forearm, but less excursion is needed. The further the loop is from the elbow center, the reverse is true. Despite intervention, some children will always use the sound hand to assist forearm lift (15).

Forearm Lock/Unlock

The basic control motions to operate the elbow lock are extension of the humerus and depression of the scapula.

This composite motion puts tension in the elbow-lock cable to lock or unlock the unit. The child must always listen for two "clicks," which indicate that the cable has cycled completely (15). For example, to unlock the elbow, the child performs the control motion and listens for the "click." The child returns his shoulder to the neutral position to allow the cable to retract. This motion produces the second "click." The child may now repeat the process to relock the elbow. If the cable does not cycle completely, the lock mechanism will not function (15).

The complex motions to lock and unlock the elbow should be taught in stages. The following methods are presented as guidelines.

1. The therapist stands behind the child and places one hand on top of the child's shoulder and the other hand on the back of the humeral section. The prosthetic elbow may be locked in the extended position. The therapist physically assists the child to move the shoulder forward while extending the humerus. The child is told to push down into the socket to depress the scapula. Tension placed on the cable unlocks the elbow. The child listens for the first "click." The child relaxes the shoulder and listens for the second "click" before repeating the process (15).

2. The therapist stands in front of the child and uses one hand to support the prosthetic forearm in 90 degrees of flexion. The elbow may be unlocked. She places the other hand on top of the shoulder. The therapist then physically assists the child to bring the shoulder forward while pushing the humerus into extension and depression. The child triggers the lock, returns the shoulder to a neutral position, and listens for both "clicks." A variation of this method is to ask the child to push the front of the shoulder into the therapist's hand when extending and depressing the humerus (15) (Figure 26-19).

If the lock does not cycle completely, the therapist will need to check the following items:

• Make sure the child understands the importance of the second "click." For both adults and children, frustration occurs when the elbow lock does not cycle and prevents the mechanism from working the next time.

• The elastic front suspensor must be tight enough to assist the return of the cable to its original position. If it is too tight, the child will not be able to pull against it to trigger the lock. Frequent inadvertent operation of the elbow usually requires the elbow lock billet to be lengthened (15).

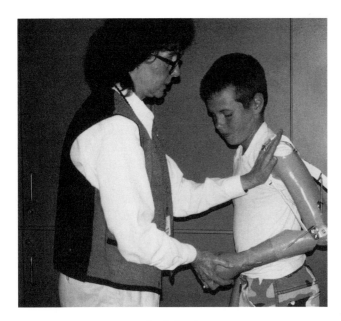

FIGURE 26-19

Child learns the control motion to lock and unlock the elbow joint.

Hands-on assistance is usually required to demonstrate the control motions. The therapist may use any variations of the methods presented to help the child understand this complex procedure.

Lift and Lock

As soon as the child can operate the lock reliably with the elbow extended, the therapist introduces another motion. Shoulder abduction maintains tension on the dual-control cable to keep the forearm in a desired position; this prevents the forearm from dropping when the humerus is extended. To practice this sequence, the child flexes the shoulder to lift the prosthetic forearm to 90 degrees using the dual-control cable. He abducts the shoulder to maintain the flexed forearm position and then quickly extends and depresses the shoulder to trigger the elbow-lock cable (15).

Initially the motions are exaggerated. Drill practice may help the child to refine this skill. One method is to present an object at a specific level and ask the child to reach out to receive it. The child must reposition the elbow each time the therapist changes the position of the object (15).

Children begin to refine forearm lift and elbow lock when they incorporate the procedure into functional activities (Figure 26-20). Providing activities at different work surface levels and in different play environments may encourage the child to change the posi-

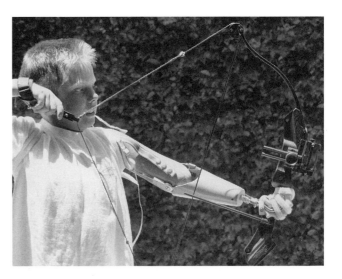

FIGURE 26-20

Patient locks elbow in extension to use prosthesis for archery.

tion of the elbow (15). The child's ability to perform the lift and lock sequence depends on the length, strength, and range of motion of the residual limb. In reality, most children avoid repositioning the elbow unless it is absolutely necessary.

Expectations of Prosthetic Wear and Use

Clinical experience shows that children who have a long transhumeral deficiency may wear and use the prosthesis to school, remove it at home, and wear it for selected periods on the weekend. The child is able to use the dual-control cable system and incorporates the prosthesis into bimanual activities.

The child with a short transhumeral limb deficiency usually has a sporadic wearing pattern. Because it is difficult to lift the weight of the prosthesis against gravity, the child uses it mainly for table-top tasks. The prosthesis is often removed for outdoor activities because it interferes with the ability to run and play.

The child with a transverse deficiency at the elbow may continue to use the prosthesis as an adult. The child with a very short residual limb will confine his limited wear and use pattern to the early school years.

UNILATERAL UPPER-LIMB AMELIA

The child with an upper-extremity amelia has the greatest need for functional restoration of the upper limb. In reality, the prosthesis does not replace the functions of a real arm, and it is difficult to fit because it covers so much of the chest area. To determine if a child will benefit from a shoulder-disarticulation prosthesis, the following questions must be asked:

- Does the family want a prosthesis for the baby?
- Will the contour and shape of the chest and shoulder area support a socket and provide stability for a prosthesis?
- Will the prosthesis interfere with the baby's gross motor development?

If the baby is a candidate for a prosthesis, it can be provided when he sits or walks independently. The factor that determines the time frame is whether the prosthesis interferes with the baby's ability to move freely (7). If possible, it is best to avoid fitting the first prosthesis when the baby enters the "terrible twos."

An endoskeletal prosthesis is preferred to decrease the weight and bulk as much as possible. The humeral and forearm segments are usually made of PVC or metal tubing, and the elbow lock is a push-button type. The humeral and forearm segments are covered with foam and stockinette to provide a soft feel and a cosmetic appearance (7,12). A chest strap secures the socket on the chest wall. The choice of TDs is the same as discussed earlier.

The loss of skin surface from which to lose body heat causes the child with a missing limb to overheat easily and to perspire profusely (7,12). The additional heat and weight generated by the shoulder-disarticulation prosthesis may interfere with a full 8 hours of wear a day. Nonetheless, the baby must wear it a consistent number of hours a day to develop a habit pattern.

Because the prosthesis has no active shoulder motion, the child cannot bring both arms to midline to clasp toys. However, it is possible to balance a large ball against the prosthesis to support it with the unaffected hand. During this period, the parents must reposition the shoulder, the forearm, and the TD to maintain the prosthesis in a functional position.

Criteria to Activate the TD and Changes to the Prosthesis

The readiness criteria to activate the terminal device are the same as described earlier. However, the cable control motion for TD operation of the shoulder-disarticulation prosthesis is more complex. The child must be able to follow directions and tolerate some frustration during the training process.

The prosthesis can be an endoskeletal or exoskeletal type. The single-control cable is added to activate the terminal device. Young children with this level of deficiency do not have the strength and range of motion to

use chest expansion or scapular abduction to operate the cable system. Therefore, the anchor for the control line is placed around the leg opposite the prosthesis in the form of a thigh cuff or thigh strap (7,12) (Figure 26-21). If the prosthesis is an exoskeletal type, a positive locking elbow replaces the push-button elbow. A nudge control is placed on the socket within reach of the child's chin. The lever on the nudge control is depressed and released to either lock or unlock the elbow (7).

TD Operation and Skill Building

The child stands to learn TD operation. The therapist stabilizes the child's pelvis, helps the child to flex the trunk, and assists shoulder-girdle elevation on the side of the prosthesis (7,12). The TD opens, and the therapist either places a toy or helps the child to place an object in the TD. The therapist also shows the child how to hold onto the object until the TD closes completely.

Trunk flexion allows the child some success with TD opening (7,12) (Figure 26-22). However, the device is not in the best position for functional activities

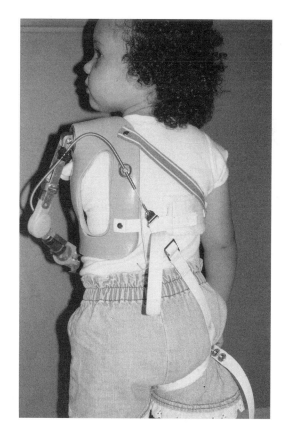

FIGURE 26-21

Endoskeletal shoulder disarticulation prosthesis with thigh-strap control.

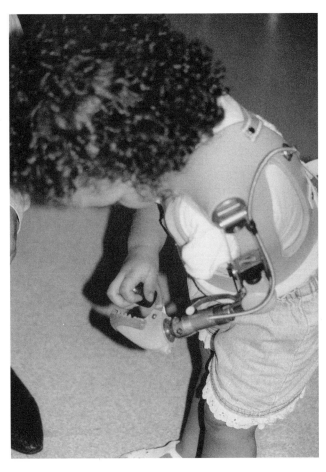

FIGURE 26-22

Child flexes trunk to open terminal device.

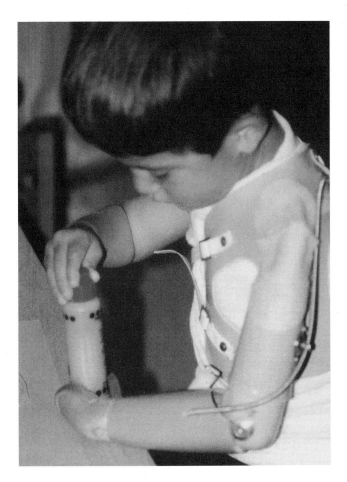

FIGURE 26-23

Child uses shoulder disarticulation prosthesis to perform activities at the midline of the body while seated at a table.

because it opens away from the midline of the body, almost at floor level. As soon as the child is able to understand another control motion, the therapist introduces shoulder elevation and trunk rotation (on the prosthetic side). This combined motion allows the TD to open at the midline of the body and also permits the child to do activities while seated at a table (7,12) (Figure 25-23). When the child sits to do activities, the control-attachment strap may become too tight or too loose, depending on the child's posture and the position of the strap. If there is too much slack in the strap and cable system, the child will have difficulty opening the TD. Too much tension on the cable will make it difficult for the TD to close completely. Therefore, the therapist must observe the child and make the necessary adjustments (7).

During this period, repetitive bimanual activities are used to help the child refine the control motion for TD operation. To use the TD effectively, all the other components must be properly positioned and adjusted.

The therapist or prosthetist should teach the parents to maintain the appropriate friction adjustment on the shoulder joint, the elbow turntable, and the wrist unit. If the friction is not adequate, the segments of the prosthesis will move during use (7). For example, a loose shoulder joint will cause the humeral and forearm segments to move into extension when the child applies any resistance to the TD. The TD moves, causing the child's work area to shift from the midline of the body to the side of the prosthesis. To avoid this problem, shoulder friction must be tight but not completely locked out. The forearm turntable and wrist can be slightly looser (7).

Once the child learns the control motion to activate the TD, the therapist is able to use imaginary and creative play to encourage a problem-solving approach to new prosthetic skills. The therapist shows the child how to position the shoulder and forearm turntable and calls attention to the best position of function for the TD. Children usually avoid prepositioning components;

there is no easy solution to help them learn this skill except for constant reminders and practice.

Learning to Lock and Unlock the Elbow

The elbow lock and unlock operation is much easier with a shoulder disarticulation prosthesis than with an above-elbow prosthesis. Most 3-year-olds are able to operate the nudge control and can learn this procedure before the dual-control cable is added (12). The child depresses the nudge-control lever with the chin to unlock the elbow. The sound hand manually positions the forearm, and the elbow is relocked (7). The lever must be positioned on the socket within reach of the child's chin. However, it must not jab the neck or face when the child turns his head.

Dual-Control Cable System for Active Forearm Lift

The readiness criteria to learn to use the dual-control cable system have already been described. However, the child with this level of limb loss must have the range of motion, the strength, and the coordination to utilize the dual-control cable and to achieve full TD opening with the elbow flexed at 90 degrees. If the child has difficulty opening the TD, it is best to continue with the single-control cable.

Teaching Forearm Lift and Elbow Lock/Unlock

The therapist unlocks the elbow and demonstrates that the same motion that opens the TD now lifts the forearm (7). A forearm stop is necessary to prevent the child from striking his face during operation. Drill activity helps the child to refine the motion to control both the speed and amount of forearm flexion.

As soon as the child has mastered forearm flexion, it is appropriate to combine lift and lock. If the child already uses the nudge control, the procedure will be easy. The child lifts the forearm to the desired position, maintains tension on the dual-control cable, and depresses the nudge control to lock the elbow (7). To lower the forearm, the child depresses the nudge control, and allows the forearm to extend.

The child refines these positioning skills by integrating them into bimanual activities (7). The therapist reminds the child to position the elbow unit and the friction components (shoulder, elbow turntable, and wrist) to place the prosthesis in the best position for the task. Changing the child's work position from sitting to standing will help him focus on the need to preposition components. As stated previously, children will preposition components only when it is absolutely necessary.

Use of the Child-Size Electric Hook

The Michigan Electric Hook for children may be used in place of a cable-operated TD at the time of initial activation. The electric hook may be beneficial if the child cannot use the cable system effectively for the following reasons:

- The child cannot or will not tolerate the thigh strap control.
- The child does not have the excursion or strength to use the cable system to achieve consistent opening of the TD, especially at the midline of the body (12,14).

The Michigan Electric Hook from Hosmer has a small motor, a modified 10X or 10P hook, and a rechargeable battery. A single-function touch pad or push button switch is used to operate the hook. The switch is placed in the top portion of the socket (Figure 26-24). The child raises his shoulder, hits the switch, and the hook opens. The child relaxes the shoulder

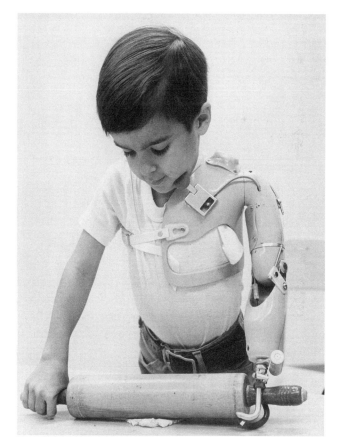

FIGURE 26-24

Shoulder disarticulation prosthesis has an electric hook and a nudge control to lock and unlock elbow.

away from the switch, and the hook closes by rubber band action (12,14).

The advantages of the electric hook are:

- The electric hook is easy to operate.
- The hook opens and closes at the same position in space thus providing a consistent work area.

The disadvantages of the electric hook are:

- The pinch force is limited by the rubber band loading, and the motor tolerates less than one full band. The limited pinch force is usually adequate for the 2-year-old, but not for the activity level of the school-age child (13,14).
- The electric hook requires more maintenance than a cable-operated hook.
- The child who initially uses a CAPP TD will need to adjust to the hook.

- The child may accidentally hit the switch during active play, causing inadvertent opening of the hook (13).

The major advantage of the electric hook is its ease of operation; the child has no difficulty learning the control motion. However, the electric hook does open and close slowly. Therefore, the therapist instructs the child to hold onto the object with the sound hand and to time the placement of the object with the closure of the hook. If continuous inadvertent operation of the hook occurs during play, the therapist should ask the prosthetist to adjust the position of the switch. The child is required to reach a little higher with the shoulder to trigger the switch, thus avoiding the accidental opening. Although children with this level of limb loss benefit from an electric hook, they rarely use other electric components, such as an elbow or wrist rotator. The function supplied by these components is offset by the increased weight to the prosthesis. When the electric

TABLE 26-1
Unilateral Upper Extremity Limb Loss Developmental Criteria for Prosthetic Intervention

TYPE OF LIMB LOSS	CRITERIA TO FIT THE FIRST INFANT PASSIVE PROSTHESIS	CRITERIA TO ACTIVATE TERMINAL DEVICE (T.D.)	CRITERIA TO ACTIVATE FOREARM LIFT AND ELBOW LOCK
Transverse deficiency below the elbow	1. Fit when baby has independent sitting balance.	1. Has 10-minute attention span. 2. Follows 2-step direction. 3. Is willing to be handled. 4. Understands that TD can hold objects. 5. Attempts to open TD with sound hand.	N.A.
Transverse deficiency at or above the elbow	1. Fit when baby sits independently or wait until walks independently. Prosthesis not to interfere with gross motor skills.	Same	1. Able to operate TD effectively. 2. Has a need to position forearm. 3. Can manually lock and unlock elbow. 4. Able to follow directions and can do drill activity. 5. Has the strength and range of motion to use dual-control cable.
Amelia	Same	1. Same criteria apply. 2. Child must be able to tolerate some frustration when learning TD. 3. Easier to learn to operate electric hook.	1. Same criteria apply. 2. If child has nudge control for elbow unit, will learn to lock and unlock before cable added for forearm lift.

hook no longer provides adequate pinch force for the child's activity level, he can resort to a cable system and thigh strap control (13).

Expectations of Wear and Use

The young child uses the shoulder disarticulation prosthesis during a specific developmental time period to perform bimanual activities. It is used at school and at home, primarily for table or desktop tasks. The child usually removes it for sports and rigorous outdoor play. Teenagers prefer not to have a prosthesis. They cite the heat, the weight, and the bulk as reasons not to wear it.

CONCLUSIONS

The prosthetic prescription and training process for the child with a unilateral upper-limb deficiency is based on principles of child development (Table 26-1). A center that has a team approach provides the best comprehensive care. For the young child, learning to use a prosthesis takes place along a developmental continuum. The role of the parents is crucial in helping the child to have a successful prosthetic experience.

The prosthetic wear and use pattern for the adult with a limb deficiency may be different from the wear and use pattern for an individual with a traumatic amputation. Nonetheless, the factors that influence long-term prosthetic use patterns are:

- The level and type of limb loss and strength of the residual limb;
- The cosmetic and functional benefit from the prosthesis;
- The patient's motivation and personal preference.

It is important to recognize that the upper extremity prosthesis is an artificial device that does not replace the functions of a real limb. Therefore, the individual who wears the prosthesis ultimately decides how and when to use it.

References

1. Patton J. Developmental approach to pediatric upper-limb prosthetic training. In: *Atlas of Limb Prosthetics*. St. Louis: Mosby, 1992.
2. Sypniewski BL. The child with terminal transverse partial hemimelia: A review of the literature on prosthetic management. *Artificial Limbs* 1972; 16:35–36.
3. Brooks MB, Shaperman J. Infant prosthetic fitting: A study of the results. *Am J Occupat Ther* 1965; 19:333.
4. Sorbye R. Upper extremity amputees: Swedish experience concerning children. In: *Comprehensive Management of the Upper-Limb Amputee*. New York: Springer Verlag, 1989; 227–229.
5. Brenner C. Fitting infants and children with electronic limbs. Detroit experience 1981 to 1990. *J Assoc Child Prosthetic Orthotic Clin* 1990; 25–30.
6. Mifsud M, AI-Temen I, Sauter W. Variety Village electromechanical hand for amputees under two years of age. *J Assoc Child Prosthetic Orthotic Clin* 1987; 22:41–46.
7. Setoguchi Y, Rosenfelder R (eds.). *The Limb Deficient Child*. Springfield, Ill.: Thomas, 1982; 95–108, 113, 114, 140–158, 180–192, 204–235.
8. Talbot D. *The Child With a Limb Deficiency: A Guide for Parents*. University of California at Los Angeles, 1979.
9. Shaperman J. The CAPP terminal device: A preliminary evaluation. *Inter Clinic Information Bull* 1975; 14:9–10.
10. Gesell A, Ilg F. *The Child from Five to Ten*. New York: Harper & Brothers, 1946; 35, 121–123, 235, 366.
11. Pulaski MS. *Your Baby's Mind and How It Grows: Piaget's Theory for Parents*. New York: Harper & Row 1978; 87–89.
12. Clarke S, Patton J. Occupational therapy for the limb deficient child: Developmental approach-unilateral upper extremity limb deficiencies. *Clin Orthopedics*, 1980; 148:47–52.
13. Patton J. Prosthetic components for children and teenagers. In: *Comprehensive Management of the Upper Limb Amputee*. New York: Springer-Verlag; 1989; 99–118.
14. Patton J, Tokeshi J, Setoguchi Y. Prosthetic components for children. In: *Physical Medicine and Rehabilitation*. Philadelphia: Hanley and Belfus, 1991; 245–264.
15. Shaperman J. Learning patterns of young children with above-elbow prostheses. *Am J Occupat Ther* 1979; 33:299–305.

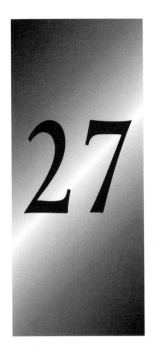

27 Pediatric Case Studies of Upper Extremity Limb Deficiencies

Yoshio Setoguchi, MD, Joanna G. Patton, OTR/L, and Joanne Shida–Tokeshi, OTR/L

The treatment approaches for the young child who has a unilateral upper extremity limb deficiency were discussed in Chapter 26. Cases I through III are examples of integrating the Child Amputee Prosthetic Project (CAPP) treatment approach with the child who has a transverse deficiency below the elbow. Prosthetic interventions using a cable-operated prosthesis and a myoelectric prosthesis will be discussed.

Children with high-level upper extremity deficiency or multiple-limb loss present a complex picture. The last two cases describe children who have severe congenital limb loss. As illustrated in case IV, children who have upper extremity anomalies with functional digits may benefit from special devices or an opposition post rather than a standard prosthesis. In case V, children who have bilateral upper extremity amelia (no arms) will develop excellent foot skills when given opportunities and encouragement. If the baby can tolerate and benefit from shoulder disarticulation prostheses, fitting may be delayed until he is walking independently.

Depending on the type and level of limb loss, prosthetic intervention may or may not be appropriate. If the child has the potential to walk, then lower extremity prostheses are usually provided when the child is ready to pull to stand. If the child's ability to stand and walk is questionable or delayed, then upper extremity prostheses may be the first option.

Prostheses are only part of the equation for children with high-level multiple limb loss. These children will always use adapted performance techniques, adapted equipment, and adaptations to the environment to be as independent as possible (1).

CASE I: TRANSVERSE DEFICIENCY BELOW THE ELBOW FITTED WITH CABLE OPERATED PROSTHESIS

Luis was initially seen at the Shriners Hospital for Children–Child Amputee Prosthetics Project (CAPP), Los Angeles at 7 months of age. He was born with a transverse deficiency of the radius and ulna (absence of the distal portion of the forearm and hand). A dimple and rudimentary nubbins remain. Both shoulder and elbow joints are normal, with full range of motion.

Luis was the result of his mother's second pregnancy, which was full term and uncomplicated. His older brother was in good health with no congenital anomalies.

Problem/Need

Luis' parents were interested in a prosthesis for their son and wanted to know what was available. They were given information about an infant prosthesis with a chest harness and a passive terminal device (TD).

At 7 months of age, Luis' development was commensurate with his age. He was able to roll and combat crawl. The team felt that Luis was not ready for a prosthesis because he was not sitting independently. His parents agreed to return to CAPP in a few months.

Prosthetic Intervention and the Training Process

Luis received his first infant passive prosthesis at 10 months. The parents requested a foam-filled infant hand for the first TD, but agreed to change to the CAPP TD 1 when he was ready for cable activation.

The family complied with the team's instructions to have Luis develop a full-time wearing pattern. They also helped him to include the prosthesis to clasp large toys and to support his body weight when creeping and pulling to stand (Figure 27-1). Luis returned several times during the year for prosthetic adjustments and to monitor his wear and use patterns.

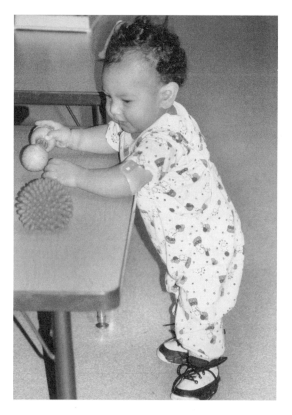

FIGURE 27-1

Infant passive prosthesis with infant passive hand.

At 2 years of age, Luis needed a new prosthesis. Although he was not ready to learn how to operate an active TD, he received a standard below-elbow prosthesis with a figure-eight harness, a single control line, and a CAPP TD 1 with soft spring. Despite an unwillingness to be handled, Luis cooperated momentarily to allow the therapist to move his arm through the control motion to teach the training techniques to his mother. During the training sessions at CAPP, Luis refused to place toys into the open TD. Because he previously wore a passive hand, it was apparent that he was unaware of the holding function of the CAPP TD. Mother was encouraged to place toys and treats inside the TD to help Luis learn this concept.

At 27 months of age, Luis was definitely aware of placing toys inside the open TD. However, he still needed verbal cues and "hands-on" assistance for all aspects of TD operation. At this point, Luis was a very active child and was more interested in gross motor activities than learning the control motion.

By 30 months of age, Luis learned to actively open the TD, but needed assistance to relax tension on the control line to close the TD. At 3 years of age, Luis' use pattern had markedly improved. However, he still required verbal reminders to preposition the TD and reposition objects inside the TD.

Outcome

At 3 years and 8 months of age, Luis demonstrates excellent gross motor and fine motor skills. He enjoys baseball and includes the prosthesis to hold a plastic bat. He is able to hit a ball with considerable force. Although Luis requires some verbal reminders to preposition the TD, he is now able to reposition objects inside the TD without assistance.

Parental influence has encouraged Luis to develop good prosthetic skills. He uses the prehensile function of the TD in a natural and spontaneous manner to perform various age-appropriate bimanual activities (Figure 27-2).

CASE II: TRANSVERSE DEFICIENCY BELOW THE ELBOW FITTED WITH CABLE-OPERATED AND MYOELECTRIC PROSTHESIS

John was initially seen at CAPP at 14 months of age. He was born with a transverse deficiency of the radius and ulna. No other congenital anomalies were present. His development was commensurate with his age level, as demonstrated by his ability to walk independently with a wide-based gait, stoop and recover his balance, eat finger foods, and say four or five single words.

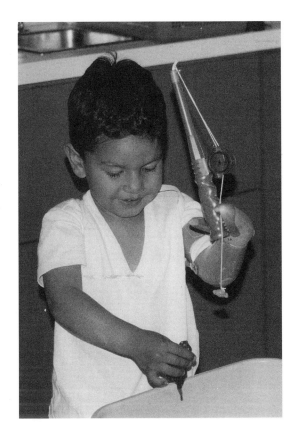

FIGURE 27-2

Use of CAPP T.D. No. 1 to perform bimanual activities.

Problem/Need

John's parents were interested in a prosthesis for their son. The CAPP team discussed the philosophy of the prosthetic program with them. As with most parents, they wanted a prosthesis that would provide both function and cosmesis.

Prosthetic Intervention and Training Process

Based on the CAPP philosophy to fit the first prosthesis when the baby achieves independent sitting balance, John was ready to receive his first infant passive prosthesis. His parents were given a choice of either the CAPP TD 1 (with no control line) or foam-filled infant passive hand. Although parents liked the appearance of the hand, they chose the CAPP TD because they could open it manually. Over time, they wanted their son to learn to push objects into the TD.

When John received his first infant prosthesis, his parents helped him develop a full-time, consistent wearing pattern (during the time he was awake). They also encouraged him to use the prosthesis to clasp large toys,

to support himself, and to stabilize objects. Although the family lives in interior Mexico, they were diligent about keeping their appointments at the CAPP clinic. When John was 28 months of age, he demonstrated the cognitive and sensory motor skills necessary to learn to actively open the TD. A cable system was added to the prosthesis and training commenced. This bright, cooperative youngster learned the control motion to operate the terminal device in 1 week. John's mother was given instructions to assist her son at home to refine the control motion and to accurately place items inside the TD with the sound hand.

John returned to the CAPP clinic in 4 months to have the fit of the prosthesis re-evaluated, to determine his level of function with the prosthesis, and to introduce additional prosthetic skills. By the age of 3, John had developed a natural and spontaneous use of the prehensile function of the prosthesis when he performed two-handed play and daily living tasks. He continued to wear the prosthesis 8 to 10 hours a day.

Because of compliance and good use with the cable-operated prosthesis, John was selected as a candidate for a myoelectric prosthesis. Mother was cautioned that an electric prosthesis usually requires more maintenance and necessitates more visits to the clinic.

John received his first myoelectric prosthesis with two state–two site Otto Bock control system and VASI 2-6 electric hand at the age of 4. He quickly learned how to separate the controls to open and close the hand before the definitive prosthesis was fabricated. Once the final prosthesis was completed, John rapidly developed good prosthetic skills and spontaneous use with his new prosthesis. He adjusted to the increased weight of the myoelectric prosthesis and continued to wear it about 10 hours a day. As growth demanded, John received new prostheses over time. A larger VASI 5-9 electric hand was issued at the age of 7 to match the size of the sound hand. Currently, he is wearing a fifth myoelectric prosthesis with the Otto Bock control system and VASI 5-9 electric hand (Figure 27-3).

Outcome

John is a bright child who demonstrates excellent problem solving and motor planning abilities. With tremendous support from his family, he continues to wear and use his prosthesis effectively on a full time basis. John is a good student who likes soccer and is learning to play various musical instruments (Figure 27-4).

A myoelectric prosthesis may require more maintenance than a cable-operated prosthesis. With instructions, parents can make routine repairs on a cable-operated system; however, routine repairs to a myoelectric prosthesis are not easily accomplished. The myoelectric prosthe-

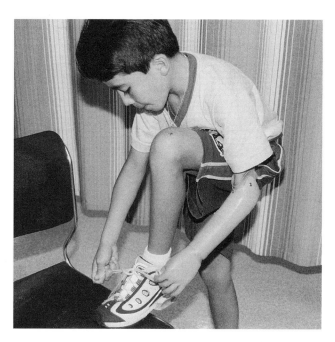

FIGURE 27-3

VASI 5-9 electric hand produces good pinch force for tying shoe laces.

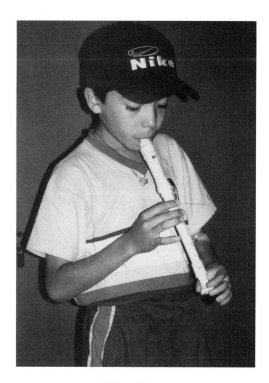

FIGURE 27-4

Myoelectric prosthesis helps patient to hold musical instrument.

sis must be returned to the prosthetist, and the family is required to make the necessary visits to the clinic to keep the prosthesis in good operating condition.

When fitting a child who lives in another country with an electric prosthesis, practitioners should be prepared to deal with problems related to mail service and customs. Some families may not have the resources for the frequent return visits that are required to maintain a myoelectric prosthesis.

CASE III: TRANSVERSE DEFICIENCY BELOW THE ELBOW FITTED WITH INFANT MYOELECTRIC PROSTHESIS

Kevin was initially seen at CAPP at 10 months of age. He was born with a left transverse deficiency of the radius and ulna, with mild subluxation of the elbow. No developmental problems or other congenital anomalies were present. No problems were reported with mother's pregnancy or delivery. At this first visit, Kevin was sitting independently, manipulating objects, and combat crawling.

Problem/Need

The parents were most interested in providing a TD that would be cosmetically appealing. They expressed that their community in Mexico would not be supportive if the device did not resemble a hand. Kevin was fitted with a passive infant prosthesis with foam-filled hand.

Prosthetic Intervention

Kevin's parents encouraged a consistent full-time wearing pattern. He developed excellent spontaneous use. A pre-flexed forearm, which kept the arm forward, assisted in his constant use of the prosthesis. Kevin used the prosthesis to support himself, to crawl, and to clasp objects. Due to extremely natural use with this passive prosthesis, Kevin was selected for an infant myoelectric fitting.

At 18 months, Kevin received his first self-suspending myoelectric prosthesis. The components included a single-site Otto Bock electrode, a second-sized Steeper SCAMP electric hand, and an internal battery recessed into the forearm. The team's goal was to observe when the child acquired the following: inadvertent opening of the hand, attention to the open hand, ability to actively open the hand, and active placement of objects into the hand. At 19 months, Kevin could not open the hand on command. He would attempt to pull the thumb open or try to push a toy into the hand (Figure 27-5). He would

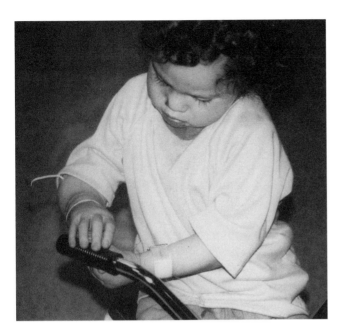

FIGURE 27-5

Child pushes SCAMP myoelectric hand onto tricycle handle.

allow objects to be placed inside the hand and participate in simple bimanual tasks.

At 20 months, Kevin was constantly pulling the prosthesis off, thus interrupting the consistent wearing pattern. A "mommy switch" was added so that a parent could open the hand by depressing this switch. This allowed Kevin to begin inserting objects into the open hand.

Kevin began opening the hand on command at about 2 years of age. Shortly thereafter, he began to insert objects into the open hand. Then problems developed with intermittent functioning of the hand, increased repair time, uncooperative behavior, and difficulty for the family to make frequent visits to the clinic from their home in Mexico. Unfortunately, to complicate matters, the family lost the myoelectric prosthesis. The team then determined that continuing with a myoelectric prosthesis would be difficult for the family.

Together with the parents, it was decided to fit Kevin with a standard body-powered prosthesis. The parents chose to try both the CAPP TD1 (Figure 27-6) and the 2-inch Steeper mechanical hand, but still seemed more interested in having a hand. Training was provided so that Kevin could develop the necessary prosthetic skills to become spontaneous using a body-powered prosthesis. Follow-through with this prosthesis has not been consistent. It continues to be difficult for the family to return to the clinic for training.

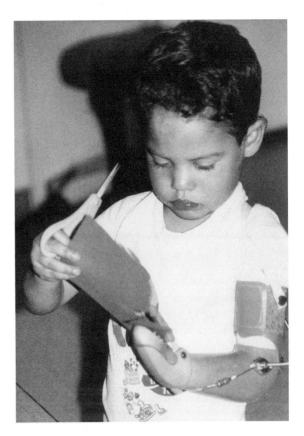

FIGURE 27-6

Child receives CAPP TD No. 1

Outcome

Kevin is currently wearing his below-elbow body-powered prosthesis about 6 hours per day. Occasionally, Kevin does not want to wear the prosthesis, and parents allow him to remove it. The 2-inch Steeper mechanical hand is worn most of the time and does not provide adequate function. Due to decreased visits to the clinic and inconsistent follow-through, Kevin demonstrates poor skills with the CAPP TD as well.

Several issues need to be considered when fitting a young child with a myoelectric prosthesis:

- Will the family be able to make the required visits for routine checks and repairs?
- Is the family able to maintain and care for this type of prosthesis?
- Is the family able to establish a consistent full-time wearing pattern and encourage bimanual use?
- Will the child be more functional with this type of prosthesis?
- Does early fitting of a myoelectric prosthesis contribute to better functional use and wearing?

- Does inadvertent opening of the hand enhance earlier awareness of the holding function?
- Do the costs of a myoelectric prosthesis outweigh the benefits (including psychological, functional, social)?

It was apparent that a good fitting, lightweight prosthesis with a pre-flexed forearm contributed to early spontaneous use with the passive prosthesis. The parents initially were very consistent with a full-time wearing pattern. However, the selection of this child as an early fitting myoelectric candidate was not ideal. For older children, our selection criteria include good spontaneous use with a body-powered prosthesis. For younger children, selection is more difficult, since the child is fitted with a passive type of prosthesis and families are beginning their journey into the world of prosthetics. The CAPP team has learned from this experience that mechanical reliability, quick repair time, commitment of the family, and accessibility to the clinic are necessary to ensure greater success.

CASE IV: BILATERAL UPPER EXTREMITY AMELIA FITTED WITH SHOULDER DISARTICULATION PROSTHESES

Robert was referred to the UCLA CAPP at 2 months of age. He was born with bilateral upper extremity amelia (no arms), but has normal lower extremities. Shoulder girdles are present and normal. No other abnormalities are present. Robert is the result of his mother's second pregnancy; pregnancy and delivery were reported normal.

Robert's parents were seen by the team and given information and guidelines concerning their child's limb deficiencies and development. At this initial visit, they were instructed not to overdress their son because:

- He has less skin surface from which to dissipate heat and may become easily overheated.
- He needs freedom to move his legs, feet, and body to explore his environment.

Robert's parents felt sad about their son's severe limb loss, but seemed able to cope with his needs. They were seen periodically by team members to monitor Robert's development, provide guidelines to encourage gross motor skills, and to provide emotional support.

Children without arms achieve normal developmental milestones but sometimes sitting and walking are delayed. Robert's growth and development progressed within normal time frames. At 5 months, he rolled from supine to prone. He began to grasp and transfer toys with his toes. Independent sitting balance was achieved at 8 months. At 10 months, Robert reached with his feet from a sitting position to grasp toys. He also began to scoot on his bottom as a method of mobility. At 13 months, Robert began to walk independently with a wide-based gait. However, he was not yet able to come to a standing position. A helmet was provided for protection and safety.

Problem/Need

At the initial visit, Robert's parents asked about "arms" for their son. They were told it was not possible to give him "flesh and blood" limbs. They were informed that prostheses could be provided at a later time.

Because Robert was walking quite well at 15 months, the CAPP team and his parents felt that prostheses would be beneficial. It was felt that the prostheses would not interfere with established gross motor skills and would allow the child to pull a toy as he walked.

Prosthetic Intervention and Training Process

Lightweight endoskeletal shoulder disarticulation prostheses were made when Robert was 17 months of age. Polyvinylchloride (PVC) tubing was used for the humeral and forearm sections. The elbow joints were nonstandard CAPP push button units. The left TD was a TRS mitt and the right was a 12P Dorrance hook. Neither TD had an active control line. Robert practiced using the right prosthesis to scribble with felt-tipped markers and to paint with a brush. These tools were secured in the 12P hook with a rubber band placed over the tip of the hook.

Robert wore his prostheses at home on a limited but consistent basis (about 2 to 3 hours per day). His mother encouraged the use of the prostheses for play activities.

Because of marital problems, Robert's mother moved out of the area and the family was lost to follow-up for almost a year. When Robert returned to CAPP at 34 months of age, he had outgrown his prostheses. He now needed a way to actively grasp an object. Exoskeletal prostheses using two Michigan electric hooks were prescribed and fabricated. Robert operated the electric hooks by hitting a touch switch located on the top of the socket. Positive locking elbows replaced the push button type. Nudge control units were mounted onto the sockets. Robert was able to hit the nudge control lever with his chin to lock or unlock the elbow.

Robert's prosthetic and therapy program was interrupted once again when the CAPP program moved locations. In the interim, his mother remarried and Robert became part of a new family. He was eventually seen at Shriners Hospital–CAPP when he was 3 years and 4 months of age.

Robert received prosthetic training to learn to use his prostheses with electric hooks. Because the electric hooks close slowly, Robert needed to learn how to time the closure of the hook for a secure grasp on objects. Robert's mother attempted to encourage her son to use the prostheses at home. However, the demands of the new family made it difficult for her to provide consistent attention.

Robert entered preschool when he was 4 years old. He found it difficult to use the prostheses for classroom activities. The electric hooks were difficult to preposition, and the prostheses limited his freedom of movement. Because Robert needed to keep up with his classmates and perform well in school, it was decided that he use his feet at school and practice with the prostheses at home.

When Robert outgrew these prostheses, the team was reluctant to provide new ones because of the intermittent wear and use pattern. However, his mother wanted Robert to learn to eat with the prostheses even though he was able to perform this activity with his feet. To help make the task easier, a Variety Ability System VV2-6 electric elbow was provided for the right shoulder disarticulation prosthesis (Figure 27-7). A rocker switch was used to control elbow flexion and extension.

Cable-operated hooks replaced the electric hooks. A thigh cuff was used as the anchor point for the single-control cable systems that operate each hook. Robert used his prostheses to eat only when his mother was available to supervise. By the time he was 7 years old, Robert refused to wear his prostheses. He and his mother frequently argued over this matter. Complex family problems and Robert's poor school performance also became apparent. Due to the family's many psychosocial problems, the social worker was asked to intervene. Robert was then referred to an outside agency for counseling. The occupational therapist suggested to his mother that the prostheses be left at CAPP to eliminate at least one source of conflict. The team felt that addressing and resolving the family problems were more important than the prostheses.

Outcome

Several months later, Robert's mother was able to relinquish the prostheses. This youngster was very happy and relieved with this decision. With counseling, Robert is more cooperative in school and is able to complete his classroom assignments. His printing with his feet has become neater and more legible (Figure 27-8). Some family tensions have been reduced, and Robert has a better relationship with his siblings.

Robert uses his feet and adapted performance techniques to complete his daily tasks. The occupational therapist provides training and adapted equipment to help Robert become more independent in dressing and personal hygiene activities. The CAPP team continues to

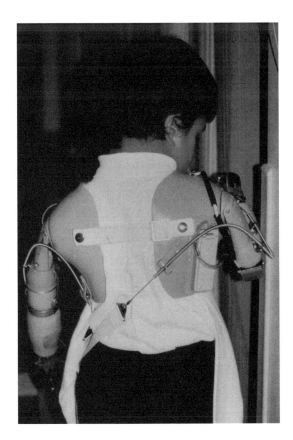

FIGURE 27-7

Bilateral shoulder disarticulation prostheses with VV2-6 electric elbow (right side).

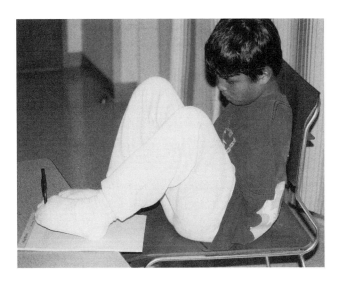

FIGURE 27-8

Child practices printing with his feet.

evaluate Robert every 6 months to monitor his needs and his progress.

CASE V: LIMB DEFICIENCIES OF ALL FOUR EXTREMITIES

Susan was born with limb deficiencies of all four extremities as part of a hypoglossia–adactylia syndrome. Limb anomalies include a right transverse deficiency above the elbow and a left partial two-digit hand (the medial digit has three normal phalanges and the lateral one has a flail phalanx). The right femur is foreshortened, with an abnormal hip joint. The fibula is absent, and there is a hypoplastic five-toed foot. Two phalanges are present on the fourth and fifth digits. The left lower extremity was first described as an amelia and later as a very short transverse deficiency above the knee.

The mother was 24 years old at the time of Susan's birth. Maternal shingles occurred during the third and fourth months of the pregnancy. Labor and delivery were uncomplicated. Susan was later seen for a genetics evaluation. Associated anomalies include bilateral nevus flamus, bilateral ear creases, micrognathia, small tongue, and partial right facial paresis.

The baby and the family were seen at CAPP for consultation when she was 6 weeks of age and then again when she was 5 months of age. Her development was commensurate with her age. Examination revealed that the right lower extremity resembled a proximal femoral focal deficiency (PFFD), Type A, with a flexed hip. The knee had a flexion contracture, but the right foot was in a good position for weight bearing. Discussion with the family focused on future prosthetic fitting for the left lower extremity and an opposition post for the left partial hand. However, the team felt that Susan was not developmentally ready for either device.

Problem/Need

Shortly after this visit, the parents sought other advice and decided to go elsewhere for care. Susan was subsequently fitted with a left opposition post and a right passive above-elbow type prosthesis with the elbow fixed at 70 to 80 degrees of flexion. She also received a Para-podium type standing brace to develop trunk and lower extremity strength.

When Susan was 13 months old, the family returned to CAPP. The parents seemed concerned and frustrated because their child was not able to use the prostheses or Para-podium. The team explained that the child was not developmentally ready for all this equipment. Because Susan recently achieved independent sitting, it was more appropriate to increase her mobility without any devices to interfere.

At 20 months of age, Susan learned to scoot on her buttocks. She also began to feed herself with a plastic spoon. The handle of the spoon was a modified ring that slipped over the left wrist.

Prosthetic Intervention, Mobility Need, and Training

At 30 months of age, Susan began to pull to stand and weight bear on the right leg. X rays showed some rudimentary femur present in the left residual lower limb, and the hip joint was not well formed. Because of the severity of the lower limb involvement, the team decided to delay lower extremity fitting. Because Susan was using her left upper extremity to perform some daily activities, the team felt she might benefit from a right upper extremity prosthesis.

Susan was fit with a right standard above-elbow prosthesis with a single control cable, an elbow lock billet, and a 10X hook. Shortly thereafter, an opposition post was made for the left partial hand. With practice, Susan developed good skills with both the prosthesis and the post. She learned to push and hold an object with the hook while she completed the more complex part of the task with the partial hand and the post.

During this period, a motorized cart was recommended and purchased by the family. It provided better mobility and a way to keep up with her peers. Susan was able to operate the joy stick control with the left partial hand.

At 2 years and 11 months of age, Susan began to bear more weight on the right leg even though the foot was in valgus. The team felt that she was ready for lower extremity fitting. A standard pylon extension above-knee prosthesis with no articulation at the knee was issued. Within 2 months, Susan was walking with the aid of a walker. A helmet was used for protection.

Over the next 2 years, Susan wore the lower extremity prosthesis for short periods during the day and continued to use the walker. Then problems with the right foot increased. The equino valgus was progressing and an ankle foot orthosis (AFO) was provided. No real improvement was seen. In addition, the child complained of pain due to the overlapping third and fourth toes. Nonetheless, Susan achieved independent walking by 5 years of age. She continued to use a wheelchair for long distances.

Other Treatment Interventions

At 5 1/2 years of age, foot surgery was scheduled. A toe transplant to the left hand was also recommended. During the surgery, a proximal neuromuscular bundle was not located and therefore, the transplant was not possi-

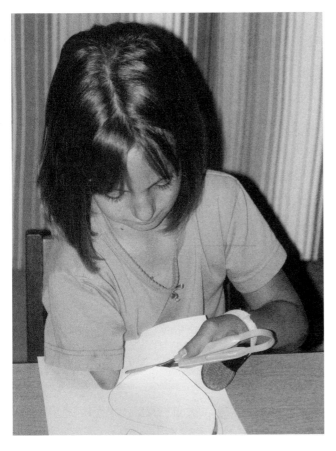

FIGURE 27-9

Patient uses opposition post to perform many bimanual activities.

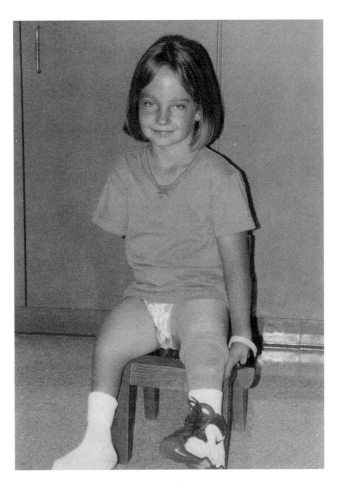

FIGURE 27-10

Lower extremity prosthesis with articulating knee joint.

ble. Reconstructive surgery to the right foot produced excellent results. Susan no longer needs an AFO and is pain free with weight bearing.

In relation to the craniofacial anomalies, Susan has had minimal intervention. The short tongue has not caused any difficulty and her speech development is normal.

Outcomes

During a $4^1/_2$ year period, Susan used a right above-elbow prosthesis to perform many bimanual activities. At age 7, she decided she no longer wanted to use it. The prosthesis was cumbersome to wear and no longer provided sufficient functional benefit. Susan has excellent function with her left partial hand and relies on her opposition post to perform many daily activities (Figure 27-9). She is independent in dressing, bathing, and completing her personal hygiene tasks.

At present, this youngster wears her left above-knee prosthesis about 10 to 12 hours a day. At age $7^1/_2$,

a knee joint was added to the prosthesis (Figure 27-10). She adapted well to the articulating knee joint and continues to have good function and stability. Susan wears the lower extremity prosthesis in the classroom, at home, and for short distances around the community. For longer distances (field trips, the mall, etc.) she uses her electric wheelchair.

Susan is a bright, motivated child who has benefited from the prosthetic intervention, support, and therapy provided by the CAPP team. Susan's mother is dedicated to assisting and encouraging her daughter to be as independent as possible.

*R*eference

1. Patton J. Upper limb deficiencies: Developmental approach to pediatric upper limb prosthetic training. In: *Atlas of Limb Prosthetics*. St. Louis, Mosby, 1992.

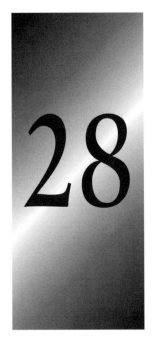

28

Follow-up, Outcomes, and Long-term Experiences in Adults with Upper Extremity Amputation

Robert H. Meier, III, MD and Alberto Esquenazi, MD

O ne of the essential elements in rehabilitation for the person with an amputation is regular, periodic follow-up visits that occur with the team. Follow-up with just the prosthetist is not usually adequate to ensure the most appropriate functional and emotional outcome once the prosthesis has been fitted. Although this process of follow-up also applies to the person with a leg amputation, it is absolutely critical to ensure the most appropriate level of prosthetic function for the upper extremity amputee. A high incidence of poor upper extremity prosthetic wearing and usage for the unilateral arm amputee is indicated in the literature. Several factors contribute to this pattern (1).

First, many individuals with an arm amputation can perform the majority of their activities of daily living (ADLs) and vocational tasks with the use of the normal arm and the residual arm. They do not need to wear a prosthesis to perform most of the activities they desire. Second, an arm prosthesis is perceived as being relatively heavy and may require harnessing and strapping that make it uncomfortable to wear and use. Third, the prosthesis may not provide a good cosmetic restoration. Fourth, the amount of function and cosmesis achieved with the prosthesis may not overcome the discomfort of wearing the artificial arm.

The major determinant in the successful wear and use of an arm prosthesis has been attributed to its comfort. Function is placed as second, and the cosmetic appearance is third. Because comfort is so important, regular follow-up should provide an assessment of comfort, and attempts to improve the comfort of prosthetic wear should be made at that time.

The level of function achieved should also be assessed at each follow-up appointment. The level attained should be compared with the ideal level expected with the level of amputation (Figures 28-1 and 28-2), the type of prosthesis provided, and any other comorbid factors that affect the use of the upper extremities.

During a follow-up appointment, an assessment of the amputee's emotional well-being should also be determined. Emotional deterioration is frequently seen after a prosthesis is fitted, the training completed, and the amputee has returned to their family and community. Follow-up sessions can look for evidence of anxiety, depression, interrupted sleep patterns, and changes in appetite. The presence of pain should be assessed routinely during these visits.

SETTINGS FOR FOLLOW-UP

The most appropriate setting for follow-up is a comprehensive outpatient amputation rehabilitation center.

TRANSRADIAL LEVEL

- Independent in ADL, donning and doffing
- Writes legibly with remaining hand
- Switch of dominance, if necessary
- Drives
- Can tie laces with one hand
- Has returned to work

- Uses a button hook
- Prepared a meal
- Adaptive equipment evaluation
- Carpentry and auto repair, if appropriate
- Wears prosthesis during waking hours
- Uses prosthesis for bimanual activities

FIGURE 28-1

This setting provides the full array of outpatient rehabilitation services under one roof and usually does not require the amputee to move from one setting to another for the necessary services. This setting is especially amputee-friendly if a prosthetic laboratory is also present in the same facility.

Providing the essential amputation rehabilitation services in one facility also assists in keeping the team

TRANSHUMERAL LEVEL

- Independent in ADL, donning and doffing
- Writes legibly with remaining hand
- Switch of dominance, if necessary
- Drives
- Can tie laces with one hand
- Has returned to work

- Uses a button hook
- Prepared a meal
- Adaptive equipment evaluation
- Carpentry and auto repair, if appropriate
- Wears prosthesis during waking hours
- Uses prosthesis for bimanual activities

FIGURE 28-2

members well informed regarding the rehabilitation plan and any changes that occur in it. Also, it allows for the most efficient flow of services and in preventing the amputee from missing key elements of their rehabilitation program.

The poorest model, because of its inefficiencies and inconvenience to the patient, is to have the array of rehabilitation services provided each in a different setting. This requires that the amputee travel from one place to another and that the information be transferred from one setting to the other. This system of information transfer often results in a breakdown or delay in information between a variety of professional service providers and their offices.

WHAT TO ASSESS AT FOLLOW-UP

A number of factors should be routinely assessed at each follow-up visit.

Outcomes Measurements

It is desirable that the team develop an outcomes measurement instrument that is used for persons with an arm amputation. A variety of functional and emotional outcome measurement instruments have been used in the past, such as the Barthel Index and the Functional Independence Measure. However, it is probably best for the team to develop an instrument that most likely fits the issues of the amputees whom they serve. In addition, the outcomes to be measured should be individualized prior to the development of the rehabilitation plan for each amputee.

An initial assessment should evaluate the same outcome elements that will be assessed at the conclusion of the initial rehabilitation plan and also during sequential follow-up visits. This type of outcomes assessment can use a predetermined list of expected functional outcomes, as seen in Figures 28-1 and 28-2, that are set for each level of unilateral or bilateral arm amputation. In using this type of outcome form, it is important for the team to indicate whether the amputee has achieved the anticipated function. If the amputee has not achieved an expected functional element, the team should decide whether this is reasonably attainable and, if so, what treatment plan should be devised to achieve this idealized function. Another type of outcomes form can be seen in Figures 28-3 and 28-4, from an OT manual printed in the 1940s from the Institute for the Crippled and Disabled in New York City. This is a listing of common daily activities that a person normally performs. In this case, the use of the prosthesis as it was incorporated into bimanual activities was rated using these forms. This outcome measure differentiates the arm amputee's

INSTITUTE FOR THE CRIPPLED AND DISABLED
400 First Avenue, New York 10, N.Y.
Single Upper Extremity Amputation - Activities of Daily Living

Name			Age	Sex		Occupation
Type of Amputation			Type of Terminal Device			
Therapist			Date(s) of Test			

RATING GUIDE
0. Impossible
1. Accomplished with much strain or many awkward motions
2. Somewhat labored or few awkward motions
3. Smooth, minimal amount of delays and awkward motions

PERSONAL NEEDS:	0	1	2	3	GENERAL PROCEDURES:	0	1	2	3
Put on shirt					Use key in lock				
Fasten buttons; cuff and front					Open and close window				
Put on belt					Play cards & shuffle				
Put on glove					Wind a clock				
Put on coat					Assemble wall plug				
Lace and tie shoes					HOUSEKEEPING PROCEDURES:				
Tie a tie									
File finger nails					Wash dishes				
Polish finger nails					Dry dishes				
Set hair					Polish silverward				
Clean glasses					Peel vegetable				
Squeeze toothpaste					Cut vegetable				
Put on a bra and fasten					Open a can				
Use zipper					Manipulate hot pots				
Hook garters					Sweeping				
Take bill from wallet					Use dust pan				
Light a match					Use vacuum cleaner				
Open pack of cigarettes					Use wet mop				
					Use dry mop				
EATING PROCEDURES:					Set up iron board				
Carry a tray					Iron				
Butter bread					Wash and wring out laundry				
Cut meat					Hang up and take down laundry				
					Thread needle				
DESK PRODCEDURES:					Sew a button				
Use dial telephone					USE OF TOOLS:				
Use phone and take notes									
Use pay phone					Layout				
Sharpen pencil					Saw				
Use ruler					Plane				
Use scissors					Sand				
Remove & repalce ink cap					Drive screws				
Fill fountain pen					Hammer				
Fold and seal letter					File				
Use card file					Drill				
Use paper clip					Power tools				
Use stapler					Gravel pit				
Wrap a package					CAR PROCEDURES:				
Type									
Write					Drive				
COMMENTS:					Change tire				
					Use jack				

FIGURE 28-3

INSTITUTE FOR THE CRIPPLED AND DISABLED
400 First Avenue, New York 10, N.Y.
Bilateral Upper Extremity Amputation - Activities of Daily Living

Name					Age	Sex		Occupation			
Type of Amputation					Type of Terminal Device						
Therapist					Date(s) of Test						

RATING GUIDE
0. Impossible
1. Accomplished with much strain or many awkward motions
2. Somewhat labored or few awkward motions
3. Smooth, minimal amount of delays and awkward motions

PERSONAL NEEDS:	0	1	2	3	EATING PROCEDURES:	0	1	2	3
Buttoning					Pulling chair from table				
Zippers					Use napkin				
Hooks					Pick up utensils				
Snaps					Drink from glass				
Lacing					Drink from cupEat with a spoon				
Tie shoe laces					Eat with a spoon				
Put on socks					Eat with fork				
Put on shoes					Cut meat				
Shorts					Eat soup				
Shirt					Eat sandwich				
Trousers					Eat potato chips				
Tuck shirt in trousers					Butter bread				
Tie necktie					Pass dishes				
Put on belt with buckle					Use salt shaker				
Blow nose					Drink from bottle				
Clean glasses					Pour liquid from pitcher				
Put on watch					Eat ice cream cone				
Wind watch									
Put on topcoat					DESK PROCEDURES				
Put on hat					Use dial telephone				
Put on overshoes					Use phone and take notes				
Use umbrella					Use pay phone				
Shave					Sharpen pencil				
Shower Lavatory procedures					Use eraser				
Lavatory procedures					Use ruler				
Brush and comb hair					Use scissors				
Set hair					Remove and replace ink cap				
Apply cosmetics					Fill fountain pen				
Squeezing toothpaste					Fold and place in envelope				
Brushing teeth					Open sealed letter				
Put on bra and fasten					Use card file				
Hook garters					Use paper clip				
Hook suspenders					Use stapler				
					Wrap package				
					Unwrap package				
					Turn pages				
					Type				
					Write				

FIGURE 28-4

ability to perform personal needs, eating, housekeeping, working at a desk, using tools, and driving. Figure 28-5 shows a form that evaluates the basic functional prosthetic skills as they are mastered in early training.

Another type of outcomes assessment has been developed at the Rehabilitation Institute of Chicago Outcomes Assessment Division. This form (Figure 28-6) is used to provide a quantification of selected prosthetic function, not all of the expected prosthetic function obtainable. Although many facilities will utilize a functional outcomes tool, an emotional outcomes tool should also be included during the follow-up visit. Another RIC-developed form measures the health-related quality of life (Figure 28-7). This is one of several quality of life scales that might be utilized to assess the emotional impact of the arm amputation, prosthetic restoration, and comprehensive rehabilitation.

The follow-up visit is ideal to assess the individual's function both with and without the prosthesis. The most efficient way to measure these gains is to develop a checklist or a visual analog scale that contains the essential outcome elements for a particular level of amputation. If the amputee has not achieved the expected functional elements, the team and the patient should first decide if this is a functional element that the patient desires to achieve. A second decision to be made is whether the level of amputation or the particular type of prosthesis will permit this specific function.

Outcomes measurement should also include the emotional adaptation to being an amputee or using the prosthesis. Several scales can be applied to assess the person's adjustment to their disability and change in body image, such as the SF-36 and the community integration questionnaire, which have been utilized in other rehabilitation outcome studies.

Interim Problems

The follow-up appointment is a good time to assess skin problems, sweating, pain, sleep pattern, appetite disturbances, or prosthetic problems.

Further Therapeutic Interventions

Probably the most frequently cited issues during a follow-up appointment is a problem with prosthetic comfort or mechanical use. Both of these complaints must be remedied immediately if the arm amputee is expected to continue to wear and use the unilateral prosthesis for function and cosmesis. A trip to the prosthetist's office should improve the prosthetic comfort. The types of pain present and the possible cause of pain should be identified. A specific pain treatment plan should be developed.

Emotional Counseling

The follow-up visit is also an important time to assess the amputee's emotional responses to the amputation and the prosthesis. The follow-up visit provides an important opportunity to assess the psychosocial adaptation to the amputation and the use of the prosthesis.

Improve Sleep Pattern

The sleep pattern of the amputee should be evaluated, and if there is any sign of a sleep disturbance, this should be treated so that the amputee gets at least 4 hours a night of uninterrupted sleep.

Amputee Education Regarding Prosthetic Rehabilitation

The follow-up appointment is also an ideal time to update the amputee's level of education regarding the latest developments in prosthetic design. This is also a good time to review the entire rehabilitation plan and reinforce the amputee's participation in this plan. On occasion, the amputee will "fall through the cracks" of the rehabilitation plan, and follow-up is an ideal opportunity to assess whether the plan is being followed in a smooth fashion. This is also a good opportunity to restate or reset the rehabilitation goals and to update or revise the entire treatment plan.

PROSTHETIC REPLACEMENT

Regular and periodic follow-up permits a regular assessment of the need for maintenance or component replacement. Once the initial shaping and shrinking have occurred, and the person is wearing a definitive prosthesis, most professionals suggest that the entire prosthesis be replaced every 3 to 5 years, depending on the frequency of use. More frequent socket changes may be necessary, but most other components should last for at least 3 to 5 years. When it is time to develop a new prescription, newly developed arm components that might be useful for the individual should be introduced and discussed.

Persons with bilateral arm amputations should always have a second set of arm prostheses for back-up should the first pair need repair that requires time away from the amputee in the prosthetic laboratory. Often, this back-up pair are a refurbished earlier pair of prostheses from earlier fittings. However, every bilateral arm amputee should have two sets of prostheses from the early days of fitting and training, because they are so dependent on a fully functional set of working prosthetic arms. The second set of arms may contain slightly differing components from the current set of prostheses, but

INSTITUTE FOR THE CRIPPLED AND DISABLED
400 First Avenue, New York 10, N.Y.
Upper Extremity Amputation - Evaluation

Name		Age	Sex	Occupation
Type of Amputation		Type of Terminal Device		
Therapist		Date(s) of Test		

RATING GUIDE
0. Impossible
1. Accomplished with much strain or many awkward motions
2. Somewhat labored or few awkward motions
3. Smooth, minimal amount of delays and awkward motions

BASIC PERFORMANCE

	0	1	2	3		0	1	2	3
Put on stump socks					Take off prothesis				
Put on prosthesis					Adjust Cineplasty pin				

BASIC MOTIONS OF OPERTATION DRILL

	0	1	2	3		0	1	2	3
Lock Elbow at 90°					Close Terminal Device				
Open Terminal Device					Unlock Elbow (Flex Forearm to mouth)				
Close Terminal Device					Lock Elbow at mouth				
Unlock Elbow (Lower forearm to extension					Open Terminal Device				
Lock Elbow in Extension					Close Terminal Device				
Open Terminal Device					Unlock Elbow (return to 90°)				

TERMINAL DEVICE DRILL

	0	1	2	3		0	1	2	3
Pick up wooden blocks					Pick up ice cream cone				
Pick up sponge blocks					Other				

TRAINING BOARD ITEMS

	0	1	2	3		0	1	2	3
Hammer and nail					Paper cup dispenser				
Padlock and key					Water faucet (round handle)				
Screen door latch					Water faucet (T-bar)				
Fountain pen					Window latch & lift				
Door chain latch					Pencil sharpener (table)				
Trunk lock (small)					Drawer pull (wood knob)				
Trunk lock (large)					Drawer pull (metal bar)				
Pencil sharpener (wall)					Drawer pull (cup handle)				
Jar and lid					Door pull (metal knob)				
Light switch (bracket type)					Door pull (spring latch)				
Light switch (toggle)					Door bolt				
Light switch (push button)					Wall bottle opener				
Light switch (rotary)					Hand bottle opener				
Electric wall plug (horizontal)					Pick up coins from table				
Electric wall plug (vertical)									

FIGURE 28-5

☐ Admission ☐ Discharge	☐ 6 month Follow-up ☐ 1 year Follow-up ☐ 2 year Follow-up	TODAY'S DATE MM DD YY / /	PATIENT ID NUMBER

UPPER EXTREMITY FUNCTIONAL STATUS

I. Please indicate your affected limb(s).

  ☐☐ Left arm ☐ Right arm ☐☐ Both arms

II. How many hours per day do currently wear a prosthesis or orthosis?

   _____ hours/per day

II. Using the scale to the right, please indicate how easily you perform the following activities.

1. Very easy
2. Easy
3. Slightly difficult
4. Very difficult
5. Cannot perform activity
NA Not applicable

IV. Do you usually perform this activity using or not using a prosthesis or orthosis?

		1	2	3	4	5	NA	Using	Not Using
1.	Wash face	☐	☐	☐	☐	☐	☐	☐	☐
2.	Put toothpaste on brush and brush teeth	☐	☐	☐	☐	☐	☐	☐	☐
3.	Brush/comb hair	☐	☐	☐	☐	☐	☐	☐	☐
4.	Put on and remove T-shirt	☐	☐	☐	☐	☐	☐	☐	☐
5.	Button shirt with front buttons	☐	☐	☐	☐	☐	☐	☐	☐
6.	Attach end of zipper and zip jacket	☐	☐	☐	☐	☐	☐	☐	☐
7.	Put on socks	☐	☐	☐	☐	☐	☐	☐	☐
8.	Tie shoe laces	☐	☐	☐	☐	☐	☐	☐	☐
9.	Full body bathing	☐	☐	☐	☐	☐	☐	☐	☐
10.	Prepare a light meal	☐	☐	☐	☐	☐	☐	☐	☐
11.	Drink from a paper cup	☐	☐	☐	☐	☐	☐	☐	☐
12.	Toileting	☐	☐	☐	☐	☐	☐	☐	☐
13.	Vacuuming floors	☐	☐	☐	☐	☐	☐	☐	☐
14.	Use fork or spoon	☐	☐	☐	☐	☐	☐	☐	☐
15.	Cut meat with knife and fork	☐	☐	☐	☐	☐	☐	☐	☐
16.	Pour from a 12 oz. can	☐	☐	☐	☐	☐	☐	☐	☐
17.	Write name legibly	☐	☐	☐	☐	☐	☐	☐	☐
18.	Use scissors	☐	☐	☐	☐	☐	☐	☐	☐
19.	Open door with knob	☐	☐	☐	☐	☐	☐	☐	☐
20.	Use a key in a lock	☐	☐	☐	☐	☐	☐	☐	☐
21.	Carry laundry basket	☐	☐	☐	☐	☐	☐	☐	☐
22.	Dial a touch tone phone	☐	☐	☐	☐	☐	☐	☐	☐
23.	Use a hammer and nail	☐	☐	☐	☐	☐	☐	☐	☐
24.	Fold a bath towel	☐	☐	☐	☐	☐	☐	☐	☐
25.	Open an envelope	☐	☐	☐	☐	☐	☐	☐	☐
26.	Stir in a bowl	☐	☐	☐	☐	☐	☐	☐	☐
27.	Drive a car	☐	☐	☐	☐	☐	☐	☐	☐
28.	Put on and take of prosthesis or orthosis	☐	☐	☐	☐	☐	☐	☐	☐

FIGURE 28-6

☐ Admission ☐ Discharge	☐ 6 month Follow-up ☐ 1 year Follow-up ☐ 2 year Follow-up	TODAY'S DATE MM DD YY / /	PATIENT ID NUMBER

HEALTH RELATED QUALITY OF LIFE

I. Please check the box in the column indicating your best response to the question.

Note: The term "physical condition" refers to the reason you use a prosthesis or orthosis.

	Not At All 1	Slightly 2	Somewhat 3	Quite a bit 4	Extremely 5
1. How much do you keep to yourself to avoid the reactions of others to your use of a prosthesis or orthosis?	☐☐	☐☐	☐☐	☐☐	☐☐
2. To what extent are you insulted by the attitudes of other people towards your physical condition?	☐☐	☐☐	☐☐	☐☐	☐☐
3. To what extent are you prevented from doing what you would like to do because of social attitudes, the law, or environmental barriers?	☐☐	☐☐	☐☐	☐☐	☐☐
4. How much does pain interfere with your activities (including both work outside the home and household duties)?	☐☐	☐☐	☐☐	☐☐	☐☐
5. To what extent do you accomplish less than you would like because of your physical condition?	☐☐	☐☐	☐☐	☐☐	☐☐
6. To what extent do you accomplish less than you would like because of emotional problems?	☐☐	☐☐	☐☐	☐☐	☐☐
7. How much does your physical condition restrict your ability to run errands?	☐☐	☐☐	☐☐	☐☐	☐☐
8. How much does your physical condition restrict your ability to pursue a hobby?	☐☐	☐☐	☐☐	☐☐	☐☐
9. How much does your physical condition restrict your ability to do chores?	☐☐	☐☐	☐☐	☐☐	☐☐
10. How much does your physical condition restrict your ability to do paid work?	☐☐	☐☐	☐☐	☐☐	☐☐
11. To what extent have you cut down on work or other activities because of your physical condition?	☐☐	☐☐	☐☐	☐☐	☐☐
12. To what extent have you cut down on work or other activities because of emotional problems?	☐☐	☐☐	☐☐	☐☐	☐☐

FIGURE 28-7

Please turn page over ↘

How often <u>during the past week</u>...	All of the Time 1	Most of the Time 2	Some of the Time 3	A Little of the Time 4	None of the Time 5
13. did you feel full of life?	☐☐	☐☐	☐☐	☐☐	☐☐
14. have you felt calm and peaceful?	☐☐	☐☐	☐☐	☐☐	☐☐
15. did you have a lot of energy?	☐☐	☐☐	☐☐	☐☐	☐☐
16. have you been happy?	☐☐	☐☐	☐☐	☐☐	☐☐

How often <u>during the past week</u>...	All of the Time 1	Most of the Time 2	Some of the Time 3	A Little of the Time 4	None of the Time 5
17. have you been very nervous?	☐☐	☐☐	☐☐	☐☐	☐☐
18. have you felt so down in the dumps that nothing could cheer you up?	☐☐	☐☐	☐☐	☐☐	☐☐
19. have you felt downhearted and depressed?	☐☐	☐☐	☐☐	☐☐	☐☐
20. did you feel worn out?	☐☐	☐☐	☐☐	☐☐	☐☐
21. did you feel tired?	☐☐	☐☐	☐☐	☐☐	☐☐
22. were you easily bothered or upset?	☐☐	☐☐	☐☐	☐☐	☐☐
23. did you have difficulty concentrating or paying attention?	☐☐	☐☐	☐☐	☐☐	☐☐

II. Please answer the following questions about work or school.

1. I am employed	☐ Full time	☐ Part time	☐ Not employed
2. I am attending school	☐ Full time	☐ Part time	☐ Not employed
3. I am currently receiving care from a... Doctor	☐ Yes	☐	☐ No
Physical therapist	☐ Yes		☐ No
Occupational therapist	☐ Yes		☐ No

FIGURE 28-7 (CONTINUED)

the key factor is that the back-up set be fully operational, achieve meaningful function, and fit comfortably.

RETURN TO VOCATIONAL AND AVOCATIONAL PURSUITS

Follow-up visits also permit an opportunity to discuss whether the arm amputee has returned to work. This discussion provides a chance to determine if it is time for the amputee to return to work, if they can return to the same work, whether they need worksite modification, or should be referred for vocational rehabilitation.

As a part of the return to work, the prior job title, work requirements, and work environment should be ascertained. It is also important to determine if the amputee would prefer to return to their previous employer, the same job, an alternate job, or pursue some further training or education.

LIFELONG FOLLOW-UP

As a team member, lifelong follow-up should be an expectation of the amputee. Although the amputee is normally a healthy individual and should feel free from systems of healthcare, he should feel invested with the team of professionals. In this manner, he can call on other team members to discuss any problems that develop and whenever he needs prosthetic replacement. This does not imply that the amputee is dependent on the team, but confers that the amputee is truly the most critical member of the team. The amputee should expect the team to provide current information regarding the latest prosthetic components and rehabilitation practices. This ongoing dialog provides a model of cooperation and cross communication that empowers the amputee to achieve at the highest level and lead an active, fulfilling lifestyle.

References

1. Meier RH. Upper limb prosthetics: Design, prescription, and application. In: Peimer C (ed.), *Surgery of the Hand and Upper Extremity*. New York: McGraw-Hill, 1996; 2453–2468.
2. Institute for Crippled and Disabled. Resource: RIC Outcomes, Allan Herriemann, PhD.

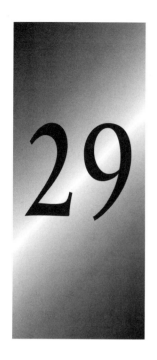

29 Return to Work Issues for the Upper Extremity Amputee

Roger Weed, PhD, CLCP, CRV and Diane J. Atkins, OTR

Upper extremity amputation has been a consequence of living since the beginning of time. Historically, the effects of war were a primary cause, and certainly some of the earlier references include pictures and accounts of primitive prosthesis design following injury sustained during wartime. One example from the American Civil War is an upper extremity prosthesis that included eating utensils. The term amputation, however, encompasses limb loss caused by trauma (e.g., burns, accidental dismemberment, electrical injury, explosion-related, etc.), disease (e.g., diabetes, cancer, cellulitis, and infection), elective surgery (due to pain such as chronic regional pain syndrome), and congenital deformities (e.g., genetic, the effect of certain medication or drugs during pregnancy). In other countries, an amputation also may be punishment for criminal behavior. However, the most common cause of amputation is related to disease and the effects the aging. This chapter, which focuses on vocational or return to work issues, is intended to include information primarily on the working age population and people with upper extremity amputations, and therefore will be limited in scope. The data is obtained from three sources: the return to work rates for persons with amputation (1), and the author's unpublished data, which was presented at the International Society for Prosthetics and

Orthotics in Amsterdam, the Netherlands, June 29, 1998 and a 2001 Netherlands Study (35).

With regard to work, according to general research, people with disabilities commonly experience a loss of, or have more difficulty in finding employment. Census research and polls conducted by the Harris Group consistently reveal that about two-thirds of people with disabilities who are of working age and report a desire to work are unable to locate employment (2,3). Of the remaining third, a little more than half are working full-time. As consultants with regard to amputation cases, the authors endeavored to locate research information about factors relating to successful return-to-work rates for people with amputation to compare these outcomes to those of people with disabilities in general. Only a few case histories and limited findings from foreign countries were identified, and they were not comprehensive statistical research projects (4,5). In response to the paucity of data at the time of the original study, the authors launched two research projects specific to amputation, and the results are reported later in this chapter.

In an effort to focus research attention on the elements associated with predicting outcome, the literature was reviewed for information that has been associated with disabilities other than amputation. Overall, several factors appear to be significant in the support of successful vocational outcome, including early referral to rehabilitation (6). In general, the higher the level of education, the better the vocational outlook. Pre-injury employment experience has been shown to be correlated with return-to-work rates in many disability classifications. Persons who were unemployed at the time of injury were less likely to be employed following injury (2, 7–11). Likewise, depending on the disability involved, more subjective factors such as employer attitudes, quality of rehabilitation, and family support, can influence rehabilitation outcome, particularly in the resumption of employment (12–15). Employers frequently have unexpressed bias toward the prospective employee with a disability (13,15). One study in workers' compensation cases revealed that 99 percent of employers would prefer not to hire workers who had a history of injury, even if there were no limitations (16). Other studies note that family support can distinctly improve outcome (12). Research centers of excellence, often partially funded by grants, presumably offer a higher quality of services and more focused rehabilitation efforts that help clients achieve higher level of independent functioning (14).

DEFINITIONS

Prior to conducting an evaluation of vocational potential, definitions specific to the industry are necessary. The definitions offered below are generally accepted, but the reader should be aware that these could vary depending on the industry. For example, *disability* in Social Security Disability Insurance (SSDI) claims specifically references the inability to perform substantial gainful activity (i.e., work). Disability for workers' compensation cases may be defined according to state law, which includes terms such as *temporary partial, temporary total, permanent partial*, and *permanent and total*. Temporary means that the injured employee is expected to improve or recover, or has not reached maximum medical improvement (MMI) (e.g., a broken arm). A person with a permanent disability is one who is not expected to regain full functioning (e.g., amputation of arm). Partial is generally understood to mean that a worker has a medical condition that interferes with working but does not prevent him or her from completing some work tasks; whereas a total disability indicates the employee cannot work at all. Disability can also be a condition that interferes with functioning from physical or mental causes (17). Many of the definitions listed below may vary depending on from which industry people with upper extremity amputations are receiving services.

- Occupational Handicap. Indicates that the client is unable to perform at a satisfactory level all of the essential requirements of an occupation.
- Employment Handicap. The difficulty a person with a disability may have in getting a suitable job because of discrimination (when there is no occupational handicap).
- Placement Handicap. Exists when the rehabilitation worker has difficulty in placing a client on a job because of the client's occupational handicap, employment handicap, or both.
- Employability. The client possesses the skills, abilities, and other worker traits necessary to perform a job; this commonly indicates that jobs exist, but there is no consideration for the number of jobs actually available in the local area nor the employment rate.
- Placeability. The ability to actually find employment; to determine placeability, the rehabilitation professional takes into account the employability factors listed above as well as the local economy and the intangible client factors such as personality and appearance. A rehabilitation plan (to include training, counseling, placement, etc.) may enhance the client's placeability expectation.
- Job Readiness. The preparation of physical, mental, emotional, and other vocational resources for entry into competitive employment; work readiness programs may include training to arrive at work on time, take breaks when appropriate, hygiene and dress, and cooperation with supervision/management.
- Work Tolerance. The ability to sustain a work effort for a prolonged period of time, to maintain a steady flow of production at an acceptable pace and level of quality, to handle work pressure, and to fulfill all of the above without acting in an unsatisfactory manner or quitting the job.
- Functional Limitation. Results when a disability interferes with or prevents a client's activity or ability to function (see Table 29-1).
- Skills. Learned or acquired tasks that can be observed and measured.
- Transferability of Work Skills. Work behaviors that are learned by doing (e.g., typing) and that may be usable in more than one occupation.
- Suitable Employment. Employment or self-employment that is reasonably attainable given the individual's age, education, previous occupation, and injury and that offers an opportunity to restore the individual as soon as practical and as nearly as possible to his average weekly earnings at the time of injury; in some states, particularly in workers' compensation claims, the only real factor considered is whether a person with a disability can physically perform a job. Suitable employment includes the client's interests, aptitudes, temperaments, and income potential.

TABLE 29-1
Functional Limitations: General

1. Mobility Limitation
   The function of getting from one location to another is limited.
2. Motility Limitation
   The inability to move an object or to do another task normally performed by using the musculoskeletal system.
3. Restricted Environment
   Bound to a place or status, or limited in activity, atmosphere, or progress.
4. Sensory Limitation
   The result of defect(s) in the transmission of information from the environment to the brain.
5. Communication Limitation
   A breakdown in the process by which information is exchanged between individuals through common symbols, signs, or behavior.
6. Pain Limitation
   When pain is continuing, unremitting, uncontrollable, and severe, it may constitute a severe functional limitation to normal living.
7. Debilitation or Exertional Limitation
   A condition in which the individual is in a weakened state for an extended time period.
8. Atypical Appearance
   Characteristics of an individual's physique and carriage that are inconsistent with what is considered acceptable by a culture.
9. Invisible Limitation
   Concealed or unapparent conditions that limit functions.
10. Substance Dependency
    Physical and/or psychological dependency.
11. Mental Limitation
    Developmentally delayed (MR) and learning disabilities.
12. Consciousness Limitation
    Unconsciousness and other defects in consciousness.
13. Uncertain Prognosis
    Involves the stress and ambiguity of those medical conditions that have an unpredictable course of termination.
14. Dysfunctional Behavior
    Emotional disorders with deviate behavior. Also behavior due to cultural disadvantages.

Source: Compiled and summarized by R. Weed from Wright, G. *Total Rehabilitation*. New York: Little Brown, 1980.

EVALUATION OF WORK CAPABILITY

In today's climate, vocational counselors serve as an instrumental member of the rehabilitation team. Vocational counselors coordinate assessments in an effort to measure a person's aptitude and achievement levels and transferable work skills. These assessments help determine the client's potential for future work activity, such as a sheltered workshop or supported employment or, in cases where work activity is not a realistic goal, to achieve their highest level of productivity or independent living. The essential premise underlying vocational rehabilitation is that involvement in work or some productive meaningful activity is the goal of a rehabilitation program (18). If return to work or productive activity is appropriate, then the steps to achieve that goal must be included in the rehabilitation plan (15).

Vocational counselors who work within the amputee arena generally are rehabilitation professionals with a minimum of a master's degree in rehabilitation counseling, hold one or more national certifications in the field of rehabilitation; and have extensive training and experience in the areas of evaluation and assessment, case management, transferable work skills, earnings capacity analysis, and job placement (15). Vocational counselors can be credentialed in a number of areas, most notably as Certified Rehabilitation Counselor (CRC) and Certified Vocational Evaluator (CVE).

Vocational counselors must be knowledgeable and stay within the accepted standards and guidelines of the particular jurisdiction for which they are preparing the rehabilitation care plan. For example, in the workers' compensation arena, the vocational counselor must work within the established definitions of disability and return to work hierarchy (15). This includes the "odd lot" doctrine that has been defined by case law as "any work that the client may be able to perform which would be of limited quantity, dependability, or quality, and for which there is no reasonably stable market for their labor activities" (19,20). In comparison, vocational counselors within the disability insurance arena, who must determine long-term versus short-term disability (LTD/STD), will be expected to provide information on the status of the client's "any/own occupation" as well as the client's vocational potential and the cost of future vocational and educational needs. Similarly, the vocational counselor within the personal injury arena will need to determine if the client has vocational potential, and to what degree. They will also need to provide information on the cost of the client's expected future vocational and educational needs in an effort to identify the vocational damages associated with the injury or disability (21).

Regardless of the specific jurisdiction, vocational counselors must be able to first determine if a client can work and, if so, what work can they perform. This determination includes providing information not only on the types of vocational activity a client can be expected to perform, but also the cost, frequency, and duration or replacement of any training or assistance (such as job coach, vocational counseling, rehabilitation technology, modified or custom-designed work station, supported employment, tuition and books, or other specialized education programs) that may be required to reach the goal (15). Depending on the severity of disability, the vocational counselor works with a variety of medical and allied health professionals in determining the client's vocational potential.

Professionals such as physicians and medical specialists, physical therapists, occupational therapists, speech/language pathologists, recreation therapists, nurses, psychologists, neuropsychologists, audiologists, counselors or other mental health professionals, and, in the case of school-age clients, school personnel, all work with the vocational counselor to provide information for a rehabilitation plan (21). Because upper extremity amputation can be a result of major trauma including electrical injury, secondary injuries may be serious. For instance, a neuropsychologist may be an important contributor to assessing cognitive and intellectual capacities in the client who has an amputation caused by electrical injury.

It is common for the vocational counselor to rely on the client's primary physician, typically a physiatrist or specialist in physical medicine and rehabilitation (PM&R), in determining a client's functional level and potential to perform vocational activity (22). In appropriate cases, the vocational counselor may request a Functional Capacity Evaluation (FCE), which may also be known as a Physical Capacity Evaluation or Functional Capacity Assessment, to objectively delineate a client's physical functioning. The FCE is expected to provide objective data regarding the client's ability to perform in various physical demand areas (i.e., lifting, standing, walking, sitting, pushing or pulling, etc.) and is usually conducted in a facility that specializes in occupational health information. The FCE provides a snapshot view of a client's abilities on one particular day (the evaluation may be conducted over 2 days) and, given the outcome of the testing, the client's work capacity from a physical standpoint is determined. It should be noted that FCEs can be controversial with regard to the "validity" of the results. However, when administered by a highly qualified professional, it is the authors' opinion that the FCE data are better than an "off the cuff" opinion by a physician. Additional factors that the vocational counselor must take into consideration in assessing a client's physical capacities is his ability to perform work activity over time (endurance), subjective complaints, test validity and reliability, and secondary gain issues (21). Potentially, part of the rehabilitation plan may include work conditioning to increase the client's strength, stamina, and endurance.

VOCATIONAL ASSESSMENT AND EVALUATION

The terms *vocational assessment* and *vocational evaluation* have been used in rehabilitation literature to generally describe the process of gathering data and determining a person's potential for work activity. Karl Botterbusch (23) defines vocational assessment as "more limited in scope" than vocational evaluation and cites the Vocational Evaluation and Work Adjustment Association (1983) definition of vocational evaluation that "incorporates medical, psychological, social, vocational, educational, cultural, and economic data." Siefker (24) noted that the two phrases "do not describe a significantly different process and can be considered synonymous." For purposes of this chapter, the phrases are used interchangeably to describe the comprehensive evaluation of a client's biographical and social history, education and work history, medical and other pertinent records (employment or personnel records, school records, parent's school records in pediatric cases, etc.), psychological/neuropsychological records, and actual vocational test results in determining vocational potential.

In compiling a rehabilitation plan, it is within the role of the vocational counselor to recommend and obtain a formal vocational assessment and evaluation, particularly in the following cases, in which the client (21):

- Is of working age (generally age 16 to 60),
- has no or unclear vocational goal,
- has no work history or a series of short sporadic jobs, or
- has not been determined permanently and totally disabled (i.e., is thought to have some vocational potential).

For clients who are catastrophically injured, it is important for the vocational evaluation to be as specific as possible and to take into account the client's personality traits, interests, aptitudes, and physical capabilities to adequately identify appropriate vocational options. In their book, *Counseling the Able Disabled,* Deneen and Hessellund (25) describe common reasons for vocational testing. Below is a modified version of their list:

- Provide information about a person's interests, mental and physical abilities, and temperament with respect to work
- Support, clarify, and document impressions gained during interviews
- Discover job interests and potential vocational objectives
- Objectively and accurately describe the client's likes, dislikes, needs, and abilities rather than rely solely on verbal interview information
- Observe and evaluate the client's physical stamina, endurance, agility, and ability as related to work performance
- Evaluate the degree that a particular impairment is a physical disability or handicap

Vocational assessments can vary depending on the particular jurisdiction in which the case is involved. For example, vocational evaluations performed for workers' compensation usually do not include personality testing in determining suitable employment. These evaluations generally focus on demonstrated interests, aptitudes, and physical capacities as well as the client's work history. It is the authors' opinion that vocational evaluations that do not consider personality should be closely scrutinized. Is there a reasonable explanation? Is it an oversight on the part of the evaluator? Is the evaluator not qualified to administer personality tests? Or, in this age of managed care, is there a deliberate attempt not to define personality traits that may have a negative effect on the client's vocational potential?

In developing a rehabilitation plan for a client with an upper extremity amputation, the vocational counselor must be able to translate the results from the vocational evaluation into the requirements for the Life Care Plan. Such requirements may include cost for training, transportation, tuition, specialized or adaptive equip-

ment, and maintenance and replacement schedules of needed equipment (24). For example, the authors were involved in identifying the costs associated with completing a master's degree and pursuing a Ph.D. for a person with triple amputation (both legs and dominant arm) who was a teacher at the time of his electrical injury. Not only were costs included in the Life Care Plan for education requirements, but also costs of transportation, prosthetic devices, maintenance and replacement, clothing allowance (due to increased wear and tear on garments as result of prosthetic use), and computer and other assistive technology needed to assist the client in attaining his vocational goal of education administrator. This case example also demonstrates that a client's ability to achieve a vocational goal is closely related to other Life Care Plan issues, such as ability to perform activities of daily living (ADLs), accessible housing and transportation, psychologic adjustment to disability, home or attendant care, wheelchair or mobility needs, and others.

In addition to having a comprehensive evaluation performed, the vocational counselor must be sensitive to how the specific tests are administered, for example: group versus individual; timed versus speeded versus untimed; paper and pencil versus computer administered versus work sample; short versus long form; normed versus non-normed; and objective versus subjective, to name a few (see Table 29-2) (21). In general, group tests are not as specific as individual tests (26,24), and speeded or timed tests are usually biased against catastrophically impaired persons. In clients who are motor and/or cognitively impaired (e.g., use prosthesis to answer questions on an answer sheet or carry out tasks), timed tests may reveal a lower score than is intellectually indicated, given that the score is based on speed rather than ability. Additionally, situational or job-specific tests that evaluate a person's ability for work activity in an actual work environment are more favorable and yield more accurate results than a work sample assessment in which job tasks are simulated. One author suggests that a client's vocational potential can be most effectively determined when the workplace is used as the primary site of all rehabilitation activity. They further indicate that no other location can be compared to the workplace for face validity and actual job activities (27).

Much has been written on the various vocational assessment tools given to persons with a disability (23,28). Table 29-3 is provided to give an overview of some of the more common or well-known tools used in the vocational assessment and evaluation of persons who are catastrophically impaired. The reader is referred to those publications referenced for a description of each test and information regarding its utility for specific populations of persons with a disability.

TABLE 29-2
Selected Issues Related to Vocational Assessment

Speeded, Timed, and Untimed Tests	Speeded and timed tests may be biased against physically impaired clients. Untimed tests may not reveal how competitive a client may be.
Individual vs. Group Tests	Generally, the group test is offered for economic reasons and is more general. Individually administered tests allow for examiner comment regarding effort and behavioral observation.
Short "Screening" vs. In-depth Testing	Vocational evaluators often use short tests for achievement, intelligence, aptitude, and interest screening. Tests such as the WRAT, Self-Directed Search, General Aptitude Test Battery (GATB), Slosson Intelligence Test, and others are not as precise as more detailed tests. Many evaluators are not qualified to administer more precise tests.
Tests vs. On-The-Job Evaluation	In order of general priority for best assessment: • on the job with an employer, • on the job based on general standard by professional evaluator, • work sample, • individually administered test, and • group test
Leaving Out Personality Factors	It is common in workers' compensation to leave out interest and personality factors when developing an opinion. Basic information with regard to interests, work values, and personality as it relates to work is recommended.

In conjunction with objective test results, the vocational counselor must take into consideration behavioral observations made during the client interview and test session. Behavioral observations are an integral part of the vocational assessment process and should always be interpreted with the actual test results and client's history (24). The qualified vocational evaluator is attuned to behavioral issues that may affect test results (i.e., pain behaviors, visual or hearing difficulties, need for medication or rest breaks, cultural issues or language barriers, and environmental issues, such as a room that is too hot or cold, or time of day). Likewise, the client's behavior may reveal areas of concern or discrepancy that may warrant further investigation (e.g., Was the client late for the testing session? What are the nonverbal behaviors? Is her appearance and grooming appropriate?). Behavior is a valid indication of how one will respond in certain situations, whether in a work environment or social/community setting (21).

In addition to behavioral observations, information about a client's abilities and skills obtained through educational and work experience may be more valid than test results (24). For this reason, a transferable skills analysis is an essential component to the vocational evaluation and to determine a client's vocational potential. Simply described, a transferable skills analysis gives a profile of the worker traits required of a specific occupation. It is used primarily for clients with a documented work history and takes into consideration the client's work experience and residual functional capaci-

ties to determine appropriate vocational options. The *Dictionary of Occupational Titles* (DOT) and *Classification of Jobs* (COJ) are necessary to compile a transferable skills analysis. (Note: Although the government's online system for occupational planning, the O*Net, is available, the data are not amenable to the transferability process.) See the "Vocational Resources" section later in this chapter for a description of these and other vocationally relevant publications.

When an individual experiences an electrical injury with resultant amputation, he also may have suffered a brain injury as well. Neuropsychologic testing helps determine how much and what kind of assistance is needed in the home, on the job, at school, and within the community. When referring for a neuropsychologic evaluation, it is prudent for the vocational counselor to know to whom she is making the referral and the credentials of the neuropsychologist. Experience has shown that the most qualified neuropsychologist not only has a Ph.D. in clinical psychology and is board certified as a neuropsychologist, but also has experience in evaluating persons across all levels of severity of brain injury and has demonstrated a common-sense approach to the evaluation and test interpretation (21).

Once a referral is made to a neuropsychologist, it is recommended that the vocational counselor provide specific questions to the neuropsychologist which, when answered, would provide information needed specifically for the Life Care Plan. The effects of brain trauma can be found in any or all aspects of one's life, including

---

TABLE 29-3
Vocational Assessment and Evaluation Tests

Intelligence:
- Wechsler Intelligence Scales (the standard of the industry)
- Stanford Binet Scales
- Slosson Intelligence Test (brief and very general)
- Raven Progressive Matrices (general reasoning ability)

Personality:
- Minnesota Multiphasic Personality Inventory (MMPI). Also in Spanish.
- 16 Personality Factors (16 PF)
- Myers-Briggs Type Indicator (MBTI)
- Personality Assessment Inventory (PAI)
- Rorschach Inkblot Test

Interest:
- Strong Campbell Interest Inventory
- Career Assessment Inventory (CAI)
- Self-Directed Search (SDS)
- Kuder Occupational Interest Inventory

Aptitude:
- Apticom (Based on the government's discontinued test, General Aptitude Test Battery)
- Armed Services Vocational Aptitude Battery (ASVAB)
- Differential Aptitude Tests (DAT)
- McCarron-Dial System
- Crawford Small Parts Dexterity
- Hester Evaluation System
- Jewish Employment Vocational Services Work Sample System (JEVS)
- Purdue Pegboard

Achievement:
- Wide Range Achievement Test (WRAT)
- Woodcock-Johnson Psychoeducational Battery
- Peabody Individual Achievement Test
- Basic Occupational Literacy Test (BOLT)

Work Sample:
- VALPAR
- TOWER

Assessment of Physical Functioning:
- Vineland Social Maturity Scale
- PULSES (Physical condition, upper limb, lower limb, sensory, excretory, support factors)
- Barthel Inventory of Self-Care Skills

*For additional information, the reader is referred to Chapter 4, in R. Weed (ed.), *Life Care Planning and Case Management Handbook, Second edition,* 2004.

---

interpersonal, vocational, educational, recreational, and ADL. It is the role of the neuropsychologist to evaluate the long-term or life-long effects of brain injury on the client's ability to function (6,15)

LABOR MARKET SURVEYS AND JOB ANALYSIS

Part of the assessment for earnings and work potential may be related to the current labor market. Obviously, a pediatric case would not include a specific employer-by-employer analysis; however, data collected by the government with regard to the future outlook of an occupation may be included. The labor market survey is designed to reveal current information about a specific job market. Questions include:

- Do jobs of a particular nature exist in the economy?
- If these jobs exist, are they available locally?
- If available locally, are these jobs open to the client?
- What do these jobs pay (including benefits)?

Once a prospective job is located, it is appropriate to conduct a job analysis. The analysis is designed to determine if job traits match the worker's traits and therefore represent a reasonable probability of successful employment. The consultant must follow specific guidelines to make sure that they are conducting the analysis according to published standards (29). Indeed, one successful malpractice lawsuit resulted when a nurse completed a "job analysis" that consisted of less than one page, and the topics covered in the analysis did not follow published standards. In fact, it appeared as if the nurse was unaware that the government and others have published standards on this topic.

For readers who may not be a vocational expert, several excellent resources are available related to performing job analyses (15,29,30).

VOCATIONAL RESOURCES

The vocational counselor has many resources available to assist in assessing a client's vocational potential and in making appropriate recommendations. A partial list of the more valuable reference materials used by the vocational counselor includes:

- *Dictionary of Occupational Titles* (DOT), 4th ed. (1991). Contains definitions of 12,741 job titles and descriptions of jobs found in the national economy. Data compiled by the U.S. Department of Labor (31). Now available in revised format on CD-ROM (32). (Also refer to the O*Net on the Internet located at http://www.doleta.gov/programs/onet/.)
- *Classification of Jobs, 2000* (COJ) (1999) (32). Contains worker trait profiles for each of the DOT job titles. The worker traits are assigned a code and rated.
- *The Enhanced Guide for Occupational Exploration (GOE)* (1991) (33). Provides descriptions of all jobs

organized within related job clusters and includes information pertaining to academic and physical requirements, work environment, salary and outlook, typical duties, skills and abilities required, and where to obtain additional information.

- *The Revised Handbook for Analyzing Jobs (RHAJ)* (1991). Gives descriptions on how to examine individual jobs to determine their suitability for a client.
- *Occupational Outlook Handbook (OOH)* (2003) (34). Clusters jobs by occupation and gives information with regard to employment potential, labor market trends, salary, requirements, and training needed to enter the occupation. This is now available online at http://stats.bls.gov/ocohome.htm.

RETURN TO WORK RESEARCH FOR AMPUTEES: STUDY 1

The first study cited in this chapter was originally published in the *Journal of Rehabilitation Outcomes* and was not restricted to people with upper extremity amputation (1). Data were gathered from two nationally recognized rehabilitation centers in the United States, one in Texas, the other in Colorado. The information collected included date of birth, date of injury or amputation, sex, description of amputation, reason for amputation, preamputation employment status (employed full time, employed part-time, or not employed) and occupation, postamputation employment status and occupation, education, and financial source for medical coverage. Because initial demographic data by the treatment programs had not been collected for research purposes, inappropriate or missing data deflated the original subject pool, thus necessitating adjustments in population parameters.

The participants were 117 amputees who had received treatment at one of the two rehabilitation centers of excellence. Among the amputees in the study (before some were eliminated because they did not meet criteria for inclusion), 17 were female (14.5%) and 100 were male (85.5%). The average age at the time of amputation for the participants was 29 years (ranging from 22 to 65 year of age). The mean age at injury or amputation was 29.6, with a range of 8 to 63 years.

With regard to education, 37.3% of amputees reported having less than a high school education and 15.3% reported having completed a high school education. Twenty-two percent of the participants had some college education, and 25.4% indicated having obtained a college degree. Based on the data collected, medical care for 52.6% of the individuals in the sample was covered by workers' compensation, and 47.4% had a coverage source other than workers' compensation. With reference to reported employment, 80.2% of people with amputation were employed pre-injury and 54.5% were employed post-injury. Regarding unemployment for people with amputation, 19.8% of the participants were not employed preinjury and 45.5% were not employed post-injury. In addition, the researchers collected information regarding source of injury and divided it into two categories, trauma and disease (see Table 29-4). As a result, the data revealed that 81.9% reported trauma as the source of injury and 18.1% attributed disease as the cause.

Due to the research focus of amputee employability, only subjects who met the age criteria of greater than or equal to 18 years of age and less than 62 years of age were included for the purpose of analysis. The selection process resulted in 92 subjects. In addition, participant level of education was collapsed into two categories, Level I and Level II, to provide a more meaningful comparison due to the small sample size represented within each original classification. Those individuals who reported having a high school diploma or less constituted Level I education. Level II education included participants who indicated attending some college or obtaining a college degree. The researchers then proceeded to create the variable employment classes, representing four categories of people with amputation employment: 1 = neither employed pre-injury nor post-injury, 2 = employment pre-injury, but not post-injury, 3

TABLE 29-4
Reasons for Primary Amputation

REASON	PERCENT*
Electrical Injury	53.3
Railroad	1.1
Burns	1.1
Cancer	3.3
Trauma (machines)	3.3
Conveyor Belt	1.1
Diabetes	3.3
Surgical	1.1
Cellulitis	1.1
Industrial	6.5
Garbage Truck	1.1
MVA	15.2
Explosion	1.1
Infection	1.1
Vasculitis	2.2
Airplane	3.3
Missing	0.8

* Percent of Selected Sample (n=92)

= employment post-injury, but not pre-injury, and 4 = employed both pre-injury and post-injury.

Among the 92 amputees with complete information, 11 were women (12.0%) and 81 were men (88.0%). The average age for the participants was 32 years of age, with a range of 18 to 61 years of age. With regard to education, 15 of the valid cases were designated as Level I education (36.6%), representing participants with a high school diploma or less, and 26 of the valid cases were included as Level II education (63.4%), representing participants with some college or a college degree. Of the selected sample, medical care for 58 amputees was covered by workers' compensation (63.7%), and 33 participants had a coverage source other than workers' compensation (36.3%). Regarding the employment of the selected participants, 4 (4.3%) amputees indicated employment neither pre-injury nor post-injury. Twenty-four (26.1%) participants reported employment pre-injury, but not post-injury. One (1.1%) person with amputation was found to be employed post-injury, but not pre-injury. Forty-six (50.0%) of the selected participants were employed both pre-injury and post-injury, and the employment status of 17 (18.5%) was unknown (Table 29-5).

The results reveal that too many variables existed to measure in a research study of this size to be as precise as the authors desired. The number and location of amputation can take multiple forms, and sample sizes were too small to obtain statistical significance on anything other than general topics.

The researchers identified significant patterns of association in reference to employment for people with amputation across the categories of education level, source of coverage, source of injury, gender, and pre-injury employment (p<.05). Twenty-three percent (23.1%) of all amputees with Level I education (high school diploma or less) were employed both pre-injury

and post-injury. In comparison, 70.8% of all amputees with Level II education (some college or college degree) reported being employed both pre-injury and post-injury (Table 29-6). Thus, the percentage of amputees employed both pre-injury and post-injury across the category of education were accounted for by 15.8% of amputees having a Level I education and 84.2% having a Level II education, as reported in this study (p<.05).

The researchers found that 61.2% of all amputees having workers' compensation were employed both pre-injury and post-injury. In contrast, of those having a coverage source other than workers' compensation, 60.0% reported being employed both pre-injury and post-injury. However, in terms of all amputees employed both pre-injury and post-injury, 66.7% had workers' compensation and 33.3% relied on a coverage source other than workers' compensation (p<.05).

Although a small sample size, 55.6% of amputees listing disease as their source of injury were employed both pre-injury and post-injury. Similarly, of those who reported trauma as their source of injury, 62.1% were employed both pre-injury and post-injury. In terms of all amputees in this study employed both pre-injury and post-injury, however, the researchers found 10.9% of these reported disease as their source of injury, in contrast to 89.1% who reported trauma as their source of injury (p<.05). Nevertheless, when solely considering post-injury employment in terms of injury source, no significant pattern of difference appears between disease and trauma.

Also, when considering employment for people with amputation across the category of gender, the reader must take note of the small number of women included in this study, compared to the number of men. With this limitation in mind, the researchers found 66.2% of men with amputation were employed both pre-injury and post-injury. In contrast, 30.0% of the women with amputation reported being employed both pre-injury and post-injury. When comparing all amputees in this study employed both pre-injury and post-injury, 93.5% were men and 6.5% were women (p<.05).

Last, the researchers found a significant pattern of association in reference to post-injury employment in

TABLE 29-5 *Amputation Employment Status*		
EMPLOYMENT STATUS	**COUNT***	**PERCENT***
Employed Pre-injury Only	24	26.1
Employed Post-injury Only	1	1.1
Employed Both Pre- and Post-injury	46	50.0
Neither Employed Pre- nor Post-injury	4	4.3
Unknown Employment Status	17	18.5
* Count and Percent of Selected Sample (n=92)		

TABLE 29-6 *Post Injury Employment Probability by Education for Amputees*	
PERCENT EMPLOYED POST-INJURY	
High school or less	Some college or college degree
23.1%	70.8%

terms of pre-injury employment. Of all the valid cases of amputees in the study, 61.3% were employed both pre-injury and post-injury, 32.0% were employed pre-injury but not post-injury, 5.3% were employed post-injury but not pre-injury, and 1.3% were neither employed pre-injury nor post-injury (p<.05). The latter two categories may be related to the age of the person. Because this study included people from the age of 18, some may not have been in the work force at the time of the injury, but did eventually become employed after treatment. A logistic regression was also conducted to identify possible predictors of post-injury employment for amputees. The researchers considered the following variables: pre-injury employment, education level, gender, and source of injury, using a forward stepwise conditional model selection. As a result, education level was identified as the only statistically significant predictor of post-injury employment, according for 16% of the variance (p=.0087).

RETURN TO WORK RESEARCH FOR AMPUTEES: STUDY 2

The second study uses unpublished data that was presented at the 1998 International Society of Prosthetics and Orthotics (ISPO) conference in Amsterdam, the Netherlands. The initial survey was sent to more than 6,600 children and adults with upper extremity limb loss. Of those, 2,239 individuals responded. After eliminating children and multiple amputations, 836 unilateral upper limb amputees were included in the study, having an average age of 46.8 years. Twenty-one percent were women and 79% were men, with the most common reason for amputation listed as farming accident followed by diabetes, burns, motor vehicle accident, industrial accident, meningiococemia, military-related, gunshot wounds, and cancer. Other trauma and other disease comprised 13.5% of the sample (see Table 29-7).

Level of amputation was most likely to be below-elbow, followed by wrist disarticulation, above-elbow, shoulder disarticulation, forequarter, partial hand, and elbow disarticulation (see Table 29-8).

With regard to type of prosthesis used, 74% used body-powered. Of those who wore a prosthesis, women were more likely to use an electric-powered version (35% electric versus 65% body) than men (23% electric versus 77% body), presumably for cosmetic purposes. No data was included to reveal people who had both electric and body-powered prosthesis.

Of interest, the amount of time an individual wore a prosthesis was significantly associated with a return to work. In addition, the amount of income was also positively correlated with the amount of time a person wore a prosthesis. As might be expected, the higher the income available to the individual, the more likely it was that they would return to work (4 to 8 times more likely). Pre-incident, 76% were employed (with some subjects either in school or too young to work at the time of injury). At the time of the study, 58.4% of upper extremity amputees were employed, with 42% earning less than $25,000, 26% earning $25,000 to 50,000, 16.6% earning $50,000 to 100,000, and 5.4% more than $100,000. No significant gender difference was noted in the rate of return to work. Of the sample, only 9.9% completed high school and 1.7% completed college. However, following amputation, there was a shift from "blue collar" to "white collar" work (e.g., carpenter and lineman to engineer or teacher). For example, pre-incident 18% were employed in professional technical occupations and post-incident, 49% were.

Of those who were unemployed, the reasons offered were early retirement (48%), in school (12%), unable to return to work (8%), pain (6%), income from settlement (3%), no need or desire to work (3%), additional expected surgeries (2%), and other (19%). Finally, as expected based on disability research, for each 10 years older a person becomes, they are 45% less likely to return to work.

TABLE 29-7 Causes of Unilateral Upper Extremity Amputation Study 2	
CAUSE	PERCENT OF SAMPLE
Farm accident	25.4
Diabetes	14.5
Motor vehicle	12.9
Other trauma	12.3
Industrial injury	8.7
Meningiococemia	5.4
Military	2.3
Gunshot wound	2.9
Other	1.2
Cancer	0.6

TABLE 29-8 Level of Amputation, Study 2	
LEVEL	PERCENT OF SAMPLE
Below-elbow	41.4
Wrist disarticulation	20.5
Above-elbow	19.8
Shoulder disarticulation	8.6
Forequarter	3.9
Partial hand	3.0
Elbow disarticulation	2.8

ADDITIONAL FOREIGN STUDY

In 2001, a study conducted in the Netherlands using a sample of 652 people with lower limb amputation revealed that 64% of the population was working at the time of the study, 31% had work experience but were not working, and 5% had no work experience. Consistent with studies in the United States, people who worked found employment in less physically demanding jobs. Of those who quit working within 2 years of the amputation, 78% reported that amputation-related factors played a role in their decision. They also commonly reported problems with obtaining work place modifications (35).

ADAPTATIONS, ACCOMMODATIONS, AND WORKSITE EVALUATION

A person with amputation will likely require some sort of adaptation for work and daily living. In most cases, the accommodation will be made through the use of various prostheses. Work-related concerns may include avoiding extreme weather or wet working conditions for a myoelectric arm and avoiding dusty, dirty, or gritty work environments for which myoelectric and certain body-powered prostheses are not designed. The job analysis should identify those problems associated with completing the "essential functions" of a job. Indeed, the Americans with Disabilities Act (ADA), PL 101-336, 1990 (36), requires *reasonable accommodation* for the person with a disability who is otherwise qualified to do the essential functions.

According to the ADA Technical Assistance Manual (37), consideration for essential functions of the job include whether:

1. the position exists to perform the function;
2. there are a limited number of other employees available to perform the function or among whom the function can be distributed; and
3. the function is highly specialized, and the person in the position is hired for special expertise or ability to perform it.

Clearly, the amount of time that one performs various tasks within the job could be considered good evidence for essential functions of the job. However, there are also occasions where an employee might perform a task only once per month (such as monthly payroll), which cannot be transferred to another individual. This could be considered an essential function of the job even though it is rarely performed.

Certainly, many individuals with disabilities can perform essential functions of the job without modification or accommodation. *Reasonable accommodation* is intended to include equal opportunity when applying for a job and to assist qualified individuals with a disability to perform essential functions of the job. A simple example is that an individual using a wheelchair should have access to apply for the employment opportunity via an accessible personnel office. In addition, the employee with a disability should also enjoy equal the benefits and privileges of employment when compared to people without disabilities.

Accommodations are considered "reasonable," in part, when they are effective. The guidelines do not require the employer to provide the "best" or most expensive option but only one which will effectively work (37). In addition, the employer is only obligated to provide reasonable accommodation when there are *known* limitations. Therefore, it becomes the responsibility of the applicant to make these issues known to the employer. If, as on some occasions, it is unknown what accommodation can be made or if it is otherwise necessary, specific documentation can be required from rehabilitation professionals, physicians, and others to verify the necessity for the accommodations. What is "reasonable" for each person is specifically assessed on a case-by-case basis and determined initially by the employer. For example, large employers may more easily be able to provide a barrier-free work site, and smaller employers might redistribute work tasks to overcome the same physical impairment (38).

Some common adaptations for upper extremity amputation are:

- Job task reassignments
- Rearrange work area for physical efficiency
- Book elevators, file carousels, or lazy Susan devices
- Clamps, jigs, clips, or other stabilizing devices
- Arm supports for wrists and hands
- Powered hand tools
- Voice-activated or voice recognition systems, including environmental controls
- Hands-free telephone adaptations
- Automated office equipment such as electric staplers, pencil sharpeners, envelope openers, manual or electronic Rolodex
- Able Office™, custom-configured work station
- Enlarged keyboards, keyguards, one-handed and alternate keyboards (see Figure 29-1)

In addition, the vocational counselor may need to problem-solve unique situations. For example, a roofer who lost his dominant arm below the elbow from an encounter with a power line had a custom-fabricated prosthesis with the roofing hammer built in (Figure 29-2).

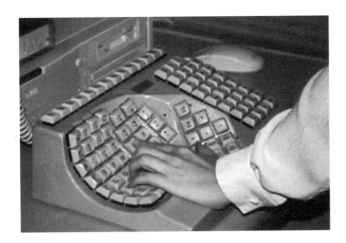

FIGURE 29-1

One hand low impact computer keyboard.

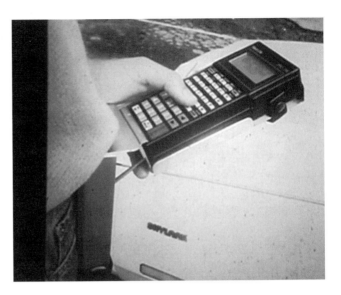

FIGURE 29-3

Calculator with belt support.

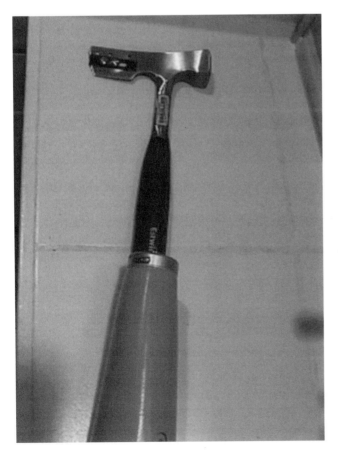

FIGURE 29-2

Roofing hammer built into prosthesis.

Another example is the automobile damage assessor who lost his nondominant arm and was able to return to work by having a custom belt-supported shelf built to hold his calculator (Figure 29-3).

For people who work with their hands, tools can become a terminal device (TD). Although they previously were available only when custom made, these TDs are now commercially produced (Figure 29-4).

In summary, accommodation and adaptations can be very helpful with regard to work for upper extremity

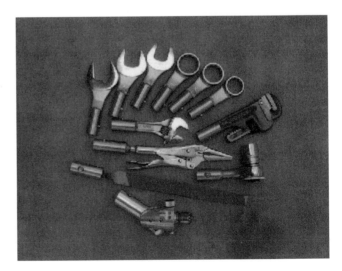

FIGURE 29-4

Texas Assistive Devices produces tools available as terminal devices.

amputees. Worksite ergonomic considerations may well overcome the client's limitations. However, most of the products commercially available are designed for recreation and daily living problems, not for work. The vocational counselor will need to develop his or her own resources with regard to rehabilitation technology in the workplace. Suggested resources are listed at the end of this chapter.

POTENTIAL COMPLICATIONS

It is probably inevitable that amputees experience complications that affect their ability to work. Many people with amputation will lose work time for medical and prosthesis fitting and maintenance. Some complications are preventable and others "just happen." Overall, potential complications in part depend on the reason for the amputation (trauma, electrical injury, diabetes, cancer, cardiovascular disease, etc.), fit of prosthesis (if one is used), work demands, living environment, quality of medical treatment, and other factors. However, common considerations for all amputees (i.e., upper and lower extremity) include (22,39):

- Psychologic adjustment to disability. In many cases, psychologic counseling will be provided while the client is an inpatient and may be continued following discharge from acute care.
- In the event of amputations where the client wears a prosthesis, the probability of occasional skin breakdown exists. This is especially true for electrocution and burn injuries, because skin loses its integrity due to the burn and tears easily. Some clients require surgical intervention to repair skin breakdown.
- Bone spurs occasionally become a problem and may require surgery.
- Phantom pain or phantom sensations are very common, at least during acute recovery, and may need medication or other treatment. Some medications impair the client's ability to operate machinery or drive.
- Osteoarthritis may be experienced in the knees and lower back, and back pain may be experienced due to an abnormal gait. The fit of the prostheses is of paramount importance to avoid these kinds of complications. In addition to proper fit, specific gait training to educate the client about proper body mechanics also will be important.
- Significant weight gain or loss affects the fit of the prosthesis and requires either adjustment or a complete refabrication of the socket.
- Complicated recoveries from other injuries may be a result of the inability for the client to manage self-care during periods of injury or illness. For example, an individual who experiences a triple amputation (bilateral upper extremity and unilateral lower extremity) may be unable to take care of himself for bowel and bladder care.
- Knee problems when not wearing the prosthesis are often a complication for bilateral below-knee amputation. It is sometimes much easier to simply walk on the knees to get around the house, such as when going to the bathroom at night or trying to get out of the house in an emergency. After years of using this method to move around, it is not uncommon for clients to experience knee problems.
- While working in hot environments or having to exert considerable effort to walk or engage in physical activity while using a prosthesis, sweating can become an irritating problem. Prostheses tend to feel heavy and awkward and require an approximate 10% increase in energy for a single below-knee amputation and much more energy expenditure with multiple amputations (40). A person with a bilateral above-knee amputation expends considerable energy simply getting from one place to another. In fact, many people with amputation may prefer to utilize a wheelchair to be able to do things more quickly. Additionally, a person with an upper extremity amputation, such as a shoulder disarticulation, requires the use of a mechanical arm or a myoelectric arm, which usually necessitates a considerable expenditure of energy. This may result in excessive sweating and irritation as well. Work in a hot environment, such as outdoors in the summer, in warm climates, or in a boiler room may become intolerable.
- Neuromas are also fairly frequent and can be quite irritating if the prosthesis impacts them. Often surgery is the treatment of choice.

CONCLUSIONS

Until recently, very little research regarding work for amputees had been published. However, the role of the vocational counselor has always been integral in exploring employment options for people with amputations. Clearly, rehabilitation efforts should include the vocational counselor as a part of the team. The vocational expert should be knowledgeable in vocational assessment, job analysis, labor market surveys, ergonomics, rehabilitation technology, job placement and, of course, amputation injury issues. Because the person with amputation can be impaired in a multitude of ways, it is a challenge to solve problems and help these people become contributing members of society. However, with the expanding field of rehabilitation technology and prosthetic design, the work future of the upper extremity amputee is bright indeed.

RESOURCES

TechKnowledge
Center for Assistive Technology and Enviromental Access
College of Architecture
Georgia Institute of Technology
Atlanta, Georgia 30332-0156
Fax 404/894-9320
404/853-9119

Breaking New Ground (farm-oriented technology)
Dept. of Agriculture and Biological Engineering
1146 ABE Building
Purdue University
West Lafayette, IN 47907
Fax 765/496-1356
765/494-1191

AgiAbility Project
National Easter Seal Society
Suite 200
700 Thirteenth Street, N.W.
Washington, DC 20005
Fax 202/737-7914
202/347-3066

Amputee Coalition of America
P. O. Box 2528
Knoxville, TN 37901-2528
Fax 423/525-7917
423/524-8772
888/AMP-KNOW

Mayer, Tommye-K (1996). *One-Handed in a Two-Handed World.*
PrinceGallison Press: Boston, MA
http://www.gis.net/princeg/ordrform.html

Texas Assistive Devices (http://www.n-abler.org, 979/798-8809)
Tools designed to upper extremity prosthesis

References

1. Weed R, Kirkscey M, Mullins G, Dunlap K, Taylor C. Return to work rates in case of amputation. *J Rehabil Outcomes Measurement* 1997, 1(4), 35–39.
2. Census Bureau. *Labor Force and Other Characteristics of Persons with Work Disability: 1981–1988.* Washington, D.C., 1989.
3. Southeast Disability & Business Technical Assistance Center. *ADA Pipeline* 1995, 4(3), 9. Atlanta: Southeast Disability & Business Technical Assistance Center.
4. Gerhards F, Florin I, Knapp T. The impact of medical, re-educational, and psychological variables on rehabilitation outcomes in amputees. *Internat J Rehabil Res* 1984, 7, 379–388.
5. Millstein S, Bain D, Hunter G. A review of employment patterns of industrial amputees: factors influencing rehabilitation. *Prosthetics Orthotics Internat* 1985, 9, 69–78.
6. Weed R (ed.). *Life Care Planning and Case Management Handbook.* Boca Raton, Fla.: St. Lucie/CRC Press, 1999.
7. CWCI. Two of three disabled employees are working three years after completing vocational rehabilitation. *California Workers' Compensation Institute Bulletin* 1989, 89(1), 1–6.
8. Greenwood R. Employment and disability: Emerging issues for the 1990s. *Switzer Monograph, 14th ed.* 1990, 9–11.
9. Kennedy E. (ed.). *Spinal Cord Injury: The Facts and Figures.* Birmingham, Ala.: The University of Alabama, 1986.
10. PSI. Controlling the effects of disability in the workplace. *Rehab Brief* 1989, 12(6), 1–4.
11. Roeschlein R, Domholdt E. Factors related to successful upper extremity prosthetic use. *Prosthetics Orthotics Internat* 1989, 13, 14–18.
12. Athelstan G. Psychosocial adjustment to chronic disease and disability. In: W Stolov, M Clowers (eds.), *Handbook of Severe Disability.* Washington, D.C.: U. S. Department of Education, Rehabilitation Services Administration, 1981.
13. Havranek J. The social and individual costs of negative attitudes toward persons with physical disabilities. *JARC* 1991, 22, (1), 15–21.
14. McMahon B, Shaw L. (eds.). *Work Worth Doing.* Orlando, Fla.: Paul M. Deutsch Press, 1991.
15. Weed R, Field T. *The Rehabilitation Consultant's Handbook* (3rd ed.). Athens, Ga.: Elliott & Fitzpatrick, 2001.
16. Brown C, McDaniel R. Perceived disability of applicants having back injuries. *J Private Sector Rehabilitation* 1987, 2(2), 89–93.
17. Dorland W. *Dorland's Illustrated Medical Dictionary* (26th ed.). Philadelphia: W. B. Saunders, 1981.
18. Marme M, Skord K. Counseling strategies to enhance the vocational rehabilitation of persons after traumatic brain injury. *J Appl Rehabil Counseling* 1993, 24(1), 19–25.
19. *Clark v. Aqua Air Industries,* 435 So. 2d 492 (1983).
20. *Crease, G. v. J.A. Jones Construction Company,* 425 So. 2d 274 (LA App. 1982).
21. Berens D, Weed R. The role of the vocational counselor in life care planning. In: R Weed (ed.), *Life Care Planning and Case Management Handbook.* Winter Park, Fla.: CRC Press, 1999.
22. Meier R. Life care planning for amputee. In: R. Weed (ed.), *Life Care Planning and Case Management Handbook.* Winter Park, Fla.: CRC Press, 1999.
23. Botterbusch KF. *Vocational Assessment and Evaluation Systems: A Comparison.* Menomonie, Wis.: University of Wisconsin Materials Development Center, 1987.
24. Siefker JM (ed.). *Vocational Evaluation in Private Sector Rehabilitation.* Menomonie, Wis.: University of Wisconsin Materials Development Center, 1992.
25. Deneen L, Hessellund T. *Counseling the Able Disabled.* San Francisco: Rehab Publications, 1986.
26. Anastasi A. *Psychological Testing,* 5th ed. New York: Macmillan Co., 1982.

27. Sbordone RJ, Long CJ (eds.). *Ecological Validity of Neuropsychological Testing.* Delray Beach, Fla.: St. Lucie Press, 1996.

28. Power P. *A Guide to Vocational Assessment,* 3rd ed. Austin, Tx.: Pro-Ed, 2000.

29. Blackwell T, Conrad D, Weed R. *Job Analysis and the ADA: A Step by Step Guide.* Athens, Ga.: E & F Vocational Services, 1992.

30. USDOI. *Revised Handbook for Analyzing Jobs.* Washington, D.C., 1991.

31. U.S. Department of Labor. *Dictionary of Occupational Titles.* Washington, D.C., 1991.

32. Field JE, Field TF. *Classification of Jobs 2000.* Athens, Ga.: Elliott & Fitzpatrick, 1999.

33. USDOI. *Enhanced Guide for Occupational Exploration.* Washington, D.C., 1991.

34. USDOL. *Occupational Outlook Handbook.* Washington, D.C, 1991.

35. Schoppen T, Boonstra A, Groothoff J, Vries J, Goeken L, Eisma W. Employment status, job characteristics, and work-related heath experience of people with a lower limb amputation in the Netherlands. *Arch Phys Med Rehabil* 2001, 82(2), 239–245.

36. PL 101-336. *Americans with Disability Act.* Washington D.C.: U.S. Government Printing Office, 1990.

37. USEEOC. *ADA Technical Assistance Manual.* Pittsburgh, Pa.: U.S. Government Printing Office, 1992.

38. Mueller J. *The Workplace Workbook: An Illustrated Guide to Job Accommodation and Assistive Technology.* Washington, D.C.: The Dole Foundation, 1990.

39. Weed R, Sluis A. *Life Care Plans for the Amputee: A Step by Step Guide.* Tampa, Fla.: CRC Press, 1990.

40. Friedman L. Amputation. In: WC Stolov, MR Clowers (eds.), *Handbook of Severe Disability* Washington, D.C.: U.S. Department of Education, Rehabilitation Services Administration, 1981; 169–188.

30 Research Trends for the Twenty-First Century

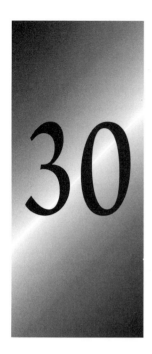

Richard F. ff. Weir, PhD, and Dudley S. Childress, PhD

When Marlon Shirley won the 100m dash at the Sydney 2000 Paralympics in a time of 11.09 seconds, he broke the existing world record for amputee sprinters by 0.24 seconds. Transtibial amputees will likely run the 100m in less than 11 second in the near future. These remarkable times are testimony to the achievements of the athletes and to the design and performance of their prostheses. Running prostheses excel because of good socket fit, good alignment, and good suspension, but the properties of these lower limb prostheses that relate most with respect to upper-limb prostheses are their proper compliance for running and the Extended Physiological Proprioception (EPP) that they exhibit. EPP as originally described by David C. Simpson at the University of Edinburgh, is literally the use of the body's own somatosensory system, often through direct extensions from the body or from a limb (e.g., the long cane in blind navigation). In the runner's case, the prosthesis is a direct extension of the shank; proprioception from the user's own knee and hip joints (including muscles) and skin sensation provide information about where the prosthesis is in space, how fast it is moving, and what forces it is experiencing. The amputee uses the artificial limb the way a tennis player uses a racquet, the way a mechanic uses a screwdriver, or the way a golfer uses a club—with skill and grace, if practiced—as a direct extension of the body. Amputees can readily use prostheses that are direct extensions of their body or of a body part in the same way; much like persons without amputations use tools that are directly extended from them. If the prosthesis is properly applied to the human body it can be used effectively, as is the case with common tools and sporting equipment (e.g., racquets, bats, sticks, clubs, etc.). Direct information from the tool to the human assists with the tool's control. In addition, one may want the extended tool to have the appropriate compliance (e.g., flexibility), as for example is provided in modern golf clubs and tennis racquets.

Designers of artificial limbs in the twenty-first century have a choice of attempting to replace the human limb with a device that is similar to the limb that was lost or to consider designing a limb that provides the kind of effectiveness and feedback exhibited by tools in the hands of good users. At least for the first couple of decades of the century, we believe practical systems for arm amputees will provide them with prostheses that are somewhat like tools; which, because of the natural somatosensory information provided, can be used with great deftness.

Osseointegration, which enables the direct attachment of prostheses to the skeletal system, is a trend that can enhance extended physiological proprioception because of rigidity of the connection between the human and the prosthesis. Osseointegration also introduces the concept of "osseoperception," through which vibratory information is conveyed directly through the connection with the bone.

The direct actuation and control of prostheses through direct connection to physiological muscle, such as in *tunnel cineplasty*—perhaps realized through *multiple miniature tunnel cineplasties*—may be used to enhance control and increase the feedback to amputees from prostheses with multiple degrees-of-freedom. Tunnel cineplasty was introduced at the beginning of the twentieth century, and although it has fallen out of favor, this control approach has been demonstrated to be effective. New surgical approaches will be needed to reinvent tunnel cineplasty in new forms.

The use of ever increasing numbers of microprocessor controls for multifunctional hands and arms will be a continuing trend in the twenty-first century. Low power, inexpensive, reliable processors are now readily available, and a continuing trend will be to use these units to assist arm amputees with control of prostheses. Microprocessors will continue to be used extensively for training purposes and to help prosthetists set system parameters easily so that their clients can be fitted more efficiently and effectively.

The development of compliant actuators *(series elastic actuators)* is a new trend in robotics that is likely to become a new trend in upper-limb prosthetics. Actuators of this kind will make it possible to construct powered fingers and artificial hands and arms that are more compliant and more functional and lifelike. In addition, such actuators should make powered prostheses more robust and durable, because shock loads on the motor drive systems will be reduced.

Other trends in design will be the expanded use of improved artificial reflexes in limbs. *Artificial reflexes* are exemplified today in the SensorHand by Otto Bock. For example, the hand automatically increases pinch force on an object that is sensed to be slipping from the grasp. Microprocessor advancements should complement this trend, enabling other artificial reflexes to be employed.

Hand replacement is a recent mini-trend, but widespread applications are not likely in the near future. *Brain signal control* of prostheses is also a distant trend that will likely take a long time to perfect for practical use. Molecular biology advances may ultimately lead to the regrowth of limbs at some distant time in the twenty-first century, but that reality is not yet a trend in the field of prosthetics.

The ultimate goal of upper-extremity prosthetics research is the meaningful, subconscious control of a multifunctional prosthetic arm or hand—a true replacement for the lost limb—but current prosthetic components and interface techniques are still a long way from realizing this goal. A true limb replacement would be a fully functioning substitute limb that is intimately connected to, and controlled almost without thought by, the amputee. The goal of such a limb replacement would be to match as closely as possible the properties and function of the original limb. Alternatively, the prosthesis as a tool can be regarded as an interchangeable device to be worn by the amputee, used as needed, and then ignored. The tool makes no pretense of trying to replace the lost limb physiologically, but is there as an aid and to help provide some of the functions that were lost. The goal of much of the research in the field is directed toward the prosthesis as a limb replacement; however, in current practice we are mostly limited to the prosthesis as a tool. The major causes of this limitation are practical ones due to the severe weight, power, and size constraints of hand–arm systems and the difficulty in finding a sufficient number of appropriate control sources to control the requisite number of degrees-of-freedom.

Of these issues, it is the lack of independent control sources that imposes the most severe impediment to the development of today's prosthetic arm systems. The current state-of-the-art, commercially available prosthetic hands are mostly single degree-of-freedom (opening and closing) devices that utilize myoelectric control. Prosthetic arms requiring multiple degree-of-freedom control use sequential control with locking mechanisms to switch control from one degree-of-freedom to the next. Generally, because vision is the primary source of feedback, the greatest number of functions that are controlled in parallel is two. Otherwise, the mental loading becomes excessive. Switch, myoelectric, or harness-and-cable are the primary modes of control for today's upper-limb prostheses. Upper-limb prosthetics research is somewhat dominated by considerations of control. Still, the importance of better actuators and better multifunctional mechanisms must not be ignored. Control is useless if effective hand and arm mechanisms are not available.

A number of the trends discussed in this chapter deal with high technology or appear to be high-tech–related approaches to the prosthetics field. However, a number of the trends may lead to simple treatments, which we believe are always desirable. In examining trends, we have taken a fairly broad perspective, and thus, we run the danger of appearing to be like many media articles today, which seem to want readers to believe that modern technology is an unalloyed godsend to amputees and that all that has gone before in prosthetics is apparently without merit. We cannot accept this notion. The prostheses currently available are well suited for amputees in many ways, and designs often rest on firm clinical foundations. For example, body-powered, cable-operated prostheses, which are often denigrated because of their simple technology, meet many of the theoretic criteria that apply to upper-limb prostheses. It is well to put potential new advances in historical perspective and to remember that users are the final arbiters concerning successful artificial limb developments. The latest news reports about new technological developments or applications may create reader excitement about their potential future applications to persons who have lost limbs, but one must always remember that media accounts may be highly speculative. It is also well to remember that solutions to all problems are not necessarily met by high technology, which of itself is not a panacea. As Fred Forchheimer, a former Swedish investigator in the rehabilitation field, has said: "The most advanced application of technology is not necessarily the same as the application of the most advanced technology."

RENEWED INTEREST IN MULTIFUNCTIONAL MYOELECTRIC CONTROL

Myoelectric control derives it name from the electromyogram (EMG), which it uses as a control input. When a muscle contracts, it produces electric potentials (the electromyogram or EMG) as a by-product of the contraction. The intensity of the EMG produced increases as muscle tension increases. If surface electrodes are placed on the skin near a muscle, they can detect this signal. This signal can then be electronically amplified and processed and used to control a prosthesis (1).

Myoelectric control has received considerable attention since it first appeared during the 1940s. However, although myoelectric control has been successful in many transradial fittings, it has failed to achieve significant success in devices requiring the simultaneous control of multiple joints or degrees-of-freedom. As generally implemented, today's myoelectric controllers use open-loop velocity control. In this scheme, the muscles send out signals to the prosthesis but receive nothing back. Constant visual monitoring, due to the open-loop nature of myoelectric control, is therefore required for effective operation. For the control of multiple degrees-of-freedom, such a control scheme places excessive mental load on the user, greatly diminishing any benefits that a multifunctional prosthesis might offer.

There have been many attempts to design fully functional arm–hand prosthesis systems. The Boston arm (2,3), the Philadelphia arm (4,5), the Edinburgh arm (6), the Sven hand (7), the Belgrade hand (8,9), and the Utah arm (10) are just a few examples of prosthetic arm systems that were developed. Although many ideas were tried and tested during the 1960s and 1970s, only a few devices made it from the laboratory into everyday clinical practice.

The Edinburgh arm, which was pneumatically powered, saw some clinical usage. It was mechanically complex and, as a result, prone to failure. Although this arm is not available today, it is important because it was an implementation of Simpson's ideas on extended physiological proprioception (EPP) and was one of the few multifunctional arm that could be controlled in a parallel fashion; that is, more than one joint could be controlled at a time. The Boston arm, developed at MIT, was the first myoelectrically controlled elbow. This elbow was extensively redesigned (11) to become the Liberty Mutual Powered elbow and is now commercially available through the Liberty Technology Company (Boston). The Utah arm is commercially available from Motion Control Inc. (Utah). In many ways, the Utah arm is an elaboration of the original Boston arm. Jacobsen, the Utah arm's developer, studied at MIT under Mann at the time of the original arm's development (12).

The Sven hand was extensively used in research, particularly in regard to multifunction control using the pattern recognition of myoelectric signals (13). The pattern recognition system they used was based on multiple EMG signals, which were processed using adaptive-weighted filters. The weights of these filters were adjusted to tailor the system to the individual user. The Philadelphia arm (4,5) also used weighted filters for the pattern recognition problem and achieved good results. The location for their myoelectrodes was based on muscle synergies associated with arm movements, instead of phantom limb sensations, as in the Sven hand. The Belgrade hand was never used clinically to any great extent but found some use as a robotics research tool as the Belgrade/USC robotic hand (14).

Multifunctional myoelectric control is an area of research that is now being revisited in the light of new technologies and tools. Ongoing research continues into the multifunctional control of artificial hand replacements using complex time, frequency, and time-frequency identification techniques to identify features in the EMG signals that describe a particular grasp pattern. Seven basic grasp patterns are used, as defined by Keller, Taylor, and Zahn (15); these have endured the test of time and are widely accepted in the field of prosthetics. These patterns are:

1. Palmar prehension (three-jaw chuck)
2. Palmar prehension (two-finger)
3. Tip prehension
4. Lateral prehension
5. Hook prehension
6. Spherical prehension
7. Cylindrical prehension

Tip, lateral, and palmar prehension are primarily the function of the thumb working in opposition to the index and middle fingers. Tip prehension, or fingernail pinch, is used mainly to grasp small objects. In lateral prehension, the thumb holds an object against the side of the index finger, as is the case when using a key. In palmar prehension (sometimes referred to as tri-digital pinch or three-jaw chuck), the thumb opposes either a single finger or two or more fingers. Palmar prehension is the grip most commonly used in daily activities. Cylindrical and spherical prehension use all the fingers of the hand to provide an encompassing grasp that firmly stabilizes the object being held. Hook prehension is achieved by flexing the fingers into a hook; the thumb is either alongside the index finger or used to lock the object held. The reduction of the function of most prosthetic hands to a single degree-of-freedom and the finding by Keller et al., that palmar prehension was the most frequently used prehensile pattern for static grasping, has meant that most prosthetic hands incorporate palmar prehension as the dominant pattern.

In the area of specific grasp pattern feature extraction, Hudgins et al. (16) and Farry et al. (17) have used neural networks to perform the pattern recognition and feature extraction. Currently, the features identified by Hudgins et al. (16) find the most widespread use. Farry et al. (18) used Hudgins' features and some of her own, using genetic programming algorithms instead of neural networks for classification. The work of Hudgins et al. (16) and the earlier work of Herberts et al. (7) demonstrated that some form of pattern recognition of myoelectric signals (adaptive filtering techniques, neural networks, genetic algorithms, fuzzy logic, etc.) could be used to control a four degree-of-freedom (DOF) hand.

Implementation of this control method requires mounting a number of electrodes (four or more) within a prosthetic socket and having an amputee visualize the phantom limb making a specific prehension pattern. The EMG signals generated at each electrode are then processed and analyzed in an on-board digital signal processor (DSP). If the EMG pattern encountered is one of those in its memory, the controller actuates the motors necessary to create the associated hand prehension pattern. Given the power and size of today's microcontrollers, programmable logic devices (PLDs) or digital signal processing chips (DSPs) and the programmable analog devices (PADs), which should be suitable for the EMG front-end signal conditioning, a multifunctional myoelectric controller ought to be feasible.

OPTIMIZING HAND FUNCTION VERSUS NUMBER OF CONTROL SOURCES

To adequately reproduce all seven prehension patterns in an artificial handlike prehensor requires three or four degrees-of-freedom (DOF). Two for the thumb, one for the index finger, and one for the remaining three fingers. This idea of limiting the function of the hand to three or four DOF turns up in many unrelated fields, where compromise must be made between function and some other variable.

Professional SCUBA diver gloves trade function for warmth to extend dive times. A mitten is warmest whereas a glove with individual fingers is the most functional. Professional SCUBA diver gloves are a compromise, having the thumb and index fingers free and the middle, ring, and little fingers together. This configuration provides the diver the basic prehension patterns of the hand while at the same time keeping the bulk of the hand warm. Consequently, the diver can work for longer periods of time before the hands become too cold for good function. In all cases, function, when compared to that of an ungloved hand, is greatly reduced due to the loss of tactile cues and the bulk of a neoprene glove. This same compromise is to be found in some shooting gloves, in which only the trigger finger has to be free.

In the area of remote manipulation, three DOFs have been used to adequately recreate the prehensile function of the hand. The SARCOS system (19) uses a three-DOF hand for the slave manipulator terminal device and limits the hand of the operator to the same three DOF when controlling the master arm. Constraining the operator's hand to the same DOF as the slave, and vice versa, enables the operator to extend his proprioception into the remotely controlled terminal device. Forces experienced by the slave are reflected back to the master and experienced by the operator.

For space suit gloves, the Direct-Link Prehensor (20,21) is an experimental design that limits the motions of the operator's hand to four DOF. It also makes use of the idea of direct extensions of body parts (extended physiological proprioception). The motivation for the project came from the problem astronauts have with their gloves, which are bulky and stiff due to the suit's pressurization. This stiffness results in limited external dexterity and excessive hand fatigue. Also, as in the case with diver's gloves, tactile sensation and manual dexterity are lost because the hand is gloved. In the case of the SARCOS terminal device and the Direct Link Prehensor, a fully functional anthropomorphic hand could not be implemented due to the complexity required. The many DOF of the natural hand were restricted to those DOF required to implement the prehension patterns of Keller et al. (15).

In the area of surgery, Beasley (22) described a surgical procedure to provide a functional four-DOF hand for persons with C5–C6 tetrapelgia. These patients retained control of four muscles distal to the elbow: the brachioradialis, extensor carpi radialis longus, extensor carpi radialis brevis, and pronator teres. The muscles had Highet's Grade IV power or better. The surgical procedure is a three-stage reconstruction that increases the involved hand's function, thus enabling the patient to have active flexion of the index and middle fingers, independent flexion of the metacarpophalangeal (MP) and proximal interphalangeal (PIP) joints, and active full digital extension, independent of wrist motion. As a result, precision prehension is possible with careful positioning of the stabilized thumb to oppose the actively flexed index and middle fingers. The result is a functional hand that retains some of its sense of touch.

In the field of neuroprosthetics, implantable four-channel functional electrical stimulators (FES) have been implanted into patients with flail arms. Through both surgery and the judicious placement of the FES electrodes, an otherwise useless limb is able to reproduce the grasp patterns of Keller et al. using four-DOF control (23).

In three of these instances, the exceptions being the surgical intervention and FES, tactile sensation was compromised either by gloves or the remote nature of the terminal device (SARCOS). Vision, proprioceptive feedback from the joints, and diffuse skin pressure were the main sources of feedback. In the case of the surgery and FES, vision and sensation (feedback) were intact but muscular function (control) was impaired. In all instances, restricting the natural hand function to the three of four DOF necessary to recreate Keller et al.'s prehension patterns was thought to maximize hand function with respect to the number of control sites available.

ARTIFICIAL REFLEXES

Alternatives to myoelectric pattern recognition have been used to automate the control process in an effort to reduce the mental burden placed on the user. In essence, these systems seek to remove the operator from the control loop and automatically respond to some external sensor input. They can be thought of as being similar to an artificial reflex loop. By putting more intelligence into the device through the use of embedded microprocessors, more and more of the decision process can be automated, taking the operator from control loop. The artificial reflexes are essentially closed loops within the mechanism or prosthesis itself. This trend of putting more on-board intelligence into prosthetic components is a trend that increases in importance in the future.

Otto Bock has a hand incorporating a microprocessor-controlled slip detector (Otto Bock Sensor-Hand). The thumb has a sensor that detects the slippage of an object grasped by the prehensor and automatically increases prehension force until it detects that the slippage has stopped. Kyberd & Chappell (24) use a system

they call "hierarchical artificial reflexes" to automate the control process. In essence, in their multifunctional hand, they take the operator "out of the loop" and use on-board processing and sensors in the hand to tell the hand what pattern to adopt. The operator only provides a conventional, single DOF open or close EMG signal. The idea is that by allowing the processor to take control, it reduces the mental loading on the operator.

COMPLIANT ACTUATORS

Another research trend of high interest is the design of compliant actuators. The primary role of the human arm is to position the hand in space so that it (the hand) can interact with the environment. Interaction with the real world is something current robotics and prosthetics actuators (DC electric motors with gear trains) do not do well. The human arm is compliant (springlike); it has "give." When the hand comes in contact with a surface, the arm gives to absorb shock and thus prevent damage to the joints. This give or compliance also stops the arm from going into oscillation or instability upon contact with hard surfaces. This phenomenon, known as *contact instability*, arises when a stiff robot arm comes into contact with a hard surface. Unless robot, environment, and the nature of the interaction between the two are precisely mathematically and mechanically defined, contact instabilities can occur, even if the mathematical representation is only slightly in error.

The human arm does not have contact stability problems due to its inherent compliance. This compliance need not be a fixed quantity, but can be varied depending on the task requirements: A stiff arm for bracing oneself against an expected blow, a relaxed arm for playing the piano. This change in arm compliance is achieved by the cocontraction of opposing muscle pairs (agonist–antagonist) that, in turn, vary joint impedance. As such, presently available body-powered wrist, elbow, and shoulder joints can be considered to have a specialized form of compliance control that can be called *two-state compliance control*. Through the use of locking mechanisms, these devices have either infinite (very high) impedance when a joint is locked or close to zero impedance when a joint is unlocked and free to be moved. When locked, such devices are free to be used as rigid extensions of the body, thus enabling the user to obtain proprioceptive cues through the device. When unlocked, the device is free to be positioned with minimal effort.

In prosthetics, Hogan (25,26) developed impedance-compliance control for the Boston elbow. It incorporated an early form of compliant control that required increased muscle activity for the lifting of increasing loads. A force transducer in the prehensor measured the static and dynamic load on the prehensor generating a second control signal, which was subtracted from the processed myoelectric signal. Thus, although the control is essentially feedforward in nature, a more natural control was thought to be possible.

Compliant actuators or actuators that would have "give" could be a boon to prosthetics because the current hard actuators tend to break if a person falls while wearing them. Shearing teeth off the output stage of gear train due to a fall is not uncommon. Toward this end, work being done by the MIT leg lab offers some interesting possibilities. They have developed a compliant actuator for robotics applications. In essence, they have introduced a force-controlled series elastic spring element between the output of a DC motor's gear reduction and the load. A local feedback loop (similar in concept to an artificial reflex), based on elasticity strain was used to create a low minimum impedance actuator (27). By inserting elasticity into the actuator, and controlling the actuator's output force with a feedback loop based on elastic strain, stability with passive loads can be assured. Robustness can be achieved because the system can absorb shock without damage.

English and Russell (28,29) have explored compliant actuators using series elasticity. They examined an actuation system, intended for use in a prosthetic arm, which mimicked the ability of antagonistic muscles in biologic systems to modulate the stiffness and position of a joint. The goal of their work was to achieve the ability to modulate joint stiffness independently of joint position and to be able to do it without using feedback control. They showed that this could be achieved using quadratic springs, or springs in which stiffness increases linearly with displacement. However, they also showed that implementing a quadratic spring was not an easy task and that the stiffness was sensitive to joint position.

An alternative approach to making robot actuators compliant was taken by Wu and Chang (30). They chose to model the muscle-reflex mechanism of primate limbs and to apply it to robotic control. They identified relevant properties of the neuromuscular system and developed a neuromuscularlike model that can accurately emulate different involuntary and voluntary movement. Their experimental results demonstrated that the emulated spindle-reflex model acts as an impedance to any changing displacement, which will enhance the needed compliant forces or torques. Due to this force-enhancement property, no external force sensor is required for sensing force feedback in this control. Both these methods offer interesting ways in which to achieve a compliant system. Pratt modifies the mechanics of the mechanism while Wu et al. wraps the mechanism in a control algorithm.

NEURAL INTERFACES

When talking to lay people about prosthetics, the conversation inevitably turns to when we will be able to connect prostheses directly to the nervous system. Most people have visions of prosthetics that stem from the media and such TV shows as "The Six Million Dollar Man," and movies such as "Star Wars" and "Robocop." Neuroelectric control, as this particular field of endeavor is known, is still a very long away from being a practical reality. Although neuroelectric control or the control of a prosthetic device by way of nerve impulses would appear to be a natural control approach, the practicality of human–machine interconnections of this kind is still problematic.

Edell (31) and Kovacs et al. (32) have conducted research concerning prosthesis connections with nerves and neurons. Edell attempted to use nerve cuffs to generate motor control signals in experimental systems. Kovacs et al. are exploring the use of integrated circuit electrode arrays into which the nerve fiber is encouraged to grow. However, nervous tissue is sensitive to mechanical stresses and this form of control requires the use of implanted systems.

A variation on this theme of peripheral neural interfaces that has recently received a lot of media attention is the use of electroencephalogram signals (EEGs). These electric signals are detected on the surface of the skull and are emitted as a by-product of the natural functioning of the brain. In what might be seen as the shape of things to come, Reger et al. (33) demonstrated a hybrid neurorobotic system based on two-way communication between the brain of a lamprey and a small mobile robot. In this case, the lamprey brain was kept alive in vitro and was used to send and receive motor control and sensory signals. Although this is a long way from any practical use in prosthetics, it does represent what the future might hold. Recently, IEEE Spectrum (34) reported on research at Duke University, where researchers had implanted an electrode array into the cerebellum of a monkey and, through the use of appropriate pattern recognition software, had it control a remote manipulator at MIT over 1,000 km away via the Internet. One of the main practical goals cited for this research is to put paralyzed people in control of artificial limbs.

In the area of functional electrical stimulation (FES), FDA approval has been granted to implant FES electrodes for the purpose of providing four-DOF control of an otherwise flail limb (23). Also in the area of FES, Loeb et al. (35) have designed and built what they consider to be a new class of implantable electronic interfaces with nerve and muscle. These devices, which they call BIONs, are hermetically encapsulated, leadless electrical devices that are small enough to be injected percutaneously into muscles (2 mm diameter by 15 mm long). They receive their power, digital addressing, and command signals from an external transmitter coil worn by the patient. This group is in the process of developing second-generation BIONs that can provide the outgoing telemetry of ongoing movements. Such devices ought to be able to be used to detect EMG signals and be used in prosthetic control.

SURGICAL INNOVATIONS

It is our belief that major advancements in upper-limb control will require additional surgical intervention to create appropriate interfaces between amputees and prostheses; interfaces that allow for sensory feedback as well as control signals. Thus, surgeons, and their willingness to perform and experiment with innovative new techniques, will be a significant trend in the future of upper-limb prosthetics development. Preservation of muscle tone and length are of paramount importance if future surgery is to be successful at creating novel physical muscle–prosthesis interfaces. Ensuring that residual muscles retain the ability to develop tension when voluntarily contracted can preserve muscle tone. This requires that either myoplasty and/or myodesis be performed at the time of initial amputation. In myoplasty, agonist–antagonist residual muscles pairs are tied off against each other. In myodesis, the residual muscle is stitched to the bone. In both cases, the residual musculature retains the ability to easily develop tension, thus reducing atrophy during the interval between initial amputation and the revisions necessary to create new muscle–tendon control interfaces. Myoplasty would generally be used on the superficial muscles, whereas myodesis could be used on the deep muscles.

The concept of *direct muscle attachment* is not new. It had its origins in Italy at the opening of the twentieth century and was brought into clinical practice in Germany by Sauerbruch around 1915 (36). The technique, called *muscle tunnel cineplasty,* fashions a skin-lined tunnel through the muscle (released at its insertion) and enables the muscle's power to be brought outside the body. A similar but alternative surgical procedure called *tendon exteriorization cineplasty* (37) uses tendon transfers combined with skin flaps to bring a tendon loop outside the body.

In Sweden, Brånemark and his team (38) have performed pioneering work in the area of *direct skeletal attachment*. These surgeons and orthopedic engineers have created interfaces for direct skeletal attachment systems for upper and lower limb amputations. Brånemark's techniques appear to have greatly diminished the infection problems that persisted in previous efforts (39).

Should direct skeletal attachment prove itself viable, it could revolutionize the prosthetic fitting of amputees.

The work of Kuiken (40) is another example of the trend to innovative surgical procedures. He advocates the use of "neuromuscular reorganization" to improve the control of artificial arms. Kuiken observed that although the limb is lost in an amputation, the control signals to the limb remain in the residual peripheral nerves of the amputated limb. The potential exists to tap into these lost control signals using nerve–muscle grafts. As first suggested by Hoffer and Loeb (41), it may be possible to denervate expendable regions of muscle in or near an amputated limb and graft the residual peripheral nerve stumps to these muscles. The peripheral nerves would then reinnervate the muscles and these nerve–muscle grafts would provide additional control signals for an externally powered prosthesis. The nerve–muscle grafts could potentially be directly attached to force sensors and provide extended physiological proprioception. Alternately, the surface EMG from the nerve–muscle grafts could serve as a traditional myoelectric control signal and be used with existing myoelectric technology. These grafts could provide *simultaneous* control of at least the terminal device and powered elbow, and possibly another degree-of-freedom such as a wrist rotation or wrist flexion–extension. In a shoulder disarticulation amputee, each of the residual brachial plexus nerves could be grafted to different regions of the pectoralis muscle.

If current surgical trends continue, hand replacement may become more widespread. However, recent news reports of the first patient to receive such a transplant are not encouraging. This patient asked to have the replacement amputated because it became an essentially flail limb. However, if solutions to tissue rejection and nerve regeneration are found, then such surgeries are likely to become more common.

In the distant future, molecular biology advances may ultimately lead to the regrowth of lost limbs in baths of the relevant proteins from cells from the amputee and attached by a team of surgeons. Alternatively, the arm may simply be grown directly from the residual limb as some starfish do when they lose a limb. Although still in the realm of science fiction, early work in this area is ongoing in Boston, where they have successfully grown ear cartilage in vitro.

PHYSIOLOGICALLY APPROPRIATE INTERFACES

Whatever the future holds, physiologically correct feedback, beyond that provided by vision, is essential if coordinated subconscious control of multifunctional prostheses is ever to be achieved. Early prostheses used a control cable connected to the artificial joint. In these systems, the amputee provided both power and control signals and transferred them to the prosthesis via the control cable. Feedback from the prosthesis was transferred back to the operator via the same control cable. The amputee retained a sense of prosthesis state through the control cable. When prosthetic arm technology moved to externally powered systems, the control modalities shifted away from cable inputs to, almost exclusively, open-loop velocity control techniques (such as myoelectric and switch control). These techniques provide little feedback beyond visual feedback. Simplicity was probably the primary reason for this reduction in feedback. The actuator of choice, the electric DC motor, is an inherently rate-controlled device (i.e., its output speed is directly proportional to the input voltage), and it can be readily controlled with on–off switches. In addition, a velocity-controlled system does not draw power to maintain a particular position.

An exception to this trend was promulgated by Simpson (42), who advocated extended physiological proprioception (EPP) to indicate that the body's own natural physiological sensors are used to relate the state of the prosthetic arm to the operator. EPP can be thought of as the extension of one's proprioceptive feedback into an intimately linked inanimate object. Consider a tennis player hitting a ball with a tennis racquet. The player does not need to visually monitor the head of the racquet to know where it will strike the ball. Through experience, the tennis player knows how heavy and how long the tennis racquet is. He knows where in space the head of the racquet is located based on proprioceptive cues from his hand, wrist, and arm.

This same EPP principle can be applied to provide proprioceptive feedback to a powered prosthetic joint. Consider parking a car that has power steering. In this instance, the driver feels, through the steering wheel, the interaction between the front wheels and the parking surface or curb. However, the user does not provide the power to turn the wheels; this comes from the engine. The driver is linked to the front wheels through the steering wheel and has extended his proprioception to the front wheels. Essentially, EPP control for externally powered prosthetic components can be thought as power-steering for prosthetic joints. The subconscious control possible with an EPP controller operating in conjunction with the proprioception of an individual's residual muscles presents the intriguing possibility of making the independent multifunctional control of a prosthetic hand or arm a reality. Suitable control muscles and EPP controllers, in conjunction with a multifunctional artificial hand, would be a step towards achieving meaningful hand prostheses control. The use of muscle (43) or tendon (37) cineplasty can be used to create miniature skin-linked muscle tunnels or tendon loops to bring muscle excursions and forces outside the body. These cineplasties do not have to be large and powerful because power is provided by the servo mechanism. Physical attachment is desired so that position, velocity, and force feedback can be achieved from the muscles' own proprioceptive apparatus. In this way, the intrinsic sensory apparatus of the residual muscle can be used to provide feedback about the servo mechanism under its control. Finally, the prosthesis could be physically attached to a person's skeleton by osseointegration (38), thus obviating the need for suspension sockets and cumbersome control harnesses and enhancing EPP and making osseoperception available.

In a prototype fitting that may presage the future, a below-elbow amputee was fitted with an externally powered hand that utilized the subject's exteriorized tendons as control input to a full EPP controller (44). The position and speed of movement of the tendon (and the muscle) directly control the position and speed of movement of the fingers and thumb of the electric hand. Movement of the flexor tendon caused the hand to close. Movement of the extensor tendon caused the hand to open. This was the first clinical fitting of a powered hand prosthesis, controlled directly by antagonist muscles (via exteriorized tendons) in a somewhat physiological manner.

CONCLUSIONS

In short, the future of what can be achieved depends to a large extent on the interactions of physicians, surgeons, prosthetists, and engineers. Physicians and surgeons need to perform innovative procedures that can be coupled with compliant engineering systems in ways that create novel human–prosthesis interfaces.

References

1. Parker PA, Scott RN. Myoelectric control of prosthesis. *CRC Critical Reviews in Biomedical Engineering* 1985; 13(4), 283–310.
2. Mann RW. Efferent and afferent control of an electromyographic proportional rate, force sensing artificial elbow with cutaneous display of joint angle. *Proc Symp Basic Problems of Prehension, Movement, Control of Artificial Limbs*, London Institution of Mechanical Engineers, 1968; 86–92.
3. Mann RW, Reimers SD. Kinesthetic sensing for the EMG controlled "Boston arm". *IEEE Transactions on Man-Machine Systems*, 1970, MMS-11(1), pp. 110–115.
4. Taylor DR, Wirta RW. Development of a myoelectrically controlled prosthetic arm. In: *Advances in External Control on Human Extremities, Proceedings of the Third International Symposium on External Control of Human Extremities*, Dubrovnik, Yugoslavia, August 25–30, 1969. Belgrade: Yugoslav Committee for Electronics and Automation (ETAN) 1970, 177–183.

5. Taylor DR, Finley FR. Multiple-axis prosthesis control by muscle synergies. In: *The Control of Upper-Extremity Prostheses and Orthoses, Proceedings of the Conference on the Control of Upper-Extremity Prostheses and Orthoses*, Göteborg, Sweden, Oct. 6–8, 1971. Herberts P, Kadefors R, Magnusson RI, Petersén I. (eds.), Springfield, Ill: Charles C. Thomas, 1974, 181–189.

6. Herberts P, Almström C, Kadefors R, Lawrence P. Hand control via myoelectric patterns. *Acta Orthopaedica Scand* 1973, 44, 389–409.

7. Simpson DC. An externally powered prosthesis for the complete arm. *Biomedical Engineering* 1969, 4(3), 106–110, 119.

8. Razic D. Kinematics design of a multifunctional hand prosthesis. In: *Advances in External Control of Human Extremities, Proceedings of the 4th International Symposium on External Control of Human Extremities*, Dubrovnik, Yugoslavia, August 28–September 2, 1972. Gavrilovic MM, Wilson AB (eds.). Belgrade: Yugoslav Committee for Electronics and Automation (ETAN), 1973, 177–183.

9. Stojiljkovic ZV, Saletic DZ. Tactile pattern recognition by Belgrade hand Prosthesis. In: *Advances in External Control of Human Extremities, Proceedings of the 5th International Symposium on External Control of Human Extremities*, Dubrovnik, Yugoslavia, August, 1974. Belgrade: Yugoslav Committee for Electronics and automation (ETAN), 1975.

10. Jacobsen SC, Knutti DF, Johnson RT, Sears HH. Development of the Utah Arm. *IEEE Transactions on Biomedical Engineering* 1982, BME-29, (4), 249–269.

11. Williams TW. Use of the Boston elbow for high-level amputees. In: Atkins DJ, Meier RH (eds.). *Comprehensive Management of the Upper-Limb Amputee*. New York: Springer-Verlag, 1989, 211–220.

12. Sears HH, Andrew JT, Jacobsen SC. Experience with the Utah arm, hand, and terminal device. In: Atkins DJ, Meier RH (eds.), *Comprehensive Management of the Upper-Limb Amputee*. New York: Springer-Verlag, 1989, 194–210.

13. Lawrence PD, Kadefors R. Classification of myoelectric patterns for the control of a prosthesis. *The Control Of Upper-Extremity Prostheses and Orthoses, Proc. Conf. Control of Upper-Extremity Prostheses and Orthoses*, Göteborg, Sweden, October 6–8, 1971. Herberts P, Kadefors R, Magnusson RI, Petersén I. (eds.). Springfield, Ill.: Charles C. Thomas, 1974, 190–200.

14. Beattie D, Iberall T, Sukhatme GS, Bekey GA. EMG Control for a robot hand used as a prosthesis. *Proc. 4th Int'l Conf. Rehabilitation Robotics (ICORR)*, Wilmington, Delaware. June 14–16, 1994. Bacon DC, Rahmin T, Harwin WS (eds.). Applied Science & Engineering Laboratories, University of Delaware, A.I. duPont Institute.

15. Keller AD, Taylor CL, Zahn V. Studies to determine the functional requirements for hand and arm prostheses. Department of Engineering, University of California at Los Angeles, 1947.

16. Hudgins BS, Parker PA, Scott RN. A new strategy for multifunction myoelectric control. *IEEE Transactions on Biomedical Engineering* 1993, 40(1), 82–94.

17. Farry KA, Walker ID, Sendonaris A. Teleoperation of a multifingered robotic hand with myoelectrics. *Proceedings of Myo-Electric Control Symposium '97 (MEC'97)*. University of New Brunswick. Fredericton, New Brunswick, Canada, August 16–20, 1993.

18. Farry KA, Fernandez MS, Abramczyk ME, Novy BS, Atkins D. Applying genetic programming to control of an artifical arm. *Proceedings of Myo-Electric Control Symposium '93 (MEC'97)*, University of New Brunswick, Fredericton, New Brunswick, Canada, August 16–20, 1993.

19. Jacobsen SC, Smith FM, Iversen EK, Backman DK. High performance, high dexterity, force reflective teleoperator. *Proc. 38th Conf. Remote Systems Technology*, LaGrange Park, Illinois, American Nuclear Society (ANS), 1990; Vol. 2, 180–185.

20. Direct-Link Prehensor. *NASA Tech Briefs* 1991, 15(12), 78.

21. Direct-Link Prehensor. Technical Support Package. *NASA Tech Briefs* 1991, ARC-11666, NASA, Ames Research Center, Moffett Field, California.

22. Beasley RW. Surgical treatment of hands for C5-C6 tetrapelgia. *Symposium on Rehabilitation After Reconstructive Hand Surgery* 1983, 14(4), 893–904.

23. Triolo R, Nathan R, Yasunobu H, Keith M, Betz RR, Carroll S, Kantor C. Challenges to clinical deployment of upper limb neuroprostheses. *J Rehabil Res Dev* 1996, 33(2), 111–122.

24. Kyberd PJ, Chappell PH. The Southampton hand: An intelligent myoelectric prosthesis. *J Rehabil Res Dev* 1994, 31(4), 326–334.

25. Hogan NJ. Prostheses should have adaptively controllable impedance. *Proceedings of the IFAC Control Aspects of Prosthetics and Orthotics*, 1982.

26. Hogan NJ. Adaptive control of mechanical impedance by coactivation of antagonist muscles. *IEEE Transactions on Automatic Control* 1984, AC-29, (8), 681–689.

27. Pratt GA. Legged robots at MIT: What's new since Raibert. *IEEE Robotic & Automation Magazine* 2000, 7(3), 15–19.

28. English CE, Russell D. Mechanics and stiffness limitations of a variable stiffness actuator for use in prosthetic limbs. *Mechanism and Machine Theory* 1999; 34, 7–25.

29. English CE, Russell D. Implementation of variable joint stiffness through antagonistic actuation using Rolamite springs. *Mechanism and Machine Theory* 1999; 34, 27–40.

30. Wu C, Chang S. Analysis and implementation of a neuromuscular-like control for robotic compliance. *IEEE Transactions on Control Systems Technology* 1997, 5(6), 586–596.

31. Edell DJ. A peripheral nerve information transducer for amputees: Long-term multichannel recordings from rabbit peripheral nerves. *IEEE Transactions on Biomedical Engineering* 1986, BME-33(2), 203–214.

32. Kovacs GTA, Storment CW, Hentz VR, Rosen JM. Fabrication techniques for directly implantable microelectronic neural devices. *Proc. RESNA 12th Conf.*, 1989, New Orleans, Louisiana, 292–293.

33. Reger BD, Fleming KM, Sanquineti V, Alford S, Mussa-Ivaldi FA. Connecting brains to robots: The development of a hybrid system for the study of learning in neural tissues. *Artificial Life Journal* 2000 (MIT Press, Cambridge, Massachusetts), 6(4), 307–324.

34. IEEE Spectrum. A mind-Internet-machine interaction: News analysis. *IEEE Spectrum* 2001, 33.

35. Loeb GE, Richmond FJR, Olney S, Cameron T, Dupont AC, Hood K, Peck RA, Troyk PR, Schulman JH. Bionic neurons for functional and therapeutic electrical Stimulation. *Proc. IEEE-EMBS* 1998, 20:2305–2309.

36. Sauerbruch F. *Die Willkürlich Bewegbare Künstliche Hand. Eine Anleitung für Chirurgen und Techniker [The voluntary controlled artificial hand. A guide for surgeons and technicians]*, 1st Edition. Berlin: Julius Springer-Verlag, 1916.

37. Beasley RW. The tendon exteriorization cineplasty: A preliminary report. *Inter-Clinic Information Bulletin (ICIB)*. New York, Committee on Prosthetics Research and Development 1966, V(8), 6–8.

38. Brånemark P-I. Osseointegration: Biotechnological perspective and clinical modality. In: Brånemark PI, Rydevik BL, Skalak R (eds.), *Osseointegration in Skeletal Reconstruction and Joint Replacement* Chicago: Quintessence Publishing 1997, 1–24.

39. Hall CW, Rostoker W. Permanently attached artificial limbs. *Bull Prosthetics Res* 1980, 10(34), 98–100.

40. Kuiken TA, Rymer WZ, Childress DS. The hyper-reinnervation of rat skeletal muscle. *Brain Res* 1995, 676, 113–123.

41. Hoffer JA, Loeb GE. Implantable electrical and mechanical interfaces with nerve and muscle. *Ann Biomedical Engineering* 1980, 8, 351–360.

42. Simpson DC. The choice of control system for the multimovement prosthesis: Extended physiological proprioception (E.P.P.) In: *The Control of Upper-Extremity Prostheses and Orthoses, Proceedings of the Conference on the Control of Upper-Extremity Prostheses and Orthoses*, Göteborg, Sweden, October 6–8, 1971. Herberts, P., Kadefors, R., Magnusson, R.I., and Petersén, I. (eds.). Springfield, Ill.: Charles C. Thomas, 1974, 146–150.

43. Brückner L. Sauerbruch-Lebsche-Vanghetti Cineplasty: The surgical procedure. *Orthopaedics and Traumatology*. Munich: Urban and Vogel, 1992, Vol. 1, No. 2, 90–99.

44. Weir RF, Heckathorne CW, Childress DS. Cineplasty as a control input for externally powered prosthetic components. *J Rehab Res Dev* 2001, 38(4), 357–363.

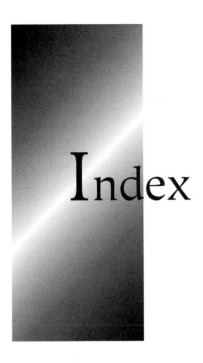

Index

Note: Boldface numbers indicate illustrations and tables.